# The Science of

# *DENTAL MATERIALS*

EUGENE W. SKINNER, Ph.D.
*Professor of Physics,*
*Northwestern University Dental School*

RALPH W. PHILLIPS, M.S.
*Professor of Dental Materials,*
*Indiana University School of Dentistry*

*Fifth Edition, Illustrated*

*W. B. Saunders Company*
*Philadelphia and London*          *1960*

# Preface

The first edition of this book was published in 1936. The present edition is the first one to be written with a co-author. The senior author wishes to express his extreme gratification for this new association and for the enthusiastic cooperation of the junior author in the preparation of this fifth edition. He has brought a fresh viewpoint and knowledge which will add much to the scientific and educational value of the text.

As in previous editions, the educational level of the book is assumed to be that of the third year liberal arts student who has completed at least the study of college physics and general and organic chemistry. His educational background and maturity are sufficient for him to be able, with the proper guidance, to form judgments as to the soundness of fundamental principles and technical procedures. We have attempted to take advantage of this predental training and intellectual ability wherever possible.

On the other hand, the text must be elementary in scope so far as the student's knowledge of dentistry is concerned. The dental phases are completely discussed in terms that the student will understand. Strictly controversial issues have been avoided as far as possible.

Some radical changes have been made in almost every chapter. A discussion with teachers of this subject has indicated that much of the success of the previous edition was related to the inclusion of many clinical applications of the basic principles described. In the present edition, the discussions of the theoretical phases have not been greatly changed, but, following the suggestions of our colleagues, the clinical applications have been considerably expanded. The principles have also been related, so far as possible, to the knowledge which the student is acquiring in other basic science courses in the dental program.

The primary changes are related to the inclusion of new concepts and facts developed since the last edition. Three new chapters have been added, covering rubber base impression materials, tarnish and corrosion as related to dental problems, and a discussion of dental burs and high speed power sources. The subjects of cavity liners, calcium hydroxide cements, dentifrices and porcelain to gold restorations are included for the first time. The material on dental amalgam has been expanded to include a critical review of the clinical restoration and the factors which control its clinical success. A similar approach has been used for other materials such as silicate cement and the gold inlay. It is hoped that with these inclusions, the subject of dental materials can be more closely coordinated with the biological and clinical sciences.

The complete presentation of the American Dental Association Specifications for Dental Materials has been omitted from this edition, since the American Dental Association now has a publication on this subject. Nevertheless, the Specifications are constantly referred to in this text. Every teacher of the subject of dental materials is urged to require his students to purchase a copy of the current edition of "American Dental Association Specifications for Dental Materials" as a companion book. The publication can be obtained for a nominal sum from the American Dental Association, 222 East Superior Street, Chicago 11, Illinois, U.S.A.

EUGENE W. SKINNER
RALPH W. PHILLIPS

# Acknowledgments

No book of this type can be written without the advice and aid of authorities in the various fields discussed. Among the many consulted, the following either contributed advice and information or read chapters concerned with their field of specialization:

Mr. John O. Semmelman and Mrs. Jean Hodson, dental porcelain; Dr. K. Dreyer Jørgensen, gypsum products; Dr. Eugene J. Molnar, rubber impression materials and zinc oxide-eugenol pastes; Dr. G. M. Brauer, Dr. Dioracy Vieira, and Dr. G. C. Paffenbarger, acrylic resin denture base material; Dr. Gunnar Ryge, soldering procedures and dental amalgam; Dr. George Von Mohr, corrosion; Dr. R. S. Lindenmeyer, dental burs; Dr. Arne F. Rommes, gold foil; Dr. Richard Earnshaw, stellite alloys and dental casting procedures; Dr. G. A. Lammie and Dr. John Osborne, dental burs; Dr. D. B. Mahler, theory of hygroscopic expansion; and Dr. B. G. G. D. Hedegård, homogenization of gold alloy.

Miss Minnie Orfanos and Miss Adele Fisher aided in the preparation of bibliographies. Mrs. Mabel Walker and staff were helpful in securing literature. Miss Marjorie Swartz assisted in reviewing the research in certain areas. Many thanks are due to Miss Gena T. Mizera, Mrs. Louise Won and Mrs. Charlene Gibson for aid in the preparation of the manuscript. As in the previous editions, Mrs. Rosamond L. Skinner patiently searched the manuscript for mistakes in English composition and similar errors.

EUGENE W. SKINNER
RALPH W. PHILLIPS

# Contents

# CHAPTER 1

# Introduction

**Historical.**   Strange as it may seem, there is comparatively little historical background for the science of dental materials and their manipulation, in spite of the fact that the practice of dentistry itself antedates the Christian era. For example, gold bands and wires were used by the Phoenicians and Etruscans for the construction of partial dentures. Gold foil has been employed for dental restorative purposes for so long a period that its origin is not known.

Modern dentistry is said to have had its beginning during the year 1728, when Fauchard published a treatise describing many types of dental restorations, including a method for the construction of artificial dentures from ivory. Somewhat later, in 1756, Pfaff first described the method for obtaining impressions of the mouth in wax, from which he constructed a model with plaster of paris. The year 1792 is important as the date when de Chamant patented a process for the construction of porcelain teeth; this was followed early in the next century by the introduction of the porcelain inlay.

It is evident, then, that many of the restorative and accessory materials of today have been in use for some time, yet little scientific information about them has been available until recently. Their use was entirely an art, and the only testing laboratory was the mouth of the long-suffering patient.

The first important awakening of interest was during the middle of the nineteenth century, when research studies on amalgam began. At about the same time there are also some reports in the literature of studies on porcelain and gold foil. These rather sporadic advances in knowledge finally culminated in the brilliant investigations of G. V. Black, which began in 1895. There is hardly a phase of dentistry which was not touched upon and advanced by this tireless worker.

The next great advance in the knowledge of dental materials and their manipulation began in 1919. During this year, the United States Army requested the National Bureau of Standards to set up specifications for the selection and grading of dental amalgams for use in federal service. This research was done under the leadership of Wilmer Souder, and a very excellent report was published in 1920.[1] The information contained in the report was received enthusiastically by the dental profession, and information along the same line was demanded for other dental materials.

At the time, the United States Government could not allocate sufficient funds to continue the work, so a fellowship was created and supported by the Weinstein Research Laboratories. Under such an arrangement, the sponsor provides the salary for research associates and a certain amount of equipment and supplies. The associates then work in the National Bureau of Standards under the direction of the staff members. They are to all intents and purposes members of the staff, supported by private interests. All findings are published and become common property under such an arrangement.

R. L. Coleman, W. L. Swanger, and W. A. Poppe were the Research Associates first appointed under this arrangement. Working under Dr. Souder, they investigated the properties of dental wrought and casting golds and accessory casting materials. This phase of the work resulted in the publication of an extensive and valuable research report.[2]

In 1928, the Dental Research Fellowship at the National Bureau of Standards was assumed by the American Dental Association, and at the present time it is administered by the Council on Research of that organization. The research carried on by the American Dental Association Research Associates in conjunction with the staff members of the National Bureau of Standards has been of inestimable value to the dental profession, and it has earned for this group an international reputation. The names of Wilmer Souder, George C. Paffenbarger and William T. Sweeney will undoubtedly live in history as the pioneer research workers who founded a new era of considerably greater research production in the field of dental materials. It was the enthusiasm of these men which prompted the organization of the first courses in dental materials to be taught in the dental schools of America and abroad. The last complete summary report[3] of their research activities was issued in 1942.

**American Dental Association Specifications.**     Although a considerable amount of the research by the American Dental Association Research Associates and their co-workers at the National Bureau of Standards is basic in nature, their primary objective is to formulate specifications for dental materials. Such specifications are essentially standards by which the value of the particular dental materials can be gauged. They present the requirements as to the physical and chemi-

.cal properties of a material which will insure that the material will be satisfactory if properly employed by the dentist. Once a specification has been formulated, the various manufacturers of the material may certify to the American Dental Association that their product meets the requirements of the particular specification. The product is then tested at the National Bureau of Standards, and if it meets the requirements of the particular specification, its trade name and the manufacturer's name are published in the *Journal of the American Dental Association.* The manufacturer is permitted to signify on the label of the product that it has been certified by the American Dental Association.

The benefit of such specifications to the dental profession has been inestimable. The dentist is provided with a criterion of selection which is impartial and reliable. In other words, if the dentist uses only those materials which meet the appropriate American Dental Association Specification, he can be assured that the material will be satisfactory. Such a statement implies, of course, that such a specification exists for the material.

An awareness by the dentist of the requirements of these specifications is important in order that he may be able to recognize the limitations of the dental material with which he is working. No dental material is perfect in its restorative role any more than an artificial arm or leg can serve as well as the original body member which it replaces.

For this and other reasons, the research in dental materials, supervised by the Council on Research of the American Dental Association, is of vital concern in the present course in dental materials. The American Dental Association Specifications for dental materials are constantly referred to in the following pages. *The discussions in this book assume that the student possesses a current copy of the* American Dental Association Specifications for Dental Materials *as a companion to this book.*

The *American Dental Association Specifications for Dental Materials* is a small book which can be purchased from the publisher, the American Dental Association, 222 East Superior Street, Chicago 11, Illinois, for a nominal sum. It is revised and published every two or three years as required to keep the contents up-to-date. It not only contains the American Dental Association Specifications in detail, but it also outlines the current dental materials research projects of the Council on Research, reviews the recent researches in the field with an excellent reference bibliography, and presents the trade names of commercial products which are currently certified to meet the requirements of the particular specification involved.

**Other Research Centers.** The work at the National Bureau of Standards has stimulated similar studies in other countries. The Commonwealth Bureau of Dental Standards has been established in Australia. Its first executive officer was H. K. Worner, and it is now under the capable direction of A. R. Docking. The Australian researchers are formulating specifications for the dental materials used in Australia.

The *Fédération Dentaire Internationale* (International Dental Federation), a world-wide organization of dentists, is actively supporting a program for the formulation of specifications on an international scale.

A number of universities in America and abroad have established laboratories for research in dental materials. In the past few years, this source of basic information on the subject has exceeded that of all other sources combined.

There have been countless contributions to this field by dental clinicians. The final criterion for the success of any material **or technic** is its service in the mouth of the patient. The observant clinician contributes invaluable information by his keen observations and analyses of his failures and successes.

Another source of information is the research laboratories of the dental manufacturers. The far-seeing manufacturer recognizes the value of a research laboratory in connection with the development and production control of his products. Unbiased information from such groups is particularly valuable.

**Scope of the Course.**     Not all of the materials used in dentistry are included in the course. For example, anesthetics and medicaments are not within the scope of this book. The science of dental materials is generally considered to comprise those materials which are employed in the mechanical procedures included in restorative dentistry, such as prosthetics, crown and bridge, operative dentistry and orthodontics. It is one of the aims of this book to introduce the materials to the beginner, and to study their physical and chemical properties as such properties are related to their proper selection and use by the dentist. It is assumed that the reader possesses a basic knowledge of physics and of general and organic chemistry.

The following chapter deals with certain concepts of engineering principles not always included in the course in college physics. Two chapters follow dealing with the chemistry and manipulation of gypsum products. Impression materials are then discussed. The chemistry of synthetic resins is presented as an introduction to a study of the acrylic resins as they are used for denture construction. Four nonmetallic dental materials used for tooth restorations are then discussed.

Before the metallic dental materials are described, a short discussion of the principles of metallography, physical metallurgy and tarnish and corrosion is presented as they can be applied to dental materials and procedures. The basic science of physical metallurgy is concerned with the properties of metals and alloys, whereas the study of metallography involves the constitution and structure of metallic substances.

Gold foil, dental amalgam and their manipulation are then de-scribed. This discussion is followed by a consideration of the gold alloys used in dentistry, and the materials and technics employed in dental casting and soldering procedures. The final chapters are concerned with the dental base metal alloys, certain technical procedures, such as abrad-ing or polishing, together with a discussion of dental burs and power sources for cutting tooth structure.

It will be observed that many branches of science will be borrowed from in the presentation of the information. The sciences of physical metallurgy and metallography have already been mentioned. Ceramics is the study dealing with the firing of pottery and porcelain. Various specialized branches of chemistry will be drawn upon. Practically all the engineering applied sciences have contributed to the subject. How-ever, in the final analysis, the subject of dental materials is a basic science in itself, with its own cultural value and principles.

**Aim of the Course.** The aim of the course is to present the basic chemical and physical properties of the dental material as they are related to its manipulation by the dentist. It is intended to bridge the gap between the knowledge obtained in the basic courses in chem-istry and physics and the dental technics. As previously noted, dental technique does not need to be an empirical process, but rather it can be based on sound, scientific principles as more information is available from further research.

In any basic science, principles should be emphasized over practice. The discussions that follow deal more with *why* the materials react as they do and *why* the manipulation variables should be observed as they are described. *How* the materials are used in the broadest sense is discussed in other dental courses. The *how* information in this course is largely limited to the material *per se*.

**Accuracy of the Technical Procedures.** As previously mentioned, no dental restoration is perfect regardless of the dental material or technic employed. Nor is any man-made structure perfect for that matter. An engineer may design some intricate type of machine but he will indicate the desired tolerance of accuracy for each part and material. He realizes that every machinist works to a certain tolerance, the degree of which, in turn, will depend upon the precision of the tools employed and the skill of the machinist.

This principle holds true in dentistry as well. Every dentist in every operation works within a certain tolerance. Unfortunately, the degree of this tolerance is unknown. Whereas the engineer may specify a tolerance of 0.01 millimeter or 0.001 millimeter for a certain structural part, as yet dental technics have not progressed to this point.

Consequently, the safest assumption to be made in such a case is to assume the required tolerance to be as small as possible. In other words, the most desirable technical procedure is the one which approaches perfection most closely.

Such is the attitude adopted in this book. An ideal situation will be assumed, and then the necessary departures from the ideal will be noted.

**Need for the Course.** One of the differences between a professional man and a tradesman is that the former possesses basic knowledge with which he can select or set up the conditions for a situation such that a prediction of eventual success of a project is reasonably assured. A riveter must be responsible for the joined beams in a bridge, but the engineer is responsible for the design of the bridge, as to where the rivets and every truss and beam are to be placed and joined, and also for the selection of the materials with which the structure is constructed. If he knew nothing about the physical and chemical properties of the steels and other metals with which the bridge is made, the structure would undoubtedly fail.

The dentist and the engineer have much in common. The dentist must analyze the stresses present in a bridge that he is to build, and be guided by such analyses in the design of the bridge. He should possess a sufficient knowledge of the physical and chemical properties of the different types of materials he is using so that he can exercise the best judgment possible in their selection. In other words, he must be in a position to know whether the dental operation requires the use of a gold alloy, a cement, or a synthetic resin, for example. Only if he knows the physical and chemical properties of each of these materials is he in a position to make such a judgment. In addition to the mechanical requirements of the materials, there are also certain physiological requirements which often complicate the situation beyond the difficulties usually encountered by the engineer.

Once the dentist has selected the type of material he should use, he must choose the material made by a certain manufacturer. It is the intention of the best dental manufacturers to cooperate with the dentist in supplying him with materials of quality in an ethical manner. The competition is keen, however, and the dentist should be in a position to evaluate the claims of the respective manufacturers in an intelligent manner. Unfortunately, there are a few unprincipled dental manufacturers who make preposterous claims and who exploit the dentist for their own profit. For his own protection and for the protection of his patient, the dentist must be able to recognize spurious practices of this sort. In addition to its other aims, the course in dental materials tries to provide the dentist with certain criteria of selection which will enable him to discriminate between fact and propaganda.

Furthermore, it is hoped that the student of dental materials will be given an appreciation of the broad scientific scope of the profession which he has chosen. Only in dentistry are the professions of medicine and engineering so closely linked.

**Limitations of Dental Materials.** In the chapters to follow, the student will become increasingly aware of the difficulties involved in producing a satisfactory dental material, or in designing a technic that is usable and practical. The requirements which are placed upon dental structures and materials in the mouth are excessive and unique. Unfortunately, too often the dentist and patient are unaware of the limitations involved and the rigid conditions imposed in the oral cavity.

First of all the dentist is limited in the design of the appliance or restoration. Access in the mouth is difficult and only a certain amount of tooth structure may be safely removed. Thus, it is a difficult task to build the structure that offers optimum resistance to stress and to caries.

Furthermore, the oral environment is ideally suited for destruction. Biting stresses on restorations may amount to thousands of pounds per square inch. Instantaneous temperature changes may be as great as 65° C. The $pH$ is rapidly fluctuating from acidity to alkalinity. The warm, humid environment of the oral cavity is most conducive to corrosion. The dental pulp and soft tissues must always be considered as they are easily injured by any irritant. These considerations, and many others, necessitate highly specialized compositions and rigid manipulative technics to assure clinical success.

Because of these most drastic conditions, the perfect restoration or ideal dental material has not yet been developed. For example, the perfect restorative material should chemically bond with the tooth, should possess physical and chemical properties essentially comparable to those of the tooth and should possess esthetic properties comparable to those of enamel and dentin. None of these characteristics is totally present in the present restorative materials.

However, dental research, and thus dental science, is moving at an accelerated pace. Probably no other area has made such far-reaching advances as has the field of dental materials. Almost phenomenal progress has been made during the last decade in most materials and techniques; yet if one visualizes the eventual application in dentistry of the research activities in the basic fields of chemistry, physics, and metallurgy, the immediate horizon is filled with possibilities which at times defy the imagination. The concepts, theories, and practice of dentistry must, and most certainly will, change with these technical advances.

Because of the complexity of problems which the oral cavity presents, the discussions in this book will often touch on other fields of science, and most certainly on the practical application of the fundamental physical and chemical properties. The dental manufacturer, research worker or dentist should not divorce the bacteriologic, pathologic or biochemical considerations from the basic chemical or metallurgical properties of the material itself. This, then, is the changing science of dental materials and progress or success can only stem from a thorough knowledge of the inherent characteristics and behavior of the materials themselves.

## Literature

1. Souder, W. H., and Peters, C. G.: *An Investigation of the Physical Properties of Dental Materials.* National Bureau of Standards Technical Paper No. 157, Washington, U. S. Government Printing Office, 1920.
2. Coleman, R. L.: *Physical Properties of Dental Materials.* National Bureau of Standards Research Paper No. 32. Washington, U. S. Government Printing Office, 1928.
3. Souder, W., and Paffenbarger, G. C.: *Physical Properties of Dental Materials.* National Bureau of Standards Circular C433. Washington, U. S. Government Printing Office, 1942.

# CHAPTER 2

# Physical Properties of

# Dental Materials

All of the phenomena to be discussed in this book are related ultimately to the physical and chemical structure of the materials concerned. All of the properties of a dental restoration are gross manifestations of a molecular, atomic or electronic nature. Since the physical properties of the materials are related to their physical structure, a discussion of the physical structure is in order.

**Classification of Solids.** For the most part, dental materials are solids, and, therefore, the solid state is of special interest. A true solid is characterized by its rigidity. Solids which may be classified as *crystalline* generally exhibit a rigidity, provided that the proper environmental conditions exist. A crystalline solid is characterized by the fact that the unit particles (molecules or atoms) are arranged in a regular fashion in space. *An arrangement of a series of points in space such that every point is situated similarly to every other point is called a space lattice.* In a crystalline solid the atoms are located in such a manner that a space lattice is formed.

On the other hand, some of the dental materials may possess a structure in which the molecules tend to be distributed at random, with no apparent regularity of arrangement. Such a structure is called *amorphous*. For example, some waxes used in dentistry exhibit an amorphous structure. One of the characteristic properties of an amorphous solid which distinguishes it from a crystalline material is that it softens under heat, without exhibiting a definite temperature for freezing or melting as a crystalline solid does. The amorphous solid seldom attains a rigidity comparable to that of a typical crystalline solid; it will flow like a liquid,

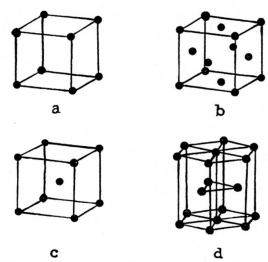

Fig. 2–1.    Unit cells of various types of space lattices: *a.* Simple cubic, *b.* face-centered cubic, *c.* body-centered cubic, and *d.* close-packed hexagonal.

slowly but completely when it is placed under a load, regardless of the temperature.

A third classification might be that of a semi-crystalline solid in which there may be groups of crystals not completely bound to each other by primary valences. In such a case, complete rigidity may be lacking and a certain amount of plasticity may be present under stress, although the main body of the material may be crystalline in character.

**Types of Space Lattice.**    There are fourteen types of space lattice possible,[1] but only four of these types will be important for study in this book. The space lattice can be pictured as made up of small prisms, each of which exhibits the full symmetry of the crystal. These prisms are known as *unit cells.* The unit cells of the space lattices of special interest are shown in Figure 2–1. The basic prism in this case is a cube with the atoms at its corners, and it is called a *simple cubic* space lattice (Fig. 2–1*a*).

If atoms are placed in the center of each face of the cube, as in Figure 2–1*b*, the type is known as the *face-centered cubic* space lattice. If an additional atom is placed at the geometrical center of the unit cell of the simple cubic lattice, the lattice is said to be of the *body-centered* type (Fig. 2–1*c*). The structure diagrammed in Figure 2–1*d* is a *close-packed hexagonal* space lattice.

A few other types of space lattice will be mentioned in connection with certain dental materials. For example, if the four-sided unit prism possesses three axes of unequal length, but mutually perpendicular to each other, the space lattice is said to be *orthorhombic.* If only one of the three unequal axes is perpendicular to the other two, the lattice is unequal length, but with all the axes perpendicular, the structure is *monoclinic.* If two of the axes are of equal length and the other is of called *tetragonal.*

Regardless of the type of space lattice, for all practical purposes the atoms of the space lattice may be considered as being suspended in space by the mutual forces existing between the atoms. If the distance between the atoms becomes too small, a repulsion will result, and the tendency will exist to restore the original distance. If the distance becomes too great, an attractive force will be active. Consequently, if an external force is exerted on a space lattice, such that the atomic spacings are increased, an atomic force will exist in opposition to the external force, which will tend to restore the original relationship of the atoms in the lattice when the external force is released. If the external force is a compressive force, the reverse situation will prevail, since the atoms will be forced closer together.

**Stress and Strain.**      The atomic forces which are internal, and which oppose the effect of the external force, are known as *stresses,* and the change in distance between the atoms is known as the *strain.* The external force which produced the change is called the *load.*

Since it is impractical to discuss atomic relationships in the testing of large structures, the stresses and strains are measured across unit dimensions. For example, the stress or force between the atoms can be defined as the resultant atomic force in a unit area of the structure. *A stress, then, is any internal force which is exerted throughout any unit area, and which resists an external force or load applied to that area.* The *strain is measured in terms of the deformation of the structure per unit dimension.* It should be noted that only the stress is a force or vector quantity, with direction and magnitude.

As an illustration, assume that a stretching force, or load, of 20 kilograms is applied to a wire 0.02 square centimeter in cross section area. The stress, by definition, will be the force per unit area, or

$$\text{Stress} = \frac{20}{0.02} = 1000 \text{ kilograms per square centimeter.}$$

In the English system of measurement, the stress is usually expressed in pounds per square inch.

If the wire were 10 centimeters long, and if it stretched 0.1 centimeter under the load, the strain, by definition, would be the change in length per unit length, or

$$\text{Strain} = \frac{0.1}{10} = 0.01 \text{ centimeter per centimeter.}$$

The accepted equivalent unit in the English system is inch per inch.

**Types of Stresses and Strains.**      As with any type of force, a stress must be defined according to its direction and magnitude. By means of their directions, stresses can be classified under three types.

*Tensile Stress.*    A tensile stress is any induced force which resists a deformation caused by a load which tends to stretch or elongate a body. A tensile stress is always accompanied by a *tensile strain.*

*Compressive Stress.*    If a body is placed under a load which tends to compress or shorten it, the internal forces which resist such a load are called *compressive stresses.* A compressive stress is always accompanied by a *compressive strain.*

*Shear.*    A stress which tends to resist a twisting motion, or a sliding of one portion of a body over another, is a *shear* or *shearing stress.* For example, if this book is closed and placed horizontally upon a table, then if it is deformed by pressing the hand on the upper cover, at the same time exerting a force parallel in direction to the cover, the pages will slip over one another and the shape of the book viewed from an end will be that of a parallelogram with two acute angles. A shear or shearing stress is thus induced in the book, which is accompanied by a *shearing strain.*

**Complex Stresses.**    It is extremely difficult to induce a pure stress of a single type in a body. For example, when a wire is stretched, the very conception of stretching connotes an internal sliding of atoms over one another. The experimentally observed stress will be predominantly tensile, but the shearing stresses and strains will also be present. Furthermore, during the deformation, the wire decreases slightly in cross section area, a condition which obviously indicates the presence of compressive stresses.

If a cylinder of plaster of paris, for example, is placed between the crushing heads of a testing machine so that the load is applied at its top and bottom, the load is resisted by compressive stresses. However, since the sides of the cylinder are not loaded, they are free to exhibit an outward deformation. Since this deformation increases the diameter of the specimen, it is equivalent to a tensile strain, and, therefore, tensile stresses must be present. Lastly, when shearing stresses are produced in the book, as previously described, it may be seen that two of the corners are moved closer together, and two are farther apart. Consequently, compressive stresses and strains are set up in the first case, and tensile in the second, in addition to the principal stress which is shear.

**Elastic Limit.**    If a small tensile stress is induced in a wire, the resulting strain will be such that the wire will return to its original length (*i.e.,* the atoms will move into their regular positions) when the load is removed. The wire is said to be *elastic* under such a loading.

If the load is increased progressively in small increments, and then released after each addition of stress, a stress value finally will be found at which the wire does not return to its original length after it is unloaded. In such a case, the wire is said to have been stressed beyond its elastic limit. *The elastic limit* of a material *is the greatest stress to which a material can be subjected, such that it will return to its original dimensions when the forces are released.* Although tensile stress was used in the illustration, the same situation can exist with any type of stress.

**Proportional Limit.**    If the wire discussed in the previous section is loaded in tension progressively in small increments until the wire ruptures, without a removal of the load each time, and if each stress is

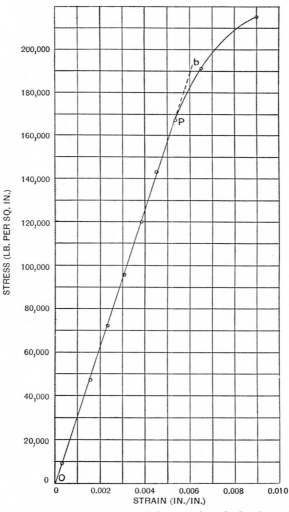

Fig. 2–2. Stress-strain curve for a stainless steel orthodontic arch wire under tension. Proportional limit, 11,700 kilograms per square centimeter (167,000 pounds per square inch); modulus of elasticity, 2,330,000 kilograms per square centimeter (33,300,000 pounds per square inch); modulus of resilience, 29.4 centimeter-kilograms per cubic centimeter (420 inch-pounds per cubic inch); ultimate tensile strength, 16,400 kilograms per square centimeter (234,000 pounds per square inch).

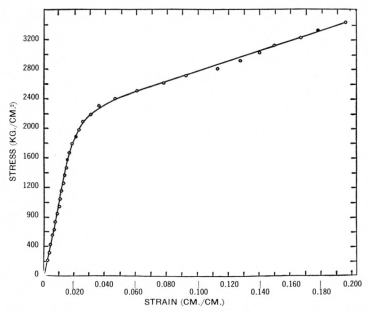

Fig. 2–3.   A stress-strain curve for tooth dentin under compressive stress. (As an exercise, the student is urged to determine the proportional limit and modulus of elasticity of the dentin from the above curve.)

plotted on a vertical coordinate and the corresponding strain is plotted on the horizontal coordinate, a curve similar to that in Figure 2–2 is obtained. It can be noted that the curve starts as a straight line but gradually curves after a certain stress value is exceeded. If a ruler is laid on the straight-line portion of the curve, and if the straight line is extended in a dotted line as shown, the stress at the point P, at which the curve digresses from a straight line, is known as the *proportional limit.*

It is a fundamental law (Hooke's law) that the stress is directly proportional to the strain in elastic deformation. Since direct proportionality between two quantities is always graphically a straight line, the straight-line portion of the graph in Figure 2–2, which was plotted from actual data, is confirmation of this law. Since the proportional limit (stress P) is the greatest stress possible in accordance with this law, it may be defined as *the greatest stress which may be produced in a material such that the stress is directly proportional to the strain.* A stress-strain curve for tooth dentin under compression is shown in Figure 2–3.

**Yield Strength.**   The conditions assumed for the definitions of elastic limit and proportional limit are not always realized under practical conditions. If the measuring instruments are sufficiently sensitive, deviations from Hooke's law, and slight permanent deformations, can be recorded at any stress when commercially processed metals and alloys are tested. Non-metallic materials, especially, are apt to be lacking in this regard. Consequently, as an approximation, it could be assumed that the first marked deviation from a direct proportionality between stress and strain might be used as a measure of the limit of direct proportionality. For example, if the strain is increased 10 to 25 per cent above previous strain increments after the addition of a certain stress, provided that all of the stress increments are equal, such a stress is indicative of the limiting stress for the direct proportionality between stress and strain. Such a stress is called the *yield strength* of the material.

Although the three terms, elastic limit, proportional limit, and yield strength are defined differently, their magnitudes are so nearly the same that for all practical purposes the terms can be used interchangeably.

**Modulus of Elasticity.** In Figures 2–2 and 2–3, if any stress value equal to or less than the proportional limit is divided by its corresponding strain value, a constant of proportionality will result. This constant of proportionality is known as the *modulus of elasticity*. Under compressive or tensile stress, it is often designated as *Young's modulus*, and when a shear stress is predominant it is sometimes called the *shear modulus* or *modulus of rigidity*.

Since the modulus of elasticity is the ratio of the stress to the strain, it follows that the less the strain for a given stress, the greater will be the value of the modulus. For example, if a wire or a similar structure is difficult to bend, considerable stress must be induced before a notable strain or deformation results. Such a material would possess a comparatively high modulus of elasticity.

The mathematical formula for the modulus of elasticity in tension which is familiar to the student of physics, is derived as follows:

$$
\begin{aligned}
\text{Let } E &= \text{Modulus of elasticity} \\
F &= \text{Applied force or load} \\
A &= \text{Cross section of the material under stress} \\
e &= \text{Increase in length} \\
l &= \text{Original length}
\end{aligned}
$$

$$
\begin{aligned}
\text{By definition: Stress} &= F/A \\
\text{Strain} &= e/l
\end{aligned}
\tag{1}
$$

$$
\begin{aligned}
\text{Then } E &= \frac{\text{Stress}}{\text{Strain}} \\
&= \frac{F/A}{e/l} \\
&= \frac{Fl}{eA}
\end{aligned}
$$

The unit for the modulus of elasticity is force per unit area.

**Flexibility.** In the case of dental appliances and restorations, a high value for the elastic limit is a requirement for the materials of which they are fabricated, since the structure is expected to return to its original shape after it has been stressed. Usually, a high modulus of elasticity is also required, since a small deformation is usually desired under considerable stress, as in the case of an inlay, for example.

There are instances, however, when a larger strain or deformation may be needed with a moderate or slight stress. For example, in an orthodontic appliance, a spring is often bent a considerable distance with a small stress resulting. In such a case the structure is said to be *flexible,* and to possess the property of *flexibility.* The *maximum flexibility* is defined *as the strain which occurs when the material is stressed to its proportional limit.* The relation between the maximum flexibility, the proportional limit and modulus of elasticity may be expressed mathematically as follows:

Let E = Modulus of elasticity
P = Proportional limit
$\epsilon$ = Maximum flexibility

From equation (1) above, $E = \dfrac{P}{\epsilon}$

or $\epsilon = P/E$ $\qquad\qquad\qquad\qquad$ (2)

**Resilience.**     Popularly, the term "resilience" is usually associated with "springiness," but technically it connotes something more than this. *Resilience is the amount of energy absorbed by a structure when it is stressed not to exceed its proportional limit.* For example, when an acrobat falls or jumps onto a trapeze net, his fall is "broken" by the resilience of the net. The net is deformed elastically by the impact, so that its energy at the time of maximum deformation is equal to the energy of the acrobat at the instant of impact. When the energy of the net is released, the acrobat is thrown into the air again, and a second impact occurs, and so on. Fortunately, part of the energy is dissipated in the form of heat, otherwise he would never stop rebounding.

By definition, work is the product of the acting force and the distance through which the force moves. When work is done upon a body, energy is imparted to it. Consequently, when a dental restoration is deformed it absorbs energy. Since it is to be tacitly assumed that the induced stress is not greater than the proportional limit, in order that the structure may not be permanently deformed, only the absorbed energy due to elastic deformation need be discussed.

When a dental restoration is deformed, the acting force is the masticating force as it acts upon the structure, and the distance through which it moves will be the deformation induced in the restoration. From the physical definition of work, it may be noted that either the amount of deformation may be large, and the applied force relatively small in magnitude, or the force may be large, and the deformation small. In either case, the resilience can be the same, provided that the values are chosen correctly. In most dental restorations, large strains are precluded because of the dangers of tooth displacement. For example, a proximal inlay might cause excessive movement of the adjacent tooth, if large strains developed. Hence, the restorative material should exhibit a type of resilience which allows stresses of considerable magnitude with but little strain. In other words, the material should possess a high modulus of elasticity.

The *modulus of resilience is the amount of energy stored up in a body, when one unit volume of a material is stressed to its proportional limit.* The modulus of resilience is determined mathematically by dividing the square of the proportional limit by twice the modulus of elasticity. The mathematical proof for this statement is as follows:

Let R = Modulus of resilience
  P = Proportional limit
  $\epsilon$ = Maximum flexibility
  E = Modulus of elasticity

Since the structure is stressed continuously from zero to P,

$$\text{the average force} = \frac{0 + P}{2} = \frac{P}{2}$$

Then, the total work done per unit volume $= R = \dfrac{P}{2} \times \epsilon$

$$= \frac{P}{2} \times \frac{P}{E} \quad \text{[from formula (2) above]}$$

$$= \frac{P^2}{2E} \tag{3}$$

The units for the modulus of resilience are expressed as energy per unit volume (centimeter-kilograms per cubic centimeter or inch-pounds per cubic inch).

**Dynamic Force.**    In all of the discussion thus far, it has been assumed that the forces and stresses were static, with no motion involved. The forces of mastication are dynamic, in that the mouth structures are subject to *impact forces,* and their effect may be different.

For example, the weight of a hammer on a table top produces no visible change in the surface of the table. Yet, if the hammer is placed in motion so that it strikes the table top, the force at impact will be much greater than the static force occasioned by the weight of the hammer alone. The magnitude of the impact force, or the stress it induced in the table, cannot be measured, but the energy received from the impact by the table can be measured. Whether or not the surface of the table will be damaged will depend upon its capacity to absorb the energy without a permanent deformation. In other words, its capacity to resist the impact elastically will be in proportion to its modulus of resilience. The analogy can, of course, be applied to a dental restoration or to any other structure. For a given material, then, the following law may be stated:

*The ability of a unit volume of a material to resist an impact without permanent deformation is directly proportional to the modulus of resilience of the material.*

A mathematical analysis of such a condition can be made with some interesting corollaries:

Let R = Modulus of resilience
 V = Volume
 K = Proportionality constant
Then, the ability to resist impact = KVR

$$= \frac{KVP^2}{2E} \text{ [from equation (3)]} \qquad (4)$$

The practical significance of the proportionality constant, K, in equation (4) is of especial interest. It represents the structural factors which are present in the design of the dental appliance. Although the proportional limit of the material used is the most important factor, the design of the structure is also important in relation to its ability to resist impact. This factor is discussed in textbooks relating to the various branches of clinical dentistry.

According to equation (4), an increase in the volume of the material will increase its ability to resist impact without permanent deformation. The two quantities are in direct proportion to each other. It can be further concluded from the same equation that the impact resistance will be decreased with an increase in the modulus of elasticity. As previously noted, however, a high modulus of elasticity is necessary in most dental restorations to provide rigidity under stress.

**Stresses during Mastication.**    During the mastication of food, the teeth are obviously subject to stress. According to the previous discussion, the mechanical properties of the teeth should be such that the loads during mastication can be successfully resisted without permanent deformation or fracture.

Some of the mechanical properties of extracted teeth have been determined under compressive stress.[1-5] It has been shown[5] that the proportional limit of a cylinder of tooth dentin from the crownal portion is approximately 1500 kilograms per square centimeter (21,500 pounds per square inch) and its modulus of elasticity is 140,000 kilograms per square centimeter (2,000,000 pounds per square inch). These properties did not vary greatly from one tooth to another, nor did they vary with the position of the dentin in the tooth crown. The properties were somewhat lower for root dentin, however.

The similar properties for enamel are much higher.[5] For cylindrical specimens of enamel from a cuspal portion of a molar tooth, the proportional limit was found to be 2,270 kilograms per square centimeter (32,500 pounds per square inch) and the modulus of elasticity was 465,000 kilograms per square centimeter (6,700,000 pounds per square inch).

As calculated from the above figures, the modulus of resilience is 8 centimeter-kilograms per cubic centimeter (116 inch-pounds per cubic inch) for tooth dentin, and 5.6 centimeter-kilograms per cubic centimeter (79.4 inch-pounds per cubic inch) for cuspal enamel. On the basis of the discussion in the last section, apparently the enamel is seven times more able to withstand energy of impact than is a similar volume of tooth dentin. Such a consideration is important structurally since the masticating stresses should be considered as dynamic rather than static in character.

A number of research studies[6-10] have been made concerning the masticating loads incurred on teeth during mastication. According to one study,[7] the maximum static force between similar opposing molar teeth exerted by different individuals varied between 11 kilograms (25 pounds) and 125 kilograms (275 pounds), with an average static biting force of 78 kilograms (170 pounds).

If it is assumed that the average force of 78 kilograms is applied to the apex of a cusp in an area equivalent to 0.04 square centimeter (0.006 square inch),* the compressive stress on the cusp in this area is calculated to be 1950 kilograms per square centimeter (28,000 pounds per square inch).

As can be noted, this stress approaches that of the proportional limit. On the other hand, had the area been selected farther toward the base of the tooth, perpendicular to the tooth axis, the stress would be less, and so on. In other words, the design of the tooth is such that the stress can be distributed in a manner which allows an overall stress resistance of considerable magnitude. This fact illustrates the design factor previously discussed, and it explains why the tooth can resist the impact energy of the dynamic forces of mastication. A sound, healthy tooth in proper occlusion with the other teeth is seldom fractured during mastication.

Further factors in the effective absorption of the energies involved are the considerations inherent in the act of chewing. Under ordinary conditions of mastication, the inelastic deformation (or toughness) of the food bolus plus the elastic resilience of the mouth structures will completely dissipate or absorb this large amount of energy without difficulty or discomfort. However, if the reader has ever had the painful experience of suddenly biting on a shot when eating wild game, he can readily testify to the enormous magnitude of the force involved even under conditions when no conscious effort is made to exert them. In such a case, most of the impact energy is transmitted to the mouth structures, and a severe pain results. The shot may be flattened, and the teeth in some cases are injured permanently. Even under conscious effort, the jaws cannot flatten the shot when a static force is used.

It should be evident, then, why the materials used for dental restorations must have sufficient strength. Not only must they be strong, but also they must have a modulus of resilience sufficiently large to absorb

---

* If it is assumed that the cusp is pointed, this area is a conservative estimate since it is equivalent to a square, two millimeters (approximately $\frac{1}{16}$ inch) on a side.

the energies involved without becoming permanently deformed. From an engineering standpoint, the construction of an inlay is quite complex in comparison to many of the problems of the structural engineer, for example. In most cases the latter may increase the bulk of his structures where resilience is needed, but the dentist does not have such an alternative; he must select a material and a design which will be satisfactory for the limited space available.

**Ductility and Malleability.**     When a structure is stressed beyond its proportional limit, it becomes permanently deformed. If the stresses are tensile in type, and if the material can withstand considerable permanent deformation without rupture, it is said to be *ductile. Ductility is*, therefore, *the ability of a material to withstand permanent deformation under a tensile load without rupture.* A metal which may be drawn readily into a wire is said to be ductile. Ductility is dependent upon plasticity and tensile strength.

*The ability of a material to withstand permanent deformation without rupture under compression,* as in hammering or rolling into a sheet, *is termed malleability.* It is also dependent on plasticity, but it is not as dependent upon strength as is ductility.

In general, ductility decreases with increase in temperature, whereas malleability increases with increase in temperature. Gold is the most ductile and malleable metal, and silver is second. Of the metals of interest to the dentist, platinum ranks third in ductility, and copper ranks third in malleability.

Ductility is commonly associated with the allowable degree of plasticity when a material is bent or contoured at room temperature, and it is quite important from a dental standpoint.

*Measurement of Ductility.*     The proper measurement of ductility is somewhat dependent upon the type of permanent deformation to which the structure is to be subjected.

Probably the simplest and most used method of measurement is to compare the increase in length of a wire or rod after fracture in tension to its length before fracture. Two marks are placed on the wire or rod, a specified distance apart which is designated as the *gauge length.* In dental testing, the standard gauge length is usually two inches (51 millimeters). The wire or rod is then pulled apart under a tensile load. The fractured ends are fitted together, and the gauge length is again measured. The ratio of the increase in length after fracture to the original gauge length, expressed in per cent, is called the *elongation.*

Another manifestation of ductility is the necking or cone-shaped constriction which occurs at the fractured end of a wire after rupture under a tensile load. The percentage decrease in cross section area of the fractured end in comparison to the original area of the wire or rod is called the *reduction in area.*

A third method for the measurement of ductility is known as the *cold bend test.* The material is clamped in a vise and bent around a mandrel of a specified radius. The number of bends before fracture are counted, and the greater the number, the greater is the ductility. The first bend is counted from the vertical to the horizontal, but all subsequent bends are counted through angles of 180 degrees.

**Flow.** Some materials will continue to flow or deform under a given load without an increase in the magnitude of the applied force. Such a condition is somewhat related to ductility, although a ductile substance does not necessarily exhibit a continuous flow under a constant load.

Flow is particularly an attribute of amorphous materials, a fact which is not surprising in consideration of their structure. Pitch is a good example of such a substance; it will fracture under a sudden blow, but if it is placed in a leaky container it will flow through the leak under its own weight. Glass tubing will bend if it is leaned against the wall or if it is laid between supports at either end.

Although flow may be measured under any type of stress, compression is usually employed in the testing of dental materials. A cylinder of prescribed dimensions is subjected to a given compressive stress for a specified time and temperature. The flow is measured as the percentage of shortening in length which occurs under these testing conditions.

**Ultimate Strength.** The ultimate strength is the greatest stress which can be induced in a body before or during rupture. Fracture under tension is properly called *ultimate tensile strength,* although *tensile strength,* or simply, *strength,* are often employed as synonymous terms. Fracture under compression is called *ultimate compressive strength,* or *crushing strength.*

It is a matter of academic interest that the strength of a material is not necessarily its stress at the instant of fracture. It is a common occurrence in the case of a ductile material for the stress to increase to a maximum value, which is designated as its strength, and then to decrease to a lower value when the fracture occurs.

**Toughness and Brittleness.** *Toughness is the total work or energy required to rupture a material.* It should be noted that *toughness* is all-inclusive in that it includes the resilience of the material as well, since the material must be stressed through its proportional limit to its fracture stress. If a stress-strain curve is plotted through the complete range, to the fracture stress, the toughness per unit volume of the material can be determined in energy units as the total area under the stress-strain curve.

*Brittleness* is generally considered to be the opposite of toughness. Toughness requires strength and plasticity, whereas brittleness connotes a lack of plasticity. In other words, the strength of a brittle substance may be near or at its proportional limit.

A brittle substance is not necessarily lacking in strength. For example

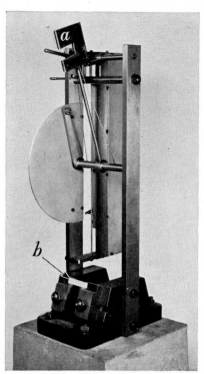

Fig. 2–4. A Charpy type impact tester. The pendulum, ready to be released, is shown at *a*, and the specimen at *b*. The impact strength is measured by the energy lost by the pendulum after impact, in comparison to its energy in a free swing.

a glass fiber may exhibit a tensile strength as high as 28,000 kilograms per square centimeter (400,000 pounds per square inch), and the strength of a quartz fiber may exceed 70,000 kilograms per square centimeter (1,000,000 pounds per square inch). Neither of these materials is ductile at room temperature.

**Impact Strength.**    *The impact strength may be defined as the energy required to fracture a material under an impact force. A Charpy-type* impact tester is shown in Figure 2–4. The pendulum, *a*, is released, and during its swing it fractures the specimen, *b*. The energy lost by the pendulum during the fracture of the specimen can be determined by a comparison of the length of its swing after the impact with its free swing when no impact occurs. The energy units are foot-pounds, inch-pounds, centimeter-kilograms, etc. Unlike most mechanical tests, the dimensions, shape and design of the specimen to be tested should be identical for uniform results.

In another type of equipment, called the *Izod impact tester*, the specimen is clamped vertically at one end. The blow is delivered at a certain distance above the clamped end, instead of at the center of a specimen supported at both ends as indicated in Figure 2–4.

**Flexure Strength.** Flexure strength, transverse strength or modulus of rupture, as this property is variously called, is essentially a strength test of a beam supported at each end, under a static load. The theory involved is beyond the scope of this textbook. The mathematical formula for computing the flexure strength is as follows:

$$S = \frac{3Wl}{2bd^2}$$

Where S = Flexure strength
l = Distance between the supports
b = Width of the specimen
d = Depth or thickness of the specimen
W = Maximum load before fracture

The units are force per unit area (pounds per square inch, kilograms per square centimeter, etc.).

**"Edge Strength."** *Edge strength* is a term sometimes applied to a tooth restorative material relating to its ability to resist mastication forces in the area of a restored cusp. So far as the stress factors are concerned, probably compressive strength best measures this property under static loading, although tensile and shear stresses are also present. With dynamic forces, the impact strength of the material may also be a factor.

It should be recognized, however, that fracture is not the only means by which a cusp can be destroyed. The cusp may disappear by virtue of its being permanently deformed. In such a case, the ductility, malleability and/or toughness of the material may be factors. Also, the cusp may wear during mastication, because of the low abrasion resistance of the dental material.

A further cause might be the dissolution of the dental material in the mouth fluids. Consequently, the term may not refer to a physical property of the material at all.

**Hardness.** Although the surface hardness of a material is a property which is difficult to define, the measurement of such a property is sometimes very significant in engineering practice. For dental purposes, the surface hardness of a material is generally measured in terms of its resistance to indentation. There are four hardness tests, any one of which may be used: the Brinell test, the Rockwell test, the Vickers test, and the Knoop test.

In the Brinell hardness test, a hardened steel ball of a specified diameter is pressed into a polished surface of a material under a specified load. The area of the surface of the indentation is computed, and divided into the magnitude of the load. The quotient is known as the *Brinell Hardness Number*, usually abbreviated B.H.N. This number is an index of hardness as defined above.

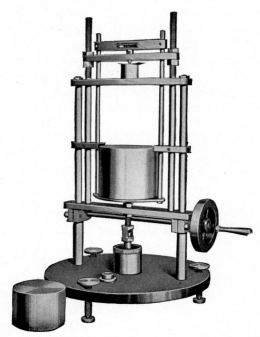

Fig. 2–5. A micro-Brinell hardness tester. The specimen to be tested may be seen on the anvil under the second top crossbar. The steel ball is in the point of the inverted cone-shaped piece, just above the specimen. The load is applied by means of the oil dash pot, resting on the bottom platform. (Courtesy of the American Instrument Co.)

The mathematical formula for the computation of the B.H.N. follows:

$$H = \frac{P}{\dfrac{\pi D}{2}\left(D - \sqrt{D^2 - d^2}\right)}$$

Where H is the Brinell Hardness Number, P the load, D the diameter of the ball, and d the diameter of the impression.

In practice, the diameter of the impression is measured accurately and the B.H.N. is determined from tables prepared for the purpose.

The Brinell tester shown in Figure 2–5, or similar equipment, is used for obtaining the Brinell hardness numbers of dental materials. This type of tester is often referred to as a "baby Brinell" instrument, because of the comparatively small diameter of the steel ball and load employed. The diameter of the ball is 1.6 millimeters ($\frac{1}{16}$ inch), and the standard load is 12.61 kilograms (27.7 pounds). The Brinell hardness number is of considerable significance in dentistry, in addition to its measurement of the resistance of a material to indentation. For example, it has been found that the B.H.N. is directly proportional to the proportional limit and ultimate tensile strength of dental gold alloys.[11]

The Rockwell hardness test is somewhat similar to the Brinell test in that a steel ball is generally used, although a diamond point may be employed under certain conditions. Instead of measuring the diameter of the impression, its depth is measured. The ball is placed initially under a static load of certain value, then the load is increased by a given amount. The increase in the depth of the impression after the second loading is measured accurately. The hardness number is registered directly on the instrument and is related to the depth of the impression. There are a number of different tests for various types of materials, with different loadings and points. The hardness number is designated according to the test employed (Rockwell C, Rockwell M, etc.).

The same principle of hardness testing as in the Brinell test is employed in the Vickers hardness test. In this test, however, instead of a steel ball, a diamond in the shape of a square base pyramid is used. The impression is square instead of round, but the method for the computation of the Vickers hardness number (V.H.N.) is the same as for the Brinell hardness number, in that the surface area of the impression is divided into the load.

The use of a spherical indenter, as employed in the Brinell hardness test, limits the testing to ductile materials. When the test is attempted on brittle materials, such as glass, porcelain or tooth enamel, the surface shatters and the impression is not definite in outline. In ductile materials, there usually is a "recovery" or decrease in the size of the impression, due to residual elastic stress, and as a result the impression exhibits a radius which is less than that of the steel ball.

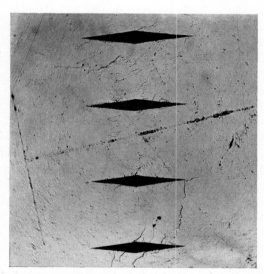

Fig. 2–6. Knoop impressions in tooth enamel. ×100.

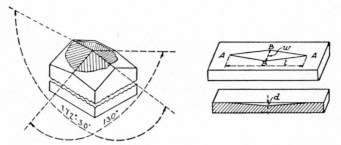

Fig. 2–7. The Knoop diamond indenting tool (*left*) and a schematic drawing of the impression (*right*).

In order to avoid such effects, the Knoop hardness test[12] employs an indenting tool to give the impressions shown in Figure 2–6. The impression is diamond-shaped or rhombic in outline, and the length of the largest diagonal is measured. Instead of the actual area, the projected area is divided into the load to give the Knoop Hardness Number (K.H.N.). The mathematical formula is

$$ I = \frac{L}{A} = \frac{L}{l^2 Cp} $$

Where I = Knoop Hardness Number
       L = Load (in kilograms)
       A = Projected area (in square millimeters)
       l = Length of the long diagonal (in millimeters)
       Cp = Constant relating l to the projected area

The indenting tool is cut from a diamond as shown in Figure 2–7. As may be noted, the longitudinal angle of the rhombus-shaped surface is 172° 30′, whereas that of the transverse angle is 130°. When the indentation is made, a cutting action occurs along the major axis of the impression, and a spreading or indenting, as with the Brinell ball, takes place along the minor axis. The stresses are therefore distributed in such a manner that only the dimensions of the minor axis will be subject to change by recovery. Since the hardness number so obtained is virtually independent of the physical properties of the material tested, the hardness of tooth enamel can be compared with that of gold, porcelain or other tooth restorative materials.

The apparatus employed for making the test is shown in Figure 2–8. The indenting tool is seen just above the anvil. The specimen is placed on the anvil under the indenter, and one of the buttons is pressed to actuate a system of relays which raises the anvil to the indenter, maintains the load on the indenter for twenty seconds, and then releases and lowers the anvil so that the specimen may be removed for the measurement of the impressions.

Regardless of the hardness test used, the higher the hardness number, the harder the surface will be.

***Relaxation.***    In the previous section, it was noted that a recovery is observed after the surface of the material has been permanently deformed by an indentation. Such an effect is commonly observed after a deformation. Not all of the atoms in the space lattice, or the molecules in the semi-crystalline or amorphous materials, are disarranged to the extent that they do not tend to attract or repel each other, and the result is a partial recovery to the original dimension. Such a condition indicates the disappearance or *relief* of certain inherent stresses and strains.

In order to explain such a phenomenon, the atomic conception of stress can be used. According to the discussion at the beginning of the chapter, a stress is present whenever the atoms of a space lattice are displaced so that the interatomic forces are not in equilibrium. When the load is removed, if the atoms resume their normal or equilibrium positions, the stress disappears and the deformation is called elastic.

On the other hand, if the stresses do not disappear when the load is removed, a condition of permanent deformation is said to exist. The same condition can exist in semi-crystalline or amorphous solids, except that the unit to be considered will be the agglomerate or the molecule.

Whenever there is a stressed condition, it is possible that the stresses

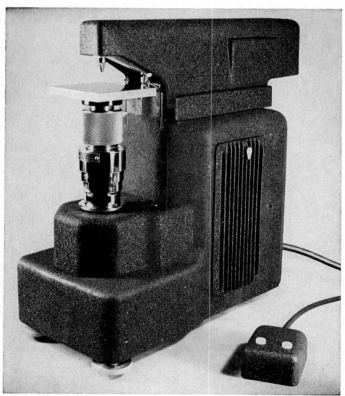

Fig. 2–8.   The Tukon tester for obtaining Knoop hardness numbers. (Courtesy of the Wilson Mechanical Instrument Co.)

may disappear, even though the material is acted upon by an external force, or after a permanent deformation. Although it has been assumed throughout the previous discussion that the positions of the atoms or molecules in a solid were stationary, such an assumption is not entirely justified. The situation is complicated because of the heat motion caused by the thermal agitation of the molecules. Each molecule vibrates about a fixed point, which is its normal position. Although the average amplitude or displacement of all of the molecules (or atoms) is determined by the environmental temperature, there will be localized deviations from this average. It can be assumed that some of the abnormal displacements of the molecules may be large, even comparable to the intermolecular distances. It is probable that such abnormal vibrations may cause the molecules under stress to return to their normal positions, and, thereby, the stress is relieved. Stress and strain relief by such a method is termed *relaxation*. It is evident that if sufficient relaxation occurs, a measurable change in dimension can be observed.

As might be expected from the theory, the higher the temperature, the more rapid the relaxation. At a constant temperature, the relaxation rate is higher at the start in comparison to the subsequent changes at a later time. Examples of relaxation, in which the relaxation may occur over a period of days or weeks before the change becomes apparent from a practical standpoint, will be given in subsequent chapters.

**Thermal Properties.**    The thermal properties of the dental materials are of important dental significance. In tooth restorations, for example, a low thermal conductivity is to be preferred to a high thermal conductivity, since the pulp and nerve supply of the tooth will be better protected from thermal shock. On the other hand, where the soft tissue is covered with a denture base (or "plate"), a high thermal conductivity seems more conducive to better health of the tissue.

Probably the thermal property most important to dentistry is the

*Table 2–1.*    *Average Expansion Coefficients (Range 20° to 50° C.)* *

| MATERIAL | LINEAR COEFFICIENT OF EXPANSION (MM./MM.°C./ $\times 10^{-6}$) |
|---|---|
| Tooth (across crown) | 11.4 |
| Silicate cement | 7.6 |
| Dental amalgam (minimum) | 22.1 |
| Dental amalgam (maximum) | 28.0 |
| Porcelain (Bayeux) | 4.1 |
| Rubber (denture, maroon base) | 56.0 |
| Rubber (denture, olive base) | 80.0 |
| Resin, vinyl (denture) | 71.0 |
| Resin, phenol-formaldehyde (denture) | 79.0 |
| Resin, methyl methacrylate | 81.0 |

* Souder and Paffenbarger, *Physical Properties of Dental Materials.* N.B.S. Circular C433.

linear coefficient of expansion, which is defined as the change in length per unit length of a material when its temperature is raised or lowered through one degree. Linear coefficients of expansion of some substances of interest in dentistry are presented in Table 2–1. As an example of the importance of this property in dentistry, a tooth restoration may expand or contract more than the tooth during a change in temperature and thus the restoration may leak or become loosened. As a specific example, according to the values in Table 2–1, a restoration made with methyl methacrylate resin will change in dimension seven times or more as much as the tooth structure for every degree change in temperature. This point will be discussed more at length in Chapter 13.

**Criteria of Selection.** Inasmuch as most of the physical properties which have been described have been obtained on specimen shapes and sizes, and under stress types which are in some cases dissimilar to mouth conditions, the question at once arises as to how dental materials can be selected by the dentist upon the basis of these properties. The engineer employs similar properties for the selection of materials for the construction of a bridge, for example, but he has an advantage over the dentist in this respect, inasmuch as he knows beforehand, at least approximately, what the expected stresses on his structure will be. Furthermore, he always multiplies these expected stress values by a "safety factor" in order that the structure may be able to withstand a certain amount of overstress.

Unfortunately, the magnitude of the forces of mastication is not known to the extent that the dentist can predict the stresses to which the restorative appliances will be subjected. General ideas as to the physical properties necessary for the materials employed can be obtained with experience, however. For example, if a certain gold alloy has given service in a certain type of dental restoration over a considerable period of time, it is reasonably certain that the alloy is satisfactory. The physical properties of the alloy can be determined, such as its proportional limit, modulus of elasticity, tensile strength, etc., and these values can serve as criteria for the selection of other materials for similar use.

The physical properties can also be used as criteria for improvement of restorative appliances. For example, a dentist discovers that a certain patient has permanently deformed a dental appliance in service. Presumably, this patient exerts large stresses in the appliance during mastication. In such a case, the logical procedure is to remake the appliance with material which possesses a higher proportional limit and Brinell hardness number.

The use of such criteria has also been valuable to the manufacturer in the development of new and improved materials. With such criteria, the success or failure of the material can largely be predicted, and the patient is saved much discomfort and ill health.

It is, also, on such a basis that the requirements of the various American Dental Association Specifications are set up. As discussed in the previous chapter, the most valuable criterion of selection for the dentist is whether or not the particular material meets the requirements of such specifications. If it does meet these requirements, the dentist can be sure that the material will be satisfactory when it is used properly.

## Literature

1. Neumann, H. H., and DiSalvo, N. A.: *Compression of Teeth Under the Load of Chewing.* J. D. Res., *36:*286–293 (April), 1937.
2. Craig, R. G., and Peyton, F. A.: *Elastic and Mechanical Properties of Human Dentin.* J. D. Res., *37:*710–718 (Aug.), 1958.
3. Stanford, J. W., Paffenbarger, G. C., Kumpula, J. W., and Sweeney, W. T.: *Determination of Some Compressive Properties of Human Enamel and Dentin.* J.A.D.A., *57:*487–495 (Oct.), 1958.
4. Stanford, J. W., Weigel, K. V., and Paffenbarger, G. C.: *Compressive Properties of Tooth Tissue and Restorative Materials.* J. D. Res., *38:*762 (July-Aug.), 1959. Abstract.
5. Stanford, J. W., Weigel, K. V., Paffenbarger, G. C., and Sweeney, W. T.: *Compressive Properties of Hard Tooth Tissues and Some Restorative Materials.* J.A.D.A., *60:*746–756 (June), 1960.
6. Black, G. V.: *Practical Utility of Accurate Studies of the Physical Properties of the Teeth and of Filling Materials.* Den. Cos., *38:*302–310 (April), 1896.
7. O'Rourke, J. T.: *Significance of Tests for Biting Strength.* J.A.D.A., *38:*627–633 (May), 1949.
8. Baker, C.: *Registration of Vertical Intermaxillary Force by the Brinell Hardness Method.* J. D. Res., *29:*256 (April), 1950.
9. Anderson, D. J.: *A Method of Recording Masticatory Loads.* J. D. Res., *32:*785–789 (Dec.), 1953.
10. Margolis, H. I., and Prakash, P.: *A New Instrument for Recording Oral Muscle Forces.* J. D. Res., *33:*425–434 (June), 1954.
11. Souder, W., and Paffenbarger, G. C.: *Physical Properties of Dental Materials.* National Bureau of Standards Circular C433. Washington, U.S. Government Printing Office, 1942, pp. 64–65.
12. Knoop, F., Peters, C. G., and Emmerson, W. B.: *A Sensitive Pyramidal-Diamond Tool for Indentation Measurements.* J. Res., Nat'l. Bur. Stand., *23:*39–61 (July), 1939.

# CHAPTER 3

# Gypsum Products: Chemistry

# of Setting. Basic Principles

A number of gypsum products are used in dentistry as important adjuncts to dental operations. Various types of plaster are used to form molds and models on which dental prostheses and restorations are constructed. When the plaster is mixed with a form of silica, it is known as *dental investment*. Such dental investments are used to form molds for the casting of dental restorations in metal; they will be discussed at length in Chapter 27. The present discussion will be confined to the essentially pure gypsum products, such as plaster, which will harden when they are mixed with water.

An excellent illustration of the importance of plaster in dentistry is its use in the preparation of a cast for an artificial denture. A mixture of plaster of paris and water is placed in an *impression tray* and impressed against the upper part of the mouth, for example. The plaster is allowed to harden or *set*, and then the impression is withdrawn. The dentist now has a life-size *negative* model of the mouth parts (Fig. 3–1). If another variety of plaster known as "dental stone" is now mixed with water, poured into the impression, and allowed to set, the hardened plaster impression serves as a mold to form a *positive* model, or *cast*, as shown in Figure 3–2. It is on this cast that the denture is constructed, without the patient being present.

## GYPSUM AND GYPSUM PRODUCTS

**Gypsum.**     Gypsum is a mineral mined in various parts of the world. Chemically, the mineral as used for dental purposes is nearly pure calcium sulfate dihydrate ($CaSO_4.2H_2O$).

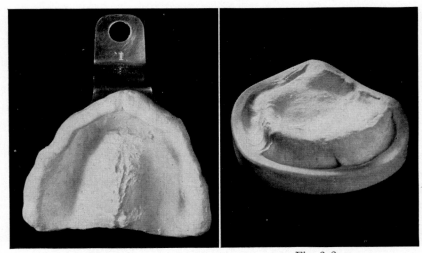

Fig. 3–1.                                    Fig. 3–2.

Fig. 3–1. An impression of an edentulous upper mouth obtained with plaster of paris. (Gehl and Dresen, *Complete Denture Prosthesis*, W. B. Saunders Co.)

Fig. 3–2. A stone cast of an upper edentulous mouth.

Different forms of gypsum have been used for many centuries for construction purposes. It is supposed that the alabaster used in the building of King Solomon's temple of Biblical fame was a form of gypsum. In spite of the fact that gypsum has been used by itself or in the form of one of its derivatives such as plaster for many centuries, there are many gaps in the knowledge of its chemistry.

**Dental Plaster.**    Plaster is the result of the calcining of gypsum. Commercially, the gypsum is first ground and then subjected to temperatures of 110° to 120° C. (230° to 250° F.). During this period, part of the water of crystallization is driven off, and the first step in reaction (1) takes place. As the temperature is raised, the remaining water of crystallization is removed, and the products are formed as indicated.

$$CaSO_4.2H_2O \xrightarrow[110°-130°C.]{\Delta} (CaSO_4)_2.H_2O \xrightarrow[130°-200°C.]{\Delta} CaSO_4 \xrightarrow[200°-1000°C.]{\Delta} CaSO_4 \quad (1)$$

| Gypsum | Plaster | Soluble | Natural |
|---|---|---|---|
| (Monoclinic) | (Orthorhombic) | Anhydrite (Orthorhombic) | Anhydrite (Orthorhombic) |

The principal constituent of the dental plasters is the calcium sulfate hemihydrate, $(CaSO_4)_2.H_2O$. The hemihydrate form possesses an orthorhombic space lattice, whereas the dihydrate is monoclinic. In fact, all of the products of calcination are of the orthorhombic form; their space lattices differ chiefly in their interatomic distances.[1]

There appear to be two different forms of the hemihydrate, depending upon the method of calcination. For example, if the gypsum is heated in a kettle in the open air to the temperatures indicated in reaction (1), a crystalline form of the hemihydrate results as shown in Figure 3–3, known as $\beta$-hemihydrate,[2] or, more popularly, as plaster of paris.

**Dental Stone.** The $\beta$-hemihydrate crystals are characterized as being somewhat irregular in shape, in contrast to the more prismatic particles shown in Figure 3–4, which are crystals of $\alpha$-hemihydrate. Alpha-hemihydrate is the product formed when the gypsum is calcined under steam pressure[2] in an autoclave, usually in the presence of water, at a temperature of 120° to 130° C. (250° to 265° F.). This type of product is the principal constituent of the dental stones, with which casts and models are made. When the $\alpha$-hemihydrate is mixed with water and reaction (1) is reversed, as described in the next section, the product obtained with $\alpha$-hemihydrate is much stronger and harder than that resulting from $\beta$-hemihydrate. The chief reason for this difference is the fact that the $\alpha$-hemihydrate requires much less gauging water when it is mixed than does the $\beta$-hemihydrate. The $\beta$-hemihydrate requires more water to float its powder particles so that they can be stirred than does the $\alpha$-hemihydrate or dental stone, because the crystals of the former are more irregular and they are considered to be porous in character.

Although all dental stones ($\alpha$-hemihydrate) require less gauging water than do the dental plasters ($\beta$-hemihydrate), there is a difference between the amounts of gauging water required by different stones. This difference can likely be accounted for on the basis of the particle size of the crystals: the larger the particle size, the less gauging water

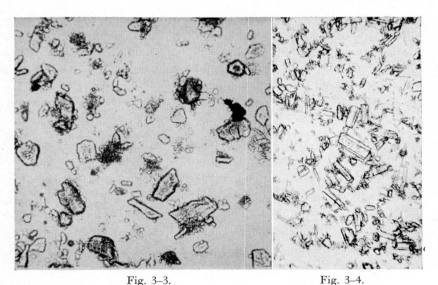

Fig. 3–3.                                    Fig. 3–4.

Fig. 3–3. Powder particles of plaster of paris ($\beta$-gypsum). ×100.
Fig. 3–4. Powder particles of dental stone ($\alpha$-gypsum). ×100.

the respective powder will require. One method by which the crystal size of α-hemihydrate can be controlled is by the incorporation of a catalyst for this purpose during the calcination in the autoclave. For example, the addition of sodium succinate (0.5 per cent or less) in the gypsum to be calcined will produce larger crystals of α-hemihydrate.[3] Other means of controlling the crystal size are by regulating the calcination procedure as to temperature, the particle size of the gypsum to be calcined, and the length of time of calcination.

**Other Gypsum Products.**     As shown in reaction (1), as the temperature is raised, or maintained in the vicinity of 130° C. (265° F.), the hemihydrate loses its water of crystallization to form a more soluble compound known as *soluble anhydrite* ($CaSO_4$).

Above 200° C. (390° F.), a relatively insoluble *"natural" anhydrite* ($CaSO_4$) is formed, which is identical with the anhydrous form of gypsum found in nature. The calcium sulfate breaks down chemically at approximately 1000° C. (1830° F.).

## SETTING OF GYPSUM PRODUCTS

**Chemistry of Setting.**     Reaction (1) can be reversed as follows:

$$(CaSO_4)_2.H_2O + 3H_3O \longrightarrow 2CaSO_4.2H_2O + Heat \qquad (2)$$

The product of the reaction is, obviously, gypsum, and the heat evolved in the exothermic reaction is equivalent to the heat used originally to calcine the product.

The different products of the calcination shown in reaction (1) are characterized by the rapidity of their reaction with water. The soluble anhydrite changes to the hemihydrate very rapidly when it is mixed with water.[4] On the other hand, the "natural" anhydrite reacts with water very slowly, if at all. The final product of the hydration is always the dihydrate (gypsum), but during hydration the anhydrous forms hydrate to the hemihydrate stage before the dihydrate is formed. The gypsum formed from the "natural" anhydrite is very hard and strong, and this anhydrite was one of the ingredients of the "slow setting stones" used in dentistry before the α-hemihydrate material was discovered. As previously noted, the chief ingredient of all modern dental plasters and stones is one of the hemihydrates.

**The Setting Reactions.**     Le Chatelier[5] was the first investigator to give a fairly complete picture of the setting of plaster. The theory is

*Table 3–1.     Solubility of Gypsum and Gypsum Products (20° C.)*

| TYPE | FORMULA | SOLUBILITY, GM./100 CC. |
|------|---------|-------------------------|
| Dihydrate | $CaSO_4.2H_2O$ | 0.2 |
| Hemihydrate | $(CaSO_4)_2.H_2O$ | 0.9 |
| Anhydrous | $CaSO_4$ | 0.3 |

based on the solubilities of the various forms of calcium sulfate involved. As can be seen from Table 3–1, the hemihydrate form is by far the most soluble of the various forms of calcium sulfate.[1]

Actually, the setting reaction is more complex than is indicated by reaction (2). Probably the stages of the reaction may be described as follows:[6]

1. When the hemihydrate and water are mixed together, a suspension of hemihydrate is formed.

2. The hemihydrate dissolves to form a solution of calcium sulfate which is heavily saturated in proportion to the dihydrate to be formed.

3. The dissolved calcium sulfate then diffuses toward nuclei of crystallization composed of gypsum (dihydrate) which were previously formed submicroscopically, or are crystals which were not previously calcined to the hemihydrate during manufacture. The dihydrate of gypsum then forms by reaction (2) and the crystal growth occurs from the nuclei as shown in Figure 3–5.

When this process is observed under the microscope in the presence of considerable water, the crystals form in burlike clusters as seen in Figure 3–5. The crystals are definitely joined at the center of the cluster, a fact which accounts in part for the strength of the dihydrate after setting. In addition, the needle-like crystals become entangled during growth, a condition which further contributes to the strength.

The situation is possibly better understood by an inspection of Figure 3–6. At two minutes (Fig. 3–6*A*) after mixing, there are mostly α-hemihydrate crystals present (see Fig. 3–4). In Figure 3–6*B* a few dihydrate crystals are evident. At 26 minutes (Fig. 3–6*C*), 10 minutes

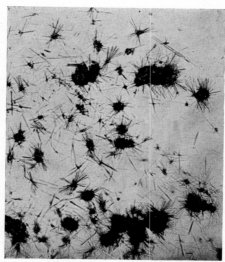

Fig. 3–5.  Gypsum crystals formed by the reaction between calcium sulfate hemihydrate and water. ×100.

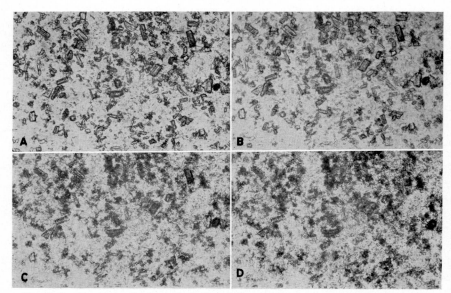

Fig. 3–6.   Stages in the setting of plaster at various times after mixing: *A.* 2 minutes; *B.* 16 minutes; *C.* 26 minutes, and *D.* 50 minutes. ×120. (Jørgensen, *Odontologisk Tidskrift*, 1953.)

later, the dihydrate crystals have almost obliterated the hemihydrate crystals. Only dihydrate (gypsum) is visible in Figure 3–6*D*, and it can be assumed that the reactions are complete.

So far as is known, the chemistry of setting is identical for both forms of the hemihydrate.

**The Water-Powder (W/P) Ratio.**    Many of the properties of a gypsum product are dependent on the ratio of the water to the powder employed. This ratio is generally computed by dividing the weight of the water used by the weight of the powder with which it is mixed. The quotient so obtained is designated as the *W/P ratio*, or water-powder ratio.

For example, if 100 grams of plaster are mixed with 60 cubic centimeters of water, the W/P ratio will be 0.6; if 100 grams of dental stone are mixed with 28 cubic centimeters of water, the W/P ratio will be 0.28, etc.

**Measurement of Setting Time.**    It is important that the dentist be able to control the time during which the reaction (2) takes place so that the product becomes hard at a convenient time after mixing. This time is known as the *setting time*. For example, in the taking of an impression, the plaster should have a short setting time so that the patient will not be unduly inconvenienced by holding the plaster in his mouth for too long a time. On the other hand, if the plaster sets too fast, the dentist will not have sufficient time to mix it with water, to place it in the impression tray, and to carry it to the patient's mouth.

The setting time is generally measured by some type of penetration test. For example, the Gillmore needles (Fig. 3–7) are often used to determine the setting time. The smaller needle weighs ¼ pound and has a point $\frac{1}{12}$ inch in diameter; the other needle weighs 1 pound and has a point $\frac{1}{24}$ inch in diameter. The water and plaster are gauged in a certain W/P ratio, and mixed together for a specified time. The mixture is spread out in a shallow container, and the surface is impressed with the point of the ¼-pound Gillmore needle. The time elapsing from the start of the mixing until the point of the ¼-pound Gillmore needle no longer will penetrate the surface is known as the *initial setting time*. When the 1-pound needle is manipulated similarly, the time elapsing from the start of mixing until the point of the needle no longer will penetrate the surface of the set plaster is known as the *final setting time.*

Another method for measuring the setting time is by means of the Vicat needle, illustrated in Figure 3–8. The rod holding the needle weighs 300 grams; the needle is 1 millimeter in diameter and 5 centimeters in length. As can be noted in Figure 3–8, the rod is supported so that the needle can be lowered to the surface of the plaster contained in the truncated cone container as illustrated. The time which elapses from the start of the mixing of the powder and the water until the needle no longer will penetrate to the bottom of the plaster is known as the setting time. Only one setting time is usually defined in this case.

For all practical purposes, the setting time obtained with the Vicat needle is the same as the initial setting time obtained with the ¼-pound

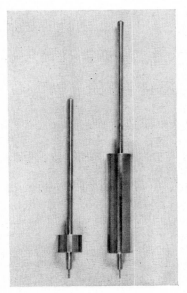

Fig. 3–7.  Gillmore needles.

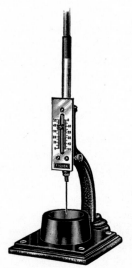

Fig. 3–8.   Vicat needle.

Gillmore needle. As a matter of fact, both tests are empirical in nature, and neither test can be related directly to the chemistry involved.

The initial setting time as given by the ¼-pound Gillmore needle and the setting time as measured by the Vicat needle are very practical. They indicate the time at which the crystallization of gypsum has proceeded to a stage at which the set plaster or stone can be subjected to small stresses, such as carving and smoothing. The crystallization generally continues for several hours.

**Control of Setting Time.**    From a practical standpoint, the setting time is related essentially to the time when sufficient crystals of gypsum are present to support the stresses induced by the ¼-pound Gillmore needle, for example. In other words, the faster the crystals are produced, the shorter will be the setting time.

As previously explained, the crystallization during setting proceeds from nuclei of crystallization. It follows, therefore, that the greater the number of nuclei of crystallization present per unit volume, the shorter the setting time will be. Consequently, any method by which the number of nuclei present in the mixture can be controlled will be effective as a control of the setting time.

*Manufacturing Process.*    The efficiency of the manufacturing process in the production of calcium sulfate hemihydrate is an important factor in the control of the setting time. If the calcination is incomplete, and considerable gypsum is left in the final product, the resulting plaster or stone will set faster than if there are fewer gypsum crystals to form nuclei of crystallization.

If natural anhydrite is present in the plaster, the time of hydration will be lengthened, and the setting time will be increased. On the other

*Table 3–2.*     *Effect of the W/P Ratio and the Mixing Time on the Setting Time of Plaster of Paris\**

| W/P RATIO | MIXING TIME (MIN.) | SETTING TIME (MIN.) |
|-----------|--------------------|---------------------|
| 0.45 | 0.5 | 5.25 |
| 0.45 | 1.0 | 3.25 |
| 0.60 | 1.0 | 7.25 |
| 0.60 | 2.0 | 4.50 |
| 0.80 | 1.0 | 10.50 |
| 0.80 | 2.0 | 7.75 |
| 0.80 | 3.0 | 5.75 |

\* Gibson and Johnson, *J. Chem. Ind.*, *51:*25T (1932).

hand, the presence of considerable soluble anhydrite may decrease the setting time, owing to its rapid rate of solution in the water.

The fineness of the plaster and stone will also be a factor. The finer the plaster, the more rapidly it will set. Not only is the solution rate increased by the increased surface of the plaster in contact with the water, but, more important, the nuclear crystals of gypsum are finer, and thus more potential nuclei of crystallization are present.

The manufacturer also can control the setting time of the gypsum product by the addition of chemicals as described later.

*Mixing.*     Within practical limits, the longer and the more rapidly the plaster is mixed, the shorter the setting time will be. Some gypsum crystals form immediately when the plaster or stone is brought into contact with the water. As the mixing begins, the formation of these crystals increases; at the same time the crystals are broken up by the mixing spatula and they are distributed throughout the mixture, with the resulting formation of more nuclei of crystallization. Thus, the setting time is decreased, as indicated in Table 3–2.

*Water-Powder Ratio.*     The W/P ratio affects the setting time. The more water used, the longer is the setting time.

Such an effect can be anticipated on the basis that the more water used, the fewer will be the nuclei of crystallization present in a unit volume of the mixture, and consequently the longer will be the setting time. The effect of the W/P ratio on the setting time[7] is exemplified in Table 3–2.

*Temperature.*     At temperatures near 0° C. (32° F.), the setting time of a given water-plaster (or stone) mixture is generally slightly greater than it is at 10° to 20° C. (50° to 70° F.). There is little effect of the temperature on the setting time at ambient room temperature. When the temperature of the mixture increases above approximately 50° C. (120° F.), a gradually increasing retardation occurs.[8] At temperatures of 97° to 100° C. above, the material will not set.

The retardation of setting at the higher temperatures is undoubtedly connected with the tendency of reaction (2) to be reversed,[6] and for the re-formation of the hemihydrate.

*Retarders and Accelerators.* Probably the most effective and the most practical method for the control of the setting time is by the addition of certain chemical modifiers to the mixture of plaster or dental stone. If the chemical added decreases the setting time, it is known as an *accelerator*; if it increases the setting time, it is known as a *retarder*.

There appears to be little relation between the chemical formulas of the modifiers added and their effect on the setting time. For example, most colloids (gelatin, glue, agar, gum arabic, dried blood, etc.) retard the setting time, whereas many inorganic soluble salts accelerate the setting time. Furthermore, a certain chemical may be an accelerator for the hemihydrate form, but a retarder for some of the anhydrite forms.[4]

Most soluble sulfates tend to accelerate the hydration of the hemihydrate, but their effect may vary with their concentration. For example, a certain plaster was mixed with water to give a setting time of 10.5 minutes. When a 3.4 per cent solution of sodium sulfate ($Na_2SO_4$) was used to replace the water in the same proportions, the setting time was reduced to 3 minutes. When either a stronger or weaker solution than this was employed, the setting time was lengthened beyond 3 minutes. When a greater concentration than 12 per cent was employed, the setting time was actually retarded beyond that of the original mixture.[7]

Potassium sulfate ($K_2SO_4$) is probably the most commonly used accelerator. It accelerates the setting time regardless of its concentration. Ferric sulfate [$Fe_2(SO_4)_3$], chromic sulfate [$Cr_2(SO_4)_3$], and aluminum sulfate [$Al_2(SO_4)_3$] are all reported to be retarders,[9] whereas the alums are generally considered to be accelerators.

As previously noted, calcium sulfate (*e.g.*, gypsum), is an accelerator for the setting time, if it is added in the solid state to provide nuclei of crystallization. A saturated solution of calcium sulfate appears to have no measurable effect on the setting time. The gypsum added to the plaster or stone for the purpose of accelerating its setting time is known commercially as *terra alba*.

The acetates and the citrates generally retard the setting time. In fact, a 10 per cent mixture of sodium citrate ($Na_3C_6H_5O_7$) in powdered silica is used commercially as a retarder for dental stones. Potassium citrate ($K_3C_6H_5O_7$) is even more effective than sodium citrate as a retarder. Borax ($Na_2B_4O_7.10H_2O$) is an excellent retarder in concentrations above 1 per cent. For example, a 2 per cent solution of borax may delay the set of a plaster for 8 to 10 hours. The tartrates are generally accelerators when used in the proper concentration. Sodium chloride ($NaCl$) is often used by the dentist as an accelerator for the setting of plaster, but it can act as a retarder if it is used in too great concentration.[10]

The theory for the action of the retarders and accelerators on the setting of plaster or stone is obscure. The mechanism of the action of borax as a retarder has been shown to be related to its absorption by the calcium sulfate during setting, with the possible formation of calcium borate.[11] The calcium borate forms a coating around the remaining hemihydrate crystals, which are thus protected from further hydration. The more concentrated the borax, the thicker the coating will be, and the longer the setting time will be prolonged. The retarding action by colloids can also be accounted for in somewhat the same manner; the colloid may also form a protective layer around the hemihydrate and inhibit the reaction.

Such a theory can be generalized to indicate that perhaps the retardation of setting is due to the adsorption of certain ions to form a surface barrier. In such a case the solution of the hemihydrate possibly is inhibited or prevented.[12] This effect can be neutralized by the accelerators which apparently can remove this barrier. In other words, the action of the accelerators may be opposite to that of the retarders, in that the former can remove or discharge protective layers, either formed spontaneously on the crystal of hemihydrate or dihydrate (nucleus of crystallization) or introduced artificially as retarders.[13]

**Setting Expansion.**    Regardless of the type of gypsum product employed, an expansion of the mass can be detected during the change from the hemihydrate to the dihydrate. Depending upon the composition of the gypsum product, this observed expansion may be as low as 0.06 per cent linear to as high as 0.5 per cent.

On the other hand, if the equivalent volumes of the hemihydrate,

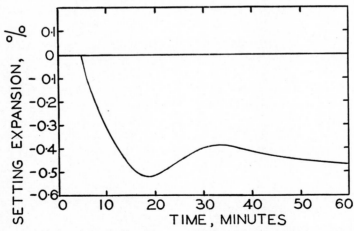

Fig. 3–9.   Dimensional changes which occur during the setting of a gypsum product. (Courtesy of A. R. Docking, Australian Bureau of Dental Standards.)

water and the reaction product (dihydrate) are compared, the volume of the dihydrate formed will be found to be less than the equivalent volumes of the hemihydrate and the water required.

The calculations are as follows:

$$(CaSO_4)_2H_2O + H_2O \longrightarrow 2CaSO_4.2H_2O$$

|           |          |                |          |
|-----------|----------|----------------|----------|
| Mol. wt.  | 290.284  | 54.048         | 344.332  |
| Sp. gr.   | 2.75     | 0.997          | 2.32     |
| Equiv. vol. | 105.556 | + 54.211 $\longrightarrow$ | 148.405 |
|           |          | 159.767 $\longrightarrow$  | 148.405 |

$$\text{Change in Volume} = \left(\frac{148.405 - 159.767}{159.767}\right)100 = -7.11 \text{ per cent}$$

It follows, therefore, that actually a volume contraction occurs during the setting.

This seemingly anomalous situation that, although a contraction can be calculated, an expansion is actually observed, can be rationalized on the basis of the mechanism of the crystallization.

As previously noted, the crystallization process is pictured as an outgrowth of crystals from nuclei of crystallization. On the basis of the entanglement of the dihydrate crystals as indicated in Figure 3–6, it is not difficult to imagine that crystals growing from the nuclei not only intermesh, but that they may also intercept each other during growth. If the growth of one crystal is interrupted by another, a stress is present at this point in the direction of the growth of the colliding crystal.

If this process is repeated by thousands of the crystals during growth, it is possible that this outward stress or thrust could produce an expansion of the entire mass, and, thus, an apparent or observed expansion can take place in spite of the fact that the *true volume* of the crystals may be less as calculated.

Although the contraction during setting is best observed experimentally by a volumetric method,[14] it can also be observed as a linear change if the hemihydrate and water mixture is allowed to react on a nearly frictionless surface, as when floated on the surface of mercury. The graph shown in Figure 3–9 was obtained in this manner.[15]

On the basis of the preceding discussion, the first part of the curve in Figure 3–9 can be interpreted as a true contraction while the dihydrate crystals were forming initially. When the crystals became sufficiently dense to impinge on one another, then their outward thrust became effective, and an expansion occurred as shown.

In practice, only the expansion in Figure 3–9 would be observed since before the period of the expansion the mass would be fluid. Only when the product of the reaction begins to crystallize or solidify can the apparent expansion be observed. In other words, had the dimensional change of the specimen been measured by ordinary methods, a setting expansion of approximately 0.12 per cent would have been reported as measured from the minimum of the curve to its maximum.

**Structure of Set Gypsum.**     Since the product of reaction (2) (gypsum) in practice is greater in *external* volume but less in *crystalline* volume, it follows that the set material is porous.

The final structure immediately after setting is, therefore, composed of interlocking crystals between which are the pores containing the excess water required for mixing as previously described.

The porosity of the set product for various W/P ratios of hemihydrate can be calculated,[12] as indicated in Table 3–3. As can be noted, the greater the W/P ratio, the greater is the porosity. Such a consideration is to be expected on the basis that there are fewer nuclei of crystallization as the W/P ratio is increased. Consequently, there is less intermeshing of the crystals of gypsum.

**Control of Setting Expansion.**     As can be noted from the experimental results presented in Table 3–4, the less the W/P ratio and the longer the mixing time within practical limits, the greater is the setting expansion.[7]

The effect of the W/P ratio on the setting expansion is to be expected on theoretical grounds. Since with the higher W/P ratios, fewer nuclei of crystallization per unit volume are present than with the thicker mixes, and since it can be assumed that the space between the nuclei

*Table 3–3.*     *Porosity of Set Gypsum as Affected by the W/P Ratio**

| W/P RATIO | POROSITY (PER CENT) |
|-----------|---------------------|
| 0.25 | 10.3 |
| 0.30 | 15.3 |
| 0.35 | 20.3 |
| 0.40 | 25.3 |
| 0.50 | 35.3 |
| 0.60 | 45.3 |
| 1.00 | 85.3 |

* Jørgensen and Posner, *J. D. Res.*, May-June, 1959.

*Table 3–4.*     *Effect of the W/P Ratio and Mixing Time on the Setting Expansion of Plaster of Paris**

| W/P | MIXING TIME (MIN.) | SETTING EXPANSION (PER CENT) |
|-----|--------------------|------------------------------|
| 0.45 | 0.5 | 0.41 |
| 0.45 | 1.0 | 0.51 |
| 0.60 | 1.0 | 0.29 |
| 0.60 | 2.0 | 0.41 |
| 0.80 | 1.0 | 0.24 |

* Gibson and Johnson, *J. Soc. Chem. Ind.*, *51:*25T (1932).

*Table 3–5.     Crystalline Shapes of Gypsum Found in Various Solutions\**

| SOLUTION | EFFECT ON SETTING EXPANSION | CRYSTALLINE SHAPE |
|---|---|---|
| Distilled Water | (Control) | Slender needle-like |
| Potassium sulfate (1%) | Reduction | Needle-like, relatively short and thick |
| Potassium nitrate (4%) | Reduction | Needle-like, short and thick |
| Potassium carbonate (1%) | Reduction | Mostly small and spheroid |
| Aluminum sulfate (4%) | None | Slender, needle-like |
| Potassium chloride (4%) | Reduction | Needle-like, short and thick |
| Rochelle salt (5%) | Reduction | Very short and massive |
| Sodium sulfate (4%) | Reduction (small) | Needle-like, short and thick |

\* Jørgensen and Posner, *J. D. Res.*, May-June, 1959.

will be greater in such a case, it follows that there will be less growth interference of the dihydrate crystals with less outward thrust resulting.

As previously related, the longer mixing time provides more nuclei of crystallization and, consequently, a greater amount of interference during growth is to be expected with increased mixing.

The most effective method for the control of the setting expansion is by the addition of chemicals. Most accelerators and retarders reduce the setting expansion markedly. For example, a 4 per cent solution of potassium sulfate may reduce the linear setting expansion from 0.4 to 0.5 per cent to 0.06 per cent,[7] when it is mixed with plaster of paris. Under such a condition, the setting time is too short for practical purposes, and borax or sodium citrate may be added to prolong the setting time and to reduce the setting expansion as well. In this manner, both the setting expansion and the setting time can be established for a given W/P ratio with no effect of mixing time on these properties.

The reason for the reduction of the setting expansion by the addition of accelerators and retarders is probably related to the morphology of the crystalline forms of gypsum obtained when solutions of these chemicals are used for mixing.[12] As can be noted from Table 3–5, whenever any of the chemicals listed in Column 1 reduced the setting expansion of the gypsum produced (Column 2), their crystalline shape differed from that obtained in water alone (Column 3). Apparently a long, slender needle-like crystal is the most effective in the production of an expansion during setting. All other types caused a reduction in setting expansion.

When terra alba is employed as an accelerator, the setting expansion is increased[16] by virtue of the additional nuclei of crystallization supplied.

**Hygroscopic Expansion.** A second type of expansion occurs when a gypsum product is allowed to set under water. It should be understood that the water involved is not that added to the hemihydrate during the mixing procedure, but that added externally during setting. This type of expansion is greater in magnitude than the setting expansion previously described, particularly in the case of the dental investments to be discussed in Chapter 27. In dental plaster and stones its linear magnitude may be only 0.1 per cent (or less)[17] higher than that of the setting expansion, but it can be a source of error in some extremely accurate dental procedures to be described.

The theory of hygroscopic expansion will be discussed in Chapter 27.

**Strength.** The strength of gypsum products is generally expressed in terms of compressive strength.

As might be expected from the theory of setting, the strength of a plaster or stone increases rapidly as the material hardens after the initial setting time. However, the free water content of the set product definitely affects its strength. For this reason, two strengths of the gypsum product are recognized, the *wet strength* and the *dry strength.* The wet strength is the strength when the water in excess of that required for the hydration of the hemihydrate is left in the test specimen. When the specimen has been dried free of the excess water, the strength then obtained is the dry strength. The dry strength may be two or more times the wet strength; consequently, the distinction between the two is of considerable importance.

The effect on its crushing strength of drying set plaster is shown in Table 3–6. It is interesting to note that relatively slight gains in strength occurred until after the sixteenth hour. Between the 8-hour period and the 24-hour period, only 0.6 per cent of excess water was lost, yet the strength doubled. A somewhat similar change in surface hardness takes place during the drying process.[18]

*Table 3–6.*    *Effect of Drying on the Strength of Plaster of Paris**

| DRYING PERIOD (HOURS) | COMPRESSIVE STRENGTH (KG./CM.²) | (LB./IN.²) | LOSS IN WEIGHT (PER CENT) |
|:---:|:---:|:---:|:---:|
| 2 | 98 | 1400 | 5.1 |
| 4 | 119 | 1700 | 11.9 |
| 8 | 119 | 1700 | 17.4 |
| 16 | 130 | 1900 | .... |
| 24 | 238 | 3400 | 18.0 |
| 48 | 238 | 3400 | 18.0 |
| 72 | 238 | 3400 | .... |

* Gibson and Johnson, *J. Soc. Chem. Ind., 51:*25T (1932).

*Table 3–7.*   *Effect of W/P Ratio and Mixing Time on the Strength of Plaster of Paris**

| W/P | MIXING TIME (MIN.) | CRUSHING STRENGTH (DRY) (KG./CM.$^2$) | (LB./IN.$^2$) |
|---|---|---|---|
| 0.45 | 0.5 | 240 | 3400 |
| 0.45 | 1.0 | 270 | 3800 |
| 0.60 | 1.0 | 180 | 2600 |
| 0.60 | 2.0 | 140 | 2000 |
| 0.80 | 1.0 | 110 | 1600 |

* Gibson and Johnson, *J. Soc. Chem. Ind.*, *51:*25T (1932).

One explanation of this effect is that probably 40 per cent or more of the strength of the set plaster is due to the cohesion of the crystals themselves in contradistinction to the strength which can be attributed to the interlocking of the crystals during growth.[4] Any excess water present presumably will reduce the cohesion of the crystals by a solution of the surface molecules. Only when this excess water is eliminated is the intercrystalline cohesion entirely effective in its contribution to the strength.

As previously noted, the set plaster or stone is porous in nature, and the greater the W/P ratio, the greater will be the porosity (Table 3–3). As might be expected on such a basis, the greater the W/P ratio, the less is the dry strength of the set material, as shown by the data[7] in Table 3–7, since the greater the porosity, the fewer crystals there will be per unit volume for a given weight of hemihydrate.

It is particularly interesting to note from Table 3–7 that the spatulation time also affects the strength of the plaster. In general, the strength will be increased with an increase in mixing time to a limit which is approximately equivalent to that of a normal hand mixing for one minute. If the mixture is over-mixed, the gypsum crystals formed are broken up, and less crystalline interlocking results in the final product.

## Literature

1. Worner, H. K.: *Dental Plasters, General Manufacture, and Characteristics before Mixing with Water.* Austral. J. Den., *46:*1–10 (Jan.), 35–46 (Feb.), 1942.
2. Haddon, C. L.: *Gypsum Plaster Products.* Chem. and Ind., *21:*190–192 (May 20), 1944.
3. Eberl, I. J., and Ingram, A. P.: *Process for Making High Strength Plaster of Paris.* Ind. Eng. Chem., *41:*1061–1065 (May), 1949.
4. Haddon, C. L.: *The Mechanism of Setting of Calcium Sulfate Cements.* Trans. Faraday Soc., *20:*337–341, 1924.
5. Le Chatelier, H. L.: *Plaster of Paris.* Ann. des Mines, pp. 346–365, 1887.
6. Jørgensen, K. D.: *Studies on the Setting of Plaster of Paris.* Odont. Tskr., *61:*305–346 (1953).
7. Gibson, C. S., and Johnson, R. N.: *Investigations of the Setting of Plaster of Paris.* J. Soc. Chem. Ind., *51:*25T (Jan. 22), 1932.
8. Worner, H. K.: *The Effect of Temperature on the Rate of Setting of Plaster of Paris.* J. D. Res., *23:*305–308 (Oct.), 1932.

9. Budnikov, P.: *Activating and Retarding Agents for the Setting of Plaster of Paris.* Kolloid Z., *44:*242–249, 1928.

10. Sodeau, W. H., and Gibson, C. S.: *The Use of Plaster of Paris as an Impression Material.* Brit. D. J., *48:*1089–1115 (Sept. 15), 1927.

11. Buchanan, A. S., and Worner, H. K.: *A Study of the Action of Borax in Retarding the Setting of Plaster of Paris.* J. Soc. Chem. Ind., *65:*23–26 (Jan.), 1946.

12. Jørgensen, K. D., and Posner, A. S.: *Study of the Setting of Plaster.* J. D. Res., *38:*491–499 (May-June), 1959.

13. Buchanan, A. S.: Plaster of Paris: *A Survey of the Literature Relating to the Composition, the Setting Reaction, and the Influence of Various Foreign Substances Therein.* Melbourne, Australia, University of Melbourne (1947), Unpublished.

14. Mahler, D. B., and Asgarzadah, K.: *The Volumetric Contraction of Dental Gypsum Materials on Setting.* J. D. Res., *32:*354–361 (June), 1953.

15. Docking, A. R., and Donnison, J. A.: *The Hygroscopic Setting Expansion of Dental Casting Investments. Part 2.* Austral. J. Den., *52:*160–166 (May), 1948.

16. Chassevant, L.: *Variation in the Volume of Plaster during and after Setting.* Rev. Materiaux Construction. Trav. Publ., Ed. C., No. 465, 188–194, 1949.

17. Hollenback, G. M.: *A Study of the Physical Properties of Elastic Impression Materials and Stones.* J. South. California D. A., *25:*20–28 (Jan.), 1957.

18. Mahler, D. B.: *Hardness and Flow Properties of Gypsum Materials.* J. Pros. Den., *1:*188–195 (Jan.-Mar.), 1951.

CHAPTER 4

# Gypsum Products:

# Technical Considerations

As described in the preceding chapter, gypsum products have many uses in dentistry. The criteria for selection of any particular gypsum product will depend upon its use, and the physical properties necessary for that particular use. For example, a dental stone is a poor material for use as an impression material; its exothermic heat during setting would be uncomfortable if not injurious to the mucous membrane of the mouth. Furthermore, if teeth are present, it would be impossible to remove the impression over the undercuts in the teeth without injury because of the high strength of the $\alpha$-hemihydrate.

On the other hand, if a strong cast is required on which to build a denture, one would not choose to employ a weak plaster ($\beta$-hemihydrate) containing considerable amounts of modifiers. If the mold or cast is to be heated to a high temperature, it is necessary to add a refractory to the plaster or stone, in order to aid in overcoming the weakening effect of the dehydration of the set product. In other words, there is no "all purpose" dental gypsum product.

**Impression Plasters.** Impression plasters are plaster of paris to which modifiers have been added. The purpose of the modifiers is twofold, (1) to regulate the setting time and (2) to control the setting expansion.

It is important from the standpoint of both the patient and the dentist that the setting time be under accurate control. The dentist should have sufficient time to mix the plaster and water, to place the mixture in the impression tray, to carry the loaded impression tray to the patient's mouth, and to place it in position against the mouth tissues. However, once the plaster is in position against the surface to be impressed, it should harden promptly so that the discomfort to the patient will not be prolonged unduly. The setting time for a given W/P ratio is determined by the addition of the proper amount of accelerator.

The setting expansion of an impression plaster should be kept as low as possible, owing to the danger of warpage of the impression, as illustrated in Figure 4–1. The impression shown diagrammatically is for the upper mouth. The flanges of the metal tray are shown at *a* and *b*. If the plaster expands against these flanges, the expansion will be confined, and the resulting stress will cause a warpage at *c*. As a result, the depth of the palate portion will be changed, and the denture or other appliance will not fit. It should be noted that the only dimensional change of practical interest occurs after the initial set; any changes in dimension which occur before the material hardens are compensated immediately by the flow of the liquid mix.

The use of an accelerator is indicated in order to reduce the setting expansion as well as the setting time. If the setting time is unduly shortened to obtain a minimum setting expansion, a retarder can be used to counteract the accelerator, and at the same time to decrease the setting expansion further. A setting expansion of approximately 0.06 per cent is the lowest that can be expected. The setting time is usually established at 3 to 5 minutes, depending upon the desired W/P ratio.

The modifiers are usually included in the plaster, ready to be dissolved in the water when the plaster and water are mixed. If desired, however, solutions containing the proper amount of modifiers can be used without changing the composition of the plaster.

When teeth are present, the plaster impression must be fractured and reassembled; otherwise, the unyielding plaster impression cannot be removed over the undercuts caused by the heights of contour of the teeth and spaces between the teeth. Consequently, a high strength is an undesirable property for an impression plaster; rather it should be brittle and relatively easy to fracture. The use of a high W/P ratio

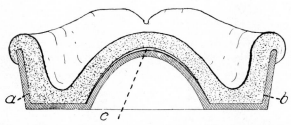

Fig. 4–1.   Warped impression due to tray flanges. The impression warps at *c* because the flanges *a* and *b* are fixed and do not allow lateral setting expansion. (Prothero, *Prosthetic Dentistry*, Medico-Dental Publishing Co.)

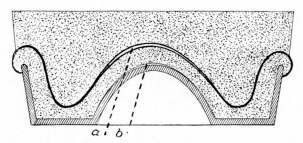

Fig. 4–2.   Warped cast due to restricted lateral setting expansion. The warpage of the impression in Fig. 4–1 may be seen at *b*. After forming the cast, a similar warpage occurred at *a*. (Prothero, *Prosthetic Dentistry*, Medico-Dental Publishing Co.)

in mixing aids in this respect, and at the same time it prevents the formation of excessive exothermic heat during the setting reaction.

Some of the impression plasters are colored and flavored to make them more palatable to the patient. The color also helps the dentist or technician to distinguish between the cast material and the impression plaster when the impression is separated from the cast.

Before the stone is poured into the impression to form the cast, the pores in the plaster impression must be sealed. Otherwise, the water and dissolved $\alpha$-hemihydrate will soak into the impression, and crystals will form so that the cast and impression cannot be separated. The impression should always be coated first with a separating medium, such as varnish or lacquer, in order to render it water-impervious. The film formed by the separating medium should be very thin in order to avoid inaccuracies from this cause.

Impression plasters sometimes contain potato starch to render them "soluble." In such a case, after the cast has thoroughly hardened, the impression and cast are placed in hot water; the starch swells, the impression disintegrates, and thus its removal from the cast is facilitated. If a starch modifier is not used, a careful and tedious dissection of the impression from the cast is often necessary to avoid injury to the latter.

***Dental Stone.***    The modern dental stones are composed chiefly of $\alpha$-hemihydrate. The modifiers amount to approximately 2 to 3 per cent of the total content. The modifiers generally consist of an accelerator and a retarder for the purpose of "balancing" the setting time and setting expansion as previously described. Coloring matter may also be added. The natural $\alpha$-hemihydrate cannot be distinguished by sight from ordinary plaster, and consequently it is of aid to have the dental stone pigmented.

The modifiers present in the various commercial dental stones vary with different manufacturers. Potassium sulfate ($K_2SO_4$) and Rochelle salt ($KNaC_4H_4O_6.4H_2O$) are present in most stones. Both of these accelerators are effective in reducing the setting expansion, and the Rochelle salt is said to reduce the strength of the final product to a less extent than does the potassium sulfate,[1] although it is less effective in reducing the setting time and expansion.

It is important that a dental stone possess a low setting expansion, particularly when it is used for the construction of a cast in a plaster impression. The reason for this becomes apparent from Figure 4–2, which represents a cross section of the impression shown in Figure 4–1 after the cast material has been poured. The discrepancy caused by the setting expansion of the impression plaster is shown at *b*. If the dental stone possesses a large setting expansion, its expansion will be inhibited by the impression and the cast will warp as shown at *a*. The total warpage is, therefore, cumulative, and the vault portion of the cast will be too high. For this reason, the setting expansion of the stone is usually limited to 0.06 to 0.12 per cent, a value which should be negligible in quantity so far as any error of practical significance is concerned.

In spite of the modifiers present, the dry crushing strengths of the dental stones may be 420 to 700 kilograms per square centimeter (6,000 to 10,000 pounds per square inch) with a low W/P ratio. The wet compressive strengths of the stones (1 hour after the initial set) are approximately 350 kilograms per square centimeter (5,000 pounds per square inch).

The stones generally fall into two classes in regard to strength; class I exhibits a dry compressive strength of 420 to 520 kilograms per square centimeter (6,000 to 7,500 pounds per square inch), whereas the class II stones may possess a dry strength of as high as 700 kilograms per square centimeter (10,000 pounds per square inch). The com-

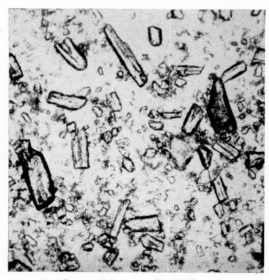

Fig. 4–3.   Powder particles of a class II dental stone. ×100.

mercial class II stones may exhibit a setting expansion of approximately 0.06 per cent, whereas the setting expansion of the class I stones is generally higher (0.10 to 0.13 per cent).

The essential difference between the two types of stone is the particle size of the $\alpha$-hemihydrate used. The type of $\alpha$-hemihydrate used in the class I stone is shown in Figure 3–4 in the preceding chapter, whereas the powder particles of the $\alpha$-hemihydrate used in the class II stones are shown in Figure 4–3. A comparison of the two figures indicates that the particle size of the class II stones is larger than that of the class I materials. As a result, a lower W/P ratio can be used to mix the class II stones. The larger crystal size of the $\alpha$-hemihydrate reduces the rate of solution and perhaps the rate at which the crystals of calcium sulfate dihydrate form. Consequently, the early wet strength of both stones may be somewhat the same; the superior strength of the class II stones becomes apparent as the crystallization is completed.

It is important that the water and powder be measured when dental stone is employed. The purpose for using dental stone instead of plaster is to attain strength, and any guessing of the proportions without measurement usually results in less than the maximum strength. For example, in the case of one particular dental stone (class I), the use of one cubic centimeter more water per 100 grams of stone resulted in a loss of dry strength of as much as 25 to 30 kilograms per square centimeter (350 to 400 pounds per square inch).[1] As a matter of fact, a thinly mixed dental stone can be weaker than a thickly mixed plaster.

**Cast Materials.** Dental stone is normally used for the construction of all types of cast. When teeth are present, they may contain cavities prepared by the dentist for the reception of inlays, crowns, etc. The preparation of an inlay or crown involves first the carving of a wax pattern which is later to be reproduced in metal. Often, the wax is carved in position on the cast. In such an event, the cast material must be very hard in order not to be abraded by the carving instrument.

The most effective manner for producing a hard surface on a cast is to employ as little water as possible in mixing the stone. Inasmuch as the $\alpha$-hemihydrate crystals are not porous and are relatively regular (Fig. 3–4), a water-powder mixture of a putty-like consistency can be vibrated into very small areas with ease.

The surface hardness of a cast made from a dental model plaster can be increased by immersing it in a 2 per cent solution of borax for several hours.[2] The more concentrated and the higher the temperature of the solution (within limits) the more borax will be taken up. Presumably a thin layer of calcium tetraborate deposited on the surface is the cause for the increase in hardness. Unfortunately, such a treatment is not effective with dental stone.[3]

The surface hardness increases more rapidly after setting than does the crushing strength, owing to the more rapid drying of the surface[4] in comparison to the interior of the cast.

The Brinell hardness number of a dry dental stone after set is approximately four times that of a hardened model plaster, mixed with a low W/P ratio.[5]

Attempts have been made to modify plaster of paris so that its strength and hardness are comparable to that of dental stone. This modification has been attempted by the addition of a retarder (borax) and an accelerator (Rochelle salt) in proportions so that the W/P ratio can be reduced as the setting time is prolonged. The strength and hardness of the plaster cast have been doubled by this means, but neither property is equal in magnitude to that of a dental stone.[1]

In some cases, a metal cast is constructed. An alloy is prepared which possesses a sufficiently low melting point that it will not harm the gypsum product when it is poured into a plaster impression in the molten condition. Since the metal is poured into the impression without pressure, the surface tension of the molten metal may cause rounded corners and a general lack of sharp detail.

**Proportioning.**    As previously noted, if a high strength is desired, as low a W/P ratio should be used as possible. However, lowering the amount of water increases the viscosity of the mix, and care must be taken to insure that the thick mixture flows into every detail when it is poured into the impression.

Since high strength not only is unimportant but also undesirable in plaster impressions, a relatively high W/P ratio can be used to provide a creamy consistency in the mix, which will flow into every detail when the impression is taken. The lowest limit of the viscosity permissible is governed by the ability of the water-plaster mixture to remain in position in the tray while the impression is being taken. The proper W/P ratio for an impression plaster is approximately 0.6 to 0.7, depending upon the plaster.

Some dental stones (class II) can be used successfully with a W/P ratio as low as 0.20. As previously noted, it is important that the water and powder be measured—preferably weighed. It is impossible to gauge a powder accurately by volume because of the packing effect. For example, the apparent density of a dental stone powder is approximately $1\frac{1}{4}$ times that of a plaster.

The packing effect of different commercial products of the same type may vary considerably from one product to another. Furthermore, the bulk of the mixed or set plaster may be entirely independent of the bulkiness of the original powder.[6] Consequently, the use of volume measurement for proportioning purposes is unreliable.

**Mixing.**    The plaster or stone is usually mixed in a flexible rubber or plastic bowl with a stiff-bladed spatula. The mid-cross section of the interior of the bowl should preferably be parabolic in shape, so

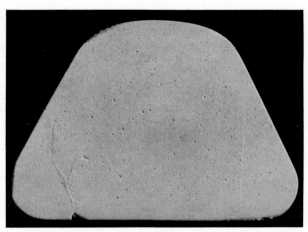

Fig. 4–4.   The surface of a set stone which was improperly mixed. Such air bubbles weaken the stone as well as impair its appearance.

there will be no corners or other discontinuities where the plaster or stone can collect and stagnate during the mixing procedure. The walls of the bowl should be smooth and resistant to abrasion. Any scratches or creases are likely to retain set plaster after the bowl has been washed. As a result, the setting time and other properties of subsequent mixes will be altered by the nuclei of crystallization unintentionally added.

The spatula should have a stiff blade. A flexible blade "drags" when it is forced through a thick mixture of stone and water, and as a result the mixing is seldom thorough. The end of the spatula blade should be rounded to conform to the shape of the mixing bowl, so that the surface of the bowl can be wiped readily by the blade of the spatula during mixing. The handle of the spatula should be of a design that can be readily grasped by the hand.

One of the great disadvantages to be avoided during the mixing of a gypsum product with water is the incorporation of air. Air bubbles in the completed cast are unsightly and produce surface inaccuracies (Fig. 4–4). They also definitely weaken the cast.

An automatic vibrator is of considerable aid in removing air bubbles during mixing, provided that the vibrations are of a high frequency and of a limited amplitude. A churning effect by the vibrator is decidedly undesirable, since violent agitation whips air into the mixture.

The water should be placed in the plaster bowl, and the powder should be sifted into the water. When the powder sinks into the water without an agglomeration of the particles, less air is carried down.

The mixture should then be held on the automatic vibrator for a few seconds, in order to remove any large air bubbles which might have been incorporated inadvertently. The actual spatulation is carried on by stirring the mixture vigorously, and at the same time wiping all of the inside surfaces of the bowl with the spatula to be sure that all of the powder is wet and mixed uniformly with the water. The mixing is continued until all of the mixture is smooth and homogeneous in texture. Further mixing is likely to break up the crystals of gypsum formed, and thus weaken the final product. The time for hand mixing is approximately 1 to 2 minutes.

The mix is then vibrated until no more air bubbles come to the surface. Some dental offices and laboratories are equipped so that the final vibration of the mix is accomplished in a vacuum in order to eliminate the air bubbles more completely.[7]

The use of a mechanical spatulator* for the mixing of plaster and stone offers considerable advantage so far as strength and porosity are concerned.[7] The rapidly moving paddles of such a device break up any air bubbles into such fine voids that the strength is not appreciably affected.

If the maximum strength is desired, the W/P ratio should not be changed during mixing. When the proportions are estimated by guesswork, the addition of more powder to a mix that is judged too thin provides essentially two mixes of plaster setting at different rates, and a weakened product always results. In the same manner, the addition of water to a too-thick mixture will cause a serious disarrangement of crystalline growth and a lack of intercrystalline cohesion. The very fact that the mix was judged to be too thick may indicate that the setting reaction has started. As repeatedly stated, *in order to obtain the maximum strength, the proportions of water and powder must be measured.*

**Construction of the Cast.** There are at least two methods for the construction of the cast. In one case, a mold for the cast is constructed. Briefly, strips of soft wax are wrapped around the impression, so that they extend approximately 1 centimeter (½ inch) beyond the tissue side of the impression. A base for the cast is formed in this manner. The process is called "boxing." The mixture of stone and water previously prepared is then poured into the impression under vibration. The mixture is allowed to run down the side of the impression, so that it pushes the air ahead of itself as it fills all tooth impressions and other concavities.

Another method is to fill the impression first as described. The remainder of the stone-water mixture is then piled on a glass plate. The filled impression is then inverted over the pile of stone, and the base is shaped with the spatula before the stone sets. Such a procedure is not indicated, however, if an easily deformed impression material has been used.

The cast should not be separated from the impression until it has thoroughly hardened. The minimum time to be allowed for setting

* See Figure 28–5.

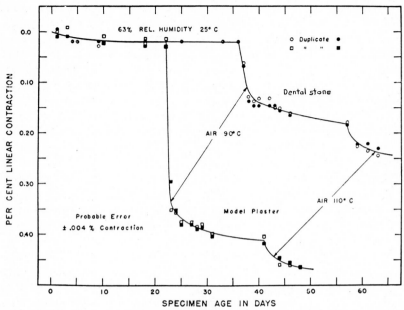

Fig. 4–5.  Dimensional changes in dental stone and model plaster stored at 25° C., 90° C., and 110° C. (Sweeney and Taylor, *J. Pros. Den.*, Dec. 1950.)

will vary from 30 to 60 minutes, depending on the rate of setting of the dental stone or plaster, and the type of impression material. The completed cast (Fig. 3–2) should be smooth, neat and accurate in every detail.

**Care of the Cast.**    If the surface of the cast is not hard and smooth when it is removed from the impression, its accuracy should be questioned. The cast is supposedly an accurate reproduction of the mouth parts, and any departure from the expected accuracy will probably result in a poorly fitting appliance. The cast should, therefore, be handled carefully and with intelligence.

Once the setting reactions in the cast have been completed, its dimensions will be relatively constant thereafter under ordinary conditions of room temperature and humidity.[8] As later outlined, however, it is sometimes necessary to soak the gypsum cast in water, in preparation for other technics. It should be remembered that the gypsum of which the cast is composed is slightly soluble in water. When a dry cast is immersed in water, there may be a negligible expansion, *provided that the water is saturated with calcium sulfate.* If it is not so saturated, gypsum may be dissolved in sufficient amount to cause a measurable reduction in its dimensions. If the stone cast is immersed in running water, its linear dimension may decrease approximately 0.1 per cent for every 20 minutes of such immersion.[9]

The safest method for soaking the cast is to place it in a water bath made for the purpose, in which plaster débris is allowed to remain constantly on the bottom of the container in order to provide a saturated solution of calcium sulfate at all times.

The effect of temperature on the storage of a plaster and a stone cast in air is shown[8] in Figure 4–5. As previously noted, storage of either set plaster or stone produces no dimensional change of practical importance. If the storage temperature is raised to 90° to 110° C. (194° to 230° F.) a shrinkage occurs as the water of crystallization is removed and the dihydrate reverts to the hemihydrate. As can be noted from the figure, the contraction of the plaster at high temperature is greater than that of the stone.

Such contractions may occur during air storage at temperatures above that of the room, as when a stone cast is dried. Probably it is not safe dimensionally to store a stone cast in air at a temperature greater than 55° C. (130° F.) for any length of time.

***Care of Gypsum Products.***    Gypsum products are somewhat sensitive to changes in the relative humidity of their environment. Even the surface hardness of plaster and stone casts may fluctuate slightly with the relative humidity of the atmosphere. For example, it has been shown[5] that the surface of a set model plaster (W/P ratio of 0.6) decreased from a B.H.N. of 4.2 to 3.4 when the relative humidity increased from 55 per cent to 72 per cent. Gypsum surfaces made with thinner mixes appear to be affected more than those with a low W/P ratio. Although the effect is small, it is worthy of note.

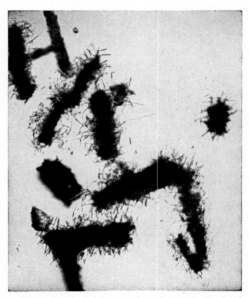

Fig. 4–6.   Powder particles after being exposed to the moisture in the air. The gypsum crystals are seen extending from the particles. (Courtesy of H. K. Worner.)

The hemihydrate of gypsum takes up water from the air quite readily. It has been shown that when the relative humidity exceeds approximately 70 per cent, the plaster takes up sufficient water vapor to start a setting reaction.[10] The first hydration probably produces a few crystals of gypsum on the surface of the hemihydrate crystal. These crystals act as nuclei of crystallization, and the first manifestation of the deterioration of the plaster is a decrease in the setting time.

As the hygroscopic action continues, more crystals of gypsum form until the entire hemihydrate crystal is covered as shown in Figure 4–6. Under these conditions, the water penetrates the dihydrate coating with difficulty and the setting time is unduly prolonged. It is, therefore, important that all types of gypsum products be stored in a dry atmosphere. The best means for storage is to seal the product in a moisture-proof metal container.

## Literature

1. Worner, H. K.: *Plaster of Paris as a Cast Material.* Austral. J. Den., *46*:84–99 (June), 1942.
2. Buchanan, A. S., and Worner, H. K.: *A Study of the Action of Borax in Retarding the Setting of Plaster of Paris.* J. Soc. Chem. Ind., *65*:23–26 (Jan.), 1946.
3. Skinner, E. W., and Gordon, C. C.: *Some Experiments on the Surface Hardness of Dental Stones.* J. Pros. Den., *6*:94–100 (Jan.), 1956.
4. Mahler, D. B.: *Hardness and Flow Properties of Gypsum Materials.* J. Pros. Den., *1*:188–195 (Jan.-Mar.), 1951.
5. Worner, H. K.: *Dental Plasters. Part II.* Austral. J. Den., *46*:35–46 (Feb.), 1942.
6. Worner, H. K.: *Dental Plasters. Part I.* Austral. J. Den., *46*:1–10 (Jan.), 1942.
7. Lindquist, J. T., Brennan, R. E., and Phillips, R. W.: *Influence of Mixing Procedure Techniques on Some Physical Properties of Plaster.* J. Pros. Den., *3*:274–285 (March), 1953.
8. Sweeney, W. T., and Taylor, D. F.: *Dimensional Changes in Dental Stone and Plaster.* J. D. Res., *29*:749–755 (Dec.), 1950.
9. Rice, W. S.: *Duplicating a Model.* CAL, *13*:4–6 (July), 1950.
10. Farmer, G. J., and Skinner, E. W.: *Effect of Relative Humidity on the Setting Time of Plaster of Paris.* Northwest. Univ. Bul., *43*:12–16 (Dec.), 1942.

# CHAPTER 5

# Impression Compound

The use of plaster of paris as an impression material was described in the preceding chapter. Plaster is, however, only one of several materials which can be used to obtain an impression.

**Classification of Impression Materials.** There are several ways by which impression materials can be classified. One way is according to the manner in which they harden. For example, plaster of paris hardens by chemical action, as do the impression pastes and the alginate and rubber impression materials to be discussed in subsequent chapters.

On the other hand, the impression compounds soften under heat and solidify when they are cooled, with no chemical change taking place. Such materials are, therefore, classified as *thermoplastic* substances. Although the reversible hydrocolloid materials to be described in Chapter 7 may not be classified strictly as thermoplastic materials, they are liquefied by heat, and they solidify, or gel, when they are cooled.

Perhaps a better way to classify the dental impression materials might be according to their use in dentistry. As previously noted, an impression made with plaster of paris cannot be removed over undercuts without the impression being fractured. If an impression of teeth is made with impression compound, the compound flows when the impression is withdrawn over the undercuts, and the tooth form is not preserved with accuracy. The same is true with an impression made with the impression pastes. Although these three types of materials can be used with certain limitations for all types of impressions, they are best adapted for obtaining impressions of edentulous mouths, and, therefore, may be classified as impression materials for use in complete denture prosthesis.

On the other hand, the hydrocolloid impression materials are best adapted for the obtaining of an accurate reproduction of tooth form, including the undercuts and interproximal spaces. Although these materials can be employed for edentulous impressions, they are used most extensively in crown and bridge, partial denture and operative dentistry, where impressions of teeth are included.

**Uses of Impression Compound.**    When the compound is used for edentulous impressions, it is softened by heat, inserted in an impression tray, and pressed against the tissues before it hardens. The bottom of the tray is sprayed with cool water until the compound hardens, after which procedure the impression is withdrawn. Such material is true *impression compound.*

Another type of compound, called *tray compound,* is used to form a tray to be used with other types of impression materials. An impression is obtained as described, and this impression may be used as a tray on which other types of impression materials may be carried to place against the tissues. For example, a mixture of impression plaster and water may be placed over the tray of compound, and an impression can be obtained in plaster. Impression pastes are used in this manner, and the hydrocolloid impression materials also can be used. In contrast to impression compound, the tray compound is somewhat more viscous when it is softened, and more rigid when it is hardened. Since the reproduction of fine detail is not important in the case of the tray compound, it generally possesses less flow properties than the regular impression compound.

Impression compound is often used in operative dentistry to obtain impressions of single teeth which contain prepared cavities. In this case, a cylindrical copper band (called a *matrix band*) is filled with the softened compound and forced over the tooth and into the prepared cavity. After the compound has been cooled, the impression is withdrawn, and a cast, or *die,* is constructed in the impression. As previously related, the contour of the tooth may not be reproduced accurately because of the flow of the compound upon withdrawal, but the form of the prepared cavity will be reproduced accurately to the smallest detail.

**Requisites for an Impression Compound.**    Desirable requisites for an impression compound are as follows:

1. It should be free of poisonous or irritating ingredients.

2. It should harden completely at, or slightly above, mouth temperature, since it is virtually impossible to chill anything uniformly in the mouth to a temperature below that of the mouth.

3. It should be plastic at a temperature which will not cause undue discomfort to the patient, and which will not be injurious to the mouth tissues. The softening temperature is, therefore, limited by practical considerations as to the maximum and minimum temperatures between which it can occur.

4. The material should harden uniformly when it is cooled, without

warpage or distortion of any sort. Lack of uniform hardening is undoubtedly a source of stress production which is later released by relaxation. Even though the material may be completely homogeneous at the time the cooling begins, so far as its composition is concerned, its low thermal conductivity may preclude a uniform cooling, particularly when it is cooled rapidly.

5. When it is soft, the material should have a consistency which will allow it to reproduce all details of crevices and other small markings, and to retain such detail after solidification. In other words, the material should be cohesive but not adhesive.

6. The material should be of such a nature that when the impression is withdrawn from the mouth it will not be deformed or fractured, and it should reproduce all undercuts completely.

7. Its surface should exhibit a smooth, glossy appearance after it has been passed through a flame.

8. After the compound has solidified, it should withstand trimming with a sharp knife without flaking or chipping. Intricate and delicate trimming of an impression is often necessary, and one should be able to trim without damage to the impression.

9. The material should not change dimension during or after removal from the mouth and it should maintain its dimensions indefinitely under reasonable conditions of storage. This requisite will be discussed more at length in a subsequent section.

**Composition.**    The formulas for the better types of impression compounds are trade secrets, and any discussion of their composition must be somewhat speculative.

One of the first substances to be used as an impression material was beeswax, and it possibly may be one of the ingredients of some of the modern products. The beeswax alone exhibits brittleness, lack of dimensional stability, and a tendency toward tackiness. In order to improve the plasticity and workability of the beeswax, certain plasticizers may be added, such as Burgundy pitch, shellac, and gutta percha.

Another combination, which probably is more representative of the modern material, is the use of stearin and Kauri resin. Stearin is the glyceride of stearic, palmitic and oleic acids, made from tallow. Its melting range is approximately 55° to 70° C. (130° to 160° F.), and it acts as an excellent plasticizer for the Kauri resin, which is easily fused at temperatures compatible with impression work. In such combinations, a filler such as French chalk is usually added, to improve the workability and texture of the compound.

In the modern impression compounds, commercial stearic acid has replaced the stearin compound. Commercial stearic acid is a combination of stearic, palmitic and oleic acids. It is graded according to its oleic acid content. The more oleic acid present, the lower are both the melting point and the hardness. The palmitic acid is a hardener.

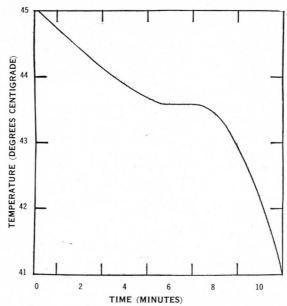

Fig. 5–1.   A time-temperature cooling curve for impression compound.

Stearic acid is more uniform than the stearin, and it provides better plasticization. It aids in the even dispersion of the filler or "extender."

The selection of the proper filler is of importance, since its texture and particle size greatly influence the workability and strength of the compound. In addition to French chalk, other fillers such as barytes or soapstone may be used.

Synthetic resins are being used considerably in compound at the present time together with natural resin. The coumerone-indene resins are the synthetic materials commonly used. Their production is more constant from batch to batch than can be depended upon with the natural resins. The coumerone-indene resins soften over a range of temperature, and they are readily plasticized with the stearic acid, previously mentioned. A high molecular weight resin can be plasticized in this manner, and its softening point will be decreased to the required range, with an increased plastic flow. Such compounds offer excellent water-resisting properties.

**Fusion Temperature.**       If some softened impression compound is wrapped around the bulb of a thermometer, and if the temperature is noted at definite time intervals during the cooling period, a curve similar to that in Figure 5–1 can be plotted. The change in rate of cooling shown by the change of slope in the curve indicates the evolution of a heat of fusion during the solidification of some of the ingredients. It is important to  note that the fusion temperature indicated in the graph is seldom the true hardening point of the compound. However, the actual impression should be completed at a temperature above this hardening point, since the compound stiffens considerably at this temperature. The impression should never be removed at this temperature, since the compound is still plastic.

Obviously, such a fusion temperature should occur above mouth temperature.

**Miscellaneous Thermal Properties.**    The thermal conductivity of these materials is very low. This property should be taken into consideration particularly during the heating and the cooling of these materials. During the softening of the material, the outside will always soften first, and the inside last. It is important that the material be uniformly soft at the time it is placed in the tray. In order to obtain a uniform softening, time must be allowed for the material to be heated uniformly throughout its mass.

It is even more important to cool the material thoroughly in the tray before the impression is withdrawn from the mouth. Usually cold water is sprayed on the tray while it is in the mouth. Such a procedure should be continued until the compound is thoroughly hardened throughout, before the impression is withdrawn. Failure to attain a complete hardening of the material before the impression is withdrawn may result in a serious distortion of the impression.

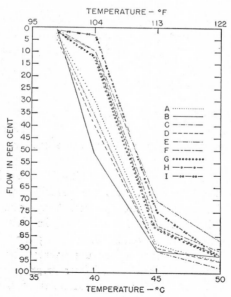

Fig. 5–2.   Flow of impression compounds at different temperatures. Curves *A, B, C,* and *D* are for impression compounds and curves *E, F, G, H* and *I* are for tray compounds. (Data from Souder and Paffenbarger, *Physical Properties of Dental Materials,* U. S. Government Printing Office.)

The linear thermal coefficient of expansion of impression compound is considerable in comparison to many other substances. For example, the average linear thermal contraction of impression compound from mouth temperature (37° C.) to a room temperature of 25° C. (77° F.) may vary between 0.3 and 0.4 per cent. According to the room temperature, then, the dimensions of the impression may be measurably different from the original dimensions in the mouth. Such an error is unavoidable and it is inherent in the technic.

However, the lower the temperature of the compound at the time the impression is obtained, the less will be the error from this source. One way to reduce the error due to thermal contraction is first to obtain an impression as usual. Then the impression is passed through a flame until the surface is softened, and a second impression is made.[1] During the second impression, the shrinkage is relatively small, since only the surface layer has been softened completely. Another modification of this technic is to spray cold water on the metal tray just before it is inserted in the mouth.[2] Thus the portion of the material adjacent to the tray will be hardened, while the surface layer is still soft. When either of these technics is employed, the impression will likely be stressed considerably, and the stone cast should be constructed before the relaxation becomes appreciable.

**Flow.**     The flow of impression compound can be beneficial or it can be a source of error. After the compound has softened and during the period it is impressed against the tissues, a continuous flow is desired; the material should flow easily to conform to the tissues so that every detail and landmark is reproduced accurately. No subsequent relaxation should occur. The viscosity or flow of the material at this stage will be a function of the temperature and of the composition of the compound.

Once the compound has solidified, any deformation should be completely elastic, so that the impression can be withdrawn without distortion or flow. Actually, such a condition cannot be realized with this type of material.

In the American Dental Association Specification No. 3 for Dental Impression Compound,[3] certain tests are described to indicate the flow of the compound at various temperatures. A cylinder of the material, 10 millimeters in diameter and 6 millimeters in altitude, is loaded at a definite temperature with a weight of 2 kilograms (4.4 pounds) for 10 minutes. The flow is designated as the shortening in length of such specimens during the test. The flow of four impression compounds and five tray compounds[4] is plotted as a function of the temperature in Figure 5–2.

According to the specification, a flow of 6 per cent is allowable for impression compound (type I) at mouth temperature (37° C.). Such an amount of flow is presumably negligible so far as its effect on the accuracy of the impression is concerned.

The specification further provides for a flow of not less than 80 per cent nor more than 85.0 per cent when the temperature of this impression compound is 45° C. (113° F.). This requirement is most important, since this is the approximate temperature at which the compound is impressed against the tissues. The amount of flow at this juncture of the technic determines the type of impression that is to be obtained in relation to the pressure on the soft tissue.

The specification requires that the flow of the tray compound (type II) shall be not more than 2 per cent at 37° C. (98.6° F.) and not less than 70 per cent nor more than 85 per cent at 45° C. (113° F.). As can be noted, the tray compound is not as plastic as the impression compound when it is softened. As a result, it can be expected that it will not record detail as readily as does the impression compound (type I).

**Distortion.** References have been made in previous sections to the induction of stresses in an impression with compound which are later relieved by relaxation and which may cause warpage or distortion. Such a condition is often unavoidable, and, therefore, the safest procedure is to construct the cast or die within the first hour after the impression has been obtained, before an appreciable relaxation can occur. Such a warpage caused by relaxation can be readily demonstrated, as shown in Figure 5–3.

One avoidable cause for warpage is the removal of the impression from the mouth before it is thoroughly cooled. If the surface of the compound is hard, but the inside is soft, a relaxation will occur immediately when the impression is withdrawn. This condition can be demonstrated easily. A piece of compound is softened, and then plunged into cold water for a few seconds. The outside will be reasonably firm, but the inside will be soft so that the piece of compound can be bent slowly into the shape of a horseshoe. When it is released, its tendency

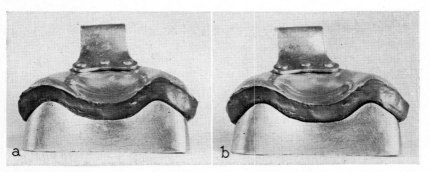

Fig. 5–3.　*a.* Fit of impression in compound on a metal mold immediately after cooling. *b.* Fit of same impression the next day.

to straighten out can be observed readily, but it will not recover its original dimensions. When such a condition is present in an impression at the time it is removed from the mouth, one cause for the warpage of the impression is evident. Such a condition is especially likely to be present if the impression is disturbed in any manner during or slightly below the fusion temperature range indicated in Figure 5–1, and above the actual hardening temperature of the compound.

**Softening of Impression Compound.** Whenever possible, compound should be softened with "dry" heat such as in an oven or similar device. Often small amounts of compound are softened over a gas flame. When a direct flame is used, the compound should not be allowed to boil or ignite so that important constituents are volatilized.

When a large amount of compound is to be softened, as when an impression is to be obtained of an entire mouth, it is difficult to heat the compound uniformly and the softening is usually better accomplished in a water bath.

There are several disadvantages in the use of a water bath. For example, if the compound is heated in the water for an excessive period of time, it may become brittle and grainy. Presumably, some of the lower molecular weight constituents are leached out by the water.

The chief disadvantage is that the plasticity of the compound may be altered by the manipulation of the compound in preparation for the impression tray. After the compound is removed from the water bath, it is usually kneaded with the fingers in order to produce a uniform plasticity throughout its mass. If water is incorporated at this stage, it apparently acts as a plasticizer. The plasticity of the compound is increased with the result that it reproduces details of the surface better, but unfortunately its flow may be doubled.[5]

If the compound is quickly dried immediately before it is handled and if it is left in the bath only until it is softened, there is no objection to the use of a temperature-controlled water bath.

The student is referred to a textbook on prosthetic dentistry[6] for the details of the preparation of the tray and the obtaining of the impression.

**Construction of the Cast.** The gypsum cast material is mixed and poured in the same manner as described for the plaster impressions, and the same precautions should be observed to avoid air bubbles.

The vault portion of the cast will not warp owing to the setting expansion of the stone or plaster as shown in Figure 4–2 in the preceding chapter. The cast material usually generates sufficient exothermic heat to soften the compound so that any setting expansion can occur unimpeded.

In fact, the compound may become sufficiently soft at this stage to allow the removal of the impression from the cast, although such a procedure should be done cautiously, so that the teeth forms, if present.

will not be fractured. The safest method for the removal of the impression is to immerse it in *warm* water until the compound has softened sufficiently to allow it to be separated easily from the cast. If the compound is overheated at this stage, it may adhere to the cast, and cause a discoloration of the stone.

## *Literature*

1. Souder, W., and Paffenbarger, G. C.: *Physical Properties of Dental Materials.* National Bureau of Standards Circular C433. Washington, U. S. Government Printing Office, 1942, p. 142.
2. Gehl, D. H., and Dresen, O. M.: *Complete Denture Prosthesis.* 4th ed. Philadelphia, W. B. Saunders Co., 1958, p. 83.
3. Paffenbarger, G. C., Stanford, J. W., and Sweeney, W. T.: *American Dental Association Specifications for Dental Materials.* Chicago, American Dental Association, 1958, pp. 20–23.
4. Souder, W., and Paffenbarger, G. C.: *loc. cit.,* p. 141.
5. Docking, A. R.: *Kneading of Modelling Compound.* Austral. J. Den., *27:*225–229, (Aug.), 1955.
6. Gehl, D. H., and Dresen, O. M.: *loc. cit.,* pp. 82–90.
7. Grossman, L. I.: *Dental Formulas and Aids to Dental Practice.* Philadelphia, Lea & Febiger, 1952, pp. 60–61.

# CHAPTER 6

# Zinc Oxide-Eugenol

# Impression Pastes

One of the dentally useful chemical reactions is that between zinc oxide and eugenol. Under the proper conditions a relatively hard mass is formed which possesses certain medicinal advantages as well as a mechanical usefulness in certain dental operations. This type of material has found a wide application in dentistry as a cementing medium, surgical dressing, temporary filling material, root canal filling, relining material for dentures, and as an impression material for edentulous mouths.

The basic composition of all of these materials is the same, mainly, zinc oxide and eugenol. Plasticizers, fillers, and other additives are incorporated as necessary to provide the desired properties for the particular use of the product.

**Impression Pastes.** Impression pastes are used as a corrective lining in a preliminary impression. For example, a preliminary impression may be taken with tray compound as described in the previous chapter. The paste is then spread over the impression with compound, and a second impression is obtained.

The paste may be supplied as a powder containing the zinc oxide, and a liquid containing the eugenol. However, many of the commercial products are dispensed as pastes in tubes. One tube is filled with a paste containing the active ingredient, zinc oxide, and the other tube contains the eugenol in a paste form. The two pastes are mixed together in the proper proportions, and the mixture is spread over the preliminary impression as described. The impression is withdrawn after the paste has hardened.

The impression pastes for edentulous mouths should be classified as impression materials which harden by chemical action.

**Chemistry.** The essential reaction between zinc oxide and eugenol is complex and not completely defined. The structural formula for eugenol is:

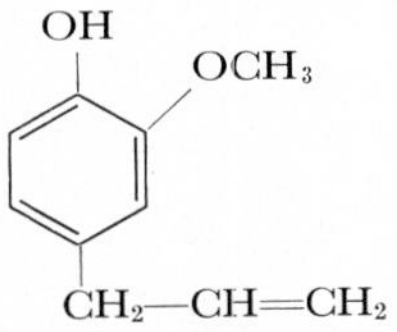

$$OH \quad OCH_3$$

$$CH_2-CH=CH_2$$

According to the available theories,[1] one of the necessary conditions for the reaction with eugenol is the presence of the methoxy group, ortho to the hydroxyl group in the benzene ring. On this basis, guaiacol and methyl guaiacol, both of which satisfy this condition, were found to react, but no other similar compounds which did not conform to this structural configuration would harden with the zinc oxide.

Not all zinc oxide powders react. For example, a dehydrated zinc oxide does not react with eugenol to form a hard mass. Such a condition infers that water may be essential to the reaction.[1]

The mechanism of the reaction appears to be a chelation process. A chelate compound, zinc eugenolate, has been identified as one of the products. Its structural formula is given as:

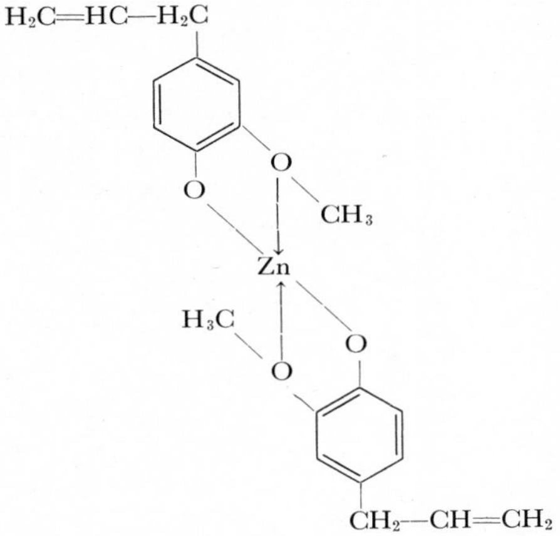

$$H_2C=HC-H_2C$$

$$O \quad O$$
$$CH_3$$
$$Zn$$
$$H_3C \quad O$$
$$O$$

$$CH_2-CH=CH_2$$

Other compounds capable of forming chelates have also been found which will form coherent products with zinc oxide.[2]

The structure of the set mass resulting from mixtures of zinc oxide and eugenol is pictured as particles of zinc oxide embedded in a matrix of long sheath-like crystals of zinc eugenolate. Any excess eugenol is likely absorbed by both the zinc eugenolate and the zinc oxide.[1]

**Composition.** Although the essential ingredients of the impression paste are zinc oxide and eugenol, certain fillers are added so that a paste will be formed before setting instead of a liquid as would be the case with the two chemicals above.

The formula in Table 6–1 represents a composition for an impression paste which has been marketed for many years.[3] It consists of a powder and a liquid. Most modern impression pastes are dispensed as two separate pastes in separate tubes. One of the tubes contains the eugenol as one of the ingredients and the other contains the zinc oxide. For example, the powder in Table 6–1 can be mixed with mineral oil, for instance, and made into a paste. An inert powder such as diatomaceous earth or talc can be incorporated in the liquid to form a paste.

As previously noted, the type of zinc oxide to be used may be critical. It should be finely divided and it should contain a very slight amount of water. Unfortunately, such water tends to reduce the shelf life (*i.e.*, ability to be stored without deterioration) of the commercial product.[4]

The addition of rosin to the paste apparently facilitates the speed of the reaction, and a smoother, more homogeneous product results. It is possible that the rosin enters the reaction in some way. Since it can be added to either, or both, liquid and powder (Table 6–1), its chemical reaction, if any, must be dependent upon the presence of both eugenol and zinc oxide together. The use of a hydrogenated rosin provides greater stability than that obtained with the natural product.

The magnesium chloride (Table 6–1) acts as an accelerator for the setting time. There are a large number of chemicals which can be used to accelerate the hardening of the impression pastes.[2, 4, 5] For example, water is an excellent accelerator. One of the problems connected with its use, however, is to incorporate it homogeneously throughout the mass of the material, since many of the ingredients are not miscible in water. This problem can be solved by the incorporation of an inert "carrier" for the water in which the water is miscible and which itself is compatible with the remaining ingredients.[6]

*Table 6–1.*   *Composition of a Zinc Oxide-Eugenol Impression Paste*

| POWDER | PER CENT |
| --- | --- |
| Zinc oxide | 80 |
| Rosin | 19 |
| Magnesium chloride | 1 |
| *Liquid* | |
| Oil of cloves or eugenol | 56 |
| Gum rosin | 16 |
| Olive oil | 16 |
| Linseed oil | 6 |
| Light mineral oil | 6 |

Other chemicals commonly used as accelerators are zinc acetate, primary alcohols, and glacial acetic acid. The accelerator can be incorporated in either paste or in both pastes.

Oil of cloves contains 70 to 85 per cent eugenol, and it is sometimes used in preference to eugenol because it reduces the burning sensation in the soft tissues of the mouth when the mixed paste is first placed in contact with them. The American Dental Association Specification for these pastes requires that the product have a maximum eugenol content of 17 per cent by weight.

The olive oil acts as a plasticizer, and it also aids in the masking of the irritant action of the eugenol.

The linseed oil and mineral oil both are plasticizers introduced to provide a smoothness and fluidity during mixing. Canada balsam and Peru balsam are often used in a similar manner. If the mixed paste is too thin or lacks body before it sets, a solid substance such as a wax or an inert powder (kaolin, talc, diatomaceous earth, etc.) may be added to one or both of the original pastes as a filler.

The variations in composition which can be used are many, and such differences may influence the choice of the dentist considerably in the selection of an impression paste.

**Setting Time.** Setting time is important since there must be sufficient time for mixing, filling the tray, and seating the impression. Once the material has been carried to the mouth in a plastic condition, only a minimum time should take place before the impression hardens. Prolonged setting may result in inaccuracy due to unavoidable movement of the tray while the paste is still soft. The composition of the paste influences the setting time. For example, within practical limits, the greater the ratio of the zinc oxide to the eugenol, the slower will be the setting time if no accelerator is present. Consequently, it is important that the proportions of the two pastes be measured before mixing. Also the smaller the particle size of the zinc oxide, the shorter will be the setting time.

The accelerating effect of the rosin on the setting time has been mentioned. It is effective in this regard provided that the rosin is in the correct proportion to the eugenol. Too much rosin may increase the setting time.[6]

The type and amount of accelerator used is by far the most important composition factor in the control of the setting time. The setting time is often affected considerably by very small changes in the amount of the accelerator present.

The setting times of a number of commercial impression pastes are shown in Table 6–2. In this table the initial setting time or the working time is defined as the time from the start of mixing until a Vicat needle no longer will penetrate to the bottom of the mixed paste. The final setting time is the time from the start of mixing until the Vicat needle either does not penetrate the surface of the set paste perceptibly, or penetrates the mass in a minimum amount.[7] The working time represents the time at which the paste begins to set and can no longer be manipulated. The final set indicates the time at which the impression can be withdrawn from the mouth.

Analysis of these data[7] and results on setting time determined on seven more recently manufactured pastes[8] indicate that these pastes fall into two general groups. One group is fast setting while the other has an initial and final set a minute or two longer. This difference has been reflected in the tentative American Dental Association Specification for zinc oxide-eugenol pastes where they have been classified in two groups, one as hard and one as soft. Setting times are measured somewhat differently but the maximum and minimum setting time limits are defined for each group.

As can be noted from Table 6–2, with the exception of material D, all of the pastes set more rapidly at 37° C. (99° F.) under water than at room temperature [25° C. (77° F.)] in the air. The setting time at 37° C. (99° F.) under water more nearly represents mouth conditions. The more rapid setting at body temperature is probably the result of both the increase in temperature and the presence of the water.

Although generally water and humidity accelerate the set, there are exceptions to this rule, for example material D. Some pastes occasionally show a retardation in set when exposed to moisture while others may be quite insensitive to it.[8] However, temperature invariably influences the setting time for all commercial products in the same way—the higher the temperature, the more rapid the set. On a hot humid day, the setting time may be so short that some of the materials cannot be used.

The setting reaction itself is exothermic. The slope of the temperature curve for most products shows a definite increase between the time of the initial and final set.

**Control of the Setting Time.**     The setting time of these materials is not as easily controlled by the operator as is the setting time of plaster of paris, for example. There are, however, at least five methods by which such a control can be effected within certain limits.

1. If the paste sets too slowly, the rate of reaction can be increased by the addition of an accelerator. As has been stated, a drop of water will usually accelerate the setting time of most of the commercially available impression pastes. However, if the paste contains a water repellent, or for some similar reason the water cannot be dispersed equally during mixing, the water may not be effective. In any event, the water should be added sparingly. Too much added water may cause a retardation in setting.[8]

Almost any primary alcohol can be added dropwise as an accelerator if the water is ineffective. If a retardation is desired, a drop of a sec-

*Table 6–2.*    *Working and Setting Times of Zinc Oxide-Eugenol*
*Impression Pastes*

| PASTE | WORKING TIME | | SETTING TIME | |
|---|---|---|---|---|
| | 25°C. (77°F.) (MINUTES) | 37°C. (99°F.)* (MINUTES) | 25°C. (77°F.) (MINUTES) | 37°C. (99°F.)* (MINUTES) |
| A | 7.5 | 2.5 | 9.0 | 4.5 |
| B | 6.5 | 2.3 | 8.0 | 4.0 |
| C | 5.0 | 5.0 | 9.5 | 7.5 |
| D | 2.0 | 3.5 | 6.0 | 6.5 |
| E | 5.0 | 4.0 | 7.5 | 5.5 |
| F | 3.5 | 3.0 | 6.0 | 5.0 |
| G | 5.0 | 3.5 | 8.0 | 6.0 |
| H | 4.0 | 3.5 | 6.0 | 5.5 |
| I | 3.5 | 2.0 | 5.0 | 3.5 |
| J | 6.0 | 4.5 | 8.0 | 6.5 |
| K | 7.0 | 6.0 | 10.0 | 9.0 |

* Specimen immersed in water.

ondary or tertiary alcohol such as glycol or glycerol can be added to the mixture before spatulation.[9]

2. When a satisfactory material sets too fast, the cause is most likely to be a high relative humidity and/or temperature. This factor is a serious problem in some parts of the country where office environment is not controlled. Cooling the spatula and mixing slab may be of some assistance.

3. The setting time can also be prolonged by the addition of certain inert oils and waxes during the mixing, such as olive oil, mineral oil, petrolatum, etc. The dilution effected in this manner decreases the ratio of the accelerator to the total volume of paste, and thereby the setting time is prolonged. However, such a practice is not entirely satisfactory since it tends to reduce the rigidity of the hardened material and, unless used with discretion, it may result in an inhomogeneous mix.

4. The setting time can be controlled in most instances by a change in the ratio of the zinc oxide paste to the eugenol paste. As to whether retardation or acceleration will be obtained depends upon which paste contains the accelerator. If the accelerator is contained in the brown, or eugenol paste, a decrease in the amount of zinc oxide paste should accelerate the setting and, conversely, an increase should retard since the total amount of accelerator will be reduced percentagewise.

It is possible, in consideration of the rosin content of each paste, and particularly in the cases where both pastes contain an accelerator, that the change in ratio of the two pastes may not be predictable in its control of the setting time.

5. The time of mixing affects the setting time to a limited extent. With most pastes, the longer the mixing time (within limits), the shorter the setting time.

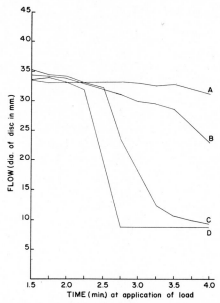

Fig. 6–1.  Flow of four commercial zinc oxide-eugenol impression pastes at various periods after mixing.

**Consistency and Flow.**  The consistency or fluidity of the paste at the time it is impressed against the tissues is of considerable importance to the type of impression desired. In order to minimize tissue displacement, most operators prefer a material that will readily flow upon insertion into the oral cavity. The tentative American Dental Association Specification for these materials makes use of a modification of the consistency test used for zinc phosphate cement to be described in a subsequent chapter. As noted in the previous chapter, the consistency of compound is dependent upon the temperature, and therefore it is likely to be difficult to control. In this respect, the impression pastes are superior in that their consistency can be regulated by the composition of the paste. The dentist can select a paste of a low or a high consistency, and, with a uniform mixing technique, he can be certain that the proper flow qualities will be present at the time the impression is to be obtained. Again, however, flow may be regulated by the mixing temperature and the humidity of the environment, even more than by the accelerator-base ratio.[10]

Not only is there a wide range of consistencies in the various commercial products, but also the flow of the freshly mixed paste varies as it is related to the time before setting. This relation is indicated by the graphs in Figure 6–1.

The results in Figure 6–1 were obtained by subjecting a freshly mixed disk of each product to a specified load at various intervals after mixing.[11] The flow of the particular paste at a specified time is expressed in terms of the spread of the disk in millimeters or increase in diameter at the various times of load application.

Possibly the better pastes (A and B) are those in which the diameter decreased the least over the period of time indicated. These materials are quite thin and their working time is apparently satisfactory.

An entirely different behavior is exhibited for pastes C and D. Although their initial consistencies are comparable, decrease in flow occurred approximately three minutes after spatulation. Thus their working time would be limited and, if a specific consistency or fluidity is desired, the time between mixing and insertion of the tray is critical. On the other hand, the reduction in flow, provided the tray was seated, might be advantageous in reducing the possibility of distortion while the impression hardens in the mouth.

Generally, there is a correlation between flow and setting time. Those materials which show a decrease in flow at various time intervals also have lower setting times and a shorter time interval between the initial and final set.

The exact degree of flow desirable for making secondary or corrective impressions is still controversial. Some operators prefer a thin impression material, believing that this will minimize tissue displacement. Others prefer a slightly stiffer material with the belief that the thin mix is more difficult to contain in the tray, produces inferior surface detail, and will be more apt to contain incorporated air.

**Rigidity and Strength.** As in the case of impressions with compound, the paste impression should be unyielding when it is withdrawn from the mouth and should resist fracture. Tests have indicated[6] that impression pastes can be compounded which will exhibit a resistance to flow at mouth temperature which is equal or superior to the similar properties of impression compound.[7]

The compressive strength of hardened zinc oxide-eugenol impression pastes may reach a maximum of 70 kilograms per square centimeter (1000 pounds per square inch) two hours after mixing.[10] There is not always a direct relationship between strength and rigidity, however.

**Dimensional Stability.** The dimensional stability of most of the impression pastes is quite satisfactory.[7] A negligible shrinkage (less than 0.1 per cent) may occur during hardening.

No significant dimensional change subsequent to hardening is to be expected with the better commercial products. The impressions can be preserved indefinitely without a change in shape due to relaxation or other causes of warpage. Such a statement assumes that the tray material is dimensionally stable.

**Tray Material.** As previously noted, a preliminary impression is often obtained with tray compound, which can be used as a tray for the impression with a paste. Such a technic is subject to the general errors of the compound impression, such as thermal changes and warpage due to relaxation. Certainly, the dimensional stability of the paste impression can be no better than that of the tray material on which it rests.

In order to obtain greater accuracy, a great many prosthodontists obtain the preliminary impression and then construct a stone cast. A tray of acrylic resin or similar material is constructed on the cast. This tray is then used for obtaining the paste impression. The details of the construction of such trays and the impression technic can be found in a textbook on denture prosthetics.[12]

**Reproduction of Detail.** One of the prime requisites of any impression material is its ability to reproduce accurately the minute detail of the oral tissues. Differences have been noted in the sharpness of detail reproduced by the various pastes.[10] It has been suggested that, in general, the pastes which set more rapidly are superior in this respect.[13] Although most pastes are readily separated, there is a tendency for some to adhere to the stone cast. Any film of paste left on the cast will naturally reduce the accuracy of reproduction. The American Dental Association Specification for this material requires that examination of a poured stone cast shall show no visible evidence of adherence of the paste to the cast or of the stone to the impression.

**Mixing Technic.** The mixing of the two pastes is generally accomplished on an oil-impervious paper, although a glass mixing slab can be used as well.

The proper proportion of the two pastes is generally obtained by squeezing two ropes of paste of the same length, one from each tube, onto the mixing slab. The orifices of the two tubes are regulated to deliver the proper amount from each tube when the lengths of the ropes are the same.

A flexible stainless steel spatula, approximately 2 centimeters (¾ inch) in width and 12 centimeters (5 inches) in length, is satisfactory for the mixing. The two ropes are combined with the first sweep of the spatula, and the mixing is continued for approximately one minute, or as directed by the manufacturer, until a uniform color is observed.

**General Considerations.** The mixture is spread over the preliminary impression, and the tray is carried into the mouth according to an approved technic, as described elsewhere.[12]

The impression should be held rigidly in position until it has thoroughly hardened. Owing to the accelerating action of the saliva on the surface of the tissues, the adjacent surface of the impression may harden first. Any disturbance of the impression at this stage will result in a warpage. Only when the material has hardened completely should the impression be removed from the mouth.

The cast can be constructed in the usual manner. As with impression compound, no separating medium is necessary.

## Literature

1. Copeland, H. I., Brauer, G. M., Sweeney, W. T., and Forziati, A. F.: *Setting Reactions of Zinc Oxide and Eugenol.* J. Research N. B. S., 55:134–138 (Sept.), 1955.
2. Brauer, G. M., White, E. E., and Moshonas, M. G.: *The Reaction of Metal Oxides with o-Ethoxybenzoic Acid and other Chelating Agents.* J. D. Res., 37:547–560 (June), 1958.
3. Kelly, E. B.: U. S. Patent No. 2,077,418 (April 20), 1937.
4. Harvey, W., and Petch, N. J.: *Acceleration of the Setting of Zinc Oxide Cements.* Brit. D. J., 80:1–8 (Jan. 4), 35–42 (Jan. 18), 1946.
5. Molnar, E. J., and Skinner, E. W.: *A Study of Zinc Oxide-Rosin Cements.* J.A.D.A., 29:744–751 (May), 1942.
6. Lawrence, G. O.: *Impression Pastes.* Austral. J. Den., 45:207–212 (Sept.), 1941.
7. Skinner, E. W., Cooper, E. N., and Ziehm, H. W.: *Some Physical Properties of Zinc Oxide-Eugenol Impression Pastes.* J.A.D.A., 41:449–455 (Oct.), 1950.
8. Vierra, D. F.: *Factors Affecting the Setting of Zinc Oxide-Eugenol Impression Pastes.* J. Pros. Den., 9:70–79 (Jan.–Feb.), 1959.
9. Molnar, E. J.: *Setting Retarders for Zinc Oxide and Eugenol Pastes.* Paper presented at the Annual Meeting of the Dental Materials Group, I.A.D.R., 1957.
10. Asgars, K., and Peyton, F. A.: *Physical Properties of Corrective Impression Pastes.* J. Pros. Den., 4:555–567 (July), 1954.
11. Clark, R. J., and Phillips, R. W.: *Flow Studies of Certain Dental Impression Materials.* J. Pros. Den., 7:259–266 (March), 1957.
12. Gehl, D. H., and Dresen, O. M.: *Complete Denture Prosthesis.* 4th ed. Philadelphia, W. B. Saunders Co., 1958.
13. McCracken, W. L.: *Impression Materials in Prosthetic Dentistry.* D. Clin. North America, November, 1958, pp. 672–684.

# CHAPTER 7

# Hydrocolloid Impression Materials:
# Theoretical Considerations

The impression materials described in the previous chapters are best suited for use in edentulous mouths, where there are no severe undercuts. Any undercuts prevent the removal of an impression without distortion or fracture of such impression materials. In the case of the plaster impression, the set plaster is fractured intentionally to remove the impression in pieces, which are reassembled. When compound or an impression paste is used for an impression of teeth, the material distorts, or flows, upon removal over the height of contour of the tooth, and the result is an inaccurate reproduction of the part.

A substance which will deform elastically when it is removed over an undercut, so that it will spring back to its original position, will produce an accurate impression of a tooth. Such a material can be obtained by using a flexible gel. The problem is to introduce a viscous fluid into the mouth on an impression tray, and to allow it to gel in position. The impression can then be removed intact, since the flexibility of the gel is sufficient to allow the impression to be withdrawn over extremely sharp undercuts, with no perceptible permanent distortion. The stone cast can be poured in the usual manner.

**Colloids.** Any solution in which the units of the solute are sufficiently large so that they will not dialyze through a suitable membrane is known as a *colloid* or a *colloidal sol*. The units of the solute or *dispersed phase* may each be aggregations of molecules, or a single large molecule. The particles are dispersed in the solvent or *dispersion medium* by virtue of the fact that they are repelled from each other by an inherent electric charge on each particle. The charge may be either positive or negative, depending upon the particular colloid. For example, the particles in an agar-agar sol are slightly charged negatively.

If the dispersed phase is of the same phase (solid, liquid or gas) as the dispersion medium, the colloid is said to be an *emulsion*. If the dispersed phase and the dispersion medium are not of like phase, the colloid is a *suspension*. Since the dental impression materials are hydrocolloids of the *emulsoid* type, in which the dispersion medium is water, only this type of colloid will be discussed.

**Colloidal Gels.** Some hydrocolloid sols possess the property of changing to a jelly or *gel* under certain conditions. If the gelation is brought about by cooling the sol, for example, the gel is *reversible* in character provided that it can be returned to the sol condition when its temperature is increased. Thus the change from the sol to the gel, and vice versa, is essentially a physical effect related to temperature. Examples of such hydrocolloids are gelatin and agar-agar.

The *irreversible hydrocolloids* are characterized by the fact that the sol is changed to the gel, but the gel cannot be reversed to the sol by any simple means. Usually the gelation is effected by a chemical reaction of some type. The alginate impression materials to be described are hydrocolloids of this type.

**Structure of the Gel.** An understanding of the mechanisms of gelation and gel structure is essential if the dentist is to appreciate the importance of certain manipulative variables and to understand the technic thoroughly. Although the internal structures of both the reversible and irreversible gels are similar, the phenomena involved are best described for the reversible type.

A gel can sustain a shearing stress without flow, and such a property clearly indicates the presence of some continuous mechanical network or structure.[1] Such a network is visualized as composed of minute, submicroscopic fibrils formed by the colloidal particles of the dispersed phase. The fibrils form a network of spaces or *micelles* in which the water is held by adsorption. The fibrils become entangled much like the twigs in a brush heap; for this reason, gels are often described as possessing a "brush-heap" structure. In the reversible type of hydrocolloid, the chains or fibrils are held together by the usual intermolecular forces or secondary valence bonds, but in the case of the irreversible hydrocolloid the bonds between the chains are of the primary valence type.

In the case of the reversible hydrocolloid, the sol and the gel possess many properties in common, with the exception of rigidity. When the temperature is raised, the chains and micelles break up, chiefly because of the increased thermal agitation of the molecules. As the kinetic energy of the molecules increases with the temperature, as evidenced in an increase in the Brownian movement, the micelles disunite and the viscosity greatly diminishes as the gel changes to the fluid sol.[2] During this period, the chains may be pictured as forming and uniting constantly, as their contact is influenced by the thermal agitation. The thermal forces predominate, however, and any adhesion which may occur on contact lacks permanence.

As the temperature decreases, the cohesive forces become more prominent and the influence of the thermal agitation decreases, until the micelles maintain a definite "brush-heap" structure. The temperature at which rigidity is attained is known as the *gelation temperature*. The gelation temperature is not analogous in all respects to a freezing point; the gel becomes more rigid as the temperature decreases below the gelation point. The gel may eventually become brittle, and lose much of its flexibility at low temperatures.

It is interesting to note that the effect of the thermal agitation on the dissociation of the chains occurs at a higher temperature as the gel is heated than does the re-establishment of the cohesion when the sol is cooled. In other words, the gelation temperature of a hydrocolloid gel is lower than its liquefaction temperature. This phenomenon is known as *hysteresis*. From a clinical standpoint, this phenomenon provides a working range for the dentist. The lower temperatures of the working range can be tolerated by the patient comfortably when the sol is impressed against the mouth tissues.

A reason for the irreversibility of an irreversible gel is now apparent. Since the chains and micelles in the irreversible gel are bonded by primary valence forces, they cannot be disrupted by thermal agitation at any temperature.

**Gel Strength.**     The strength of a gel is fundamentally related to the "brush-heap" density, and the concentration of the dispersed phase. The two factors are by no means independent, since the greater the concentration of the dispersed phase, the greater will be the number of micelles or "brush-heap" density. On the other hand, as noted in the previous section, in a reversible hydrocolloid the "brush-heap" density also increases as the temperature decreases below the gelation temperature for a given concentration of the dispersed phase.

The strength of the gel can also be increased by the addition of certain modifiers such as fillers and chemicals. The fillers usually consist of fine powders of an inert substance. The powder particles may be imagined to be "caught" in the micelle network in such a manner that the brush heap is rendered more rigid with less flexibility. The effectiveness of the filler in increasing the strength of the gel is definitely related to the size, shape and density of its particles. The filler also acts to increase the viscosity of the sol when the reversible hydrocolloid is liquefied.

The effect of the chemicals which may be added to control the strength of the gel is related to the ionization effects of the chemical on

material has been liquefied, it must be sufficiently viscous not to flow out of the tray, even though the tray is inverted when it is placed in the mouth. Furthermore, it must have sufficient viscosity so that it will flow through the perforations in the tray (Fig. 7–1) to a slight extent, without continuing to flow to an extent that all of the material runs out. On the other hand, its viscosity must not be so great that it will not readily penetrate every detail of the teeth and soft tissues to be impressed.

The agar sol by itself is likely to be too fluid for this purpose, and the use of fillers and other modifiers is employed as previously described. As noted in the previous section, the incorporation of borax definitely increases the viscosity of the sol.

The viscosity of five commercial reversible hydrocolloid impression materials in the sol condition as influenced by the temperature is shown in Figure 7–3. All of the materials increase in viscosity as the gelation temperature is approached. The beginning of the molecular cohesion to form the micelle structure can be noted by the rather abrupt change in the slope of the curves toward the horizontal, as the temperature decreases. This increase in viscosity probably may be attributed to a bonding of the agar-agar molecule at first only by secondary attractive forces at widely separated points which is then followed by further bonding by non-localized secondary attractive forces as the temperature drops.[9]

A study of Figure 7–3 indicates that there is a noteworthy difference between the materials in the viscosity of the sols as affected by the

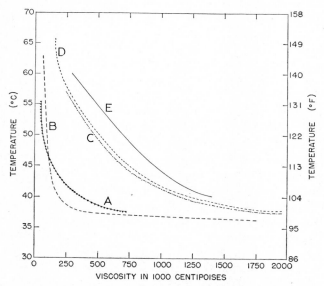

Fig. 7–3. Viscosity of the sols of five commercial reversible hydrocolloid impression materials as influenced by the temperature. (Courtesy of Coe Laboratories, Inc.)

decrease in temperature. The change in viscosity with decrease in temperature in the case of materials *A* and *B* is small, compared with the large change which occurs with materials *C, D,* and *E.* No change of practical interest occurs in the case of material *B* until its temperature is approximately 6° C. (10° F.) above its gelation temperature.

The greater viscosity and its slow increase with decrease in temperature in the case of materials *C, D,* and *E* are probably due to the fact that these materials contain a borate compound of some nature. Presumably the viscosity of the sol in the case of materials *A* and *B* is governed by means of fillers or thermoplastic substances or both. Since the material in the impression tray is usually at a temperature slightly above the gelation temperature at the time it is impressed against the tissues, the viscosity of the material at such temperatures is an important consideration.

**Gelation Temperature.**    The temperature at which the hydrocolloid impression material sets to a gel is of importance to the dentist. If the material gels at too high a temperature, it is possible that injury may result to the mouth tissues involved, or the surface of the sol may gel when it contacts the tissues and a severe surface stress may develop. If the gelation temperature is too far below that of the mouth temperature, it will be difficult or even impossible to chill the material to a temperature sufficiently low to obtain a firm gel adjacent to the mouth tissues.

The temperature of gel formation is best determined for dental purposes by a determination of the temperature at which a cylindrical object such as a thermometer bulb can be imprinted into the material and withdrawn so that a clean, clear-cut hole is left in the gel. A metal tube with a 10 millimeter bore and a wall thickness of approximately 1 millimeter is prescribed for this purpose in the American Dental Association Specification No. 11. According to this specification, the gelation temperature must not be less than 37° C. (98.6° F.) or more than 45° C. (113° F.). Most modern reversible hydrocolloid impression materials exhibit a gelation temperature between 36° C. (97° F.) and 42° C. (108° F.).

**Gelation Time.**    Gelation of reversible hydrocolloid is, of course, a function of both temperature and time. As indicated above, the lower the temperature, the more rapid will be gelation. Also the longer the sol is held at a given temperature, the greater will be the viscosity of the sol. Numerous publications have stressed the importance of leaving the tray in the mouth until the gelation has proceeded to a point where the gel strength is sufficient to resist deformation or fracture.[10] The minimum time is five minutes and, provided that care is exercised to avoid movement of the tray, a longer gelation time will do no harm.

**Dimensional Stability.**    As previously noted, gels are invariably subject to changes in dimension by syneresis and imbibition, according to their environment. Once the impression is removed from the mouth and carried into the air at room temperature, syneresis usually starts immediately, with a resulting shrinkage of the gel. Since the impression must be exposed to the air for sufficient time to construct the cast, some shrinkage is bound to occur.

The effects of imbibition and syneresis on dimensional stability have been studied by numerous investigators. These investigations have included the dimensional change of the materials when floated on mercury,[11] when laid in a trough,[12, 13] when confined in an impression tray,[10, 14] as determined by the fit of a master tapered die in the reproduced stone model,[15] and by the fit of castings fabricated on stone dies.[14] All such investigations have emphasized the distortion which may result from fluctuations in water content within the impression.

Typical examples of the changes observed are the curves shown in Figure 7–4. The curves indicate the dimensional changes of six commercial materials which are listed by the code letters *A, B, C, D, E,* and *F.* The gelled materials were allowed to remain in air for 60 minutes, after which they were immersed in water for the succeeding 3 hours.[12]

As can be noted, all of the materials shrank in air, but the shrinkage of some of the materials was much greater than others. For example, material *F* shrank 1.0 per cent, whereas material *A* shrank only 0.18 per cent in the same time and under the same environmental conditions. The difference is largely due to differences in gel concentration and chemical composition of the materials.

When the specimens were subsequently immersed in water, all but one of the materials (*D*) returned to within 0.1 per cent of their

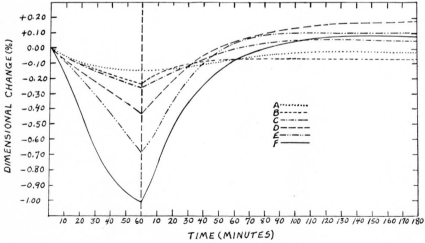

Fig. 7–4.   Linear contraction in air (31 to 42 per cent relative humidity) and subsequent expansion in water of six reversible hydrocolloid impression materials.

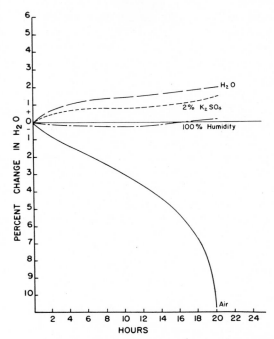

Fig. 7–5.   Percentage change in water content by weight of a reversible hydrocolloid impression material in various storage media.

original size (Fig. 7–4). However, it should not be inferred from these data that contraction due to syneresis can be compensated for by reimmersion in water. Although the average linear change might be within 0.1 per cent of the original size, the expansion is not uniform in all parts of the impression.[10] Because of differences in bulk and degree of residual stress present, one would not expect it to expand exactly to the same magnitude or direction in all areas.

Had the specimens used in the experiment been allowed to dry for longer than 60 minutes, or had the relative humidity been lower so that they would have dried faster, the shrinkage would have been greater. However, in the experiment it was found that the specimens began to warp when they were exposed to the air for only one hour. Furthermore, subsequent imbibition resulted in further warpage. It is clear that the impression should be exposed to the air for as short a time as possible if the best results are to be obtained.

**Storage of the Impression.**    Various media, such as a 2 per cent solution of potassium sulfate or 100 per cent relative humidity, have often been suggested as environments in which to place the impression in order to prevent dimensional change. It is true that if the actual change in water content of the gel is measured, it is quite small in certain environments. Results obtained in four different media may be seen for one commercial product in Figure 7–5. These data are typical of most materials and they indicate that a relative humidity of 100 per cent best preserves the normal water content.[16] In fact, the change in water content in a water saturated atmosphere is negligible. Unfortunately, there is however, some water lost, as indicated in Figure 7–5, and the loss occurs mainly in the exposed top surface of the gel while the water on the interior remains the same. Consequently, a contraction due to syneresis occurs in the top layer and a distortion of the impression results.

It has been suggested that a bath of some type might eventually be developed for maintaining exact equilibrium conditions. If the osmotic pressure between the bath and the impression material were equal, then the water change would be negligible. Such a condition would probably never be realized under practical conditions. The osmotic pressure would fluctuate with the composition of the material and thus this balance would likely be impossible for the manufacturers to control from one lot of material to another.

Furthermore, there is evidence that the relaxation of the internal stresses that are inherent in the impression may be of equal importance to water fluctuation during storage. Such relaxation of stress produces distortion regardless of storage environment.[17]

When all factors are considered, it is evident that there is no satisfactory method for the storage of a hydrocolloid impression. Consequently, the stone cast should be constructed routinely as soon as the impression is removed from the mouth.

**Mechanical Properties.** According to the American Dental Association Specification No. 11 for Hydrocolloidal Impression Material, the compressive strength of these materials should not be less than 2000 grams per square centimeter (28.4 pounds per square inch). In other words, if the material exhibits a compressive strength of at least 2000 grams per square centimeter under the conditions of test, it will be satisfactory. Presumably, the material will not fracture upon removal if it meets this requirement. Some commercial materials of this type exhibit compressive strengths well above this minimum value.

The stress-strain relationships of the hydrocolloid impression materials are not linear over any portion of their stress-strain curve. Although the slope of the curve is a general indication of its stiffness under static loading, it is doubtful that true values for the modulus of elasticity and proportional limit can be obtained. The greater the rate of loading the specimen, the closer the stress-strain curve approaches a straight line. In other words, when a low rate of loading of the specimen is employed in testing, the amount of flow or permanent deformation is relatively great, and vice versa. Translated into practical terms, this fact has considerable clinical importance. It demonstrates the necessity of deforming the impression rapidly when it is removed from the mouth or model if the original dimensions are to be preserved. The impression should never be removed by a teasing or weaving method but rather by a sharp jerk in a direction as nearly as possible parallel to the long axes of the teeth. A slow removal of the impression is a common cause for inaccuracy.

The amount of deformation which these materials can withstand is not primarily dependent on their high strength. Actually the strain at the point of rupture more truly measures the ability of the material to resist rupture than does compressive strength.[18]

In practice, the permanent deformation of the material after stressing is measured as the percentage deformation, or *set*, that occurs in a cylindrical specimen 1.27 centimeters (0.5 inch) in diameter and 1.91 centimeters (0.75 inch) in height after a 12 per cent strain is applied for one minute. According to the current American Dental Association Specification No. 11, this set should not exceed 3.0 per cent.

Repeated loading of a gel apparently increases its stiffness. For example, when a cylinder of the material (1.27 $\times$ 1.91 centimeters) was stressed from 200 grams per square centimeter to 2000 grams per square centimeter, and then allowed to remain unstressed for an hour, the strain was 5 to 7.5 per cent less when the procedure was repeated at the end of an hour.[3] In other words, when a hydrocolloid impression is to be removed from the mouth, and thereby placed under strain, it should be strained suddenly and only once; otherwise, repeated strain might increase the difficulty of removing the impression because of its increase in stiffness and the resulting likelihood of fracture.

Regardless of the type of loading, the relaxation of the gel is never complete, and it does not return entirely to its original dimension after deformation. The permanent deformation remaining is called the set, as mentioned earlier. It should, of course, be as small as possible. Although these materials are classified as elastic, they are not perfectly so. However, the amount of permanent deformation is clinically negligible provided the material is adequately gelled, removed with a sharp jerk, and undercuts present in the cavity preparation are minimized. The greater the strain to which the impression material is subjected, the greater will be the distortion or set.

## Literature

1. Lewis, W. K., Squires, L., and Broughton, G.: *Industrial Chemistry of Colloidal and Amorphous Materials.* New York, The Macmillan Co., 1942, pp. 223–249.
2. Kendrick, Z. V.: *The Physical Properties of Agar Type Hydrocolloid Impression Material.* J.A.D.A., *40:*575–584 (May), 1950.
3. Paffenbarger, G. C.: *Hydrocolloid Impression Materials: Physical Properties and a Specification.* J.A.D.A., *27:*373–388 (March), 1940.
4. Jones, W. G. M., and Peat, S.: *The Constitution of Agar.* Chem. Abs. *36:*4097 (July 20), 1942.
5. Wood, E. F.: *Agar in Australia.* Bulletin 203, Melbourne, Council for Scientific and Industrial Research, 1946.

6. Stangerberg, J. W. H., Crowell, W. S., and Gross, C. V.: *Plastic Hydrocolloid Composition and Method of Making.* U. S. Patent 2,165,680 (July 11), 1939.
7. Preble, B.: *Dental Impression Composition.* U. S. Patent 2,234,383 (March 11), 1941.
8. Skinner, E. W., and Gordon, C. C.: *Some Experiments on the Surface Hardness of Dental Stones.* J. Pros. Den., *6:*94–100 (Jan.), 1956.
9. Ferry, J. D.: *Protein Gels, Advances in Protein Chemistry,* Vol. IV. New York City, Academic Press, Inc., 1948, pp. 10–12.
10. Phillips, R. W., and Ito, B. Y.: *Factors Influencing the Accuracy of Reversible Hydrocolloid Impressions.* J.A.D.A., *43:*1–17 (July), 1951.
11. Hampson, E. L.: *The Effects of Environment on the Dimensional Stability of Reversible and Irreversible Impression Materials.* Brit. D. J., *99:*371–380 (Dec.), 1955.
12. Skinner, E. W., Cooper, E. N., and Beck, F. E.: *Reversible and Irreversible Hydrocolloid Impression Materials.* J.A.D.A., *40:*196–207 (Feb.), 1950.
13. Luster, E. A.: *Dimensional Change of Agar-Agar Gel on Immersion in Various Sulphate Solutions.* J. D. Res., *30:*281–289 (Apr.), 1951.
14. Skinner, E. W., and Hoblit, N. E.: *A Study of the Accuracy of Hydrocolloid Impressions.* J. Pros. Den., *6:*80–86 (Jan.), 1956.
15. Hollenback, G. M.: *A Study of the Physical Properties of Elastic Impression Materials and Stones.* J. South. California D. A., *25:*20–28 (Jan.), 1957.
16. Swartz, M. L., Norman, R. D., Gilmore, H. W., and Phillips, R. W.: *Studies on Syneresis and Imbibition in Reversible Hydrocolloid.* J. D. Res., *36:*472–478 (June), 1957.
17. Gilmore, H. W., Phillips, R. W., and Swartz, M. L.: *The Effect of Residual Stress and Water Change on the Deformation of Hydrocolloid Impression Materials.* J. D. Res., *37:*816–823 (Sept.), 1958.
18. Cresson, J.: *Suggested Revisions for Testing Dental Elastic Impression Materials.* J. D. Res., *28:*573–582 (Dec.), 1949.

CHAPTER 8

# Hydrocolloid Impression

# Materials (Continued):

# Technical Considerations

## IRREVERSIBLE HYDROCOLLOID IMPRESSION MATERIALS

During World War II, the importation of agar-agar from Japan was stopped. Since the domestic sources had not been developed at that time, the supply of agar-agar became so depleted that it was allocated entirely to the medical profession for bacteriologic purposes. At that time the irreversible alginate type of hydrocolloid impression material was developed as a substitute, and is still being used with excellent results, particularly for partial denture and orthodontic impressions. Actually, at the present time, its general use far exceeds that of the reversible type.

**Chemistry.** The chief ingredient of the irreversible hydrocolloid impression materials is one of the soluble alginates. An alginate is a salt of alginic acid which is extracted from marine kelp. It is generally conceded to be a linear polymer of the sodium salt of anhydro–beta–$d$-mannuronic acid with the following structural formula:[1-3]

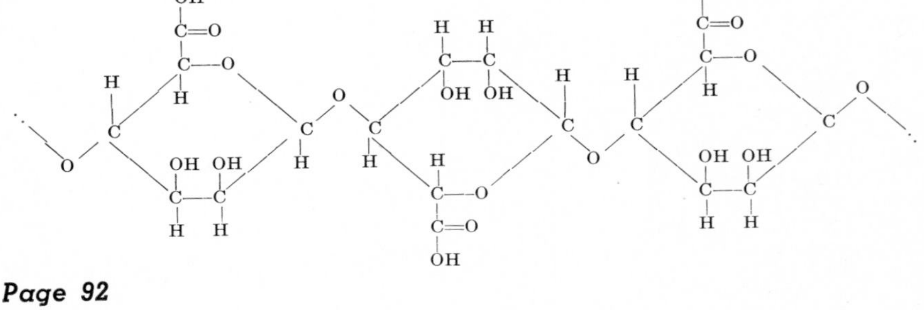

Alginic acid is insoluble in water, but some of its salts are not. The acid can be changed to an ester salt very readily, since the carboxyl groups are free to react. Most of the inorganic salts are insoluble, but the salts obtained with sodium, potassium, ammonium and magnesium are soluble in water.[4] Both sodium and potassium alginates are used quite extensively in dental impression materials.

The soluble alginates dissolve in water, and they form viscous sols at relatively low concentrations. The viscosity of the sol for a given concentration increases with the molecular weight of the alginate.

The problem from a dental standpoint is to place the viscous sol of the soluble alginate, contained in an impression tray, against the mouth tissues, and while it is in position, to change it to a gel so that it will hold its form when it is withdrawn from the mouth. This change is effected by a chemical reaction in which the soluble alginate is changed to an insoluble gel form.

There are a number of methods for the production of this change but the simplest and best understood method is to cause the soluble alginate to react with calcium sulfate to produce the insoluble calcium alginate. Practically, such a reaction must take place in the mouth, and, therefore, it must be delayed while the impression material is mixed with water, placed in the impression tray, and carried to the mouth. The reactions are best illustrated by a typical example.

Calcium sulfate is an excellent compound for the production of a calcium alginate when it reacts with potassium or sodium alginate in aqueous solution. The production of the calcium alginate can be delayed, however, by the addition of a third soluble salt to the solution, with which the calcium sulfate will react in preference to the sodium alginate to form an insoluble calcium salt. Thus, the reaction between the calcium sulfate and the soluble alginate is prevented so long as any of the added salt is left.[5]

The added salt is known as a *retarder*. There are a number of soluble salts which can be used, such as sodium or potassium phosphate, oxalate, or carbonate. The calcium sulfate is known as the *reactor*.

For example, if suitable amounts of calcium sulfate, potassium alginate and trisodium phosphate are mixed together in proper proportions in water, after they become dissolved partially or totally, the following reaction will take place:

$$2Na_3PO_4 + 3CaSO_4 \rightarrow Ca_3(PO_4)_2 + 3Na_2SO_4 \qquad (1)$$

When the supply of trisodium phosphate is exhausted, the calcium ions begin to react with the potassium alginate to produce calcium alginate as follows:

$$K_nAlg + \tfrac{n}{2}CaSO_4 \rightarrow \tfrac{n}{2}K_2SO_4 + Ca_{\frac{n}{2}}Alg \qquad (2)$$

**Composition.** A possible formula for an alginate impression material based upon the above reactions is as follows (per cent by weight):

| | |
|---|---|
| Potassium alginate | 12 per cent |
| Diatomaceous earth | 70 |
| Calcium sulfate (dihydrate) | 12 |
| Trisodium phosphate | 2 |

The exact proportion of each chemical to be used varies with the type of raw material. Particularly the amount of retarder (trisodium phosphate) must be adjusted carefully to provide the proper gelation time. In general, if approximately 15 grams of the above powder is mixed with 50 cubic centimeters of water, gelation will occur in about 6 to 8 minutes at normal room temperature.

The purpose of the diatomaceous earth is to act as a filler. The filler, if added in proper amounts, can increase the strength and stiffness of the alginate gel, produce a smooth texture, and insure a firm surface that is not tacky. Without a filler, the gel formed lacks firmness, and exhibits a sticky surface covered with a syneretical exudate.

The functions of the remaining ingredients have already been explained. Any type of calcium sulfate can be used as the reactor. The dihydrate form is generally used, but under certain circumstances the hemihydrate is said to produce an increased shelf life of the powder, and a more satisfactory dimensional stability of the gel. If an insoluble gypsum anhydrite is used, the gelation reaction can be retarded by virtue of the insolubility of the reactor, and no other type of retarder may be needed.[5]

One of the disadvantages of the preceding formula is that a soft surface is apt to appear on the cast due to the retardation of setting as described for the reversible hydrocolloid impression materials. Additional ingredients are often added to prevent such a condition. For example, the addition of sodium silicofluoride ($Na_3SiF_6$) or potassium silicofluoride in proper amount to the above formula will cause a decrease in the $p$H of the gel, and a better stone surface results.[6] Another metallic salt can be added such as lead silicate which greatly increases the gel strength. Presumably, the acidity increases sufficiently during the reaction in the presence of the sodium silicofluoride so that the lead salt may go into solution and produce a lead alginate in addition to the calcium alginate as shown in reaction (2).

There are a number of different fluorides used in commercial alginate impression materials such as zinc fluoride,[7] potassium ferric fluoride,[8] potassium and/or sodium zinc fluoride,[9] and potassium titanium fluoride.[10] It is claimed that each fluoride compound imparts certain unique properties to the gel not contributed by the other salts. In most of the commercial products these additions are made to the essentially basic formula previously described and, as previously stated, their chief contribution is to act as hardeners for the stone surface.

**Shelf Life.** Alginate impression materials deteriorate rapidly at elevated temperatures. Materials which were stored for one month at 65° C. proved to be unsuitable for dental use, either failing to set at all or setting much too rapidly.[11] Even at 50° C. there was evidence of deterioration, probably due to depolymerization of the alginate constituent. Thus alginate impression materials should be stored at cool temperatures and never for any prolonged period at any temperature above 37° C.

The alginate impression material is dispensed to the dentist in individually sealed packages with sufficient powder pre-weighed for an individual impression, or in bulk form in a can. The individual packages are preferred since there is less chance for contamination during storage, and the correct powder-water ratio is assured since plastic cups are provided for the measurement of the water.

If the bulk package is employed, the lid should be firmly replaced on the container as soon as possible after each use so that a minimum amount of moisture contamination will occur. Furthermore, the proper proportion of alginate powder should be weighed and not measured by volume as many manufacturers direct. As discussed in the case of dental stone (page 53), a powder cannot be measured accurately by volume.

**Gel Structure.** As described in the preceding chapter, the fibrils forming the micelles in an alginate gel are assumed to be held together by primary valence bonds rather than by intermolecular forces as in the case of the reversible hydrocolloids. Presumably, when the alginic acid is changed to a soluble salt such as sodium alginate, the cation is attached at a carboxyl group to form an ester or salt. When the insoluble salt is formed by the reaction of the sodium alginate in solution with a calcium salt, for example, the calcium ion may replace the sodium to form a cross-linked molecular complex. Such a complex or network presumably forms the brush-heap structure of the gel.

Actually, if the reaction goes to completion, the calcium alginate produced is a formless coagulum, with which it is impossible to produce an impression. Very likely, sufficient calcium ions go into solution to produce a desirable amount of cross-linkage. Further solution of the calcium salt may be prevented by the formation of a dense sheath around the reactor particle as the reaction progresses.

The final structure of the gel is, then, possibly an indeterminate brush-heap network composed of partially cross-linked molecules of calcium alginate. The unreacted alginate sol, excess water, and particles of filler can be pictured as being entangled in such a network to produce a gel structure of a type which can be used for obtaining impressions.

**Control of Gelation Time.** The time of gelation measured from the beginning of mixing until the gelation occurs is of interest, since

*Table 8–1.*      *Effect of Temperature on Gelation Time*

| TEMPERATURE (°C.) | (°F.) | GELATION TIME (MINUTES) |
|---|---|---|
| 6 | 43 | 7.8 |
| 10 | 50 | 6.2 |
| 15 | 59 | 5.5 |
| 20 | 68 | 4.5 |
| 25 | 77 | 4.0 |
| 30 | 86 | 3.5 |
| 35 | 95 | 2.8 |
| 40 | 104 | 2.5 |
| 45 | 113 | 2.0 |
| 50 | 122 | 1.8 |

sufficient time must be allowed for the dentist to mix the material, to load the tray, and to place it in the patient's mouth. A prolonged gelation time is tedious for both the patient and for the dentist. On the other hand, a premature gelation which begins before the filled impression tray is placed in position in the mouth will result in a distorted and generally useless impression. Once the gelation starts, it must not be disturbed, as any fracturing of the fibrils will be permanent. A fractured gel cannot be joined again unless it is re-gelled. Probably the optimum gelation time is between 3 and 7 minutes at a room temperature of 20° C. (68° F.).

There are several methods for the measurement of gelation time, but probably the best method for the dental practitioner is to observe the time from the start of mixing until the material is no longer tacky or adhesive when it is touched with a clean, dry finger. Working time, the minimum interval necessary for mixing and filling the tray, may be measured by a penetration test. The proposed American Dental Association Specification for the alginate type of hydrocolloid specifies that by this test the working time should not be less than two minutes.

As previously related, the gelation time is best regulated by the amount of retarder added. However, such a method of control is not feasible for use by the dentist, since the action of the retarder is critical, and its addition is better regulated by the manufacturer. The gelation time of some commercial products can be altered by changing the W/P ratio and mixing time, but such changes are apt to impair certain properties of the gel.

The best method for the dental practitioner to control the gelation time is to alter the temperature of the water used for mixing the alginate material.

The effect of the temperature of the water on the gelation time of a commercial product[12] is shown in Table 8–1. It is evident that the higher the temperature, the shorter is the gelation time. If the flow of the material is plotted against the temperature of the mixing water, the same relationship is found, *i.e.*, the higher the temperature, the less is the duration of flow.[13] Flow is an important characteristic of the material since it is one of the properties which controls the accuracy of reproduction. The impression material should be fluid enough to move into intimate contact with the tissues if it is to reproduce them accurately. The importance of using the proper temperature for the water is evident. In hot weather special precautions should be taken to provide cool water for mixing so that a premature gelation will not be obtained.

Some commercial materials exhibit greater sensitivity to temperature changes than others. The change in gelation time per degree centigrade between 20° C. (68° F.) and 30° C. (86° F.) in the case of the material used for obtaining the data in Table 8–1 is 0.1 minute, or 6 seconds per degree centigrade (3 seconds per degree Fahrenheit). Some commercial materials have been found to exhibit as much as 20 seconds change in gelation time for every degree centigrade change in temperature. In such a case, the temperature of the mixing water should be regulated carefully within 1° to 2° C. of a standard temperature (usually 20° C. or 70° F.) so that a constant and reliable gelation time can be obtained. Obviously, the manufacturer should inhibit the effect of temperature on his product as much as possible. From this standpoint, the ideal material would be one that would permit ample working time yet gel rapidly as it contacts the warm oral environment.

**Strength.** As noted in the preceding chapter, the crushing strength of a reversible hydrocolloid impression material should be at least 2000 grams per square centimeter. With proper manipulation, the strength of the alginate impression materials may be greater than that of the agar materials. In fact, the proposed American Dental Association Specification for alginate type hydrocolloid requires a minimum strength of 3,500 grams per square centimeter (50 pounds per square inch).

The composition of the alginate material can radically affect its gel strength. As previously noted, the type of reactor used can influence the strength considerably. The type and amount of the soluble alginate

*Table 8–2.    Increase in Compressive Strength of an Alginate Gel from the Time of Gelation*

| TIME FROM GELATION (MINUTES) | COMPRESSIVE STRENGTH (GM./CM.²) |
|---|---|
| 0 | 3,400 |
| 4 | 7,800 |
| 8 | 8,300 |
| 12 | 7,200 |
| 16 | 7,500 |

used is of considerable importance, as well as the nature of the other ingredients and their proportions.

All of the manipulative factors affect the gel strength, and these factors are under the control of the dentist. For example, if too much water or too little water is used in mixing, the final gel will be weakened. The proper W/P ratio should be employed as specified by the manufacturer.

The time for mixing the powder and water should be noted with a timepiece. For example, it has been shown[12] that the strength of the final gel can be reduced 50 per cent if the mixture is insufficiently mixed. Insufficient spatulation results in failure of the ingredients to dissolve sufficiently so that the chemical reactions can proceed uniformly throughout the mass. Overmixing gives equally poor results, since any calcium alginate gel formed during prolonged spatulation will be broken up, and the strength will, therefore, be impaired. The directions supplied with the product should be adhered to in all respects.

The mix itself should be stirred vigorously at approximately 200 to 225 r.p.m. Even after thorough spatulation, the smoothness of the final material will differ with various brands of alginate.[14] However, a smooth, creamy mixture should be expected when the better commercial products are employed. The better products have a small particle size, passing a U. S. Standard Sieve No. 20, and thus mix smoothly.

Although the stress-strain relationships of the alginate impression materials are approximately the same as those specified for the reversible hydrocolloid materials, the set of the alginate materials is likely to be slightly higher than that found with the other type.

The strength of the alginate gel increases for several minutes after the initial gelation. As can be noted from Table 8–2, the gel strength of the particular impression material investigated actually doubled during the first 4 minutes after gelation, and it did not increase in strength appreciably after the first 4 minute period. It is clearly indicated from such data that the alginate impression should not be removed from the mouth for at least 2 to 3 minutes after the gelation has occurred.

Although the tendency invariably is to remove the tray prematurely, there is also a disadvantage in leaving the alginate in the mouth too long. As pointed out in the previous chapter, reversible hydrocolloids show no apparent deleterious effect even when held in the mouth for as long as ten minutes. However, with a few alginate materials it has been shown that if the impression is held for five, rather than two or three, minutes after gelation a definite distortion results.[15]

**Surface Reproduction.** The accuracy of any model produced from an impression material is obviously a function of its inherent accuracy. This accuracy of reproduction is dependent not only on the dimensional behavior of the materials involved but also on the surface condition of both the impression and model. Surface accuracy involves the duplication of surface detail and is governed by the interfacial relationship between the impression material and the model material.

The proposed American Dental Association Specification for alginate type hydrocolloid includes a test for detail reproduction. To meet the specification, the alginate must reproduce a line 0.0015 inch in width.

**Dimensional Stability.** The dimensional stability of eight different alginate impression materials in air and in water is shown in Figure 8–1. The materials were mixed according to the directions of the manufacturer, and the changes in linear dimensions were measured in air and subsequently in water; the experimental conditions were identical with those described for the similar experiment using the reversible materials (Fig. 7–4, p. 87).

The dimensional changes occurring with the alginate gels is characterized by a slight initial expansion. The expansion can probably be attributed to a continued imbibition of the residual free water by the gel after the initial gelation.[12]

Some of the irreversible impression materials apparently do not lose water by evaporation as readily as do the reversible materials (*cf.* Fig. 7–4), since their contraction in air is not as great. This observation is corroborated by the fact that the loss of water by weight in air is not as

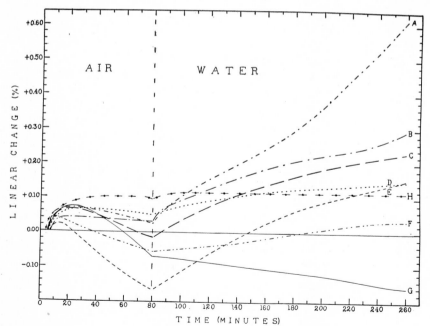

Fig. 8–1. Change in dimension of various alginate impression materials in air and in water.

great with the alginate materials as it is with the reversible hydrocolloid materials.[16]

When the specimens were immersed in water after having been exposed to the air for 80 minutes, the effect of the resulting imbibition on the dimensional change was somewhat erratic (Fig. 8–1). All of the materials except material *G* exhibited a certain amount of swelling, but only four of them (materials *D, E, H* and *F*) maintained their original dimension within 0.1 per cent. Consequently, storage in water is never indicated for impressions obtained with the alginate materials.

The dimensional stability of the alginate gel is probably influenced by other factors than syneresis and imbibition. For example, the formation of the insoluble alginate is generally accompanied by a contraction. If the reaction (2) (p. 93) is prolonged, it is conceivable that the gel might continue to contract even though it is immersed in water, as in the case of material *G* (Fig. 8–1). Likewise, as pointed out in Chapter 7, the relaxation of stress in the impression is accompanied by dimensional change.

Some of the alginate gels currently used in dentistry exhibit excellent stability in an atmosphere of 100 per cent humidity. Consequently, if the alginate impression must be preserved, it should be placed in a humidor. However, as with the reversible materials, the cast should be constructed immediately after the impression is obtained for the most accurate results. There is no adequate method for storage of any of the hydrocolloid impression materials.

## TECHNICAL CONSIDERATIONS

Hydrocolloid impression materials are used extensively in modern dental practice. Not only are they used for the obtaining of impressions of the entire mouth, but also they are employed for impressions of individual teeth containing prepared cavities for the insertion of inlays. Since the two types of materials have much in common, they will be discussed together.

**Selection of a Tray.** The proper selection of a tray is of considerable importance to the accuracy of the impression. The type of tray to be selected will depend upon many considerations. Only those considerations related to the proper manipulation of the material will be discussed.

It is imperative that some type of impression tray be used in which the gel can be locked mechanically. Unlike impression compound, for example, the hydrocolloid material usually exhibits no adhesive properties whatever. Consequently it must be retained mechanically in the tray so that the impression can be withdrawn over the undercuts around the teeth.

A type of perforated tray which has been quite successful in this regard is illustrated in Figure 7–1, p. 82. When the reversible impression material is placed in the tray in the sol condition, it is pushed through the perforations slightly. After gelation, the material which has passed through the perforations, or *retentions*, acts to retain the gel in the tray when the impression is removed. A similar type of tray is employed with alginate impressions, except that the water circulating coils are omitted.

The design of this type of tray is most important. Unless the impression material is firmly retained in the tray, the impression will be distorted when it is removed from the mouth. The proper retention of the impression will be affected by the number of perforations, their location and distribution in the tray, and their size.

Too many or too large perforations may allow too much of the liquefied material to leak out while the impression is being placed in position. As an upper impression, for example, is placed in position against the tissues, there should be a certain amount of light pressure exerted on the material by the tray to force it into intimate contact with the tissues. If there are too many or too large perforations, a reverse pressure may be more effective in forcing the sol through the retentions. Such a situation is likely to be more troublesome in the case of the alginate materials than with the reversible type.[17]

In fact, as shown in Figure 8–2, it is possible to use unperforated trays with the reversible hydrocolloids. The impression material tends to lock itself to the overhanging rims of the tray as well as to the compound or wax stops that are used at the open ends of the tray. The real purpose of these stops, however, is to aid in maintaining stability during the critical period of gelation. These reinforcements are also helpful to prevent the tray from being pressed down onto the teeth themselves.

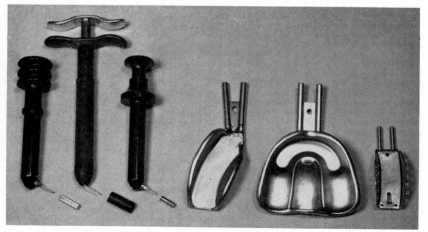

Fig. 8–2. Armamentarium for use in obtaining impressions with reversible hydrocolloid impression material. Three types of syringes for injection of the material into prepared cavities are shown at the left. On the right are various types of water-cooled trays.

If maximum accuracy is to be attained, at least a one-eighth inch layer of hydrocolloid should separate the tray from the tooth.[18, 19] Bulk is necessary for accuracy.

*"Wash" Impressions.* One method for overcoming a reverse flow of material is to form a special tray with compound or similar material, and to use the impression material as a "wash" or corrective material,[20] as described in the case of the zinc oxide-eugenol impression pastes (see page 68). If such a technic is employed, special care should be taken that sufficient bulk of the hydrocolloid material is present between the compound and the tissues. Otherwise, the impression may be distorted or fractured upon removal. Also, the surface of the compound or resin must be roughened or otherwise treated to provide retention for the gel. One method is to paint the surface of the preliminary impression with a solvent, such as chloroform, and then to press cotton fibers which act to retain the gel quite effectively into the sticky surface.

The "wash" impression method provides a certain advantage over the use of the perforated metal tray in that a more uniform distribution of the gel is assured at the time the impression is obtained. A uniform distribution of the material in the tray at the time the impression is obtained can also be an important factor in preventing subsequent distortion of the impression. For example, the greatest bulk of material in a commercial impression tray is apt to be in the vault or palate portion of an upper impression. During any subsequent syneresis this portion may shrink more in actual volume (not percentage volume) than the smaller amount of material over the ridges. As a result, the height of the vault or palate portion of the cast will be less than the original dimension, and the denture or palatal bar may not fit.

*Impressions of Prepared Cavities.* Cavities are prepared in carious teeth for the reception of artificial restorations of some sort, such as inlays or crowns. When hydrocolloid impressions are obtained from such prepared cavities, special care must be taken to insure that complete detail is obtained accurately. Either reversible or irreversible hydrocolloid may be used for this purpose with equal accuracy,[21] but the sharper cavity detail and superior stone surface lend the advantage to the reversible hydrocolloid.

No attempt will be made to outline the indirect technic in detail but only the fundamental steps involved. There are many excellent publications on the detailed procedure[18, 19, 22-25] for both the reversible and irreversible hydrocolloids.

Proper armamentarium for the boiling, storage, and tempering of reversible hydrocolloid is essential. The dental office should be organized for the technic. Various types of conditioners for preparation and storage of the hydrocolloid material are available; one type is shown in Figure 8–3.

The first step is to produce a fluid sol in the tube of hydrocolloid gel. Boiling water is a convenient means of liquefying the material. A minimum of ten minutes boiling is essential and there is no evidence that longer periods are harmful. Whenever the material is re-liquefied after a previous use it is more difficult to break down the agar lattice-work, so approximately three minutes should be added each time the material is re-boiled.

After it has been liquefied, the material may be stored in the sol condition until ready for use. A storage temperature between 63° C. (145° F.) and 69° C. (155° F.) is ideal. Lower temperatures may permit premature gelation and a viscous material will result.

The material which is used to fill the tray must be cooled or "tempered." The purpose of this is to increase the viscosity of the hydrocolloid so that it will not flow out of the tray and to reduce the temperature and thus prevent discomfort to the patient. Therefore, the tray (Fig. 8–2) is filled and placed into the "tempering" bath of the conditioner. Various combinations of temperatures and times may be employed[18] but a satisfactory one[22] is to cool the material for approximately ten minutes at a temperature of 46° C. (115° F.). The time may be varied for the batch or brand of hydrocolloid and for the particular viscosity preferred by the operator.

While this tray material is being cooled, the cavity preparation is finished. In order to secure maximum detail, the most common method for obtaining the impression is to fill the prepared cavity with the hydrocolloid by ejecting it from a specially constructed syringe as shown in Figure 8–2. The sol, taken directly from the storage compartment, is first ejected at the base of the preparation and then is carried distal-mesially over the cavity (Fig. 8–4). The needle is held

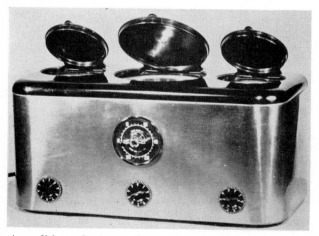

Fig. 8–3. A conditioner for impressions with reversible hydrocolloid. Compartment at the left is a bath for boiling, the center bath is for storage, and the bath at the right is for "tempering."

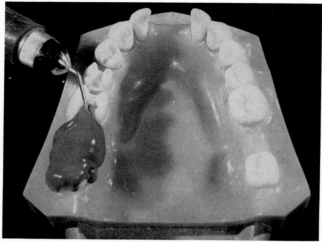

Fig. 8–4.  Filling a prepared cavity with a reversible hydrocolloid impression material.

close to the tooth, beneath the surface of the ejected material, in order to prevent a trapping of air bubbles.

When the entire technic is properly standardized, by the time the cavity preparations and adjoining teeth have been covered, the tray material is cooled to the proper temperature and viscosity and is ready to be carried to the mouth to form the bulk of the impression. The water soaked outer layer of hydrocolloid is first scraped off. Failure to remove that layer may prevent a firm union between the tray material and the hydrocolloid which has been previously injected into the cavity preparation.

The tray is immediately brought into position, seated with passive pressure. The sol in the tooth bonds to the hydrocolloid in the tray to form a homogeneous impression.

Gelation is accomplished by circulating cool water, approximately 16° C. to 21° C. (60° F. to 70° F.), for not less than five minutes. Care must be exercised to prevent any movement of the tray during the time that the gel is forming. After gelation, the impression is withdrawn in one piece.

**Distortion During Gelation.**    There are always certain strains introduced during gelation. As can be noted from Figure 7–4, page 87, the reversible hydrocolloid materials contract initially after gelation by syneresis. If the material is held rigidly by the retentions in the impression tray, such a contraction of the material may be manifested by an expansion of the space or area occupied by the impression. Owing to the elasticity of the gel, such an effect will be more pronounced the thinner the layer of the gel. For example, it is conceivable that portions of the impression near the tray may be enlarged, but other areas farther removed from the tray may exhibit a contraction, because the gel in the latter region may be less influenced by the retentions. The result is likely to be an over-all distortion of the impression. Since a varying bulk of impression material will aggravate such a condition, another advantage for a uniform distribution of the gel between the tray and the mouth tissues is evident. As mentioned earlier, compound reinforcements are advantageous for this purpose.[26]

The stresses introduced by the two types of impression materials may differ because of the method by which the gelation takes place. In the case of the reversible hydrocolloid impression materials, the gelation begins adjacent to the cool tray and continues to the warmer mouth tissues. Since the sol is a poor thermal conductor, a rapid cooling may cause a concentration of stress near the tray when the gelation first takes place. Consequently, water at approximately 20° C. (68° F.) is more suitable for cooling the impression[18, 19] than is ice water, for example.

On the other hand, in the case of the alginate impression materials, the gelation begins adjacent to the mouth tissues because of the higher temperature in this area. Regardless of where the gelation begins, if the impression is not held rigidly in position during the gelation period, considerable stress will be induced. If the tray is moved even slightly, the shearing action between the gelled portion and the sol or partly gelled region will induce stresses which later may relax to produce a distortion.

**Distortion During Removal.** The brush-heap structure of the gel is of such a nature that a sudden force is always resisted without distortion or fracture more successfully than a force which is applied slowly. Consequently, when the impression is removed, it is necessary to remove it suddenly, with a jerk, rather than to "tease" it out, as might be done with an impression in compound or plaster. The removal is accomplished in a direction as nearly as possible parallel to the long axes of the teeth.

**Distortion During Relaxation.** As previously noted, hydrocolloid gels are subject to dimensional changes brought about by syneresis and imbibition, regardless of whether they are of the reversible or the irreversible type. In addition to these causes for dimensional instability, as pointed out previously, hydrocolloid gels are also notable for the fact that stresses can be induced readily in them. After the load is removed, almost complete relaxation of the stresses occurs over a period of time. Such a relaxation in a hydrocolloid impression is likely to produce a distortion after removal which may bring about a serious inaccuracy. One type of this distortion can be brought about by the exertion of pressure on the tray during the gelation period. The tray should be held under passive pressure.

The gel will also be stressed in any regions where dimensional changes have been restrained, and a subsequent relief or relaxation will likely result in a distortion of the impression. Consequently, the

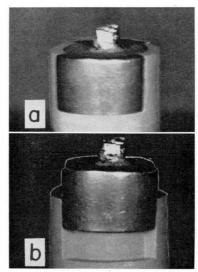

Fig. 8–5. *a.* Fit of a master casting on a stone die constructed immediately after the impression of the master die was removed. *b.* Fit of same casting when the die was constructed one hour after removal of the impression.

dental stone cast should be constructed as soon as possible after the impression has been obtained, not only to prevent troublesome effects due to imbibition and syneresis, but also to minimize the possible distortions due to relaxation of stress.[16]

The importance of the immediate construction of the cast cannot be overemphasized. A vivid example of the dangers involved can be seen in Figure 8–5. The master gold casting was constructed on a steel die. An impression of the die was obtained as previously described. When the casting was fitted on a stone die constructed within 15 minutes after the impression was obtained, the fit was excellent (Fig. 8–5a). An impression permitted to stand only one hour in air resulted in the inaccuracy shown in Figure 8–5b.

**Surface Hardness of the Cast.** A hard surface on the cast is very important to the accuracy of the entire technic, so that the surface will not be disturbed in subsequent operations. One method for obtaining a hard surface is to electroplate the hydrocolloid impression with copper[27] and then to reinforce the electroplated layer with dental stone. Unfortunately, most plating procedures for hydrocolloid impressions produce measurable distortion.

If the surface of the stone cast is to be employed for the construction of the dental restoration, every possible precaution must be taken to insure a maximum surface hardness. The slightest chalkiness or porosity in or near the reproduced prepared cavity will result in a serious inaccuracy. The irreversible hydrocolloids are of special concern since, although they produce a good stone set, it is not equal to that of the reversible hydrocolloids or the rubber base impression materials[14, 15, 28] to be discussed in the next chapter. As noted in a previous chapter, the first consideration in obtaining a hard surface on the stone cast is to employ a low W/P ratio.

The principal reason for the decrease in the surface hardness of a stone cast obtained from a hydrocolloid impression is the effect of the hydrocolloid on the setting reaction of the stone. A hydrocolloid is an excellent retarder for the setting of a gypsum product. Consequently, the surface of the cast in contact with the gel may set very slowly or not at all. It is not uncommon to separate a stone cast from a hydrocolloid impression after sufficient time has elapsed for the material to harden and to find the surface of the cast soft and rough in appearance, as shown in Figure 8–6. Such a surface is totally unfit for use in an accurate dental technic. The amount of these surface imperfections depends upon the particular combination of hydrocolloid material and dental stone employed.

Even though the surface of the stone may appear to be satisfactory, the hardness of the surface may be affected nevertheless. As can be noted from Table 8–3, not all gypsum products are affected in the same manner.[29] Of the five products, the surface of the model plaster was affected the least, but the hardness of plaster is so low that its use as a die material is not indicated. The two stone bases are sometimes used in dental stones. The hardness of one (No. 1) was not greatly affected, but the hardness of the other (No. 2) was radically reduced.

The first two products are commercially available dental stones of

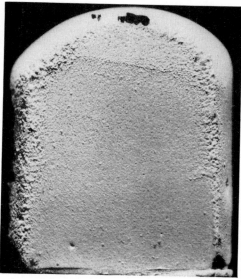

Fig. 8–6. A stone surface obtained after the stone had set in contact with the surface of a reversible hydrocolloid impression material.

*Table 8–3.* *Effect of a Reversible Hydrocolloid Impression Material on the Surface Hardness of Five Gypsum Products*

| GYPSUM PRODUCT | CONTROL *<br>(K.H.N.) | IN CONTACT WITH<br>REVERSIBLE HYDROCOLLOID<br>(K.H.N.) |
|---|---|---|
| Class I stone | 24.6 | 23.9 |
| Class II stone | 51.8 | 32.4 |
| Stone base No. 1 | 35.2 | 34.9 |
| Stone base No. 2 | 60.4 | 29.3 |
| Model plaster | 7.0 | 8.1 |

* Gypsum product allowed to set in contact with a glass surface.

Class I and Class II. Whereas the hardness of the Class I stone was not greatly affected by the hydrocolloid gel, that of the Class II stone was reduced considerably. Since the Class II stone is especially recommended and employed for the construction of dies in hydrocolloid impressions, its reduction in hardness is a matter of concern.

**Use of Hardening Solutions.** One method for the prevention or the minimizing of a soft stone surface is to immerse the impression in a hardening solution.

There are at least three different methods by which the hardening solution may increase the hardness of the stone surface: (1) Its action may be that of an accelerator for the setting time of the gypsum product, to overcome the retarding action of the gel surface on the setting of the dental stone. (2) It may react with the surface of the gel in such a manner as to produce a surface layer which will reduce or prevent syneresis, and therefore eliminate the retarding action of the gel. (3) It may react with the stone surface directly so as to increase its hardness. Of the three possible reactions, it would seem that as a first consideration the hardener should be an accelerator for the setting of the stone, regardless of what other action it may have.

Unfortunately, the use of hardening solutions has not been standardized. The effectiveness of the solution in increasing the hardness of the stone surface appears to depend upon the chemical employed in the solution and its concentration in reference to the characteristics of the gel used for the impression. Examples of various chemicals employed in hardening solutions are potassium sulfate (Fig. 8–7), manganous sulfate, potash alum, and zinc sulfate. A recommended concentration is 2 per cent.[29]

It has been shown that the hardening solution may affect the dimensional stability of the hydrocolloid impression.[18, 30] This effect varies with the chemical employed, its concentration, and the composition of the gel.[31] For this reason, the hydrocolloid impression should not be immersed in the hardening solution for more than 10 to 15 minutes, since only the surface layer of the gel need be saturated with the solution. Usually, a period of five minutes is sufficient to provide such a saturation. This treatment may be done while the stone mix is being prepared. The solution of potassium sulfate may be reused until it becomes unduly contaminated.

In the past most alginate impressions required immersion in a hardening or fixing solution before the stone was poured. However, the formulas of the alginate products have now been adjusted so that this procedure is no longer essential. Although zinc sulfate has been suggested as the ideal hardening solution,[32] the effect is probably dependent on the exact composition of the alginate and should be so specified by the manufacturer.

Immersion of the die either in water or oil after it has set reduces surface hardness, strength, and abrasive resistance.[33] Although immersion of set plaster in a saturated solution of borax increases hardness as much as 140 per cent,[34] this treatment has no effect on stone.[29] Likewise the addition of hardening solutions to the stone itself does not increase hardness when it is allowed to set in contact with a hydrocolloid gel.

**Other Factors.** The stone cast, or die, should be kept in contact with the impression for at least 30 minutes, or, preferably, 60 minutes before the impression is separated from the cast. Even though a hardening solution of the proper type is used, the setting time of the stone in contact with the impression material will probably be increased, and sufficient time should be allowed for the stone to set.

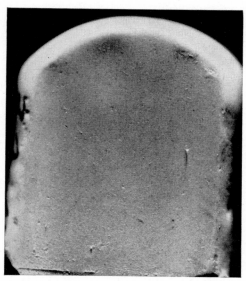

Fig. 8–7. Stone surface obtained in the same manner as that in Figure 8–6 except that the hydrocolloid impression was immersed in a solution of potassium sulfate (2 per cent) just before the stone mix was poured.

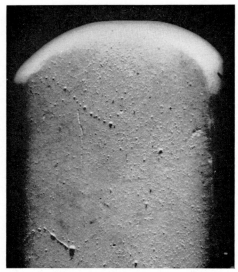

Fig. 8–8.   Surface of stone separated 18 hours after the stone mix was poured against a reversible hydrocolloid impression material.

It is possible, however, to allow the stone to remain in contact with the hydrocolloidal gel for too long a time. The stone surface shown in Figure 8–8 is an example of what may happen if the cast is allowed to remain in contact with the hydrocolloid impression overnight. Such a condition can sometimes be avoided if the impression is treated with a hardening solution before the cast is prepared.[35]

After the impression has been filled with stone, it may be placed back in either the humidor or 2 per cent potassium sulfate while the stone hardens. For some reason, somewhat superior stone surfaces are obtained if the stone hardens in an atmosphere of approximately 100 per cent relative humidity. In any event, the filled impression should never be immersed in water while the stone sets.

A rough stone surface will result if excess water has collected on the surface of the impression at the time the stone mixture is poured. However, the surface of the impression should not be dried completely, or the gel will adhere to the surface of the cast upon its removal.[35] The surface of the impression should be shiny but with no visible water film or droplets at the time the cast is constructed.

A poor surface on the cast will result whenever the hydrocolloid material is not well mixed in the sol condition. Some years ago the use of a mixing syringe was essential but now most brands of the materials are well blended by the manufacturer. As previously noted, the alginates should be mixed vigorously for the recommended time in order to insure a homogeneous mixture.

Surface imperfections may be minimized by use of a mechanical vibrator when pouring the stone. Only mild vibration should be used, however. Vacuum equipment for mixing the stone is also superior to hand spatulation. In any event, the stone should be added slowly and in small quantities.

## Literature

1. Hirst, E. L., Jones, J. K. N., and Jones, W. O.: *The Structure of Alginic Acid. Part I.*, J. Chem. Soc., pp. 1880–1885, 1939.
2. Steiner, A. B., and McNeeley, W. H.: *Organic Derivations of Alginic Acid.* Indust. Eng. Chem., *43:*2073–2077 (Sept.), 1951.
3. Nelson, W. L., and Cutcher, L. H.: *Properties of d-Mannuronic Acid Lactone.* J. Am. Chem. Soc., *54:*3409–3412 (Aug.), 1932.
4. Steiner, A. B.: *Manufacture of Glycol Alginates.* U. S. Patent 2,426,125 (Aug. 19), 1947.
5. Wilding, S. W.: *Material for Taking Impressions for Dental or Other Purposes.* U. S. Patent 2,249,694 (July 15), 1941.
6. Noyes, S. E.: *Dental Impression Composition.* U. S. Patent 2,425,118 (Aug. 5), 1947.
7. Meyer, H. G.: *Dental Impression Compositions.* U. S. Patent 2,623,808 (Dec. 30), 1952.
8. Grumbine, R. S.: *Dental Impression Composition.* U. S. Patent 2,837,434 (June 3), 1958.
9. Cresson, J.: *Dental Impression Material.* U. S. Patent 2,769,717 (Nov. 6), 1956.
10. Fink, A.: *Dental Impression Material.* U. S. Patent 2,652,312 (Sept. 15), 1953.
11. Pfeiffer, K. R., Harvey, J. L., and Brauer, G. M.: *Deterioration During Storage of Alginate Hydrocolloidal Dental Impression Material.* U. S. Armed Forces M. J., *5:*1315–1320 (Sept.), 1954.
12. Skinner, E. W., and Pomes, C. E.: *Alginate Impression Materials: Technic for Manipulation and Criteria for Selection.* J.A.D.A., *35:*245–256 (Aug. 15), 1947.
13. Nealon, F. J.: *The Effect of Temperature on the Flow of Alginates.* J. Pros. Den., *3:*814–817 (Nov.), 1953.
14. Phillips, R. W., and Price, R. R.: *Some Factors Which Influence the Surface of Stone Dies Poured in Alginate Impressions.* J. Pros. Den., *5:*72–79 (Jan.), 1955.
15. Phillips, R. W., Price, R. R., and Reinking, R. H.: *Use of Alginate for Indirect Restoration.* J.A.D.A., *46:*393–403 (April), 1953.
16. Gilmore, H. W., Phillips, R. W., and Swartz, M. L.: *The Effect of Residual Stress and Water Change on the Deformation of Hydrocolloid Impression Materials.* J. D. Res., *37:*816–823 (Sept.), 1958.
17. Jordan, L. G.: *Alginate Impression Materials.* J.A.D.A., *32:*985–986 (Aug.), 1945.
18. Phillips, R. W.: *Factors Influencing the Accuracy of Reversible Hydrocolloid Impressions.* J.A.D.A., *43:*1–17 (July), 1951.
19. Mann, A. W.: *A Critical Appraisal of the Hydrocolloid Technique: Its Advantages and Disadvantages.* J. Pros. Den., *1:*727–732 (Nov.), 1951.
20. McCracken, W. L.: *Impression Materials in Prosthetic Dentistry*, D. Clin. North America, November 1958, pp. 671–684.
21. Skinner, E. W., and Hoblit, N. E.: *A Study of the Accuracy of Hydrocolloid Impressions.* J. Pros. Den., *6:*80–86 (Jan.), 1956.
22. Thompson, M. J.: *A Standardized Indirect Technic for Reversible Hydrocolloid,* J.A.D.A., *46:*1–18 (Jan.), 1953.
23. Sears, A. W.: *Hydrocolloid Impression Technique for Inlays and Fixed Bridges.* D. Digest, *43:*230–234 (May), 1937.
24. Fusayama, T.: *Indirect Inlay and Crown Technic Using Alginate.* J.A.D.A., *54:* 74–77 (Jan.), 1957.
25. Pfeiffer, K. R., and Jeffreys, F. E.: *A Complete Bridge Technic Utilizing the Alginate Hydrocolloids.* J.A.D.A., *40:*66–74 (Jan.), 1950.

26. Tylman, S. D.: *Reversible and Irreversible Hydrocolloid Impression Materials.* D. Clin. North America, November 1958, pp. 713–726.
27. Dwight, O. D.: *Copper Plating of Reversible Hydrocolloid Impressions.* J. D. Res., *28:*456–459 (Oct.), 1949.
28. Hollenback, G. M.: *A Report on the Physical Properties of Alginate Impression Materials.* J. South. California D. A., *25:*21–27 (July), 1957.
29. Skinner, E. W., and Gordon, C.: *Some Experiments on the Surface Hardness of Dental Stones.* J. Pros. Den., *6:*94–100 (Jan.), 1956.
30. Skinner, E. W., and Pomes, C. E.: *Dimensional Stability of Alginate Impression Materials.* J.A.D.A., *33:*1253–1260 (Oct.), 1946.
31. Kendrick, Z. V.: *The Physical Properties of Agar Type Impression Material.* J.A.D.A., *40:*575–584 (May), 1950.
32. Fusayama, T., and Hosoda, H.: *Surface Reproduction of Elastic Impressions.* J. D. Res., *38:*929–939 (Sept.), 1959.
33. Peyton, F. A., Leibold, J. P., and Ridgley, G. V.: *Surface Hardness, Compressive Strength and Abrasion Resistance of Indirect Die Stones.* J. Pros. Den., *2:*381–389 (May), 1952.
34. Buchanan, A. S., and Worner, H. K.: *A Study of the Action of Borax in Retarding the Setting of Plaster of Paris.* J. Soc. Chem. Ind., *65:*23–26, 1946.
35. Phillips, R. W., and Ito, B. Y.: *Factors Affecting the Surface of Stone Dies Poured in Hydrocolloid Impressions.* J. Pros. Den., *2:*390–400 (May), 1952.

CHAPTER 9

# Rubber Impression Materials

In addition to the hydrocolloid gels discussed in the last two chapters there is still another type of elastic impression material which is soft and rubber-like in nature, technically known as an *elastomer*. These materials are also classified as synthetic rubbers in contrast to natural rubber. Although these rubbers are often classified as colloid gels, in contrast to the hydrocolloid gels, they are *hydrophobic* (water hating) instead of *hydrophilic* (water loving) as are the other types of gels.

The rubber impression materials are two component systems, in that a polymerization occurs by a condensation reaction in the presence of certain chemical reactors. There are two types of rubber bases employed as dental impression materials. The base for one type is a polysulfide compound[1], and a silicone[2, 3] base is employed for the other type.

**Chemistry (Polysulfide Rubber).** The process of changing the rubber base product, or liquid polymer, to a rubber-like material is generally known in industry as *vulcanization* or *curing*. Both terms originated in connection with the production of rubber by heating the natural rubber gum, or latex, with sulfur. By analogy, the two terms have been carried over into the synthesis of the rubber-like molecule even though in some cases no sulfur is present.

The basic ingredient of the liquid polymer is a polyfunctional mercaptan or polysulfide polymer with the average structural formula:[1]

$$HS(R—S—S)_{23}—R—SH$$

where R is assumed to be:

$$C_2H_4—O—CH_2—O—C_2H_4$$

At this stage, the material for dental purposes is a liquid polymer, and it is polymerized or cured to the polysulfide rubber by a reaction with some type of a reactor.* Usually lead peroxide ($PbO_2$) and sulfur are employed. The lead peroxide is the polymerizing agent and the sulfur provides better physical properties.[4]

When the lead peroxide is mixed with the polysulfide polymer, the rubber polymer is formed:

$$2HS—(R—S—S)_{23}—R—SH + PbO_2 \longrightarrow$$
$$—S(R—S—S)_{23}—R—S—Pb—R(S—S—R)_{23}—S— + 2H_2O \quad (1)$$

Sulfur then probably reacts as follows:

$$—S—(R—S—S)_{23}—R—S—Pb—S—R(S—S—R)_{23}—S— + S \longrightarrow$$
$$—S(R—S—S)_{23}—R—S—S—R(S—S—R)_{23}—S— + PbS \quad (2)$$

A slight temperature rise occurs during the reaction.

In dentistry, the mixing of the two components is accomplished outside the mouth, but the curing occurs with the impression tray in place in the mouth. As will be shown, certain modifications are made in composition so that the process can be effected easily.

The end product is a rubber material of adequate elasticity and strength which can be removed over undercuts quite readily.

**Chemistry (Silicone Rubber).**     The base for the formation of a silicone rubber is some type of an organosilicone such as poly(dimethyl siloxane):

$$H_3C—\underset{\underset{CH_3}{|}}{\overset{\overset{CH_3}{|}}{Si}}—O\left[\;\underset{\underset{CH_3}{|}}{\overset{\overset{CH_3}{|}}{Si}}—O—\underset{\underset{CH_3}{|}}{\overset{\overset{CH_3}{|}}{Si}}—O—\underset{\underset{CH_3}{|}}{\overset{\overset{CH_3}{|}}{Si}}—O—\underset{\underset{CH_3}{|}}{\overset{\overset{CH_3}{|}}{Si}}—O—\right]_n \underset{\underset{CH_3}{|}}{\overset{\overset{CH_3}{|}}{Si}}—CH_3$$

If this material, a liquid, is heated with benzoyl peroxide ($C_6H_5$—$COO)_2$, a reaction occurs between one of the methyl radicals in the chain and a similar methyl group in an adjacent chain. Thus, the two polymers are cross-linked with benzoic acid formed as a by-product. A synthetic rubber results which has found extensive application in industry.

When the room temperature vulcanization method is employed, other reactive silicone types containing reactive terminal groups, are included with a poly(dimethyl siloxane) and the structure of the end product is not the same as that for the heat-cured type.[2]

The cure is effected with a type of organometal compound and some type of an alkyl silicate. One of the preferred organometals is tin octoate (tin caprylate, $Sn[CH_3(CH_2)_6CO_2]_2$), and a type of ethyl silicate is usually employed. In certain instances, hydrogen may be evolved in copious amounts which deleteriously affects the surface of the stone cast as shown in Figure 9–1. Many methods have been tried to minimize this troublesome effect. One method is to introduce a hydrogen acceptor such as an aldehyde or chromium oxide, or both.[4]

* Oftentimes erroneously called a catalyst. As can be noted in the reactions, this chemical becomes part of the final polymer.

The most successful solution to the evolution of hydrogen during cure is to employ a specific type of silicone base. For example, if a poly(dimethyl siloxane) of the following type is used,

$$HO - \left[ \begin{array}{c} CH_3 \\ | \\ -Si-O- \\ | \\ CH_3 \end{array} \right]_n -H \tag{3}$$

under the proper conditions, a vulcanization without hydrogen evolution can be effected, with tin octoate as the reactor in the presence of a poly(ethyl silicate).[5] The reaction is presumably effected by a cross linking through the terminal hydroxyl groups.[4]

**Composition.** A chemical analysis of a domestic polysulfide rubber impression material resulted in the identification of the ingredients[6] as shown in Table 9–1.

*Table 9–1.* *Composition of a Polysulfide Rubber Impression Material**

| COMPOSITION | PER CENT |
|---|---|
| BASE | |
| Polysulfide polymer | 79.72 |
| Zinc oxide | 4.89 |
| Calcium sulfate | 15.39 |
| ACCELERATOR | |
| Lead peroxide | 77.65 |
| Sulfur | 3.52 |
| Castor oil | 16.84 |
| Other | 1.99 |

* Pearson, *Brit. D. J.*, Aug. 2, 1955.

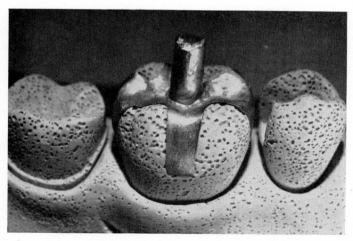

Fig. 9–1. Stone die is pitted because of the evolution of gas from the silicone rubber impression.

It is not known whether the formula given in Table 9–1 is typical, but it is sufficiently complete so far as the present discussion is concerned. Very likely, many commercial products include stearic acid as a control for the curing rate and an odor-masking agent, otherwise the odor before and during curing may be quite obnoxious.

Commercially, these products are dispensed as two pastes, in a manner similar to that for the zinc oxide-eugenol impression pastes (Chapter 6). In fact, these two types of impression material have much in common so far as mixing technic and general manipulations are concerned.

The base material in Table 9–1 is a paste. The polysulfide polymer is a liquid and is plasticized to a paste form by the addition of the two inert fillers or extenders, zinc oxide and calcium sulfate, indicated in Table 9–1.

Silica of a fine particle size is also employed in most materials of this type as a reinforcing agent. The fine silica apparently enters the semicrystalline structure as a reinforcing agent to enhance the elastic properties and strength. Titanium dioxide may also be added to lighten the color.[4]

The other tube is known as the "accelerator," since it is assumed that the curing time can be accelerated or retarded according to the amount of accelerator used. This point will be discussed in a following section.

It should be noted that when the term *accelerator* is employed, the paste or liquid to be added to the base paste is inferred, whereas the term *reactor* refers to the chemical in the accelerator which produces the cure.

Since both the lead peroxide and sulfur are powders, a plasticizer such as castor oil or, preferably, a liquid rubber plasticizer is added to provide a paste. The color of the base is white or tinted, but the color of the accelerator paste is always a blackish brown because of the lead peroxide reactor. If the base is not this color, some other type of reactor has been used.

Although no specific quantitative analysis of the silicone impression materials is available, the ingredients employed are fairly well known by analogy with known principles employed in heat vulcanization of silicone rubber.

The *gum* as received by the manufacturer is already in the form of a paste containing the poly(dimethyl siloxane) and the poly(ethyl silicate). Since both of these latter compounds are liquids, a finely divided inert silica filler is employed. The selection of a filler is most critical as a reinforcing agent since the intermolecular attractions between the silicone polymers is much less than that in the synthetic rubber compounds. As a result, the influence of the filler on the strength of a silicone rubber is much more critical than with the polysulfide rubbers. Its particle size should approach that of the silicone polymer macromolecule. The average diameter of the silica particles may be as small as 10 to 20 millimicrons. There appears to be an optimum particle size according to the manufacturing method. If the particle size is too small, the filler may agglomerate or separate.[7] As before, a titanium dioxide filler may also be used as a whitener.

Although the accelerator for the silicone materials can be supplied as a paste, it is usually supplied as a liquid. As previously mentioned tin octoate is generally employed as the reactor. In order to aid visually in securing a homogeneous mix of the paste and the accelerator liquid, the latter is usually colored with a dye.

**Spatulation.** The polysulfide rubbers are mixed as described for the zinc oxide-eugenol pastes (p. 76). The proper lengths of the two pastes are squeezed onto a mixing pad. The brown paste is smoothed flat with a flexible, stainless steel spatula so that both sides of the blade are covered. This procedure provides greater ease in cleaning the blade later, since the brown paste is less adhesive than the white.

The brown paste is then spread into the white paste and the mixture is spread out over the mixing pad. The mass is then scraped up with the spatula blade and again smoothed out. The process is continued until the mixed paste is of *uniform color* with no streaks of the base appearing in the tan colored paste. A uniform mixture is of utmost importance to an accurate impression. The mixing should be completed in approximately one minute or less.

If both the base and accelerator for the silicone rubber impression materials are supplied in paste form, the mixing procedure is the same as for the polysulfide rubber material. As previously noted, however, the reactor is usually supplied in the form of a colored oily liquid. When the base paste is dispensed from the tube, a certain length is extruded onto the mixing pad and the liquid is placed beside the rope of paste with a stated number of drops per unit length of paste, according to the directions supplied by the manufacturer of the product.

Sometimes the silicone base paste is supplied in a jar and the proper quantity is measured by volume in a measuring cup. The accelerator is dispensed by drops according to the volume of the paste.

In any case, the paste is picked up with the spatula and smoothed into the liquid and the mixing is continued as previously described. The process is continued as before until a complete blending is attained as indicated by an even color throughout the mass.

Regardless of the type of the rubber, whether polysulfide or silicone, it should again be emphasized that the curing will not be complete throughout the mass if the mixture is not homogeneous. In such a case, a distorted impression will result.

**Setting Time.** The setting time can be defined as the time elaps-

*Table 9–2.      Working Time and Setting Time of Rubber Impression*
*Materials*

| MATERIAL | WORKING TIME (MIN.) | | SETTING TIME (MIN.) | |
|---|---|---|---|---|
| | 25°C.(77°F.) | 37°C.(98.6°F) | 25°C.(77°F.) | 37°C.(98.6°F.) |
| POLYSULFIDE TYPE | | | | |
| A | 9.0 | 2.0 | 12.5 | 4.5 |
| B | 5.0 | 2.5 | 9.0 | 4.5 |
| C | 9.0 | 3.5 | 12.5 | 6.0 |
| SILICONE TYPE | | | | |
| F | 3.5 | 3.0 | 7.5 | 5.0 |
| G | 3.5 | 2.0 | 6.0 | 4.0 |

ing from the beginning of mixing until the cure has advanced sufficiently that the impression can be removed from the mouth with a minimum of distortion. It should be noted that the setting time does not correspond to the curing time. Actually the curing may continue for a considerable time after setting. Particularly the silicone rubber impression materials may continue to polymerize for two or more weeks after mixing.[8]

Although there are many methods for the measurement of the setting times of these materials, probably the most satisfactory method is by the use of some type of penetrometer. The test described for obtaining the setting times of zinc oxide-eugenol impression paste (p. 71) can be applied to the setting of these pastes as well, as shown in Table 9–2,[9, 10] As noted in Chapter 6, the working time represents the limit of time during which the paste can be manipulated and seated in the mouth.

As can be noted from the table, the polysulfide rubber impression materials are quite sensitive to temperature during curing, but the silicone materials are less sensitive to such a change.

Although the setting time of the silicone rubber materials compares favorably with that of the polysulfide rubber materials, the working time of the former is apt to be too short for some dental operators.[11]

The setting time of the polysulfide rubber can be controlled by the temperature of the mixing slab or pad. Acceleration can be effected by an increase in temperature and a retardation by a decrease in temperature, provided that the temperature does not approach the dew point of the environment. If water collects on the mixing slab, an acceleration may occur.

The effect of the temperature on the cure of the polysulfide rubber is quite marked. The rate of reaction is approximately doubled with every temperature rise of 10° C. (18° F.), at least between temperatures of 20° C. (68° F.) and 70° C. (158° F.).[12] Thus, variations in room temperature may markedly influence the setting time.

As previously noted, water in small amount accelerates the setting of the polysulfide rubber. The addition of a drop of water during mixing is a practical method for the acceleration of the cure. Although a high relative humidity during mixing may cause a decrease in working time, the effect is not great.[12]

Retardation of cure can be effected by the addition of a drop or two of oleic acid during the mixing.[10, 12]

Within certain limits, the accelerator paste can sometimes be employed for the control of the working and setting time.[10, 12] Theoretically, the greater the amount of the paste added to the base paste, the shorter the setting time should be. The degree to which the control can be effective depends upon the formulation by the manufacturer.[9] Furthermore, any marked change in the ratio of the two pastes may impair the mechanical properties of the rubber.[9, 13]

Although a change in the ratio of the accelerator paste to the base paste is not considered good practice with the polysulfide impression materials, this procedure appears to be the sole method for the control of the working and setting times of the silicone materials. So far as is known, the proportions of accelerator to the paste may vary widely with suitable elastic and other properties still being achieved.[14] However, the retardation obtained by a reduction of the accelerator may be more marked than is the acceleration obtained by increasing the accelerator beyond a certain limit.[15] Attempts to dilute the accelerator chemical with a low viscosity poly(dimethyl siloxane) resulted in an incomplete cure, and frequently a tacky surface occurred on the impression.[11]

The setting time can be estimated by the dentist by occasionally prodding the material in the mouth with a blunt instrument. When it is firm and returns to position readily, it can be assumed that the material has set sufficiently for removal. The disappearance of tackiness as determined with the finger is not an adequate test for the setting time.[13]

**Elasticity.** A number of methods have been proposed for the measurement of the elastic properties of these materials.[3, 9, 12, 16] One accepted method is to measure the properties of strain and set. In the test for set, a cylinder of the material is compressed 12 per cent of its altitude and then released. The set is computed as the percentage of permanent deformation after stress.

The cylinder is then subjected to a compressive stress of 100 grams per square centimeter and then a stress of 1000 grams per square centimeter. The percentage linear deformation which occurs between the two stresses is designated as the strain and it is presumably a measure of the stiffness of the material.

A second method has been employed for the determination of set as described in the present American Dental Association Specification No. 11 for reversible hydrocolloid impression material.[17] In this test,

*Table 9–3.*     *Elastic Properties of Rubber Impression Materials*

| MATERIAL | STRAIN (PER CENT) | SET (PER CENT) |
|---|---|---|
| POLYSULFIDE TYPE | | |
| A | 6.1 | 2.6 |
| B | 6.4 | 4.0 |
| C | 13.3 | 6.9 |
| SILICONE TYPE | | |
| F | 11.6 | 1.6 |
| G | 5.1 | 0.8 |

after the strain has been determined the cylinder is unstressed, and then the stress of 100 grams per square centimeter is re-applied. The percentage difference of the altitude between the first stressing at 100 grams per square centimeter and the second application of the same stress is designated as the set.

With either method it is assumed that the set value is an indication of the permanent deformation of the impression which can be expected when it is removed from the mouth over undercuts.

The values for strain and set (second method),[10] shown in Table 9–3, were obtained with cylinders of material which had been allowed to remain at 37° C. (98.6° F.) for three minutes after setting at room temperature as indicated in Table 9–2. With the exception of the comparatively large value for set in the case of material C, the properties shown are comparable to the similar requirements of the specification for the reversible hydrocolloid impression materials.[17] Material C is intended for use with a syringe for injecting prepared cavities as described in a later section. Consequently, it can be assumed that the elastic properties of these materials are quite similar to those of the reversible hydrocolloid impression materials.

As can be noted from Table 9–3, the set property for the silicone rubber impression materials is lower than that of the polysulfide rubber materials. This quality is apparently inherent in the silicone materials in that they permanently deform less readily under stress than do the polysulfide rubbers.[8, 16] Probably the difference is not of practical importance. When the set is determined by the first method described, it is lower than the similar values given in Table 9–3.

As might be expected, the elastic properties of the rubber impression materials improve with time of curing.[8, 11–14] In other words, the longer the impression can remain in the mouth before removal, the more accurate it will be after removal.

The strength of the rubber impression materials is entirely adequate. For example, if a cylinder of a material used for the data in Table 9–3 is loaded sufficiently in compression, it will usually flatten out without fracture and will return to a cylindrical shape when the stress is released.

**Dimensional Stability.**    Since both types of rubber materials are water repellent, changes in dimension due to syneresis and imbibition are not to be expected. However, a shrinkage is generally expected during a polymerization reaction and consequently a dimensional change during curing should be anticipated, particularly with the slowly curing silicone rubber impression materials. Moreover, certain by-products of the condensation reactions, particularly in the case of the silicone rubbers, may cause additional shrinkage as they volatilize. Also the low molecular weight polymers and even the plasticizer may evaporate and further shrinkage may occur for the same reason. Still another factor, particularly after the removal of an impression over an undercut, might be a contraction by stress relaxation. It can be assumed that a distortion of the impression will result whatever the cause of the contraction.

Many investigations have been published concerning the dimensional stability of these products.[8, 10, 13–16, 18, 19] In general, the results of the various investigations agree at least as to the order of magnitude of the changes which occur during cure, and the results presented in Table 9–4 are probably typical.

A method by which the dimensional changes during cure of the rubbers can be studied is that the freshly mixed rubber can be floated on the surface of mercury and its dimensional changes can be observed with a comparator microscope focused on a marker, or markers, attached to the surface of the rubber as described for the determination of the setting expansion of gypsum products (p. 42). The results in Table 9–4, columns two and three, were obtained in this manner.

A second method is to confine the material in some manner, as in an impression tray, and to observe the changes quantitatively as in the previous method. This method more nearly approximates clinical conditions, since, as will be discussed later, it is imperative that the impression material be held rigidly in the tray at the time the impression

*Table 9–4.*    *Dimensional Stability of Rubber Impression Materials*

| MATERIAL | FREE | | CONFINED IN A TRAY | |
|---|---|---|---|---|
| | 30 MIN. (PER CENT) | 3 DAYS (PER CENT) | 30 MIN. (PER CENT) | 3 DAYS (PER CENT) |
| POLYSULFIDE RUBBER | | | | |
| A | −0.05 | −0.13 | 0.00 | −0.13 |
| B | −0.03 | −0.11 | | |
| SILICONE RUBBER | | | | |
| C | −0.06 | −0.87 | −0.01 | −0.40 |
| D | −0.08 | −3.04 | 0.00 | −0.81 |
| E | −0.05 | −0.37 | +0.04 | −0.13 |

is removed from the mouth. The results shown in columns four and five (Table 9–4) were obtained in this manner with the use of special testing equipment.[20]

Certainly it can be stated from the results presented in Table 9–4 that the rubber materials are much more stable dimensionally than are the hydrocolloid impression materials (Figs. 7–4 and 8–1). However, it is evident that all of the materials change dimensionally with time and that such a change is greater in magnitude for the silicone rubber impression materials than for the polysulfide rubber materials.

Although the dimensional change during curing is reduced when the material is confined (Table 9–4), it still is worthy of consideration from the standpoint of accuracy, particularly for the dental operations which require a minimum tolerance of error.

Very likely, the stone die or cast should be constructed within the first hour after the removal of the impression from the mouth if the available accuracy is to be maintained,[21, 22] particularly when a silicone rubber material is employed.

**Thermal Properties.**    Although both types of rubber materials are good heat insulators, it is estimated that the conductivity of the silicone rubbers is twice that of ordinary rubber.[23]

The average linear coefficient of thermal expansion for eleven commercially available polysulfide rubber impression materials has been determined as $150 \times 10^{-6}$ per °C.,[12] whereas the same property for three silicone rubber materials averaged $200 \times 10^{-6}$ per °C.[24]

The practical interpretation of such results is that when an impression using a polysulfide rubber is removed from the mouth at a temperature of 37° C. (98.6° F.) to a room temperature of 20° C. (68° F.) the impression should shrink 0.26 per cent linearly. Similarly, the silicone rubber impression should contract 0.34 per cent. Such a dimensional change is beyond the limits of clinical tolerance, and the subsequently fabricated dental structures would not fit. Very likely, the thermal shrinkage is greatly inhibited by the adhesion of the rubber to the impression tray as noted in connection with the curing shrinkage. Certainly, it has not been reported as of significance in research investigations on accuracy of fit.[9, 18, 19]

**Shelf Life.**    Although a segregation of the ingredients of the accelerator pastes for the polysulfide rubber materials has been reported,[12] it is suspected that the fault was due to a lack of blending during manufacture. So far as is known, this type of rubber material properly manufactured, does not deteriorate appreciably in the tubes during storage under normal environmental conditions.[9]

Such is not the case with the silicone rubber impression materials.[23] The silicone gum from which the paste is made may stiffen in the tube.[3] Under normal conditions of temperature its shelf life is about eight months. Continuous exposure of the silicone paste to the air accelerates the stiffening. For this reason, the tube should be kept tightly closed with the screw cap provided when not in use.[3]

The tin octoate reactor also deteriorates with age. Its shelf life in a closed container is at least four months at 21° C. (70° F.). Under no circumstances should it be stored above 27° C. (80° F.) for an extended period. An excessive exposure of some of the commercially available reactors to air results in the formation of a solid substance. Presumably, the liquid stannous octoate is changed to the solid stannic form.[4]

Because of their limited shelf life, it is best not to maintain a large supply of the silicone impression materials in storage in the dental office. It has been suggested that any material on hand, particularly the reactor, should be stored in a cool place[3] in order to prolong the shelf life. Whenever a new package of the material is received, it should be tested for setting time immediately. If it does not behave properly, it should be returned to the dental dealer.

**Miscellaneous Properties.** The storage medium for a rubber impression is not critical, but, as previously stated, a long storage time is not indicated because of the distortion occasioned by a continued curing. The water sorption of the materials is negligible.[12] However, if the tray material is of a plastic type which may imbibe water and change in dimension, the impression should not be stored in a moist environment.[18]

Spherical indentations sometimes appear on the surface of an impression obtained with a polysulfide rubber material. Such indentations appear on the surface of the stone die as convexities or nodules as illustrated in Figure 9–2. Presumably, this effect is due to the collapse of a void near the surface.[18] Such voids are probably the result of air bubbles trapped during mixing. Such depressions are not generally observed on the surface of silicone rubber impressions. However, since

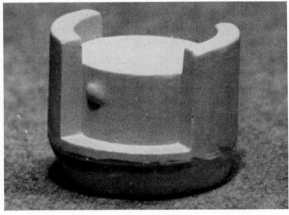

Fig. 9–2. Nodule on a stone die due to a collapse of a void in the polysulfide rubber impression.

such imperfections usually do not appear for a number of hours after the impression is removed from the mouth, they should not be troublesome if the dentist constructs the stone die within the first hour as previously suggested.

Unlike the hydrocolloid impression materials, the rubber impression materials do not materially affect the hardness of the stone surface.[10] A smooth, hard stone surface on the die can be expected when the rubber impression materials are used, unless hydrogen gas is evolved during the curing of the silicone rubber impression.

As previously noted, the evolution of gas during the curing of a silicone material may cause a pitted surface on the stone die (Fig. 9–1). Several methods have been suggested for avoiding such trouble with commercial products which present this problem,[3, 19] but the usual method is to delay the pouring of the stone until the gas evolution has subsided. Since such a procedure may require a delay of one[14] to forty-eight hours,[3] it is not feasible in consideration of the lack of dimensional stability of the silicone materials. Very likely, if the gas evolution is troublesome, the dentist should discard the particular product in favor of a material which does not exhibit this fault.

At first thought, it might be considered that the lead-containing polysulfide rubber impression material might be toxic. Tests have shown that this is not likely to be the case,[6] at least during the limited time the material is in the mouth while an impression is obtained.

Although the reactor, tin octoate, used in the curing of the silicone rubber materials is toxic, the final product is non-toxic.[4]

The choice between a polysulfide or a silicone base rubber impression material will be governed by the particular characteristics preferred by the operator. In general, it may be said that the silicone materials have the advantage of superior color, odor, and similar esthetic properties. They are also cleaner to handle. On the other hand, they are inferior to the polysulfide rubbers from the standpoint of shelf life. Impressions of equal accuracy, as with hydrocolloid, can be secured with either material with the proper technic.

## TECHNICAL CONSIDERATIONS

The rubber impression materials can be described as a universal type of impression material. They can be employed for any type of dental impression required by the dentist. However, they are primarily intended for impressions of the hard tissue where elasticity is a necessary prerequisite. Their use for multiple impressions (impressions of several teeth at the same time) for crown and bridge construction, and for impressions of single teeth will be discussed so far as the technic applies to the proper manipulation of the materials. A description of the complete clinical technic can be found in the dental literature.[25, 26]

**Accuracy of Fit.** In the previous sections the various properties of the rubber materials have been discussed with respect to their contributions to the accuracy of the impression. In the last analysis, however, the dental appliance finally fabricated should fit satisfactorily in the mouth. Sometimes certain factors involved in the technical procedures are not evident in the basic quantitative determinations. Consequently, studies concerned with the accuracy of the fit of the final dental appliance are necessary for the proper evaluation of the particular dental materials involved.

For such evaluations of the usefulness of the materials in connection with the fabrication of dental gold inlays and crowns, the steel master dies shown in Figure 9–3 are often used. An accurately fitting crown is cast in gold to fit the die on the left, and a mesio-occluso-distal inlay is cast to fit the die on the right. If an impression is obtained with a rubber impression material, for example, of either master die and if a stone die is prepared, in the impression, the master castings can be fitted to the stone dies and the accuracy of fit can be compared with that of the casting on the master die.

In such a test, any dimensional change of the stone during setting or subsequently is ignored in estimating the accuracy of the impression material itself. Such an assumption is possibly justified if a class II stone is employed with a definite W/P ratio and technic. It will be recalled (p. 52) that the setting expansion of such stones is negligibly small.

It is much more difficult to fabricate gold alloy castings to fit the dies shown in Figure 9–3 than to fit a clinical case because of the lack of tapering walls in the former case. However, any procedures which are sufficiently accurate for these dies will undoubtedly satisfy the clinical requirements.

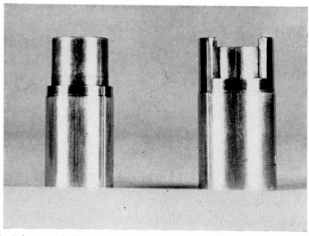

Fig. 9–3.   Stainless steel dies to represent a shoulder-crown preparation (*left*) and a cavity prepared for a mesio-occluso-distal inlay (*right*).

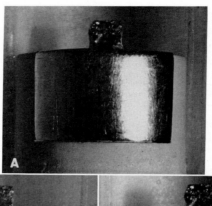

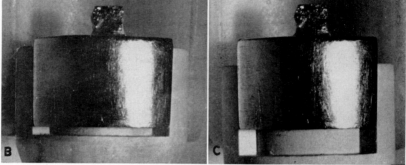

Fig. 9–4. The greater the thickness of the wall of the rubber impression from which the above stone dies were constructed, the poorer the fit of the casting. Wall thickness, *A*. 0.5 mm., *B*. 2.0 mm., *C*. 4.5 mm.

**Preparation of the Tray.**   The methods for proportioning and mixing the rubber impression materials have already been discussed.

Like the zinc oxide-eugenol impression pastes, the rubber materials are used as "wash" or corrective lining impression materials. The use of a tray compound as described in Chapter 6 is not advisable in this case. The plasticizers employed in the rubber impression pastes may soften the surface of the compound. As a result, the impression is likely to be distorted because of a lack of adequate support for the rubber.

As can be concluded from the fit of the master castings shown in Figure 9–4 on the stone dies constructed from rubber impressions with different bulk, the less the distance between the impression tray and the master die (Fig. 9–3, right), the more accurate is the impression.[18] This fact has been demonstrated by many investigators.[8, 9, 13, 14, 18, 19] It should be noted that this finding is directly opposite to that recommended for the hydrocolloid impression where a greater bulk of material produced better accuracy than did the smaller bulk. Not only should the bulk be less with the rubber impression materials but it should also be evenly distributed.[18] In general, the optimum thickness for the impression is 2 to 4 millimeters.

Although stock impression trays are available which can be contoured closely to the mouth parts, a better method is to construct a tray with a plastic material, such as a self-curing resin which will be described in a subsequent chapter. A rough impression is obtained of the mouth using any convenient impression material. A stone cast is constructed. The important parts of the cast are covered with two thicknesses of base plate wax or asbestos which is later overlaid with the uncured resin. When the resin has cured, it can be used as a tray. The impression material then occupies the space left by the base plate wax. Thus, a uniform bulk of impression material is provided with a minimum thickness.

**Adhesion to the Tray.** The next problem is concerned with the adhesion of the rubber impression material to the tray. As with the hydrocolloid impression materials, complete adhesion to the tray is imperative when the impression is removed from the mouth. Otherwise, a distorted impression will result.

Although perforated trays similar to those used for hydrocolloid impressions would be satisfactory from this standpoint, they are not as convenient or practical as the custom built resin tray just described. Adhesion can be obtained by the application of an adhesive to the plastic tray, previous to the insertion of the impression material. The adhesive then forms a tenacious bond between the rubber material and the tray.

The adhesive employed with the polysulfide rubber impression materials is a butyl rubber cement. The base for the adhesive employed with the silicone rubber materials usually contains poly(dimethyl siloxane) or a similar reactive silicone and ethyl silicate. The poly (dimethyl siloxane) acts as an adhesive for the rubber, and hydrated silica forms from the ethyl silicate to form a physical bond with the impression tray.[4] In either case, a slightly roughened surface on the tray will increase the adhesion.

**Multiple Impressions.** As with the hydrocolloid impression materials, an impression of a number of teeth can be obtained at one time with the use of a syringe (p. 104).

The problem is somewhat different with the rubber impression materials than with the reversible hydrocolloid impression materials. In the latter case, the sol will remain fluid as long as the temperature is held above the gelation point. In the case of the rubber materials, a thickening of the mix occurs as the curing proceeds. Although the consistency may be such that an impression with the tray can be effected, the rubber may be too thick to be extruded from the syringe. The working time for the syringe material may be two to four minutes less than that indicated in Table 9–2.[11]

Such a working time may be satisfactory with the polysulfide rubber materials, but it will usually be too short when the silicone rubbers are employed.

In order to overcome such a situation, some manufacturers have provided rubber materials with two consistencies, one consistency for use with the tray, and the other with a thinner consistency for use with the syringe. The syringe type also is given longer working and setting times.

Material C in Tables 9–2 and 9–3 is a syringe type. As can be noted, the material exhibits a longer setting time than the other materials (Table 9–2), but its set is higher than the tray types (Table 9–3). For this reason, this type of material is not recommended for use as a tray impression, but when a small amount is injected into the prepared cavity and reinforced with the tray type material, it is satisfactory.

The method of employing both the syringe and tray types of rubber materials is often referred to as the *double mix* technic because two separate mixtures are required with two separate mixing pads and spatulas. Usually the tray material is mixed first.[25] The tray is filled with a uniform thickness of material and set aside.

The material for the syringe is then mixed, the syringe is filled and the material injected into the prepared cavities as described for the hydrocolloid impression materials (p. 103). The filled tray is then carried to place.

The procedure should be timed so that neither the tray nor the syringe material have cured to a point where they will not cohere when they are brought together.

The stiffness of the material at the time the impression is seated influences the accuracy, particularly in the case of the silicone materials.[19] If the material has cured beyond a certain point, deformation will occur upon removal of the tray and a smaller die will result. As the viscosity of the material increases before seating, the resulting stone die will invariably become smaller. Ideally each commercial material has an optimum time at which it should be carried to the mouth.

Not only is the double mix method more accurate than the single mix technic, but also there is less chance for bubble formation as previously described.[18, 19]

**Removal of the Impression.**        Under no circumstances should the impression be removed until the cure has progressed sufficiently to provide sufficient elasticity that a distortion will not occur. One method for the determination of the time of removal is to inject some of the syringe material into an interproximal space not in the area of operation. As previously noted, this material can be prodded with a blunt instrument from time to time, and when it is firm and returns completely to its original contour, the impression can be removed.

From a practical standpoint, the curing rate of the rubber impression material should not be so slow that the time before removal from the mouth is unduly long. It is estimated that with a satisfactory rubber material the impression should be ready to be removed within at least ten minutes from the time of mixing, allowing six to eight minutes for the impression to remain in the mouth.[27]

For the same reasons presented in the case of the hydrocolloid impression materials, the rubber impression should be removed suddenly, with a jerk.[12]

**Single Impressions.** The technic for single impressions is similar to that for multiple impressions except that only one tooth is involved.

The "tray" employed is usually a copper matrix band which is a short copper tube, approximately 30 gauge (Brown and Sharpe) in thickness, with a length and diameter suitable for encompassing the particular tooth involved.

The band should be fitted to the tooth and then reinforced with compound. Otherwise the impression will be squeezed with the fingers when it is removed from the tooth and a distortion will occur. The reinforcement can be obviated if a copper "shell" is employed, which is essentially a copper band with one end closed with the same gauge of copper metal, to form a cup-shaped receptacle.

The adhesive is applied to the band and the band is filled with the previously mixed rubber material. The prepared cavity is injected as usual with the syringe, and the filled band is pressed to place. The same precautions in removal are observed as previously described for the multiple impressions. Either a syringe or a tray type material can be used, but usually only one type is employed.

**Stone Die.** As previously noted, the stone die should be constructed shortly after the impression has been removed from the mouth in order to avoid a distortion due to the warpage of the rubber material. In this respect, the quantitative results shown in Table 9–4 can be correlated with the fit of the master castings shown in Figures 9–5 and 9–6. The impressions were filled with stone at the times indicated after removal from the master die.

As can be noted, a slight discrepancy in fit occurred even though the stone was poured within two hours (Fig. 9–5). The fits at later times are obviously unsatisfactory.

As noted previously, the stainless steel master dies are more difficult to fit than a practical case, and, therefore, the conditions for fit on this die may be somewhat exaggerated from a clinical viewpoint. This fact is illustrated by the fit of the master castings for a practical case shown in the upper row of photographs in Figure 9–6 which were constructed in a polysulfide rubber impression. It is evident that the time factor is not as critical in this case. However, a close inspection will show that the master casting on the die does not fit when constructed six hours after the removal of the impression.

In the lower row (Fig. 9–6) is shown the fit of a master casting on stone dies constructed from silicone impressions at the same times after

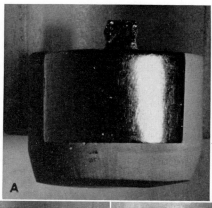

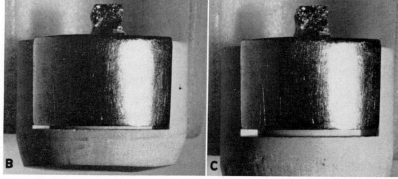

Fig. 9–5.   Fit of a master casting placed on stone dies constructed from a polysulfide rubber impression of the master steel die (Fig. 9–3) at varying periods after removal from the mouth. *A.* Poured immediately; *B.* Poured in 2 hours; *C.* Poured in 24 hours.

removal as for the top row. As can be noted, the fits are very poor after the first hour. It is evident that the dimensional stability of the silicone rubber impression materials is inferior to that of the poly-sulfide rubber materials as indicated quantitatively in Table 9–4.

It should be evident from the pictorial data shown in Figures 9–5 and 9–6 that the stone die should be constructed *within one hour* after the impression is removed. Otherwise, the dentist cannot be sure that his accuracy is within the allowable tolerances.

**Miscellaneous Technics.**     Under no circumstances should the rubber impression material be allowed to thicken appreciably before the tray or band is seated. Owing to the compressive stresses induced in the partially set material, the impression will "spring back" upon removal, and the dies will be too small.[9, 19]

For much the same reason, it is difficult to repair a rubber impression by the addition of more material and then to re-seat the impression. The added material is cushioned by the induction of compressive stress in the already cured rubber. When the impression is removed, the stresses are released. As a result, a small die or cast results.[10] Only if the original impression is vented with holes drilled in strategic areas can this effect be minimized. In such a case, it is hoped that any excess added material will be vented. The safest method is to obtain a new impression when bubbles or similar defects appear.

It is possible to construct successive stone dies or casts from impressions obtained with polysulfide rubber, when duplicate stone dies are needed. The successive dies will be of essentially the same accuracy as the first die constructed.[18] Such does not appear to be the case, however, when silicone rubber impression materials are used.[19] The second or third stone die constructed from the same silicone rubber impression may not be as accurate as the first due to the lack of dimensional stability of the impression material.

**Reproduction of Detail.**    The necessity for the impression material to reproduce the finest detail of the mouth parts is, of course, self-evident.

This property was tested, for example, by placing a series of Knoop indentations, graded from 422 microns to 34 microns in length, in a

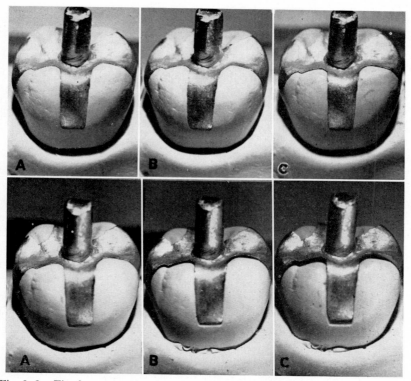

Fig. 9–6.   Fit of a master casting for a practical case. Upper row, from a polysulfide rubber impression, lower row, from a silicone rubber impression. Stone poured at *A*. 10 minutes, *B*. 6 hours, and *C*. 24 hours.

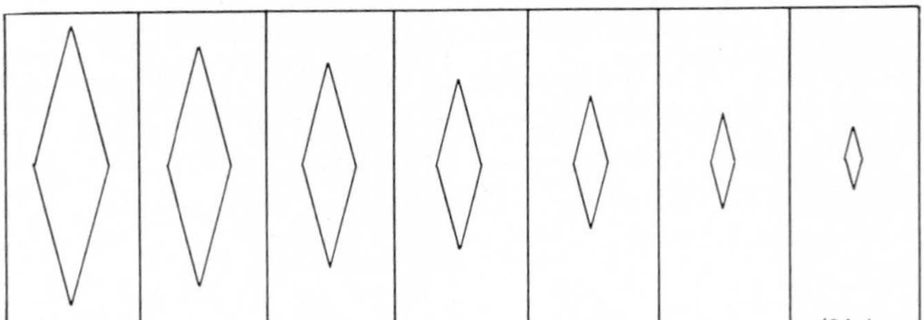

| Material | (422μ) | | | | | | (34μ) |
|---|---|---|---|---|---|---|---|
| HYDROCOLLOID A | | | | | | | 100 |
| HYDROCOLLOID B | | | | | | 96 | 80 |
| ALGINATE A | | | 94 | 87 | 61 | 30 | 2 |
| ALGINATE B | | | | 87 | 65 | 31 | 7 |
| POLYSULFIDE RUBBER A | | | | | | | 100 |
| POLYSULFIDE RUBBER B | | | | | | | 100 |
| SILICONE A | | | | | | | 100 |
| SILICONE B | | | | | | | 96 |
| SILICONE C | | | | | | | 98 |

Fig. 9–7. Reproduction of detail. Below each schematic drawing of a Knoop impression is shown the percentage reproduction of the particular impression in the indicated impression material.

stainless steel test block.[28] Each impression material was applied in turn to the surface of the test block, and the number of impressions of the indentations reproduced in repeated trials were counted. The results are tabulated in Figure 9–7 as the percentage reproduction of each Knoop indentation shown diagrammatically at the top of the Figure.

The first two materials listed are reversible hydrocolloid impression materials, and apparently they reproduced the smallest impressions easily. It is evident that the alginate impression materials were the poorest in this respect. The rubber impression materials were equal to the reversible hydrocolloid gels in their ability to reproduce fine detail.

When dental stone is formed over such test impressions, the finest detail is not always reproduced.[28, 29] In other words, the rubber impression materials are able to reproduce detail more accurately than can be transferred to the stone die or cast.

The clinical significance of such measurements is not entirely evident. In the first place, it is possible that the surface interaction between the impression materials and the stainless steel test block may not be the same as between the impression material and the mouth tissues. Probably this difference is particularly important in the case of the alginate impression materials, and it might account for their inadequacy in this respect as shown in Figure 9–7. Furthermore, it is possible that the detail obtained with the rubber impression materials on the steel block might be greater than that obtained in the mouth, because of the property of water repellence exhibited by these materials.

Secondly, the tolerances required for accurate dental work in this respect are not known. However, it is logical to assume that the greater the detail reproduced, the better will be the impression or stone die.

## *Literature*

1. Jorezak, J. S., and Fetts, E. M.: *Polysulfide Polymer.* Ind. Eng. Chem., *43:*324–338 (Feb.), 1951.
2. Meals, R. N., and Lewis, F. M.: *Silicones.* New York, Reinhold Publishing Corporation, 1959, p. 96.
3. McLean, J. W.: *Silicone Impression Materials.* Brit. D. J., *104:*441–451 (June 17), 1958.
4. Molnar, E. J.: Personal Communication.
5. Berridge, C. A.: *Room Temperature Curing Organo-Polysiloxane.* U.S. Patent 2,843,555. July 15, 1958.
6. Pearson, S. L.: *A New Elastic Impression Material: A Preliminary Report.* Brit. D. J., *99:*72–76 (Aug. 2), 1955.
7. Meals, R. N., and Lewis, F. M.: *loc. cit.,* pp. 36, 41.
8. McLean, J. W.: *Silicone Impression Materials, A Research Report.* Den. Practitioner, *9:*56–63 (Nov.), 1958.
9. Skinner, E. W., and Cooper, E. N.: *Desirable Properties and Use of Rubber Impression Materials.* J.A.D.A., *51:*523–536 (Nov.), 1955.
10. Skinner, E. W.: *Use and Criteria of Selection of Rubber Impression Materials.* Ann. Den., *16:*79–91 (Sept.), 1957.
11. Myers, J. E., and Peyton, F. A.: *Chemical and Physical Studies of the Silicone Rubber Impression Materials.* J. Pros. Den., *9:*315–324 (March–April), 1959.
12. Jørgenson, K. D.: *Thiokol as a Dental Impression Material.* Acta Odont. Scandinavica, *14:*313–334 (Nov. 4), 1956.
13. Fairhurst, C. W., Furman, T. C., Schallhorn, R. V., Kirkpatrick, E. L., and Ryge, G.: *Elastic Properties of Rubber Base Materials.* J. Pros. Den., *6:*534–542 (July), 1956.
14. Tomlin, H. R., and Osborne, J.: *Some Observations on Silicone Materials.* Brit. D. J., *105:*407–412 (Dec. 2), 1958.
15. Anderson, J. N.: *Silicone Base Impression Materials.* M.D.S. Thesis, University of Sheffield, 1957, p. 84.
16. Ostlund, S. G.: son.: *Some Properties of Rubber Base Materials.* Sart. Odont. Tider., *65:*94–104 (1957).
17. Paffenbarger, G. C.: *Hydrocolloid Impression Materials: Physical Properties and a Specification.* J.A.D.A., *27:*373–388 (March), 1940.
18. Schnell, R. J., and Phillips, R. W.: *Dimensional Stability of Rubber Base Impressions and Certain Other Factors Affecting Accuracy.* J.A.D.A., *57:*89–98 (July), 1958.
19. Gilmore, W. H., Schnell, R. J., and Phillips, R. W.: *Factors Influencing the Accuracy of Silicone Impression Materials.* J. Pros. Den., *9:*304–314 (March–April), 1959.
20. Hollenback, G. M.: *Study of Physical Properties of Elastic Impression Materials and Stones.* J. South. California D. A., *25:*26 (Jan.), 1957.
21. Phillips, R. W.: *Physical Properties and Manipulation of Rubber Impression Materials.* J.A.D.A., *59:*454–458 (Sept.), 1959.
22. Skinner, E. W.: *The Properties and Manipulation of Mercaptan Base and Silicone Base Impression Materials.* D. Clin. North America, November 1958, pp. 685–697.
23. Meals, R. N., and Lewis, F. M.: *loc. cit.,* pp. 60–61.
24. Anderson, J. N.: *The Dimensional Stability of Three Silicone-Base Impression Materials.* D. Practitioner, *8:*568–572 (Aug.), 1958.

25. Sturdevant, C. M.: *Impressions for Indirect Inlays.* J.A.D.A., *54:*357–366 (March), 1957.

26. Sturdevant, C. M.: *Mercaptan Rubber Impression Technique for Single and Multiple Restorations.* D. Clin. North America, November 1958, pp. 699–711.

27. Phillips, R. W.: *Elastic Impression Materials—A Summary of a Recent Conference and Analysis of the Current Status and Recent Research.* J. Pros. Den., *8:*650–656 (July), 1958.

28. Ayers, H. D., Phillips, R. W., Dell, A., and Henry, R. W.: *Detail Duplication Test Used to Evaluate Elastic Impression Materials.* J. Pros. Den., *10:*374–381 (March), 1960.

29. Fusayama, T., and Hosoda, H.: *Surface Reproducibility of Elastic Impression Materials.* J. Pros. Den., *9:*929–939 (Sept.-Oct.), 1959.

# CHAPTER 10

# Chemistry of the

# Synthetic Resins

There is probably no other single class of substances which has influenced modern living during the present century more than have the synthetic plastics. By definition synthetic plastics are nonmetallic compounds, synthetically produced (usually from organic compounds) which can be molded into various forms and then hardened for commercial use.[1] Clothing, building materials, household appliances, electronic equipment and almost every line of human endeavor have some items or parts constructed of a plastic of some form. The term "plastic" includes fibrous, rubber-like, and resinous or hard, rigid substances. All of these materials have certain chemical similarities in that they are composed of polymers or complex molecules of high molecular weight. The particular form and morphology of the molecule determines to a large extent whether or not the plastic is a fiber, a rubber-like product or a resin.[1]

The field of the giant molecules, or the high polymers as the chemist calls them, is one of the most exciting of all areas in science. Their discovery and historical development is one of the most fascinating stories in chemistry.[2, 3] Originally they were literally laboratory nuisances, the waxy, sticky residues left after certain organic reactions. It was only during the last 30 or 40 years that these resinous materials, composed of giant molecules, attracted the attention of the chemist and thus the entire field of plastics was born. The impact on dentistry of current research in this field is difficult to envision, but probably nowhere else may one anticipate as far-reaching or significant effects as upon dental practice

**Classification of Resins.**     Synthetic resins are usually molded in some manner under heat and pressure into useful articles. If the resin is molded without chemical change, for example, by softening it under heat and pressure and by cooling it after it has been molded, the resin is classified as *thermoplastic.* On the other hand, if a chemical reaction takes place during the molding process, so that the final product is chemically different from the original substance, the resin is classified as *thermoset.* Thermoplastic resins are fusible, and usually they are soluble in organic solvents. Thermoset resins are generally insoluble and infusible.

**Dental Resins.**     Although the dentist uses all forms of plastics in one way or another, the type most closely related to the restoration of missing teeth or tooth structure is that of the synthetic resins. The resins are employed for the restoration of missing teeth and missing tooth structure (restorations) and for the construction of dentures. The denture base (the part of the denture which rests on the soft tissues of the mouth) is customarily made of a resin and often the denture teeth as well. The optical and color properties of the resins thus employed are so excellent that the restoration will often escape detection.

The particular synthetic resin most used currently in dentistry is an acrylic resin, poly(methyl methacrylate). Consequently, the properties and use of this particular resin will be stressed.

However, there are so many different types of synthetic resins, and more types are being developed constantly, that the dentist cannot afford to limit his knowledge to one specific resin. Rather he should possess some knowledge of the fundamental concepts of resin chemistry, so that he can better evaluate new developments in this field as they occur. For this reason, the present chapter is devoted largely to a brief review of the fundamentals of resin chemistry.

**Requisites for Dental Resin.**     The reason the present-day dental resins are more or less limited to poly(methyl methacrylate) is that this is the only resin which has so far been developed which will provide routinely the essential properties for use in the mouth without deterioration.

Ideal requisites for a dental resin are as follows:

1. The material should exhibit a translucence or transparency such that it can be made to duplicate esthetically the mouth tissues which it is to replace. It should be capable of being tinted or pigmented to this end.

2. There should be no change in color or appearance of the material subsequent to its fabrication whether it is in or out of the mouth.

3. It should neither expand, contract nor warp during processing nor during subsequent normal use by the patient. In other words, it should be dimensionally stable under all conditions.

4. It should possess adequate strength, resilience and abrasion resistance to withstand all normal usage.

5. It should be impermeable to the mouth fluids to the extent that it will not become unsanitary or disagreeable in taste or odor. If used as a filling material or cement it should chemically bond to the tooth itself.

6. Food or other matter taken into the mouth should not cling to the resin so that the restoration cannot be cleansed in the same manner as the mouth tissues.

7. The resin should be tasteless, odorless, non-toxic and non-irritating to the mouth tissues.

8. It should be completely insoluble in the mouth fluids or in any substances taken into the mouth, with no evidence of corrosive attack.

9. It should have a low specific gravity and a relatively high thermal conductivity.

10. Its softening temperature should be well above the temperature of any hot foods or liquids taken into the mouth. If the appliance can be easily removed from the mouth, ideally the resin should be capable of withstanding the temperature of boiling water for purposes of sterilization, with no evidence of warping or other change.

11. In case of unavoidable breakage, it should be possible to repair the resin easily and efficiently.

12. The fabrication of the resin into a dental appliance should be easily effected with simple equipment.

No resin has yet been found which will meet all of the above requirements. The conditions in the mouth are most disadvantageous to the life of any substance; only the most chemically stable and inert materials can withstand such conditions without deterioration.

## POLYMERIZATION

The constitution of a polymeric substance is customarily described in terms of its structural units, as is implied by the etymology of the term *polymer* (*i.e.*, "many members"). Polymerization occurs by a series of chemical reactions by which the macromolecule or *polymer* is formed from a simple molecule known as a *monomer*. Basically, the polymer is made up of a particular recurring, simple structural unit, which is essentially related to the monomer structure. The structural units are connected to each other in the polymer molecule by covalent bonds. In some cases, the molecular weight of the polymer molecule may be as high as 50,000,000. Any chemical compound possessing a molecular weight in excess of 5000 is considered to be a macromolecule.[4]

The molecules within the final polymer invariably consist of molecular species which vary in degree of polymerization, generally over a considerable range. Usually, however, the *average degree of polymerization* may be found by dividing the total number of structural units by the total number of molecules.[3] Another method of expressing the degree of polymerization is by the *number average molecular weight* which represents the mass of the sample divided by the number of mols it contains. The number average molecular weight for various commercial dental polymer powders[5] varies from 3,500 to 36,000 while the same products after curing show average molecular weights from 8,000 to 39,000. Polymerization is never entirely complete and the per cent of residual monomer has a pronounced effect on the molecular weight. For example, with 0.9 per cent residual monomer in a sample of resin polymer having an original number average molecular weight of 22,400, the molecular weight of the resultant cured resin[5] was approximately 7,300.

Polymerization can be effected by either a series of condensation reactions, or by simple addition reactions. If the polymerization is effected by condensation reactions, the process is known as a *condensation polymerization.* If the polymerization is brought about by an addition reaction, an *addition polymerization* takes place.

**Physical Properties.** The physical properties of the polymer are greatly influenced by almost any changes in temperature, environment, composition or molecular weight and structure. In general, the higher the temperature, the softer and weaker the polymer becomes. When a thermoplastic resin becomes sufficiently soft to mold, it is said to have reached its *softening temperature* or *molding temperature.*

The strength of the resin is affected by the degree of polymerization.[5] Generally, a resin possesses mechanical strength only when its degree of polymerization is relatively high, in the neighborhood of 150 to 200 recurring units.[6] The strength of the resin increases quite rapidly with increase in degree of polymerization until a certain molecular weight is attained which is characteristic for the given polymer. Above this molecular weight, there is not a great change in strength with further polymerization. The number average molecular weight is very significant as an indication of the relation of the molecular weight to strength. The value for the number average molecular weight is lowered markedly by the presence of a relatively few molecules with a low degree of polymerization, which weaken the resin considerably.

Complex side chains on the monomer molecule generally produce a weaker resin with a lower softening temperature in comparison to the similar properties of a polymer which possesses a straight chain structure. If the chains are cross-linked, however, the strength is increased, and the resin is generally infusible.

**Condensation Polymerization.** The reactions producing condensation polymerization progress by the same mechanism as similar chemical reactions between two or more simple molecules. The primary compounds react with the formation of by-products such as water, halogen acids, ammonia, etc. These spontaneous and random reactions occur again and again, to produce the macromolecule.

The construction of polymers by the condensation method is rather slow and tends to stop before the molecules have reached a truly giant size because as the chains grow they become less mobile and numerous. Products such as nylon have acquired their valuable properties when they reach a molecular weight of 10,000 to 20,000. However, to build molecules with molecular weights in the hundreds of thousands or millions by condensation is very difficult.

Several condensation resins have been used in dentistry in the past for the construction of denture bases. The principal resin so employed was a phenol-formaldehyde resin known popularly as "Bakelite," named after its inventor, L. H. Baekeland.

The reactions for this resin are very complicated, and little is known regarding the final structure. The first reactions are between phenol and formaldehyde to form an alcohol of some type. For example:

$$
\underset{\text{OH}}{\bigcirc} + CH_2O \rightarrow \underset{\text{OH}}{\bigcirc}\!-\!CH_2OH
$$

(1)

The alcohols can then react by condensation to form the macromolecules, possibly as follows:

$$
\underset{\text{OH}}{\bigcirc}\!-\!CH_2OH + \underset{\text{OH}}{\bigcirc}\!-\!CH_2OH \rightarrow \underset{\text{OH}}{\bigcirc}\!-\!CH_2\!-\!\underset{\text{OH}}{\bigcirc}\!-\!CH_2OH + H_2O, \text{ etc.}
$$

(2)

When it is considered that various types of mono- and di-alcohols can be formed in reaction (1), it can be understood that the reaction products indicated by (2) become cross-linked and, eventually, the compounds become so complicated that it is virtually impossible to identify their final chemical structure.

When the molecular weight is relatively low, the material is known as a *resole*. At this stage it is thermoplastic and alcohol-soluble. It can be molded at this stage and reacted further under heat to a *resite*, which is its final form. In the resite stage it is both insoluble and infusible.

Although the product as used for denture bases was translucent and strong, it proved to be chemically unstable in the mouth. It gradually discolored, possibly by oxidation. In all probability, the curing procedure employed was not controlled properly.

At present, there is no condensation resin employed extensively in dental procedures. However, such a situation may change, and the dentist should be familiar with the basic concepts of condensation polymerization.

**Addition Polymerization.** All of the resins employed extensively in dental procedures at the present time are produced by *addition polymerization*. As a matter of fact, this type of polymerization is so common that often the term "polymerization," when used alone, is understood to indicate addition polymerization.

Unlike condensation polymerization, there is no change in composition during addition polymerization; the macromolecules are formed from smaller units, or monomer, without change in composition, since the monomer and the polymer have the same empirical formulas. In other words, the structure of the monomer is repeated many times in the polymer.

As opposed to condensation polymerization, the addition method can produce giant molecules of almost unlimited size. Starting from an active center, it adds one monomer at a time and rapidly builds a chain which, in theory, can go on growing indefinitely as long as the supply of building blocks holds out. The process is simple but not easy to control.

One of the requisites of a polymerizable compound appears to be the presence of an unsaturated group. Since many of the polymerization resins are derived from ethylene, an ethylene derivative can be used for purposes of illustration:

$$\begin{array}{c} \text{H} \quad \text{H} \\ | \quad\quad | \\ \text{C}=\text{C} \\ | \quad\quad | \\ \text{H} \quad \text{R} \end{array} \qquad\qquad (3)$$

Theoretically, R can be almost any radical that one might choose. For example, it can be hydrogen, and the original ethylene gas can be polymerized under heat and pressure to polyethylene.

**Activation of Polymerization.** The exact mechanism of polymerization reactions is still somewhat obscure, but for the purposes of the present discussion it can be assumed that the reactions are initiated by activated molecules. For example, structure (3) above becomes activated, and the double bonds "open up":

$$\begin{array}{c} \text{H} \quad \text{H} \\ | \quad\quad | \\ -\text{C}-\text{C}- \\ | \quad\quad | \\ \text{H} \quad \text{R} \end{array} \qquad\qquad (4)$$

This activated molecule then "collides" with another molecule, and the second molecule becomes activated:

$$\begin{array}{ccccc} \text{H} \ \text{H} & & \text{H} \ \text{H} & & \text{H} \ \text{H} \ \text{H} \ \text{H} \\ | \ | & & | \ | & & | \ | \ | \ | \\ -\text{C}-\text{C}- & + & \text{C}=\text{C}- & \rightarrow & -\text{C}-\text{C}-\text{C}-\text{C}- \\ | \ | & & | \ | & & | \ | \ | \ | \\ \text{H} \ \text{R} & & \text{H} \ \text{R} & & \text{H} \ \text{R} \ \text{H} \ \text{R} \end{array} \qquad (5)$$

The process continues, and the polymer is finally formed:

$$
\begin{array}{c}
\text{H} \quad \text{H} \quad \text{H} \quad \text{H} \quad \text{H} \quad \text{H} \quad \text{H} \quad \text{H} \quad \text{H} \quad \text{H} \\
| \quad | \quad | \quad | \quad | \quad | \quad | \quad | \quad | \quad | \\
\cdots - \text{C} - \text{C} - \text{C} - \text{C} - \text{C} - \text{C} - \text{C} - \text{C} - \text{C} - \text{C} - \cdots \\
| \quad | \quad | \quad | \quad | \quad | \quad | \quad | \quad | \quad | \\
\text{H} \quad \text{R} \quad \text{H} \quad \text{R} \quad \text{H} \quad \text{R} \quad \text{H} \quad \text{R} \quad \text{H} \quad \text{R}
\end{array} \qquad (6)
$$

The polymerization can be pictured as a series of chain reactions such as takes place during an explosion. The process occurs very rapidly, almost instantaneously. The reactions are exothermic, and considerable heat is evolved.

The polymerization procedure outlined above demonstrates the formation of the simplest of all polymers, the *linear polymer* in which the structural units are connected one to another in linear sequence. It might be represented simply by the type formula:[3]

$$
\text{M}' - \left[ - \text{M} - \right]_{x-2} \text{M}'' \qquad (7)
$$

where the principal structural unit is represented by M and x is the degree of polymerization. The *terminal* units are M' and M''. All structural units except the terminal ones must be bivalent.

The structural units of the polymer may be connected together in a manner as to form a *nonlinear* or *branched* polymer. In this type some of the structural units must possess a valence greater than two. A typical branched polymer in which the branching unit is represented by Y might be indicated by:

$$
\begin{array}{c}
\text{M}' \\
| \\
\text{M} \\
| \\
\text{M} \\
| \\
\text{M}' - \text{M} - \text{M} - \text{Y} - \text{M} - \text{M} - \text{Y} - \text{M} - \cdots \\
| \\
\text{M} \\
| \\
\text{M} \\
| \\
\cdots - \text{M} - \text{Y} - \text{M} - \cdots
\end{array} \qquad (8)
$$

Highly ramified molecular structures may then be formed by further propagation of the branched structure.

The original activation of the monomer molecules can be effected by ultraviolet light and other active rays, heat, or by an energy transfer from another activated compound, such as a catalyst or accelerator. Since the last-named method is the one employed in dentistry, it will be discussed at length.

The activation of the ethylene derivative (3) above by another activated compound $R_1 \cdot$* can be written as follows:

$$
\begin{array}{c}
\text{H} \quad \text{H} \qquad\qquad \text{H} \quad \text{H} \\
| \quad | \qquad\qquad | \quad | \\
R_1 \cdot + \text{C} = \text{C} \rightarrow R_1 - \text{C} - \text{C} \cdot \\
| \quad | \qquad\qquad | \quad | \\
\text{H} \quad \text{R} \qquad\qquad \text{H} \quad \text{R}
\end{array} \qquad (9)
$$

* Represents the activated condition.

or if M represents $\begin{matrix} H & H \\ | & | \\ C & = & C \\ | & | \\ H & R \end{matrix}$ the reactions can be diagrammed as follows:

$$R_1 \cdot + M \rightarrow R_1M \cdot \qquad (9')$$

The reaction then progresses:

$$\begin{aligned} R_1M \cdot \quad + M &\rightarrow R_1MM \cdot \\ R_1MM \cdot + M &\rightarrow R_1MMM \cdot \\ R_1M_{n-1} \cdot + M &\rightarrow R_1M_n \cdot \end{aligned} \qquad (10)$$

where $n$ is any integral number.

It should be noted that the activating chemical $R_1$ is not a catalyst, as the latter term is usually defined, since it definitely enters into the chemical reaction and becomes part of the final chemical compound. It probably might better be termed an *initiator*.[7]

This method of polymerization then is dependent upon the formation of *free radicals*. A free radical is a compound with an unpaired electron, usually a fragment of a larger molecule which has been split by heating.[8] This unpaired electron makes the radical very reactive. The conventional symbol C=C, of course, represents two pairs of electrons. When a free radical encounters a double bond, it may pair with one of the electrons in the extra bond, leaving the other member of the pair free. Thus the monomer itself then becomes a free radical.

A number of substances capable of generating free radicals are potent accelerators for the polymerization of poly(methyl methacrylate) resins. The most commonly employed is benzoyl peroxide which decomposes at relatively low temperatures to release free radicals. Other aromatic peroxides, particularly *p*-chlorobenzoyl peroxide, are especially suitable for the auto-polymer systems.[9]

The decomposition of benzoyl peroxide, between 50° and 100° C., may be represented as:

$$(R\text{-}COO)_2 \longrightarrow 2R\text{-}COO \cdot \longrightarrow 2R \cdot + CO_2$$

where $R \cdot$ is the usual symbol for the activated condition.

**Stages in Polymerization.**   The polymerization process can be described as occuring in four stages: (1) initiation, (2) propagation, (3) termination, and (4) chain transfer.

*Initiation.*   The initiation or induction period is the time during which the molecules of the initiator become energized or activated and start to transfer their energy to the monomer molecules. This period is greatly influenced by the purity of the monomer. Any impurities present which can react with the activated groups can increase the length of this period. The higher the temperature, the shorter is the length of the initiation period.

The initiation energy for the activation of each monomer molecular unit is given as 16,000 to 29,000 calories per mol in the liquid phase.[10]

*Propagation.* The propagation reactions are illustrated by reactions (9) and (10) above. Since only 5000 to 8000 calories per mol are required once the growth has started, the process continues with considerable velocity. Theoretically the chain reactions should continue, with the evolution of heat, until all of the monomer has been changed to polymer. Actually the polymerization is never complete.

*Termination.* The chain reactions can be terminated either by direct coupling or by the exchange of a hydrogen atom from one growing chain to another.

The termination by direct coupling can be illustrated in terms of the diagrammatic reaction (10) above. Let $R_1M_n$ represent a polymer of $n$ monomer units, and $R_1M_m$ signify a polymer of $m$ monomer units. Then:

or
$$R_1M_n\cdot + R_1M_m\cdot \rightarrow R_1M_{m+n}$$
$$R_1M_n\cdot + R_1M_m\cdot \rightarrow R_1M_n + R_1M_m \tag{11}$$

In other words, both molecules become deactivated by an exchange of energy.

Another means by which such an energy exchange can be effected is by the exchange of a hydrogen atom, for example:

$$R_1M_n{-}\underset{\underset{H}{|}}{\overset{\overset{H}{|}}{C}}{-}\underset{\underset{R}{|}}{\overset{\overset{H}{|}}{C}}\cdot + R_1M_m{-}\underset{\underset{H}{|}}{\overset{\overset{H}{|}}{C}}{-}\underset{\underset{R}{|}}{\overset{\overset{H}{|}}{C}}\cdot \longrightarrow R_1M_n{-}\underset{}{\overset{\overset{H}{|}}{C}}{=}\underset{\underset{R}{|}}{\overset{\overset{H}{|}}{C}} + R_1M_m{-}\underset{\underset{H}{|}}{\overset{\overset{H}{|}}{C}}{-}\underset{\underset{R}{|}}{\overset{\overset{H}{|}}{C}}{-}H \tag{12}$$

where $R_1M$ and R have the same significance as in reaction (9′) above. As before, $m$ and $n$ represent numbers of monomer molecules linked in the chain.

*Chain Transfer.* Although chain termination can result from *chain transfer*, the process differs from the termination reactions described in that the active state is transferred from an activated radical to an inactive molecule, and a new nucleus for further growth is created.

For example, a monomer molecule may be activated by a growing macromolecule in such a manner that termination occurs in the latter:

$$R_1M_n{-}\underset{\underset{H}{|}}{\overset{\overset{H}{|}}{C}}{-}\underset{\underset{R}{|}}{\overset{\overset{H}{|}}{C}}\cdot + \underset{\underset{H}{|}}{\overset{\overset{H}{|}}{C}}{=}\underset{\underset{R}{|}}{\overset{\overset{H}{|}}{C}} \longrightarrow R_1M_n{-}\underset{}{\overset{\overset{H}{|}}{C}}{=}\underset{\underset{H}{|}}{\overset{\overset{H}{|}}{C}} + H{-}\underset{\underset{H}{|}}{\overset{\overset{H}{|}}{C}}{-}\underset{\underset{R}{|}}{\overset{\overset{H}{|}}{C}}\cdot \tag{13}$$

Thus, a new nucleus for growth results.

In the same manner, an already terminated chain might be reactivated by chain transfer, and continue to grow:

$$R_1M_m{-}\underset{\underset{H}{|}}{\overset{\overset{H}{|}}{C}}{-}\underset{\underset{R}{|}}{\overset{\overset{H}{|}}{C}}\cdot + R_1M_n{-}\underset{}{\overset{\overset{H}{|}}{C}}{=}\underset{\underset{R}{|}}{\overset{\overset{H}{|}}{C}} \longrightarrow R_1M_m{-}\underset{}{\overset{\overset{H}{|}}{C}}{=}\underset{\underset{R}{|}}{\overset{\overset{H}{|}}{C}} + R_1M_n{-}\underset{\underset{H}{|}}{\overset{\overset{H}{|}}{C}}{-}\underset{\underset{R}{|}}{\overset{\overset{H}{|}}{C}}\cdot \tag{14}$$

**Inhibition of Polymerization.** As noted in the previous section, the polymerization reactions are not likely to result in a complete exhaustion of the monomer, nor do they always form polymers of high molecular weight. Impurities in the monomer often inhibit such reactions.

Any impurity in the monomer which can react with free radicals will inhibit or retard the polymerization reaction. It can react either with the activated initiator or any activated nucleus, or with an activated growing chain to prevent further growth. The presence of such inhibitors influences the length of the initiation period markedly, as well as the degree of polymerization.

For example, the addition of hydroquinone in small amount to the monomer will inhibit polymerization if no initiator chemical is present, and it will definitely retard the polymerization in the presence of an initiator. With hydroquinone and quinone inhibitors (*e.g.*, benzoquinone), the initiation period is directly proportional to the amount of inhibitor added.[11, 12]

The presence of oxygen often causes a retardation of the polymerization, since the oxygen can react with the free radicals. It has been shown that the reaction velocity and the degree of the polymerization are less if the polymerization is accomplished in the open air in comparison to the higher values obtained when the reaction is carried on in a sealed tube,[12] for example. The influence of oxygen on polymerization is governed by many factors, such as concentration of oxygen, temperature, and light.[3]

It is common commercial practice to add a small amount (approximately 0.006 per cent) of hydroquinone to the monomer in order to aid in the prevention of polymerization during storage.

**Copolymerization.** When two or more monomers are mixed, it is possible that the polymer formed may contain units of all of the monomers originally present. Such a polymer is called a *copolymer* and its process of formation is known as *copolymerization*.

Copolymerization is best illustrated with two monomers, although it is possible to have more than two monomers involved. For example, two monomers consisting of ethylene derivatives might possess the following structural formulas:

$$
\begin{array}{cc}
\begin{array}{c}
\text{H} \quad \text{H} \\
| \quad\; | \\
\text{C}=\text{C} \\
| \quad\; | \\
\text{H} \quad \text{R}_2
\end{array}
& (15)
\end{array}
\qquad
\begin{array}{cc}
\begin{array}{c}
\text{H} \quad \text{H} \\
| \quad\; | \\
\text{C}=\text{C} \\
| \quad\; | \\
\text{H} \quad \text{R}_3
\end{array}
& (16)
\end{array}
$$

where $R_2$ and $R_3$ are two different radicals. It is conceivable that after the polymerization in the usual manner the following copolymer might result:

$$\ldots-\overset{\overset{\displaystyle H}{|}}{\underset{\underset{\displaystyle H}{|}}{C}}-\overset{\overset{\displaystyle H}{|}}{\underset{\underset{\displaystyle R_2}{|}}{C}}-\overset{\overset{\displaystyle H}{|}}{\underset{\underset{\displaystyle H}{|}}{C}}-\overset{\overset{\displaystyle H}{|}}{\underset{\underset{\displaystyle R_3}{|}}{C}}-\overset{\overset{\displaystyle H}{|}}{\underset{\underset{\displaystyle H}{|}}{C}}-\overset{\overset{\displaystyle H}{|}}{\underset{\underset{\displaystyle R_2}{|}}{C}}-\overset{\overset{\displaystyle H}{|}}{\underset{\underset{\displaystyle H}{|}}{C}}-\overset{\overset{\displaystyle H}{|}}{\underset{\underset{\displaystyle R_3}{|}}{C}}-\ldots \quad (17)$$

The copolymer structure shown in equation (17) is, however, highly idealized, since the occurrence of alternately placed radicals in the chain would seldom occur. It is more likely that their position will be at random—a matter of probability.

As a matter of fact, the composition of the copolymer seldom corresponds to the composition of the original monomer mixture. If the monomer given in formula (15) above is designated as *A*, and if the formula given in (16) is called *B*, then the composition of the copolymer will depend upon the relative reactivities of the different molecules and the molecules of the same composition. For example, if the tendency of monomer *A* to polymerize is so great that it polymerizes independently of *B*, no copolymerization will occur, and the resulting resin will be a mixture of two polymers. Such a condition seldom or never occurs. On the other hand, *A* and *B* may exhibit a greater tendency to polymerize together than to polymerize separately. In such a case, all of the monomers present might enter into the copolymer with no independent polymerization taking place.

In the majority of cases, the final resin consists of a mixture of polymers and copolymers with varying degrees of polymerization or copolymerization. Not all monomers will copolymerize sufficiently for practical purposes, and therefore every combination must be tried before the results can be known. Nevertheless, copolymerization may alter the physical properties of the resulting resin considerably from those of the resins formed individually from the monomers involved. Many useful resins are manufactured by copolymerization. The effect of copolymerizing is often compared to the alloying of metals by the metallurgist to produce useful metals of different properties.

Methyl methacrylate and acrylic and methacrylic esters all copolymerize readily, with little inhibition between monomer pairs. For example, small amounts of ethyl acrylate may be copolymerized with methyl methacrylate to alter the flexibility of the denture.

*Cross-linkage.* Formation of chemical bonds between linear polymer molecules, commonly referred to as *cross-linking*, can also lead to infinite networks of molecules. Vulcanite, through the action of sulfur and other chemicals, is an excellent example of a process of this type. Generally speaking, cross-linkage provides a sufficient number of cross-links, or bridges, between the linear macromolecules to form a three-dimensional network that alters the solubility, strength, and water sorption of the resin. For example, cross-linkage has been made use of widely in the manufacture of acrylic teeth in order to increase their craze resistance. It will be recalled that the soluble alginate molecules became cross-linked to form the gel network in the gelation reaction. Also, cross-linkage occurs during the heat vulcanization of silicone rubber (page 114).

**Plasticizers.**     Plasticizers are often added to resins to reduce their softening or fusion temperatures. For example, it is possible to plasticize a resin which is normally hard and stiff at room temperature to a condition where it is flexible and soft. Plastic handbags, raincoats, etc., are often made from resins of this type. Often the plasticizer is added in relatively smaller amounts than would appreciably affect the flexibility of the resin at normal room temperatures. Although the softening temperature of the resin is somewhat reduced, in the case of dental resins, the function of the plasticizer is to increase the solubility of the polymer in the monomer.

The action of the plasticizer is the partial neutralization of the secondary valence bonds or intermolecular forces which normally prevent the resin molecules from slipping past one another when the material is stressed. Its action may be considered analogous to that of a solvent, since it penetrates between the macromolecules. It is usually an insoluble high-boiling compound. Its molecular attraction to the polymer should be extremely great so that it will not volatilize or otherwise leach out during the fabrication or the subsequent use of the resin. Since such a condition is seldom completely realized in practice, plasticizers are used sparingly in dental resins.

As might be expected from the theory, plasticizers usually reduce the strength and hardness of the resin, as well as the softening point.

### TYPES OF RESINS

As previously mentioned, in order for a synthetic resin to be useful in dentistry it must exhibit exceptional qualities in regard to its chemical and dimensional stability, and yet it must possess properties which render it relatively easy to process, strong, hard, and not brittle. A few resins of possible interest to the dentist will now be studied.

**Vinyl Resins.**[13]     Like most polymerization resins, the vinyl resins are derivatives of ethylene. Ethylene ($CH_2{=}CH_2$) is a simple molecule yet it is this monomer which has made possible a great bulk of the present polymer derivatives. At elevated temperatures, it is believed that the ethylene reacts with oxygen to form a peroxide, which then decomposes into a free radical and initiates polymerization.

Two of the derivatives of ethylene of special interest are, vinyl chloride:

$$\begin{array}{cc} H & H \\ | & | \\ C & = C \\ | & | \\ H & Cl \end{array} \qquad (18)$$

and vinyl acetate:

$$
\begin{array}{cc}
H & H \\
| & | \\
C & = C \\
| & | \\
H & O \\
& | \\
& C=O \\
& | \\
H & - C - H \\
& | \\
& H
\end{array}
\tag{19}
$$

Vinyl chloride polymerizes in the usual manner to form poly(vinyl chloride):

$$
\cdots - C - C - C - C - C - C - \cdots
\tag{20}
$$

Vinyl acetate forms poly(vinyl acetate) on polymerization:

$$
\cdots - C - C - C - C - C - C - \cdots
\tag{21}
$$

Poly(vinyl chloride) is a clear, hard resin, which is tasteless and odorless. It darkens when exposed to ultraviolet light and, unless it is plasticized, it discolors when it is heated near its softening point for molding purposes.

On the other hand, the poly(vinyl acetate) is light- and heat-stable, but it exhibits an abnormally low softening point ($35°$ to $40°$ C.). When monomers of vinyl chloride and vinyl acetate are copolymerized in varying proportions, many useful copolymer resins result. A copolymer of approximate composition vinyl chloride 80 per cent and vinyl acetate 20 per cent was once used for the construction of denture bases. The resin was excellent for this purpose in every respect, except that the molecular weight distribution could not be controlled.[14] The average molecular weight was so high that the molding temperature employed was not sufficient to soften the resin thoroughly during molding. As a result, many permanent stresses and strains were induced. Instead of being released by relaxation, the stresses acted to reduce the endurance limit of the resin, and the dentures fractured along the midline of the anterior ridge and palate region after they had been in service for a time.

**Polystyrene.** When a benzene radical is attached the vinyl grouping, styrene, or vinyl benzene, results:

$$
\begin{array}{c}
\text{H} \quad \text{H} \\
| \qquad | \\
\text{C}{=}\text{C} \\
| \qquad | \\
\text{H} \quad \text{C}_6\text{H}_5
\end{array}
\tag{22}
$$

Such a monomer polymerizes to polystyrene (polyvinyl benzene) by addition in the regular manner:

$$
\cdots\cdots{-}\overset{\displaystyle\text{H}}{\underset{\displaystyle\text{H}}{\text{C}}}{-}\overset{\displaystyle\text{H}}{\underset{\displaystyle\text{C}_6\text{H}_5}{\text{C}}}{-}{-}\overset{\displaystyle\text{H}}{\underset{\displaystyle\text{H}}{\text{C}}}{-}\overset{\displaystyle\text{H}}{\underset{\displaystyle\text{C}_6\text{H}_5}{\text{C}}}{-}{-}\overset{\displaystyle\text{H}}{\underset{\displaystyle\text{H}}{\text{C}}}{-}\overset{\displaystyle\text{H}}{\underset{\displaystyle\text{C}_6\text{H}_5}{\text{C}}}{-}\cdots\cdots
\tag{23}
$$

Polystyrene is a clear resin of the thermoplastic type. It is stable to light and many chemical reagents, although it is soluble in certain organic solvents. It is being used for the construction of denture bases to a limited extent.

It can be copolymerized with a number of resins. Its copolymer with divinyl benzene is of interest in that a cross-linked polymer is formed. For example, as little as one mol of *p*-divinyl benzene copolymerized with 40,000 mols of styrene results in a cross-linked polymer which is insoluble and infusible.[15]

**Acrylic Resins.** The acrylic resins are derivatives of ethylene, and contain a vinyl group in their structural formula. There are at least two acrylic resin series which are of dental interest. One series is derived from acrylic acid, $CH_2{=}CHCOOH$, and the other from methacrylic acid, $CH_2{=}C(CH_3)COOH$. Both of these compounds polymerize by addition in the usual manner.

Although the polyacids are hard and transparent, their polarity, caused by the carboxyl group, causes them to imbibe water. The water tends to separate the chains and to cause a general softening and loss of strength. Consequently, they are not used in the mouth.

The esters of these polyacids are, however, of considerable dental interest. For example, if R represents any ester radical, the formula for a polymethacrylate would be:

$$
\tag{24}
$$

When it is realized that theoretically R can be almost any organic or inorganic radical, it is evident that thousands of different acrylic resins are capable of formation. Such a consideration does not include the possibilities of copolymerization, which are also very great.

*Table 10–1.*     *Softening Temperatures of Polymethacrylate Esters*

| POLYMETHACRYLATE | SOFTENING POINT (°C.) |
|---|---|
| Methyl | 125 |
| Ethyl | 65 |
| *n*-Propyl | 38 |
| Isopropyl | 95 |
| *n*-Butyl | 33 |
| Isobutyl | 70 |
| *sec*-Butyl | 62 |
| *tert*-Amyl | 76 |
| Phenyl | 120 |

The effect of esterification on the softening point for a few of the polymethacrylate compounds[16] is shown in Table 10–1. The softening point is often expressed as the $T_g$ value.[3] $T_g$ is the transition point to a glass or, more simply, it is the approximate temperature at which the polymer changes from a hard and more or less brittle material to a "rubbery" or liquid one. This temperature range is invariably quite narrow for the amorphous polymers such as the poly(methyl methacrylates).

Generally, until the side chain becomes quite long, the longer the side chain, the lower is the softening temperature. For example, poly (methyl methacrylate) is the hardest resin of the series presented, with the highest softening temperature. Ethyl methacrylate possesses a lower softening point and surface hardness; *n*-propyl methacrylate is still softer, and so on. If an isomer of a straight chain esterifying agent is used, it is interesting to note that the softening temperature is increased above that of the normal straight chain compound. For example, the softening temperature of poly(isopropyl methacrylate) is greater than that of poly(ethyl methacrylate), yet the softening temperature of poly(*n*-propyl methacrylate) is only 38° C. (Table 10–1). As the molecular weight of the straight chain alkyl groups increases further, the softening point continues to decrease until the liquid state is attained at room temperature. For example, poly(dodecyl methacrylate) [monomer, $CH_2=C(CH_3)COOC_{12}H_{25}$] is a viscous liquid at room temperature. Some resins, such as addition polymers of isobutylene, may be liquid at temperatures as low as −70° C.

Apparently the effect of esterification with an aromatic alcohol definitely increases the softening point, even though the molecular weights of the aromatic and aliphatic esterifying compounds may be nearly the same; this fact is illustrated by the relatively high softening point of poly(phenyl methacrylate) as given in Table 10–1.

*Methyl Methacrylate.*     Poly(methyl methacrylate) by itself is not used in dentistry to a great extent in molding procedures. Rather, the liquid monomer, methyl methacrylate, is mixed with the polymer which is in the powdered form. The monomer partially dissolves the polymer to form a plastic dough. This dough is packed into the mold, and the monomer is polymerized by one of the methods previously discussed. Consequently, the monomer, methyl methacrylate, is of considerable importance in dentistry.

Methyl methacrylate[16] is a clear, transparent liquid at room temperature, which boils at approximately 100.8° C. (213.4° F.). Its melting point is —48° C. (—54.4° F.). Its density is 0.945 grams per cubic centimeter at 20° C. (68° F.). The heat of polymerization is 12.9 K. cal./mol. It exhibits a high vapor pressure, and it is an excellent organic solvent. Although the polymerization of methyl methacrylate can be initiated by ultraviolet light or heat, it is commonly polymerized in dentistry by the use of a chemical initiator as previously described.

The conditions for the polymerization of methyl methacrylate are not critical, provided that the reaction is not carried out at a too rapid rate. The degree of polymerization will vary with the conditions of polymerization such as the temperature, method of activation, type of initiator used and its concentration, purity of chemicals, and similar factors. A volume shrinkage of 21 per cent occurs during the polymerization of the pure monomer.

*Poly(Methyl Methacrylate).* Poly(methyl methacrylate) is a transparent resin of remarkable clarity; it transmits light into the ultraviolet range to a wave length of $0.25\mu$. It is a hard resin with a Knoop Hardness Number of 18 to 20. Its tensile strength is approximately 600 kilograms per square centimeter (8500 pounds per square inch), and its density is 1.19 grams per cubic centimeter. Its modulus of elasticity is approximately 24,400 kilograms per square centimeter (350,000 pounds per square inch).

The resin is extremely stable; it will not discolor in ultraviolet light, and it exhibits remarkable aging properties. It is stable chemically to heat; it will soften at 125° C. (260° F.), and it can be molded as a thermoplastic material. Between this temperature and 200° C. (400° F.), depolymerization takes place. At approximately 450° C. (850° F.), 90 per cent of the polymer will depolymerize to the monomer. When the polymer has a molecular weight above 650,000, it will degrade to a lower polymer at the same time that it evolves monomer.

Poly(methyl methacrylate), in common with the acrylic resins, exhibits a tendency to retain water either by imbibition or surface absorption. Since both absorption and adsorption are involved, the term *sorption* is usually used to include the total phenomenon. It has been reported that typical dental methacrylate resins show an increase of approximately 0.5 per cent by weight after one week in water.[17, 18] Higher values have been reported[19] for a series of methyl methacrylate polymers. The sorption of water is nearly independent of temperature from 0 to 60° C. but is markedly affected by the molecular weight of the polymer. The greater the molecular weight, the smaller is the weight increase. Sorption is reversible if the resin is dried.

Since it is a chain polymer, it can be expected that it will be soluble in a number of organic solvents, such as chloroform and acetone.[17]

*Epoxy Resins.* Another resin family of recent interest to dentistry is the epoxy resin. These thermosetting resins may be cured at room temperature and possess unique characteristics in terms of adhesion to various metals, wood and glass, chemical stability, and strength.[20]

The epoxy-resin molecule[21] is characterized by the reactive epoxy or ethoxyline groups:

$$\underset{-C\!-\!\!-\!\!-\!\!-\!\!-C-}{\overset{\displaystyle O}{\triangle}}$$

which serve as terminal polymerization points. In this group, the ring is in a somewhat unstable condition and prone to open and combine with compounds having an available hydrogen. Cross-linkage is easily accomplished.

In its simplest form the epoxy molecule is represented by the diglycidyl ether of bisphenol A:

$$CH_2\text{———}CH\text{—}CH_2\text{—}O\text{—}\bigcirc\text{—}\underset{CH_3}{\overset{CH_3}{C}}\text{—}\bigcirc\text{—}O\text{—}CH_2\text{—}CH\text{———}CH_2$$

The epoxy resin, which is often a viscous liquid at room temperature, may be cured by use of a reactive intermediate to join the resin chains. The primary cross-linking agents are polyfunctional primary and secondary amines, such as diethylene triamine, $\underset{H}{\overset{H}{\diagdown}}N\text{—}R'$.

Other agents such as polybasic acids, boron trifluoride[22] and certain anhydrides may also be employed although the amines are the most common.

Several modified epoxy resins have been introduced as denture base materials.[23] The mixed resin is poured into the flask and a low temperature, 120° F., cure is used. Although certain advantages have been claimed, the problems of color stability and patient sensitivity are still present. Certain of the amine curing agents have been reported as irritating while others seem to be quite mild.[24]

The possible use of an epoxy resin as a restorative material has also been suggested.[25] When fused quartz is used as a filler, the thermal coefficient of expansion can be reduced to a point where it approximates that of the tooth crown. The marked adhesion of this type of resin to the surfaces of most materials suggests the possibility of coordinate or covalent bonding between the resin and the prepared tooth surface. However, such a bond has not as yet been demonstrated.

## Literature

1. Mark, H.: *Intermolecular Forces and Mechanical Behavior of High Polymers.* Ind. Eng. Chem., *34*:1343–1348 (Nov.), 1942.
2. Mark, H. F.: *Giant Molecules.* Scientific American, *197*:80–90 (Sept.), 1957.
3. Flory, P. J.: *Principles of Polymer Chemistry,* Ithaca, Cornell University Press, 1953, pp. 3–56.
4. Konigsberger, C.: *Organic Chemistry,* in Houwink, R.: *Elastomers and Polymers.* New York, Elsevier Publishing Co., Inc., 1950, Vol. I, p. 32.
5. Caul, H. J., and Schoonover, I. C.: *A Method for Determining the Extent of Polymerization of Acrylic Resins and Its Applications for Dentures.* J.A.D.A., *39:* 1–9 (July), 1949.
6. Dean, R. B.: *Modern Colloids.* New York, D. Van Nostrand Co., Inc., 1948, p. 114.
7. Konigsberger, *loc. cit.,* p. 53.
8. Natta, G.: *How Giant Molecules Are Made.* Scientific American, *197*:98–104, (Sept.), 1957.
9. Rose, E. E., Lal, J., and Green, R.: *Effect of Peroxide, Amine and Hydroquinone in Varying Concentrations on the Polymerization Rate of Polymethyl Methacrylate Slurries.* J.A.D.A., *56*:375–381 (March), 1958.
10. Konigsberger, *loc. cit.,* p. 47.
11. Goldfinger, G., Skeist, J., and Mark, H.: *The Mechanism of Inhibition of Styrene Polymerization.* J. Phys. Chem., *47*:578, 1943.
12. Yanagawa, T., and Yoshida, T.: *Organic Glasses: I. Polymerization Velocity of Methyl Methacrylate.* J. Soc. Chem. Ind. (Japan), *45: Suppl. Binding,* 412, 1942.
13. Schildknecht, C. E.: *Vinyl and Related Polymers.* New York, John Wiley & Sons, Inc., 1952.
14. Schoonover, I. C., and Sweeney, W. T.: *Some Properties of Two Types of Resins Used for Dentures.* J.A.D.A., *25*:1487–1500 (Sept.), 1938.
15. Staudinger, H., and Heuer, W.: *Highly Polymerized Compounds. XCIII. The Breaking up of the Molecular Fibers of the Polystyrenes.* Ber., *67*:1164, 1934.
16. Powers, P. O.: *Synthetic Resins and Rubbers.* New York, John Wiley & Sons, Inc., 1943, p. 150.
17. Tylman, S. D., and Peyton, F. A.: *Acrylic and Other Synthetic Resins Used in Dentistry.* Philadelphia, J. B. Lippincott Co., 1946, p. 118.
18. Peyton, F. A., and Mann, W. R.: *Acrylic and Acrylic-Styrene Resins: Their Properties in Relation to Their Uses as Restorative Materials.* J.A.D.A., *29*:1852–1864 (Oct.), 1942.
19. Brauer, G. M., and Sweeney, W. T.: *Sorption of Water by Polymethyl Methacrylate.* Modern Plastics, *32*:138–144 (May), 1955.
20. Shell Chemical Corporation: *Epon 828 in Casting Applications.* Technical Bulletin SC:52–14.
21. Lee, H., and Neville, K.: *Epoxy Resins. Their Application and Technology.* New York, McGraw-Hill Book Co., Inc., 1957, p. 6.
22. Booth, H. S., and Martin, D. R.: *Boron Trifluoride and Its Derivatives.* New York, John Wiley & Sons, Inc., 1949, p. 219.
23. Kydd, W. L., and Wykhuis, W. A.: *A Modified Epoxy Resin as a Denture Base Material.* J.A.D.A., *56*:385–388 (March), 1958.
24. Lea, W. A., Block, W. D., and Cornish, H. H.: *The Irritating and Sensitizing Capacity of Epoxy Resins.* A.M.A. Arch. Dermat., *78*:304–308 (Sept.), 1958.
25. Bowen, R. L.: *Use of Epoxy Resins in Restorative Materials.* J. D. Res., *35*:360–369 (June), 1956.

# CHAPTER 11

# Denture Base Resins:

# Technical Considerations

A complete acrylic denture for the upper mouth is shown in Figure 11–1. The artificial teeth are seated on the *denture base*, the part of the denture which retains the artificial teeth and rests on the soft tissues of the mouth. The denture base resin is tinted to imitate the natural gum tissues as closely as possible.

The better the fit of the denture base, the better will be the retention of the denture in the mouth, and the greater will be the comfort to the patient. Consequently, considerable attention will be given to the discussion of methods of improving the fit and the dimensional stability of the denture. There are, of course, many factors other than the fit of the denture base which determine its efficiency in function, but the fit is basically very important. The maximum biting force of a patient wearing an artificial denture may be only 15 per cent of the force exerted by a person with natural dentition.[1] Thus close adaptation of the denture base to the oral structures is imperative to prevent even further loss of chewing efficiency.

The artificial teeth are constructed either of porcelain or of resin, tinted to simulate the human teeth. Acrylic dentures can often be constructed so lifelike in appearance as to defy detection except by trained observers.

**General Technic.** Considerable discussion of the processing technic will be given in subsequent sections. Briefly, the process consists first of the construction of the base plate in wax on the stone cast. The artificial teeth are then placed in position in the wax.

The cast, with the wax base plate, is seated in freshly mixed dental

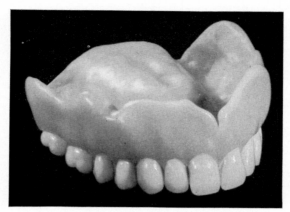

Fig. 11–1.  A complete upper acrylic resin denture.

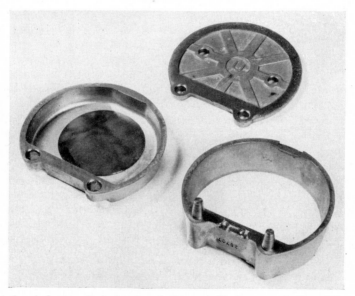

Fig. 11–2.  A denture flask showing the lower half, the upper half, and the cover.

stone or plaster in the lower half of a denture flask. Such a flask is shown in Figure 11–2. It consists of three parts: a lower half, an upper half, and a cover. The three parts fit together accurately when they are placed in contact with each other.

The upper half of the flask is placed in position and is also filled with plaster or stone. The cover is pressed on, and the flask is held under pressure until the stone sets. When the two halves are separated, the teeth will remain in the upper half, since they are retained in the stone or plaster. The wax is removed, and the *mold space* remains in which the denture base material is to be molded. After it has been molded the denture is removed from the flask and finished as shown in Figure 11–1.

The denture base is sometimes cast in metal, but the technic employed is entirely different than that used for the acrylic resin denture base. The metallic denture base materials will be discussed in subsequent chapters.

**Historical.** *Vulcanite.* The search for a satisfactory non-metallic denture base material has been long and arduous.[2] The first non-metallic material used with success was vulcanite (hard rubber). Rubber is an unsaturated polymer of isoprene:

$$\ldots-C=C-C-C-C=C-C-C-C=C-\ldots$$

The rubber was supplied to the dentist in a plastic sheet form, impregnated with sulfur. The plastic sheet was cut up and packed into the mold space. When the material was cured under heat (160° C., or 320° F.) and pressure, the rubber became *vulcanized, i.e.,* the sulfur united with the rubber to produce a saturation of the double bonds. A hard, rigid material resulted which was thermoset by classification.

The vulcanite dentures exhibited excellent fit, dimensional stability, strength and tissue tolerance, but they were totally lacking in esthetic qualities. Hard rubber is definitely opaque to light, and no amount of tinting can produce the translucence so necessary to a successful imitation of the human soft tissue.

Consequently, the search for a denture base material centered around the property of translucence in addition to the usual properties of adequate strength, dimensional stability, etc.[3]

*Cellulose Products.* As early as 1870, cellulose products were tried as denture base materials. They were of two types, cellulose acetate and cellulose nitrate. The denture bases were molded by a thermoplastic process, and, in order to obtain the proper molding plasticity, it was necessary to plasticize the cellulose products considerably. Although the molded product exhibited a lifelike appearance and possessed satisfactory physical properties at the start, it gradually warped and discolored in use. The plasticizers leached out, and in many cases the denture base disintegrated.

It is interesting to note that, in spite of the previous failures with this material, it was again used during and immediately after World War I, with the same disappointing results.

*Phenolic Resins.* The unsuccessful use of the thermosetting phenolic resins ("Bakelite") for denture bases has already been discussed (p. 139). The denture bases made from the phenol-formaldehyde resin gradually discolored during use in the mouth. This discoloration was thought to be due to a chemical instability brought about by an improper curing procedure. Very likely the proper processing of a phenolic resin is too critical for use in the dental laboratory.

*Vinyl Copolymer Resins.* As described on page 146, the vinyl copolymer resins, processed by a thermoplastic method, were unsatisfactory because the degree of polymerization was not adequately controlled in the manufacturing process. The molding temperature employed was too low for a proper molding, and the resulting processing strains produced a low endurance limit. The dentures fractured during service, particularly in the anterior palate region.

*Acrylic Resin.* The modern denture base material is an acrylic resin—poly(methyl methacrylate):

$$\begin{array}{c}
\text{H} \quad \text{CH}_3 \quad \text{H} \quad \text{CH}_3 \quad \text{H} \quad \text{CH}_3 \quad \text{H} \quad \text{CH}_3 \\
| \quad | \quad | \quad | \quad | \quad | \quad | \quad | \\
\cdots -\text{C}-\text{C}-\text{C}-\text{C}-\text{C}-\text{C}-\text{C}-\text{C}- \cdots \\
| \quad | \quad | \quad | \quad | \quad | \quad | \quad | \\
\text{H} \quad \text{C}=\text{O} \quad \text{H} \quad \text{C}=\text{O} \quad \text{H} \quad \text{C}=\text{O} \quad \text{H} \quad \text{C}=\text{O} \\
| \quad \quad | \quad \quad | \quad \quad | \\
\text{O} \quad \quad \text{O} \quad \quad \text{O} \quad \quad \text{O} \\
| \quad \quad | \quad \quad | \quad \quad | \\
\text{CH}_3 \quad \quad \text{CH}_3 \quad \quad \text{CH}_3 \quad \quad \text{CH}_3
\end{array}$$

The resin is transparent. It can be colored or tinted to almost any shade and degree of translucence. Its color and optical properties are stable under all normal conditions, and its strength and other physical properties are adequate. The properties of acrylic resins are not ideal, of course, any more than the properties of any other dental material are ideal. However, it is the combination of desirable characteristics which have made them so acceptable.

One decided advantage of poly(methyl methacrylate) as a denture base material is the ease with which it can be processed in comparison to the other materials used previously. Although poly(methyl methacrylate) is a thermoplastic resin, in dentistry it is not usually molded by thermoplastic means. Rather, the liquid (monomer) methyl methacrylate is mixed with the polymer, which is dispensed in the form of a powder. As will be discussed in detail in a subsequent section, the monomer plasticizes the polymer to a doughlike consistency which can be easily molded initially in the mold space, prepared as previously described. The monomer is subsequently polymerized and the resulting denture base is composed of a solid, homogeneous resin. The polymerization can be effected either by heating the polymer-monomer mixture, usually in a water bath, or by chemical activation at room temperature.

## HEAT-CURING DENTURE BASE ACRYLIC RESINS

**Composition.** The monomer is generally pure methyl methacrylate with a slight amount of hydroquinone (0.006 per cent or less), which aids in the inhibition of polymerization during storage.

The polymer usually consists of a powder composed of small spherical particles, as shown in Figure 11–3. The spheres (*pearls* or *beads*) can be polymerized from monomer which has been heated in some non-polymerizing liquid. For example, the monomer can be dispersed in water by a vigorous stirring; a small amount of benzoyl peroxide is added. As the water is heated, the monomer polymerizes to form the pearls as shown (Fig. 11–3). Usually some inert substances such as talc or gelatin (called *stabilizers*) are added to prevent the cohesion of the pearls as they form.

The composition of the final product is essentially poly(methyl methacrylate). Often, however, a copolymer with some other softer acrylic resin, such as ethyl acrylate ($CH_2=CHCOOC_2H_5$) is produced. The additional resin is usually present in a minor amount. Occasionally the poly(methyl methacrylate) is plasticized with some inert, high-boiling substance such as butyl phthalate [$C_6H_4(COOC_4H_9)_2$]. If the plasticizer content is less than approximately 8 to 10 per cent, the properties of the denture resin are not adversely affected, provided that a proper plasticizing procedure has been followed. The use of too much plasticizer in denture resins, however, may result in deterioration of the resin in the mouth fluids.[4]

The pigment can be incorporated in the pearl during the initial polymerization, or it can be added after the polymerization by an impregnation into the pearls by means of a ball mill, for example. When the latter method is employed, the pigment is ground into the surface of the pearl. The pigment can be seen clinging to some of the polymer particles in Figure 11–4. The unpigmented pearls are part of the transparent powder which has been blended with the pigmented material to produce the proper shade.

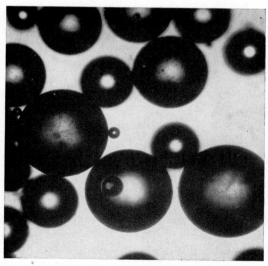

Fig. 11–3. Polymer pearls, high-lighted to show detail. The pearls are actually transparent.

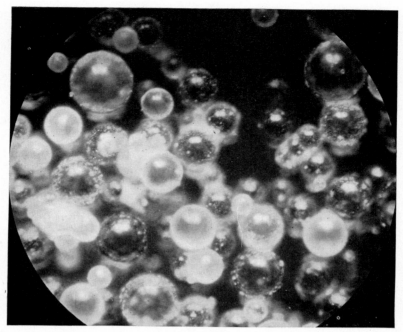

Fig. 11–4. Polymer particles with coloring pigment clinging to some of the pearls. The unpigmented clear pearls are blended with the pigmented particles to provide the proper shade. (McLean, *Dental Practitioner*, Feb., 1951.)

Most modern acrylic resin denture base materials contain a cross-linking agent such as glycol dimethacrylate:

$$CH_3—C—C—O—CH_2—CH_2—O—C—C—CH_3$$

This chemical contains two polymerizable bonds, and it can cross-link with other groups in at least two directions when it is polymerized. When it is used as a copolymer with methyl methacrylate, a more insoluble and infusible resin results compared to the similar properties of poly(methyl methacrylate) alone. The cross-linking agent is incorporated in the monomer, about 1 to 2 per cent in amount.

Usually the monomer and the polymer are combined immediately before the mixture is to be placed in the denture mold. However, the polymer and monomer can be pre-mixed by the manufacturer and supplied to the dentist in the form of a flexible sheet or gel, ready to be packed into the mold. Unfortunately, in spite of the added inhibitor, the pre-mixed material may harden in its container during storage and, therefore, it possesses a short shelf life.

At least one denture resin is dispensed in the gel form exclusively.

This particular material contains vinyl resin in addition to poly (methyl methacrylate). Instead of the employment of poly (methyl methacrylate) for the solid component of the monomer-polymer mixture, a copolymer of vinyl chloride and vinyl acetate is used. The vinyl copolymer is processed to a plastic gel by saturation with methyl methacrylate monomer. The resulting gel is packed into the mold space and the resin is polymerized by heat in the usual manner. The resulting resin is a mixture of methyl methacrylate and (predominantly) vinyl copolymer resin.

Polystyrene is sometimes used to process denture bases. A cylinder of polystyrene of the proper molecular weight distribution is softened under heat and forced into the mold space under pressure by a process known as *injection molding*. In other words, advantage is taken of the thermoplastic property of the resin.

Because most of the denture resins are acrylic resins and are supplied in the form of a powder (polymer) and a liquid (monomer), the technic employed with this type of resin will be discussed in detail.

**Preparation of the Mold.** As previously noted, the stone cast with the wax base plate and teeth in position is embedded in some type of an investing medium (either plaster or, preferably, stone) in the lower half of the flask. After the investing material hardens, it is coated with some type of *separating medium* so that the stone or plaster mixture to be poured into the upper half of the flask will not adhere to that in the lower half.

After the investing material has set in the top half, the flask is heated sufficiently to soften the wax, and then the halves are separated. The wax is completely removed from the mold. Any residual wax is flushed out with boiling water containing an ordinary household detergent in proportions of 1 tablespoonful to 1 pint of water.[5]

During its processing, the resin must be carefully protected from the gypsum surfaces in the mold space for two reasons: (1) Any water incorporated into the resin from the gypsum during processing will definitely affect the polymerization rate and the color of the resin. The denture produced will craze readily because of the stresses formed by the evaporation of water after the processing, particularly if the resin is not cross-linked. (2) Dissolved polymer and free monomer must be prevented from soaking into the mold surface. If any liquid resin penetrates into the investing medium, portions of the gypsum material will be joined to the denture after polymerization with the result that it will be virtually impossible to separate the investing material from the resin.

**Monomer-Polymer Ratio.** Although it is not critical, the proper ratio of monomer and polymer may be of considerable importance to the structure of the final resin[6] in many instances. In general, the more polymer used, the less will be the reaction time of the polymer and

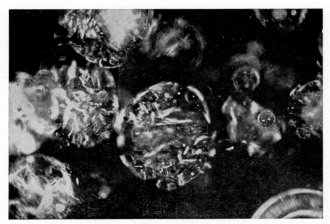

Fig. 11–5. The outer layer of the polymer pearl, saturated with monomer, is slough-ing off and dissolving in the surrounding monomer. (Courtesy of H. M. Vernon.)

monomer. Furthermore, the resin will tend to shrink less during proc-essing if less monomer is used.

However, sufficient monomer must be employed to wet each polymer pearl thoroughly. In order to obtain the proper proportions, it has been suggested[6] that the liquid be placed in a mixing jar, and that the powder be added until all of the liquid is taken up by the powder. The mixing jar is then tapped or vibrated to bring any excess monomer to the surface, and more polymer is added until the liquid is saturated. The approximate proportions of polymer to monomer are generally three to one by volume or two to one by weight.

**Monomer-Polymer Reaction.** The function of the monomer in the polymer is to produce a plastic mass which can be packed into the mold. Such a plasticization is accomplished by a partial solution of the poly-mer in the monomer. No polymerization is expected to occur at this stage.[7]

At least four stages can be identified during the reaction of the powder and liquid:

*Stage 1.* The polymer gradually settles into the monomer and a somewhat fluid, incoherent mass is formed.

*Stage 2.* The monomer attacks the polymer. This is accomplished by the penetration of the monomer into the polymer; the layer of polymer so penetrated sloughs off and either goes into solution or is dispersed in the monomer. The photomicrograph shown in Figure 11–5 pictures such an attack on the polymer by the monomer. The layer of polymer containing the monomer is tacky, and this stage is characterized by a stringiness if the mixture is touched or pulled apart.

*Stage 3.* As the monomer diffuses into the polymer, and the mass becomes more saturated with polymer in solution, it becomes smooth

*Table 11–1.* *Influence of Monomer-Polymer Ratio on the Time to Reach the Dough Stage**

| POWDER (GRAMS PER 10 CC. OF LIQUID) | TIME TO REACH THE GEL STAGE (MIN.) |
|---|---|
| 15 | 100 |
| 20 | 52 |
| 25 | 33 |
| 30 | 12 |

* Peyton, *J.A.D.A.* May, 1950.

and doughlike. It is no longer tacky, and it does not adhere to the walls of the mixing jar. It consists of undissolved polymer particles suspended in a plastic matrix of polymer dissolved or dispersed in the monomer. This stage is often called the *dough* or the *gel stage*. While the mixture is in this stage it is packed into the mold.

*Stage 4.* The monomer seemingly disappears, by evaporation and by further penetration into the polymer. The mass becomes more cohesive and rubber-like. It is no longer plastic, and it cannot be molded by the methods used in dentistry.

**Dough-forming Time.** Different powders require different lengths of time to reach the dough stage (stage 3). As previously stated, the more monomer used, the longer will be the time required. However, as can be noted from the results[6] presented in Table 11–1, the time to reach the dough stage is by no means in direct proportion to the amount of monomer used with a given amount of polymer.

The higher the temperature of the mixing jar, the shorter will be the time from the start of mixing to the formation of the dough. If the dough-forming time is impractically long, the mixing jar may be heated in warm water, provided that moisture is not allowed to contact the resin. Under no circumstances should the jar be heated above approximately 55° C. (130° F.), since polymerization accelerates at a temperature slightly above this temperature. The disadvantage of heating the mixture is that the working time, or the time that the material remains in the dough stage, is shortened.

The degree of polymerization of the polymer powder used greatly affects the rate of solution of the polymer in the monomer. In general, the higher the molecular weight of the polymer, the longer the dough-forming time will be. Often a powder consisting of a blend of various molecular weights is employed in order to shorten the monomer-polymer reaction time, and at the same time to maintain to a considerable extent the physical properties contributed by the high molecular weight portion.

As previously mentioned, the polymer powder may be a copolymer of methyl methacrylate with a small amount of other more soluble acrylic resins. For example, poly(ethyl acrylate) is more soluble in methyl methacrylate than is poly(methyl methacrylate). Consequently, the solubility of the powder can be increased by a copolymerization with ethyl acrylate.

The solubility can also be increased by the addition of a plasticizer. In fact, the dough-forming time can be reduced by an increase in the solubility of the polymer in the monomer regardless of the means employed.

Another factor which influences the dough-forming time is the size of the polymer particles. Since more area is presented for solution, the smaller the particle size of the polymer, the more rapid is the solution of the polymer in the monomer, and the shorter the dough-forming period. However, this factor is apt to be of minor importance in comparison to some of the other factors mentioned.

According to the American Dental Association Specification No. 12 for denture base resin, stage 3 must be attained in at least 20 minutes from the start of mixing at a mixing temperature of 23° C. (73.4° F.).

**Working Time.** The *working time* is the time elapsing between stage 2 and stage 4, or, in other words, the time that the material remains in the dough form. According to the American Dental Association Specification No. 12, the dough should be moldable for at least 5 minutes.

As already indicated, the working time is affected by the temperature; the lower the temperature, the longer is the working time. Some commercial denture resins can be preserved in a moldable condition in a refrigerator for many hours. An objection to such a storage is that unless special precautions are taken, moisture condensation on the resin occurs when the material is removed from the refrigerator for use, and moisture contamination results.

There are a number of methods for increasing the time of the dough stage at room temperature. For example, it can be reasoned that a blend of molecular weights might prolong such a stage; the lower molecular weight fraction might conceivably result in an early dough stage, and as the monomer diffuses more slowly into the pearls of higher molecular weight, the dough stage might be prolonged.

**Trial Closure.** It is very important that the mold be filled properly at the time the resin is polymerized; consequently the mold is packed with dough in several stages.

At the time the resin dough is inserted in the mold, the temperature of the latter should not be higher than 55° C. (130° F.) in order to prevent excessive evaporation of the monomer. Also the resin may start to polymerize when it comes in contact with the mold. The stiffer resin then will not flow readily during trial packing and may even distort the mold. A mold at room temperature is preferable, since the working time will be longer at the lower temperature.

The resin is rolled into a ropelike mass, bent into a horseshoe shape and placed in the upper half of the flask as shown in Figure 11–6. A piece of thin polyethylene or water-saturated cellulose sheet is placed over the resin and the mold space. The purpose of such a sheet is to prevent the adhesion of the resin to the lower mold surface when the two halves of the flask are pressed together.

When the lower half is pressed against the upper half, it is very important that the pressure be applied slowly so that the dough will be spread evenly throughout the mold space. When further application of pressure meets with considerable resistance, the two halves are separated. If too much material has been placed in the mold, it will be found to have overflowed onto the *land* surrounding the mold space, as shown in Figure 11–7. The excess material is called the *flash*. If a flash does not occur, it is possible that there was insufficient dough in the mold at the start; consequently, more resin is added, and the process is repeated.

The flash is carefully removed, and another trial closure is made; usually the flask can be closed entirely during the second trial closure, although care should be used not to force the closure unduly. The trial closures are repeated until no flash is observed. Large pressures are not needed. Only sufficient pressure during closure for metal to metal contact is required. The separating plastic sheet is then removed, and the two halves are closed under considerable pressure, which is maintained until the denture has been processed.

Ideally the flask should be permitted to rest in the clamp under pressure for a considerable time before curing in order to permit the monomer to saturate the polymer thoroughly and flow into all the intri-

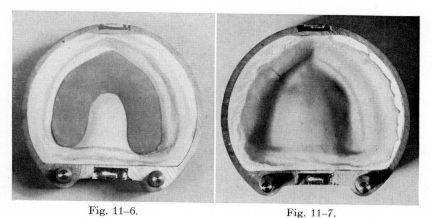

Fig. 11–6.        Fig. 11–7.

Fig 11–6.   Resin in place in the upper half of the flask, ready for the trial closure to begin.

Fig. 11–7.   After the first trial closure, a flash of material generally is found to have spread over the land surrounding the mold space.

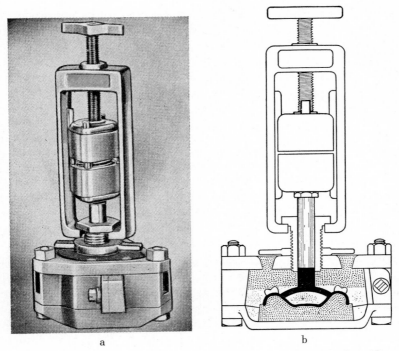

a                                    b

Fig. 11–8.  *a*. Pryor injector flask and press. *b*. Diagrammatic cross section. (Courtesy of the Hanau Mfg. Co.)

cacies of the mold.[8] One hour is a practical time although overnight is better.

Extreme care should be exercised to avoid overpacking the mold. No excess should be added after the final trial pack. To do so will produce a distorted mold and an opening of the bite.[9]

The trial closure is a very important step in the processing procedure; a properly filled mold results in a much better fit of the denture.

**Injection Packing.**  The mold can be filled by injecting the dough into the mold, and the trial closures can be eliminated. Equipment for such a procedure is shown in Figure 11–8*a* and *b*.

In practice, the mold is first incompletely filled with the prepared dough. The equipment is assembled as shown in Figure 11–8*a*, and excess dough is placed in the reservoir, located immediately below the piston. As the handle at the top is turned, a coiled spring is activated, which in turn exerts pressure on the piston to force the dough into the mold. As can be noted from the figure, the two halves of the flask are held together by bolts.

The general preparation of the mold is the same as that previously outlined, but no trial closure is necessary, since there will be no flash if the proper injection pressure is employed. The chief advantage of this method of processing is that the human element can be eliminated in the proper filling of the mold. However, there is no difference in the final result when either the injection or the compression method is used properly.[9]

**Initial Heating.** The polymerization reaction becomes rapid at temperatures above 60° C. (140° F.). During the heating of this material to that temperature, a thermal expansion of the resin occurs. Since the linear coefficient of expansion of poly(methyl methacrylate) is 0.000081 millimeter per millimeter per degree centigrade, a noteworthy expansion can be expected during the initial heating.

In the injection technic, such an increase in volume can be compensated for by a back pressure on the piston, but in the case of the denture molded by compression, no such relief is possible. A little thought will show that the pressure of the resin on the mold will depend upon the ratio of the area of the denture base to its volume. For example, a thin denture base will exert less pressure on the investing medium during thermal expansion than will a thicker base of the same area, inasmuch as the greater bulk of the latter will increase in volume more than will the former, when both are heated over the same temperature range.

It has been estimated that the maximum pressure on the mold surface exerted by the resin in a mold of average size is 29 kilograms per square centimeter (420 pounds per square inch).[10] In most instances, such pressures are less than the proportional limit of the investing medium, and no permanent deformation of the mold space should be expected under normal conditions. However, if a permanent deformation of the investing material does occur, a warpage of the denture will result.

In order to safeguard completely against a warpage during this

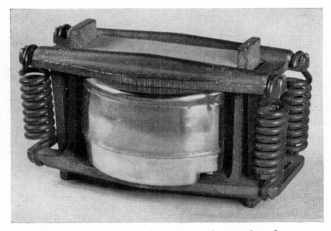

Fig. 11–9. A flask under pressure in a spring clamp.

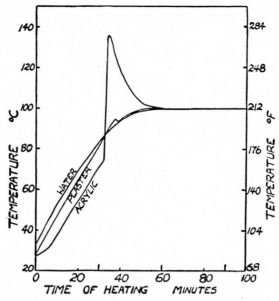

Fig. 11–10.   Temperature-time heating curves for the water bath, investing plaster, and acrylic resin during the polymerization of a one inch cube. (Tuckfield, Worner and Guerin, *Austral. J. Den.*, March, 1943.)

period, some dentists prefer to employ a spring clamp on the flask during curing, as shown in Figure 11–9. An objection to the use of a spring clamp is that if the halves of the flask are allowed to separate during the initial heating, a flash will be produced by the leakage of the soft plastic dough from the mold. As a result, the vertical dimension of the denture will be increased. However, such an error is preferable to a distortion or fracture of the investing medium which might be caused by the pressure of the resin during thermal expansion. The use of a strong spring clamp on a flask may be particularly indicated in the cases of exceptionally bulky dentures; otherwise it is probably better to maintain the flask under a constant static pressure of considerable magnitude throughout the curing cycle.

**Polymerization.**   As previously noted, the dental resins usually contain benzoyl peroxide, $(C_6H_5COO)_2$. When the temperature of the dough increases above 60° C. (140° F.), the molecules of benzoyl peroxide decompose to form free radicals. A free radical reacts with a monomer molecule, and a new free radical is formed, which in turn becomes attached to another monomer molecule, and the chain reaction is thus propagated until a termination occurs.

The principal factor which governs the rate of polymerization is the rate at which the free radicals of the benzoyl peroxide are released, and, in the reaction under discussion, this factor is largely determined by the temperature. An increase in temperature also increases the rate of polymerization because of the increased kinetic energy of the monomer molecules and the resultant increase in chemical reactivity.

The presence of the polymer in the monomer is another factor which is conducive to an increase in the rate of polymerization. Furthermore, the effect of the polymer is more pronounced at higher temperatures than it is at lower temperatures.

Generally, the lower the temperature of the polymerization, the greater will be the molecular weight of the polymer, although the time required to complete the reaction may be greatly lengthened. Although this rule holds in the processing of dental resins, the other factors enumerated may also affect the polymerization to an appreciable extent, and higher temperatures with shorter curing times are often equally effective.

**Temperature Rise.** The polymerization reaction is exothermic, and the amount of heat evolved may be a factor in the proper processing of the denture. A one inch cube of acrylic resin dough was invested in a denture flask in the usual manner, and the temperature changes in the water bath, the investing plaster, and the resin were observed and plotted[7] as in Figure 11–10.

As can be noted from Figure 11–10, the temperature of the water and the plaster increased from room temperature to 100° C. (212° F.) in 60 minutes. The temperature of the acrylic resin increased at the same rate as the other two materials until a temperature slightly above 70° C. (160° F.) was reached, when it began to increase at a rapid rate. At this temperature, sufficient molecules of benzoyl peroxide were activated to produce the chain reaction, and to cause the temperature of the interior of the resin to rise considerably above the temperature of the boiling water at which the resin was polymerized.

**Internal Porosity.** The general effect of the temperature rise above 100° C. (212° F.) is to produce a porosity in the interior of a thick piece of the resin. The boiling point of the monomer is very slightly higher than that of the water. Although the rate of polymerization is extremely rapid, it is not instantaneous, and if the temperature rises above the boiling point of the residual monomer or some of the very low molecular weight polymers, these components may boil with the production of bubbles, as shown in Figure 12–3C in the next chapter.

This type of porosity will not be present on the surface of a denture. The reason is that the exothermic heat can be conducted away from the surface of the resin into the investing medium, and the temperature in this region is not likely to rise above the boiling point of the monomer. In the center of a thick portion, however, the heat cannot be conducted away with sufficient rapidity, and, therefore, the temperature in the center portion may rise considerably above the boiling point of the monomer.

Porosity of this type may occur in the thick ridge portions of an

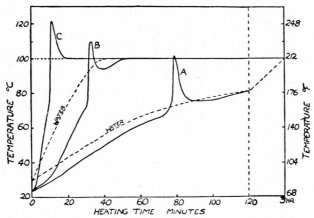

Fig. 11–11. Temperature changes in acrylic resin cured at different rates. (Tuckfield, Worner and Guerin, *Austral. J. Den.*, March, 1943.)

acrylic resin denture, but never in the thin palate portions of an upper denture, for example. If the resin section is thin, the exothermic heat can be conducted away with sufficient rapidity to prevent the formation of bubbles.

**Curing Cycle.** The *curing cycle* is the technical name given to the heating process employed in the polymerization of the monomer in the denture mold. The curing cycle presented in Figure 11–10 is unsatisfactory because of the large amount of exothermic heat evolved. One way to prevent the internal porosity is to decrease the rate of polymerization by heating the resin more slowly.

Different curing cycles are graphed in Figure 11–11, and the resin specimens obtained in each case are shown in Figure 12–3 in the next chapter, with the same letter designations as in Figure 11–11. When the flask was plunged directly into boiling water, the change in the temperature of the resin is shown by curve *C*; considerable internal porosity was present after the polymerization, as might be expected (specimen *C*, Fig. 12–3).

When the water was heated in forty minutes from room temperature to the boiling temperature (curve *B*, Figure 11–11), the temperature rise of the resin above 100° C. (212° F.) was not so pronounced, but since the boiling temperature of the monomer was exceeded, at least a certain amount of porosity could be expected to occur (specimen *B*, Figure 12–3). When the water was heated so slowly that three hours was required to reach 100° C. (212° F.), no porosity occurred, since, as shown by curve *A*, the temperature of the resin did not exceed that of the boiling point of the monomer at any time (specimen *A*, Fig. 12–3).

The curing cycle presented by curve *A* would be generally unsatisfactory for a denture base, since the temperature of the mold presumably never reached 100° C. (212° F.). In the case of an upper denture, the thicker ridge portions would be polymerized satisfactorily, owing to the temperature rise brought about by the magnitude of the exothermic heat. The temperature of the thinner palate portion would never approach 100° C. (212° F.) and the degree of polymerization would be less in this region. As a result the strength of the thinner palate portion would be less than it should be.[11, 12] The graph of a curing cycle which should result in a properly polymerized denture base without internal porosity is shown in Figure 11–12. The denture base is polymerized at 65° C. (150° F.) for 90 minutes, during which period the thick portions of the denture are cured without the occurrence of porosity due to the boiling of the monomer. Then the flask is boiled in water for one hour in order to polymerize the thin portions adequately.

There are many successful variations of the curing cycle shown in Figure 11–12. It is the practice in some dental laboratories to heat the flasked denture base in water at a temperature of 60° to 70° C. (140° to 160° F.) for nine hours or overnight. Such a curing cycle produces adequate strength in all parts of the denture base, but if, following this cycle, the flask is placed in boiling water for 30 minutes, the strength of the thin portions will be increased[11] as previously noted. This latter method is preferable certainly for very thin dentures or partials where the bulk of the resin is small. Likewise it can be easily controlled and standardized.

It is to be noted that regardless of the exact curing cycle employed, care is exercised to polymerize the resin reasonably slowly and to terminate the cycle with a period of time at 100° C. (212° F.). Only then can maximum polymerization occur to provide the greatest strength possible. The importance of the boiling phase of the cycle to the residual monomer content of the finished denture[13] is shown in Table 11–2. It is apparent that a 48-hour cure would be required at 70° C. to achieve approximately the same residual monomer level with that of a denture that was cured only one and one-half hours at 70° C. followed by boiling for one hour.

*Table 11–2.* *Residual Monomer Content in Various Areas of a Denture with Different Curing Cycles**

| | RESIDUAL MONOMER | |
|---|---|---|
| CURE | LABIAL (PER CENT) | BUCCAL (PER CENT) |
| 8 hours at 70°C. | 2.50 | 2.55 |
| 24  "    "    " | 1.36 | 1.33 |
| 36  "    "    " | 1.24 | 1.23 |
| 48  "    "    " | 0.75 | 0.69 |
| 1½ hrs. at 70°C. + 1 hr. at 100°C. | 0.63 | 0.69 |

* Smith, *Brit. D. J.*, Aug. 5, 1958.

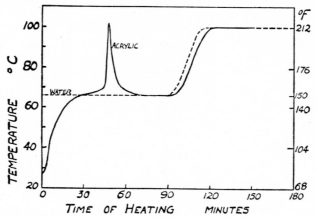

Fig. 11–12.  A recommended curing cycle to avoid internal porosity. (Tuckfield, Worner and Guerin, *Austral. J. Den.*, March, 1943.)

Another investigation showed a number average molecular weight of 13,000 for a resin polymerized for four hours at 70° C. (160° F.) as compared to 48,000 for the same material cured three hours at 70° C. (160° F.), followed by one hour at 100° C. (212° F.).[14]

The flask should be cooled slowly from the boiling water temperature. If the flask is placed directly into tap water, warpage of the denture due to the differential thermal contraction of the resin and gypsum mold will result. Cooling overnight is ideal. However, removing the flask from the water bath, bench cooling it for 30 minutes and then placing it in cold tap water for 15 minutes is generally satisfactory.

After deflasking and polishing, the denture is stored in water until it is delivered to the patient.

## CHEMICALLY ACTIVATED DENTURE BASE ACRYLIC RESINS

**Chemistry.**    Instead of using heat to activate the benzoyl peroxide, a chemical activator can be employed, so that the polymerization can be completed at room temperature. For example, a small amount of tertiary amine such as dimethyl-*p*-toluidine [$CH_3C_6H_4N(CH_3)_2$] can be added to the monomer, before the monomer and polymer are mixed as described for the heat-curing resins. After mixing, free radicals are formed from the benzoyl peroxide by a reaction with the dimethyl-*p*-toluidine, and the polymerization reaction presumably proceeds as previously described. These resins, first used for dental purposes in Germany during World War II,[15] are known variously as "self-curing," "cold cure," or "autopolymer" resins, to distinguish them from the resins polymerized when heat is employed for activation. It should be noted that the fundamental difference between the two types of resins is the method of the activation of the benzoyl peroxide. As a general rule, not as great a degree of polymerization can be attained with a chemical activator as when the activation is effected by heat.[14]

The type and concentration of both the activator and initiator influence the rate and degree of polymerization. There appears to be a maximum useful concentration of the amine at approximately 0.75 per cent while the maximum concentration for the peroxide is 2.0 per cent.[16] As with the heat-cured resins, the rate of polymerization is influenced by the particle size of the polymer. The smaller the particle size, the more rapid is the polymerization.

The color stability of the self-curing resins is apt to be inferior to that of the heat-cured type owing to the subsequent oxidation of the tertiary amine. This condition can be minimized by the addition of certain stabilizing agents to prevent such oxidation, or the polymerization may be consummated by the use of a more stable activator. In particular the sulfinic acid derivatives,[17] such as *p*-toluene sulfinic acid, appear to be quite good from this standpoint.

**Technical Considerations.** The technic employed for the processing of the self-curing denture resins is essentially the same as that previously described for the heat-curing resins. The same procedure is used in the mixing of the monomer and polymer. The same precautions must be observed in the preparation of the mold.

The monomer-polymer reactions, in the case of the self-curing resins, are likely to be complicated by a polymerization reaction which may begin before the dough stage is reached. The working time for the self-curing resins is invariably shorter than for the heat-cured materials.[18] A lengthy initiation period before the polymerization begins is desirable so that there will be plenty of time for the trial closures. The production of a flash during the processing of this type of resin is apt to cause an increase of the vertical dimension of the denture as described for the heat-curing resins. It should be noted that insofar as the importance of the proper filling of the mold is concerned, the technical considerations for the two types of resins are identical.

One method to prolong the initiation period is to decrease the temperature of the mixing jar. Such a procedure would delay the solution of the polymer in the monomer, and would prolong the dough-forming time. The material will, in most instances, remain in the dough form longer, and the working time will be increased. There are many methods by which the initiation period can be prolonged by chemical means. Unfortunately, the resin is apt to exhibit inferior strength properties if its initiation period is too prolonged by such methods. At best the transverse strength will be approximately 80 per cent of that for the heat-cured resins.[18, 19] In any event, if the resin meets the requirements of the American Dental Association Specification No. 12, the dough will be workable for at least 5 minutes.

In the case of the self-curing resins with the minimum working time,

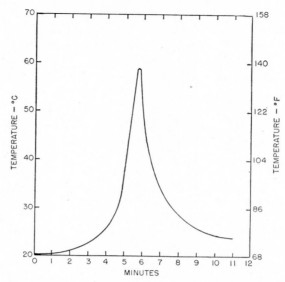

Fig. 11–13. Temperature change of a self-curing denture resin during polymerization. First observation three minutes after monomer and polymer were mixed.

it is doubtful that more than two trial closures can be made. Considerable care must be taken to insure that the proper amount of resin is employed, so that only the minimum number of trial closures will be necessary. Undoubtedly, the injection technic could be used to considerable advantage in the processing of self-curing denture bases, since no trial closure is needed in this instance, and the operation can be completed well within the 5-minute period.

**Time and Temperature for Processing.** Although it is not necessary to process the self-cured denture resins by the conventional heat cycle, that step has been suggested as a means of polymerizing the resin further in order to increase the strength. However, the heat curing cycle then eliminates certain of the advantages of the self-cured resin. The somewhat better initial fit of the self-cured denture[20, 21] and its reduced internal stress would be negated.

Inasmuch as no significant thermal expansion of the self-curing resin is to be expected during the processing, there is no need for the spring clamp such as was described for the processing of the heat-cured resin. Consequently, the use of a rigid bench clamp or similar device is advocated for use during the final closure of the flask and the subsequent curing.

The time to be allowed for the curing before the denture is removed from the flask will vary with different materials. Undoubtedly the initial hardening of the material will occur within 20 to 30 minutes after the final closure of the flask, but it is doubtful that the polymerization will be complete. A better dimensional stability of the denture base will be insured if the flask is held under pressure for 2 to 3 hours, or overnight. As previously mentioned, the polymerization of the self-curing resins is never as complete as that of the heat-curing type; 3 to 5 per cent of the self-curing resin is composed of free monomer, in comparison to approximately one-tenth as much free monomer that may be found in a resin processed in boiling water.[14] Consequently, it is most important that the polymerization reaction of the self-curing resins be as complete as possible before the pressure on the flasked denture is released. Otherwise, a subsequent warpage of the denture may occur in service.

The exothermic temperature change of a sphere of self-curing resin approximately 5 centimeters (2 inches) in diameter is shown in Figure 11–13. The curve is very similar to that shown in Figure 11–10, except that the temperature at the time of activation is that of the room. As in the case of the heat-curing resins, the temperature of the bulky portions will be higher at their center than at their surfaces because of the poor thermal conductivity of the resin. It is to be expected, therefore, that the thinner portions of the denture will be less polymerized and, therefore, will be weaker than the thick portions. Only in a bulk not likely to occur in denture bases will the exothermic heat be sufficient to cause the monomer to boil; consequently, no porosity due to boiling monomer is to be expected in the processing of a denture with the self-curing resins.

## *Literature*

1. Manly, R. S., and Vinton, P.: *A Survey of the Chewing Ability of Denture Wearers.* J. D. Res., *30:*314–321 (June), 1951.
2. Robinson, H. C.: *Reminiscences of Denture Materials.* Brit. D. J., *66:*68–71 (Jan. 16), 1939.
3. Taylor, W. D.: *Consideration of the Newer Denture Materials.* J.A.D.A., *21:*861–868 (May), 1934.
4. Tylman, S. D., and Peyton, F. A.: *Acrylics and Other Synthetic Resins Used in Dentistry.* Philadelphia, J. B. Lippincott Co., 1946, pp. 55–60.
5. Schoonover, I. C., Fischer, T. E., Serio, A. F., and Sweeney, W. T.: *Bonding of Plastic Teeth to Heat-Cured Denture Base Resins.* J.A.D.A., *44:*285–287 (March), 1952.
6. Peyton, F. A.: *Packing and Processing Denture Base Resins.* J.A.D.A., *40:*520–528 (May), 1950.
7. Tuckfield, W. J., Worner, H. K., and Guerin, B. D.: *Acrylic Resins in Dentistry, Part II.* Austral. J. Den., *47:*1–25 (March), 1943.
8. Sweeney, W. T.: *Acrylic Resins in Prosthetic Dentistry.* D. Clin. North America, November 1958, pp. 593–602
9. Grunewald, A. H., Paffenbarger, G. C., and Dickson, G.: *The Effect of Molding Processes on Some Properties of Denture Resins.* J.A.D.A., *44:*269–284 (March), 1952.
10. Taylor, P. B.: *Acrylic Resins: Their Manipulation.* J.A.D.A., *28:*373–387 (March), 1941.
11. Harman, I. M.: *Effects of Time and Temperature of Polymerization of a Methacrylate Resin Denture Base.* J.A.D.A., *38:*188–203 (Feb.), 1949.
12. Caul, H. J., and Schoonover, I. C.: *A Method for Determining the Extent of Polymerization of Acrylic Resins and Its Application for Dentures.* J.A.D.A., *39:* 1–9 (July), 1949

13. Smith, D. C.: *The Acrylic Denture Base.* Brit. D. J., *105:*86–91 (Aug. 5), 1958.
14. Taylor, P. B., and Frank, S. L.: *Low Temperature Polymerization of Acrylic Resins.* J. D. Res., *29:*486–492 (Aug.), 1950.
15. Blumenthal, L. M.: *Recent German Developments in the Field of Dental Resins.* Fiat Final Report No. 1185, Department of Commerce, Office of Technical Services, Washington, D. C., May, 27, 1947.
16. Rose, E. E., Lal, J., and Green, R.: *Effect of Peroxide, Amine and Hydroquinone in Varying Concentrations on the Polymerization Rate of Polymethyl Methacrylate Slurries.* J.A.D.A., *56:*375–381 (March), 1958.
17. Brauer, G. M., and Burns, F. R.: *Sulfinic Acid Derivatives as Accelerators in the Polymerization of Methyl Methacrylate.* J. Pol. Sci., *19:*311–321 (Feb.), 1956.
18. Caul, H. J., Sanford, J. W., and Serio, A. F.: *Properties of Self-curing Denture Base Resins.* J.A.D.A., *44:*295–298 (March), 1952.
19. Stanford, J. W., Burns, C. L., and Paffenbarger, G. C.: *Self-curing Resins for Repairing Dentures: Some Physical Properties.* J.A.D.A., *51:*307–315 (Sept.), 1955.
20. Mowery, W. E., Burns, C. L., Dickson, G., and Sweeney, W. T.: *Dimensional Stability of Denture Base Resins.* J.A.D.A., *57:*345–353 (Sept.), 1958.
21. Skinner, E. W., and Jones, P. M.: *Dimensional Stability of Self-curing Denture Base Acrylic Resin.* J.A.D.A., *51:*426–431 (Oct.), 1955.

# CHAPTER 12

# Denture Base Resins: Technical Considerations (Continued). Acrylic Resin Teeth

When a resin is employed in a situation requiring precision of dimension, one of the properties to be given first consideration is its dimensional stability. As noted in the previous chapter, the fit of the denture in the mouth of the patient is of prime consideration. Consequently, any change in the dimension of the denture base, either during its processing or during its function in the mouth, is of considerable importance. Since the acrylic resins exhibit certain unavoidable dimensional changes, the dentist should appreciate these limitations so that he will not expect the impossible. Also, he should understand the variables which can minimize inaccuracy of fit and subsequent distortion.

**Curing Shrinkage.** When methyl methacrylate monomer is polymerized, the density changes from 0.94 gram per cubic centimeter to 1.8 grams per cubic centimeter.[1] This change in density is reflected in a volumetric shrinkage of 21 per cent. If the conventional powder-liquid method of processing with heat is employed, as outlined in the previous chapter, approximately one-third of the volume of the dough is monomer; consequently the calculated volume shrinkage of the dough should be 7 per cent. It can also be calculated that the acrylic denture base should shrink linearly approximately 2 per cent during the processing. It is evident that a shrinkage of such a magnitude cannot occur in practice, if the denture is to fit.

Actually, the observed linear curing shrinkage is much less than 2 per cent. There may be a number of reasons for this seeming discrepancy, but the most likely cause is that the observed shrinkage may be thermal and not due to polymerization. As the resin shrinks thermally in the mold during tthe cooling of the denture *base*, near the curing temperature it is quite soft and the pressure in the mold causes it to contract at the same rate as the cast. During some stage of the curing, it attains sufficient rigidity that it contracts independently of the cast The temperature at which this change occurs is known as the *transition temperature*. Other physical properties of the resin, such as thermal expansion, density, and refractive index, also are changed markedly at this temperature. Consequently, only from the transition temperature to the room temperature can a true thermal contraction exist.[2] Since the transition temperature varies with different commercial denture base materials, the observed curing shrinkages can be expected to vary as well.

As a specific example, let it be assumed that the transition temperature of a denture resin is 75° C. (167° F.). If the resin denture is cooled to a room temperature of 20° C. (68° F.) in the flask, the thermal contraction can be calculated.[2] The generally accepted value for the linear coefficient of expansion of poly(methyl methacrylate) is $81 \times 10^{-6}$ per degree centigrade. Consequently,

$$(75 - 20)\ 81 \times 10^{-6} = 0.0044 \text{ mm./mm.} = 0.44 \text{ per cent}$$

This value is in general agreement with the linear shrinkages as observed across the posterior ridge portion of an actual denture. It is on this basis that it has been claimed that the curing shrinkage is more nearly related to the thermal shrinkage than to any effect of the polymerization shrinkage.[3] Actual linear curing shrinkage values have been reported for various commercial denture base materials as ranging from 0.2 to 0.5 per cent.[2, 4-6]

A curing shrinkage in a maxillary denture is often evidenced by a discrepancy in the palate region as shown in Figure 12–1. Presumably, during cooling the resin shrinks toward the areas of the greatest bulk, which in this case are the ridge portions of the denture base. Such a shrinkage causes a tensile stress to occur in the thinner palate region. When this stress is relieved, the resin is pulled away from the palate. As evidenced by the self-curing resin denture base in Figure 12–2, in which case a negligible amount of thermal shrinkage occurred, the fit of the denture base is much better.

The better fit of the self-curing resin could be anticipated if only on the basis that the cure is carried out at a lower temperature than the heat-cured resin. Thus, the thermal contraction would be less. The superior initial fit of the self-cured resin denture has often been reported.[1, 3, 7, 8]

Possibly the dimensional changes of the mold materials themselves may influence the final dimensions of the denture base.[9, 10] However, probably the minor and less effective dimensional changes within the mold materials themselves are masked by the more complex and significant changes which occur during the processing procedure.[11]

**Porosity.** It was previously noted that internal porosity may develop in the thick portion of a denture base, caused by the boiling of the monomer or of the low molecular weight polymers, when the temperature of the resin increases above the boiling point of these phases. It should be noted that in some cases such a type of porosity might occur at a temperature lower than the boiling point of the pure monomer. For example, if any water becomes entrapped in the gel

Fig. 12–1.

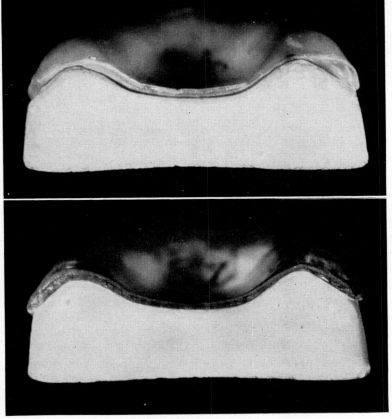

Fig. 12–2.

Fig. 12–1. An upper denture base constructed with a heat-curing resin, showing a characteristic palate discrepancy.

Fig. 12–2. An upper denture base constructed with a self-curing resin, no discrepancy is visible.

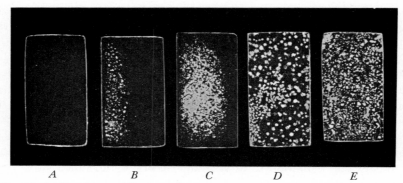

|     |     |     |     |     |
| --- | --- | --- | --- | --- |
| *A* | *B* | *C* | *D* | *E* |

Fig. 12–3. Specimens of heat-cured resins showing different types and degrees of porosity. *A.* Properly cured, no porosity. *B.* Too rapid rate of heating, area with no porosity was near the wall of the metal flask. *C.* Too rapid rate of heating. *D.* Insufficient mixing of monomer and polymer. *E.* Insufficient pressure during curing. (Tuckfield, Worner and Guerin, *Austral. J. Den.,* (March), 1943.)

before or during polymerization, the boiling point of the monomer may be lowered. Other inclusions might also cause a similar effect. A conservative heating cycle for the heat curing resins is always desirable in order to be sure that such porosity is avoided.

This type of porosity may not occur equally throughout the section involved. For example, the specimen *B* shown in Figure 12–3 exhibits a porosity only near one edge. The specimen was flasked so that the edge which is clear was nearer the metal wall of the flask. It is apparent that the metal in the flask conducted the exothermic heat away from this area with sufficient rapidity to prevent the occurrence of porosity. For this reason, the thick lingual posterior area of a lower denture base, for example, is more apt to exhibit porosity than is the buccal portion, since the latter is generally nearer the metal flask.

A second cause for porosity in an acrylic denture base is a lack of homogeneity in the dough or gel at the time of the polymerization. Although the dentist may follow the directions carefully in the preparation of the dough, complete homogeneity of the mass is difficult to attain without an extensive mixing procedure not generally feasible in the dental laboratory. It is probable that some regions will contain more monomer than others. These regions will shrink more during polymerization than the adjacent regions, and such a localized shrinkage would tend to produce voids.

There is another factor which can produce a localized porosity. Some of the polymer particles will be attacked more rapidly than the others because of possible differences in molecular weight, composition and size, as discussed in the previous chapter. When the polymerization begins, those portions with the greater amount of polymer in solution will polymerize first. During the subsequent shrinkage, the resin in the slower polymerizing portions will be drawn toward the more rapidly polymerizing sections, and again a porosity due to localized shrinkage will result.

It is for these reasons that the resin should not be packed before it reaches the dough stage. When such a contraindicated procedure is followed, the inhomogeneity is so great that a porosity occurs similar to that shown in specimen *D*, Figure 12–3. The voids are usually larger than those formed by too rapid polymerization (specimens *B* and *C*, Fig. 12–3), and they appear on the surface of the specimen as well as internally.

Such porosity can generally be avoided with the heat-curing resins if the filled flask is held under pressure for a minimum of 2 to 3 hours after the final closure. This procedure permits a better diffusion of the monomer and a closer approach to an equilibrium of the monomer-polymer reaction, before the polymerization begins. It is evident that the possibility of this type of porosity can be eliminated if the pre-mixed gel furnished by the manufacturer is used.

This latter type of porosity is likely to be quite prevalent in the case of the self-curing acrylic resins. The initiation period is usually so short that there is little opportunity to establish equilibrium conditions. Such porosity can be reduced in these resins by the control of some of the other factors mentioned, such as the degree of polymerization, curing under pressure,[12] pearl size and composition of the polymer powder. Even at best the porosity of the self-cured resin may be greater.

A third type of porosity, exemplified by specimen *E* in Figure 12–3, is caused by a lack of adequate pressure during the polymerization, generally brought about by a definite lack of dough or gel in the mold at the time of the final closure. The bubbles are not spherical, and they are usually smaller than those of the previous type (specimen *D*), but they are larger than those caused by too rapid curing. This type of porosity as well as the preceding type may be in such abundance as to cause the resin to appear white. A pigmented resin may appear lighter in color for this reason. On the other hand, as mentioned in the last chapter, care must be exercised to avoid any excess resin after the final trial pack.

**Water Sorption.**      Poly(methyl methacrylate) absorbs water quite readily. The amount of water retained depends on the number of polar groups in the polymer.[13] The water presumably enters the resin between the macromolecules, and forces them slightly apart, although some water is sorbed by the polymer itself.[14] The action of the water in this respect is not unlike that of a plasticizer. Although the amount of water imbibed is not great, a measurable swelling of the resin may occur. It has been determined that acrylic resins expand linearly at the rate of 0.23 per cent for each 1 per cent increase in weight of water sorbed.[15] The major portion of such swelling is virtually completed after an immersion in water at body temperature (37° C.) for about one week. Perceptible increases in dimension can be detected, however, for a period of six weeks or longer.

One method for the measurement of the water sorption is to obtain the increase in weight of the resin per unit of surface area exposed to the water. Such a method is specified in the American Dental Association Specification No. 12. A disk of material is prepared with a diameter of 50 millimeters (1.97 inches) and a thickness of 0.5 millimeter (0.02 inch). The disk is first dried to constant weight, and then it is stored in water for 24 hours. According to the Specification, the gain in weight by the resin during this treatment must not be greater than 0.7 milligram per square centimeter. There is no apparent difference between the heat-curing or the self-curing resins in this regard.[16, 17]

The dimensional change occurring in the resin during water imbibition can be measured. Such a measurement probably is proportional to the amount of water imbibed by the resin only if the specimen is free of stress. Measurements of strips of denture resin presumably stress-free have indicated that the increase in dimension brought about by water sorption is, for all practical purposes, equal to the curing shrinkage of the specimens.[2] Similar measurements on acrylic dentures indicate, however, that such a swelling does not compensate for the curing shrinkage.[18, 19]

The variations in the exact dimensional changes occurring in clinical cases can be explained on the basis of (1) the degree of residual stress, to be discussed in the next section, and (2) the amount of water in the resin when the processing was completed. As mentioned in Chapter 11, the water sorption of poly(methyl methacrylate) is independent of the molecular weight at all temperatures below 70° C. (158° F.).[14]

If allowed to dry, the resin will lose water and contraction will result. Thus, if the patient does not keep the denture in water at all times when not in use, a distortion may result. The denture will then not fit properly until it has re-sorbed the water lost and returned to its normal contour.

**Solubility.**    Although the denture base resins are soluble in many solvents, they are virtually insoluble in most fluids with which they will come in contact in the oral cavity.

When the disk employed for the determination of the water sorption as described in the preceding section is dried out the second time, any loss of weight observed would presumably be a measure of its solubility in the water during the test. According to the American Dental Association Specification No. 12, such a loss in weight must not be greater than 0.04 milligram per square centimeter of surface. Such a loss is negligible from a clinical standpoint. The solubility of the self-curing resins is slightly higher than that of the heat-curing resins.[16] The difference is not of practical importance, however.

## EFFECTS OF PROCESSING STRESSES

It is axiomatic that whenever a natural dimensional change is inhibited, the structure involved will be placed under stress, with certain portions strained as a result of the stress. If such stresses are present in the final form of the structure, they will likely be relaxed in time, and a warpage may result.

There are three established methods by which processing stresses can be detected experimentally in acrylic dentures.[20] The stresses can be relieved if the denture is heated above the transition temperature of the resin, as for example, if the denture is immersed in boiling water.[21] The resulting distortion and warpage observed presumably is proportional to the amount of stress released.

Inherent stresses can also be detected by means of polarized light[22] if the resin is clear. Such stresses are indicated in the specimen shown in Figure 12–4. A third method is to subject the resin specimen to a solvent, such as methyl methacrylate. Any stresses will produce a crazing as the solvent attacks the strained area if a cross-linking agent is not present. The presence of a cross-linking agent definitely minimizes the release of stresses induced during the fabrication of a denture. Thus, many of the possible warpages to be described in the subsequent discussions, which are due to the release of stress, may be considerably reduced with such a resin composition.

Methods for measuring stress in the denture, when subjected to masticatory forces, have also been evolved. Surface stress can be determined by the use of strain gauges. These small resistance wire fila-

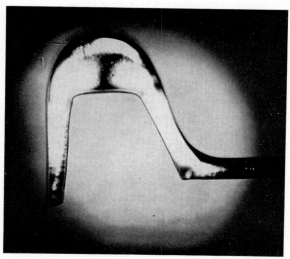

Fig. 12–4.   Processing stresses in a specimen of acrylic resin as seen in polarized light. The dark areas are not under stress but the light areas are.

ments can be cemented onto the surface of the denture and the stress determined by the alteration in the current passing through the gauge.[23] Brittle lacquers may also be painted on the denture and the relaxation of stress can be detected by a cracking of this coating.[23] The following discussion, however, will be primarily concerned with the stresses inherently present in the denture base itself and not those induced by external forces.

**Stresses Induced before Polymerization.**    It is possible that the major portion of processing stresses are first introduced during the dough-forming stage. In a previous section it was shown that a localized shrinkage can occur during polymerization because of the inhomogeneity of the original monomer-polymer mixture. Such localized conditions of shrinkage result in the induction of stress in the areas. In fact, porosity is always accompanied by a certain amount of stress.[22]

It is logical to assume that any type of inhomogeneity in the dough at the time processing begins will result in the creation of processing stress. As the temperature of the resin increases during the processing, the dough becomes more plastic, and such stresses can be relieved to some extent by the flow of the resin. Such a relief is more apt to take place when the resin is cured under heat; any relief of this nature in the case of the self-curing resins will be dependent on the exothermic heat of polymerization.

Undoubtedly, stresses are induced in the resin during its initial heating to the polymerization temperature. The thermal expansion of the dough will induce a considerable degree of compressive stress by the confinement of the resin in the mold. Some of the stresses induced during this period will also be relieved by the flow of the resin while it is plastic.

**Polymerization Shrinkage.**    As previously noted, a polymerization shrinkage of as much as 7 per cent by volume can be expected during the polymerization of the denture. Since such an amount of shrinkage is not observed in the final denture base, it may be concluded that the polymerization shrinkage was inhibited in some manner.

It has been suggested[24] that this type of shrinkage can be reduced in the case of the heat-curing resins (1) by the adhesion of the resin to the walls of the mold and the resistance offered by the shape of the mold, (2) by the relief of the compressive stresses induced in the resin during the initial heating, and (3) by a flow of the resin brought about by the relief of the stresses in the investing medium.

There will be a certain amount of resistance to the shrinkage caused by the adhesion of the resin to the walls of the mold. Such a fact is evidenced by the observation that the thinner the specimen of material, the less is the observed curing shrinkage.[4] Furthermore, it can be reasoned that the shape of the mold might offer a certain amount of resistance to the shrinkage, particularly during the earlier stages of the polymerization.

The second factor is concerned with the compressive stresses introduced into the resin dough during the initial thermal expansion. These stresses will be relieved during the polymerization shrinkage, and a certain amount of shrinkage compensation will result therefrom.

The third factor is closely allied to the preceding consideration, in that the investing medium may have been stressed during the initial thermal expansion, and the flow of the resin caused by the relaxation of these stresses would also contribute to the shrinkage compensation.

In any event, the polymerization shrinkage is not an important factor in the curing shrinkage observed with the heat-cured resin denture base. This fact is evidenced by the consideration that the observed curing shrinkage of a denture base constructed with a self-curing resin is low (approximately 0.1 per cent).[8] Presumably, approximately the same amount of polymerization shrinkage occurs with both types of resin, yet the curing shrinkage of a heat-cured denture base is greater than that of a self-cured denture base. Such an observation further confirms the previous conclusion that the thermal contraction of the heat-cured resin is the chief cause for the observed curing shrinkage with this type of material.

Furthermore, an experiment comparing the stress relief which occurred in an acrylic resin cured at room temperature with the stress relief of the same resin, polymerized at 100° C. (212° F.) showed that the processing stresses in the former were only one-fifth to one-third of the latter.[22, 25] Such an observation indicates that most of the processing stresses are derived from sources other than the polymerization shrinkage.

**Thermal Contraction.** It has been shown that the shrinkage during the cooling of a heat-cured denture base is not always the same in all directions. Although the differences appear to vary with various denture resins, in general the shrinkage across the posterior is greater than that between the anterior cuspid areas and the anteroposterior ridge distances.[26] Since a true thermal contraction would result in a uniform change throughout the denture, it can be assumed that the normal thermal change was inhibited by one or more of the foregoing factors.

As previously noted, above the transition temperature the resin is soft and contracts at the same rate as the cast. Since the linear coefficient of expansion of the stone and the resin differ,[2] it follows that stresses will be introduced in the denture at this stage, not all of which will be relieved by flow. These stresses will likely remain after the denture cools below the transition temperature. Any stresses incurred below the transition temperature when the denture contracts independently of the cast should be elastic in nature and will be relieved when the denture is removed from the flask. However, the partial relaxation of the more permanent stresses may result in a warpage of the type shown in Figure 12–1, as well as the unequal thermal contraction in various areas.

Such a discrepancy can be reduced. One way is to lower the transition temperature. The amount that this temperature can be reduced is limited by the practical consideration of the temperatures encountered in the mouth. The denture base must be rigid at all times during service, and its transition temperature should be higher than any temperatures likely to occur in the mouth. The lowering of the transition temperature can be accomplished by a modification of the composition of the resin as previously described for the control of the monomer-polymer reaction time.

Another method is to polymerize the resin below the transition temperature, near or at room temperature, as in the case of the self-curing resins. The only thermal contraction which occurs during the processing of the self-curing resins is the result of the cooling after the evolution of the exothermic heat. Although the temperature during this period may rise momentarily above the transition temperature in the bulkier portions of the denture, no marked thermal changes of the mold are likely to take place, and the processing stresses and the observed curing shrinkage are kept to a minimum.

Stressed areas are generally present around the necks of porcelain teeth; they are caused by the differential thermal contraction between the porcelain and the resin during the cooling of the heat-cured denture base. In the early days, an unmodified methyl methacrylate resin was used, and it was not uncommon to find that the posterior porcelain teeth had fractured during the processing. Such fractures were generally produced by the pressure on the teeth at their points of contact, caused by the thermal contraction of the resin around the teeth. Such a condition is seldom experienced with the modern modified denture acrylic resins.

**Water Sorption.**     Undoubtedly, the swelling due to the imbibition of water into the acrylic resin denture is inhibited by the presence of processing stresses. As a matter of fact, an initial contraction may sometimes be observed when the denture base is initially immersed in water. Such a distortion is likely to be more prevalent in a denture base cured under heat than in one fabricated with a self-curing resin.

The changes in dimension which occurred after two heat-cured acrylic resin dentures were immersed in water[27] are shown in Figure 12–5. As can be observed, both the volume (curve $A$) and the weight (curve $B$) increased in a regular manner as might be expected. The change in linear dimension, as measured between the posterior ridge portions, was manifested as a contraction initially. In one denture, the subsequent swelling in water produced sufficient expansion to overcome the initial contraction (curve $C_1$), but in the case of the other denture (curve $C_2$)

the dimensions did not increase sufficiently to restore its original dimensions during the period of observation (six weeks).

Undoubtedly the changes in dimension indicated by curves $C_1$ and $C_2$ in Figure 12–5 are caused by a relaxation of stress brought about by the water imbibition, since similar dentures stored in air showed no such distortion. The comparatively large distortions measured in this denture may have been caused by the fact that the mold was overfilled with resin at the time of the final closure. Similar observations made under conditions of proper mold content[18, 28] indicate a similar lack of dimensional stability during water sorption, but of less magnitude.

**Crazing.** Crazing of a resin consists of the formation of small cracks, which may vary in size from microscopic dimensions to a size that is readily visible to the unaided eye. In some instances, the crazing in a clear resin is evidenced as a hazy or foggy appearance rather than as individual cracks. In any event, whenever such a crazing occurs, it produces a weakening effect on the resin and reduces the esthetic qualities of the denture. Cracks formed on crazing may indicate the beginning of a fracture.

Crazing may occur under mechanical stress, or as the result of an attack by a solvent. The crazing appears to occur in poly(methyl methacrylate) only when a tensile stress is present. The crazing cracks appear at right angles to the direction of the tensile stress. The modern concept is that crazing is an actual mechanical separation of the polymer

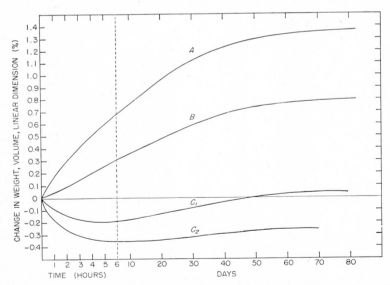

Fig. 12–5.   Changes in volume (curve *A*), weight (curve *B*), and linear dimension across the "heels" (curves $C_1$ and $C_2$) of two acrylic resin dentures during immersion in water for 80 days.

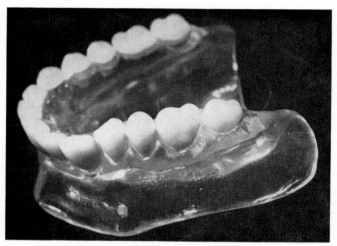

Fig. 12–6.   Crazing cracks around the porcelain teeth in an experimental denture.

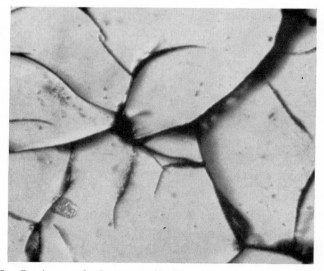

Fig. 12–7.   Crazing cracks in an acrylic denture resin which was processed in a mold lined with a tinfoil substitute, and then immersed in methyl methacrylate for 15 seconds. ×75. (Courtesy of C. W. Fairhurst and G. Ryge, Marquette University.)

chains or groups of chains under tensile stress.[29] Crazing usually starts on the surface in a region where the polymer molecules are oriented at right angles to the direction of the applied tensile stress. It then gradually penetrates inward. Such a type of crazing is visible around the porcelain teeth in the experimental denture shown in Figure 12–6. The tensile stress was probably induced by the contraction of the resin around the tooth during the cooling of the denture after it had been processed under heat. The direction of the crazing cracks is radial to the tooth, as predicted by the theory. It is not known how prevalent such crazing is in practical cases, since the pink color of the denture base obscures such cracks.

Although crazing by solvent action also indicates the presence of surface stresses, the crazing cracks are more randomly oriented than those shown in Figure 12–6. The solvent attack results in V- or Y-shaped cracks as illustrated in Figure 12–7. The solvent enters the surface of the resin along the lines or surfaces of strain, in which minute invisible crazing cracks were probably already present. The crazing can appear in the presence of even weak solvents, such as alcohol. However, as previously noted, cross-linking of the resin reduces this fault considerably.

**Mold Lining.** As outlined in a previous chapter, the walls of the denture mold should be lined with some substance which will prevent the penetration of the monomer into the surrounding investing medium, as well as the leakage of water into the acrylic resin during the curing. When linear methyl methacrylate polymer (*i.e.*, not cross-linked) comes in contact with water during processing at elevated temperatures, the resin is susceptible to crazing. Sorption of water at higher processing temperatures is greater than at room temperature. Consequently, such sorption causes the surface of the resin to become supersaturated with water when the specimen cools. Evaporation of this excess water then sets up stresses which eventually are released by the formation of craze cracks.[30]

It has been the custom to burnish thin sheets of tinfoil over the surface of the mold. However, such a process is apt to be somewhat difficult and time-consuming. As a result, a number of preparations have been offered as a substitute for tinfoil.

The nature of the tinfoil substitutes is generally some type of film-forming material which is painted on the mold surface after the wax base plate has been removed, just before the mold is to be filled with resin. For example, a solution of an alginate can be used, such as sodium, potassium or ammonium alginate. Presumably the soluble alginate reacts with the plaster or stone to form a film of calcium alginate.

Unfortunately, such films are not entirely water impervious, and the resin sorbs water at the higher temperatures with heat-curing procedures and a warpage of the denture results. Also, crazing is sometimes encountered.

Although a number of research studies have demonstrated the disadvantages of such a mold lining material,[31–34] it is used in the great majority of denture cases processed in the commercial dental laboratories. Nevertheless, the denture will exhibit better dimensional stability if tinfoil is employed for the mold lining in the processing of a heat-cured denture. When a self-curing resin is used, however, the tinfoil substitutes appear to be satisfactory.[32]

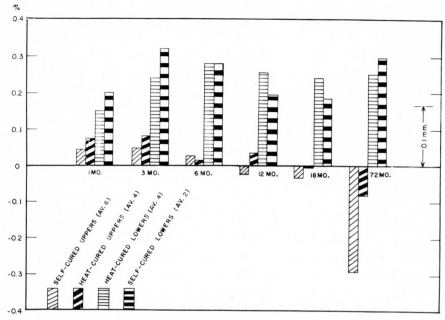

Fig. 12–8.    Dimensional change of a series of acrylic resin dentures in service for six years. (Sweeney, *D. Clin. North America*, November, 1958.)

**Clinical Significance of Stress Relaxation.**    It is apparent from the foregoing that every denture contains a certain amount of residual stress, contributed by variables associated with the curing procedure and water sorption. As has been indicated earlier, probably the greatest distortion of the denture occurs at the time the cured denture base is removed from the cast and the stress is released.[21]

However, the denture does continue to change dimensionally over a long period of time. The linear change[35] of a series of upper and lower clinical dentures processed with both heat-cured and self-cured resins may be seen in Figure 12–8. The dentures were measured across the posterior at the times indicated.

It is apparent, from these data, that the distortion is generally in the magnitude of 0.1 to 0.2 millimeter (0.2 to 0.3 per cent), depending on the resin and the type of denture. Upper dentures tended to change less in dimension than lowers, although, according to the average data (lower left, Figure 12–8), there was little difference regardless of the type of denture or the acrylic resin employed. When the dimensional change was measured in three planes,[36] or on the entire contour of the denture,[36-39] distortion in certain areas was somewhat greater but in general it was within the magnitude indicated in Figure 12–8.

The clinical significance of such distortions is unknown. However, since dimensional stability and accuracy of fit are essential to patient comfort and preservation of occlusal relationships, every care must be exercised by both dentist and patient to minimize distortion.

## MISCELLANEOUS TECHNICS

**Repair of Acrylic Resin Dentures.** If an acrylic denture is fractured in service, it can be repaired. Other sources[40-41] should be consulted for a detailed account of the technic involved. Essentially the technic involves the fastening of the fractured parts together with wax or by other means. A stone cast is then constructed in the denture base. The cast with the denture is invested in a flask as usual. After the wax has been flushed out, acrylic resin repair material is packed in the space remaining, and it is cured in the usual manner.

If the repaired portion is heat-cured, any boiling of the denture is likely to cause a considerable warpage of the denture by the release of processing stresses. Repeated curing of the denture at 100° C. (212° F.) results in a distortion as illustrated in Figure 12–9. Consequently, the cure should be effected at a lower temperature, less than 75° C. (167° F.), and the time should be prolonged for as long as nine hours, or overnight. If the repair is completed with the use of a self-curing resin, a better fit can be obtained, but the repair will be somewhat lacking in strength, in comparison to that obtained with the heat-curing resin.

The repair is weaker than the original resin, regardless of how the

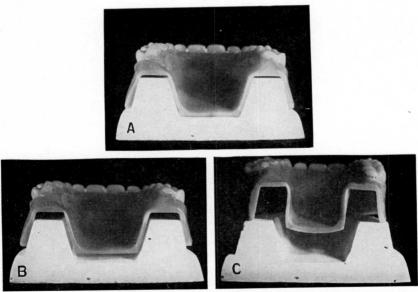

Fig. 12–9. *A.* Experimental denture on master cast after original curing. *B.* Same denture on same cast after recuring in a flask at 100° C. (212° F.) for ½ hour. *C.* Same denture on same cast after recuring nine times in same manner. (Courtesy of H. K. Worner, University of Melbourne.)

repair is made. Such a situation can result from the lower degree of polymerization due to the method of curing.[42]

Another suggestion is that the weakness of the repaired area may be due to the shape of the edges of the denture base to which the repair is joined. The edges at the fracture are generally trimmed back in order to provide bulk for the repair material. The edges are then usually rabbeted to provide a greater area for the union between the repair material and the denture base. If sharp angles are avoided in such preparations of the edges, a stronger repair may result.[43] The sharp edges cause a concentration of stress in the resin during polymerization or during cooling, which weakens it.

The self-cured resins, because of their ease of use and better fit of the repaired denture, are generally employed for the average repair. If the denture is properly constructed so that there is no undue trauma in localized areas, the reduced strength of the self-cured resin is probably not a clinical problem. Color stability may be inferior with certain products;[17] however, any material which meets American Dental Association Specification No. 13 for denture self-curing repair resin will be satisfactory.

**Relining and Rebasing.** Because of tissue changes which take place during the wearing of the denture, it often is necessary either to reline or to rebase the denture in order to restore the proper retention and function. If the denture is to be relined, an impression of the tissues can be obtained, using the denture as an impression tray. A cast is then constructed, and the denture and cast are invested in a flask as usual. The halves of the flask are separated, the impression material is removed, and new acrylic resin is cured against the old by the compression molding technic.

As in the case of denture repair, a low curing temperature for the relining process is necessary in order not to distort the denture if a heat-cured denture is used. In any event, the denture base is likely to be warped toward the relined side because of the processing shrinkage of the relining material. Such warpage is not so pronounced when the self-curing resins are employed in this manner, and better results can be expected if the proper technic is employed.[44]

Certain types of resins are available which can be used for relining dentures directly in the mouth. The better types are plasticized self-curing resins. Unfortunately, most of these resins are more susceptible to deterioration in the mouth fluids and have inadequate color stabilities as compared with either the self-curing or heat-cured resins.[12] For this reason, they should be considered only as temporary expedients until the conventional rebasing technic can be employed.

Probably the most satisfactory method for the restoring of the fit of the denture is to *rebase* it. Essentially the same flasking technic can often be employed as for the relining. After the halves of the flask have been separated, the denture base is softened under heat and removed from the teeth, which remain embedded in the plaster in the upper half of the flask. An entirely new denture base is then processed in the usual manner. However, if the old denture base resin possesses too high a softening temperature to be removed readily, a more complicated technic can be employed as outlined in textbooks on prosthetic dentistry.[45] The rebased denture is generally more stable in function with a better fit than is the relined denture.

## ACRYLIC RESIN TEETH

The use of acrylic resin teeth in dentures to replace the usual porcelain tooth has gained considerable favor during recent years. The Knoop hardness number of the acrylic resin teeth is for all practical purposes no greater than the hardness number of a heat-cured acrylic resin denture base. A minimum Knoop hardness of 15 is required in American Dental Association Specification No. 15 for Plastic Teeth. Although a satisfactory *in vitro* method for measuring abrasion resistance of artificial teeth has not yet been evolved,[46] clinical observations definitely indicate that the acrylic teeth exhibit more abrasion during function than do either the porcelain teeth or the natural teeth. Such an abrasion of the acrylic tooth is considered beneficial by some authorities as a means of the perpetuation of balanced occlusion.[47] Others, however, feel that excess wear is not desirable.

The resin teeth possess certain advantages over porcelain teeth in esthetic qualities and greater resistance to shock. Their low modulus of elasticity reduces the objectionable "clicking" often experienced by denture wearers. Furthermore, a definite chemical bond between the tooth and the resin can be effected during processing. It is estimated that the processing stresses introduced in the acrylic resin denture base by the resin teeth are approximately one-fourth the amount produced by similar porcelain teeth.[22]

The composition of resin teeth is essentially poly(methyl methacrylate) copolymerized with a cross-linking agent as described for the denture base materials. Usually a greater amount of cross-linking is employed in the acrylic resin teeth than in the similar denture base material in order to reduce the tendency of the teeth to craze during the construction of the denture and to produce a certain amount of increase in strength and hardness.

If the cross-linked copolymer is not used, trouble is often experienced with crazing of the teeth when they are in contact with the monomer-polymer dough. Also, during the setting of the teeth in the wax model base plate, it is often the practice to smooth the wax with a flame. Such a technic should be employed cautiously when any type of acrylic teeth is present, since the surfaces of the teeth may be melted or burned. In such a case, surface stresses will be induced during cooling and crazing is more likely to occur in service.[25, 48]

American Dental Association Specification No. 15 includes a craze test. In an evaluation[49] of eleven brands of acrylic teeth, only five products were found to be craze resistant after undergoing a conventional curing cycle. However, if water was prevented from contacting them during heating, all teeth were craze resistant. The relationship of water sorption and crazing was discussed earlier.

Union between the acrylic resin teeth and the heat-cured denture base can be easily produced, provided that the surface of the tooth resin is completely clean. The slightest film of wax will prevent such a union.[50] It is extremely important that the mold be flushed thoroughly with a detergent solution as previously described (page 159) in order to remove all of the wax. Although the cleansing of the teeth is equally important when a self-curing resin is used, a chemical union can be effected only by a modification of the chemical properties of the resin-tooth surface.

## PHYSICAL PROPERTIES

**Strength.**     The strength of the acrylic resin denture base materials may fluctuate considerably according to the composition of the resin, the technic of processing, and the subsequent environment of the denture. The stress properties of the resin are generally measured by means of a transverse test, as described in the American Dental Association Specification No. 12. A specimen of dimensions 2.5 millimeters (0.0984 inch) in thickness, 10 millimeters (0.3937 inch) in width and approximately 65 millimeters (2.559 inches) in length is subjected to a transverse loading at a specified rate. Typical stress-strain curves obtained by this method are shown in Figure 12–10. Since no straight-line portion of the curves is discernible, usually the deflection obtained at designated loads is employed as a measure of the stress-strain properties of the resin, rather than the usual proportional limit and modulus of elasticity. These relationships are described in detail in the Specification.

The interpretation of the lack of a straight-line portion in the stress-strain curve is that a plastic flow of the resin is produced during the loading in addition to an elastic deformation. When the load is released, the stresses are relaxed slowly, and the structure may never recover completely from the original deformation.[51]

It has been repeatedly stated that the lower the degree of polymerization of a given solid polymer, the less will be its strength. In this respect, the curing cycle employed with a heat-curing resin is most important. The transverse stress-strain curves shown in Figure 12–11 indicate the progressive weakening and decrease in rigidity of the resin as the curing time was reduced, when the curing temperature was held constant at 71° C. (160° F.).[52]

Owing to the lower degree of polymerization attained and to the residual monomer retained, the maximum strength and rigidity of the self-curing resins is lower than that of the heat-curing type. It is for this reason that the self-curing resins are given a different classification in the American Dental Association Specification No. 12 for Denture Base Resin.

As can be noted from Figure 12–10, the strength and rigidity of the resin is reduced after the sorption of water.[53] It is of further interest that its strength and rigidity are less if the resin is stressed under water than when it is stressed in air.

The properties of the resin may also be reduced by the finishing of the denture with abrasives and polishing agents. The heat from the polishing wheel, for example, may cause a warpage of the denture by a release of processing stresses.[11] Excessive heat incurred during polishing or abrading may cause a partial depolymerization with a resulting decrease in the degree of polymerization, and a decrease in strength and rigidity.

As discussed in the previous chapter, the exothermic heat evolved during the polymerization varies according to the bulk of the denture.

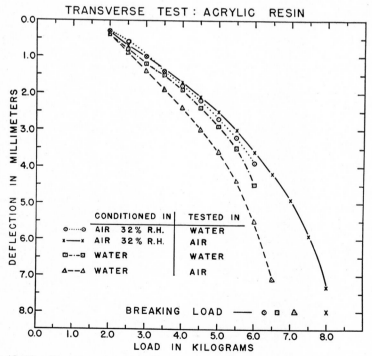

Fig. 12–10.   Transverse stress-strain curve for a typical acrylic resin denture base material, showing the influence of different conditioning procedures and testing environments. All specimens were conditioned for 3 days as indicated before testing. (Swaney, Paffenbarger and Caul, *J.A.D.A.*, Jan., 1953.)

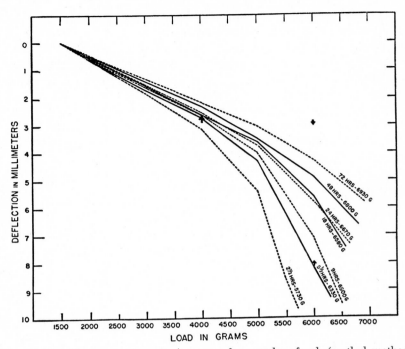

Fig. 12–11. Transverse stress-strain curves for samples of poly(methyl methacrylate) cured for different times at 71° C. (160° F.). The curing time and transverse load at fracture are noted on each curve. (Harman, *J.A.D.A.*, Feb., 1949.)

On this basis, it can be expected that the bulkier portions of the denture may exhibit greater strength than the thinner portions. This fact can be proved by a determination of the properties of standard test specimens prepared from sections of a test sample with different thicknesses,[52] as indicated in Figure 12–12. In other words, the ridge portions of an upper denture may be stronger than the palate portions.

The stress-strain curve of an acrylic resin under tensile stress is similar to that obtained under a transverse test in that no portion of the curve is a straight line. However, if certain assumptions are made for the calculations, the approximate values for the tensile properties of the dry, heat-cured resin tested in air are: modulus of elasticity, 24,000 kilograms per square centimeter (340,000 pounds per square inch); proportional limit, 275 kilograms per square centimeter (3900 pounds per square inch), and tensile strength, 525 kilograms per square centimeter (7500 pounds per square inch).[54] The self-curing resins generally exhibit tensile properties lower than those for the heat-curing resins.

The tensile strength of resin is much lower than that of alloys used for denture castings but it seems adequate, judging by the small amount of breakage of dentures experienced in service. Such fracture is more likely due to low fatigue strength.[1]

Because of superior tensile strength and fatigue resistance, nylon (a thermoplastic polyamide polymer) has been used as a denture base material. However, at the present time, lack of dimensional stability and technical problems in fabrication make it inferior to acrylic resins.[55–56]

**Miscellaneous Properties.** The Charpy impact strength of an acrylic resin denture base, cured under heat activation, is approximately 10 to 13 centimeter-kilograms per square centimeter, whereas that for a self-curing resin is in the neighborhood of 8 centimeter-kilograms per square centimeter.

The Knoop hardness number of a self-curing resin is approximately 16 to 18, whereas that for a resin cured under heat may be as high as 20. Such differences are of academic interest only.

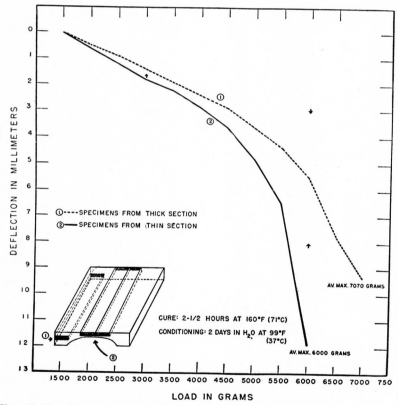

Fig. 12–12. Transverse strength and rigidity of poly(methyl methacrylate) as affected by the thickness of the prepared sample. Specimens No. 1 prepared from the thicker portions of the block (lower left corner) exhibited a greater strength and rigidity than did specimens No. 2 prepared from the thinner portions. (Harman, *J.A.D.A.*, Feb., 1949.)

The color stability of the resin is usually tested by an exposure to ultraviolet light. The heat-cured resins generally exhibit good color stability. The resins cured by chemical activation are sometimes not as color stable as the former type, but this deficiency can be minimized as previously described.

**Denture Cleansers.**     A wide variety of agents are used by patients for cleaning artificial dentures.[57-58] In approximate order of preference, they include dentifrices, proprietary denture cleansers, soap and water, salt and soda, household cleansers, bleaches, and vinegar. Either immersion in the agent or, more generally, brushing of the denture with the cleanser is employed.

The most common commercial denture cleansers are the immersion type and are usually marketed as a powder. Their composition[57] includes alkaline compounds, detergents, flavoring agents, and sodium perborate. When the powder is dissolved in water the perborate decomposes to form an alkaline peroxide solution which in turn decomposes to liberate oxygen. The oxygen bubbles supposedly then act mechanically to loosen the dèbris.

The household bleaches (hypochlorites) also effectively remove certain types of stain. They do not influence the color of the denture. However, due to their effect on the metal, hypochlorites should not be employed with any base metal appliance.[59]

The influence of abrasive agents on acrylic resin has been investigated.[57-58] The tooth brush itself has little effect on the surface of the resin. Salt, soda, soap and most commercial dentifrices are not harmful. However, household cleansers, used by approximately 10 per cent of all patients,[58] are definitely contraindicated. Prolonged use of such agents may affect the fit of the denture and the rough surface produced makes maintenance of a clean surface most difficult. The patient should be warned accordingly.

**Allergic Reactions.**     Possible toxic or allergic reactions to poly (methyl methacrylate) have long been postulated. Theoretically, chemical irritation could occur from either the polymer, the residual monomer, the benzoyl peroxide, hydroquinone, or pigment. All of these ingredients have been subjected to biological evaluation from this standpoint.

It is probable that true allergic reactions to acrylic resins are seldom seen in the oral cavity.[60-61] The residual monomer, approximately 0.5 per cent in a well processed denture,[62] is the usual component singled out as an irritant. If the monomer content in the denture is measured after storage in water, it is found that the free monomer at the surface of the denture is leached out within seventeen hours.[62-63] The remainder of the monomer is not readily extracted. Even if some of it were made available under continued stressing of the denture, the evidence suggests that it would wash away rapidly.

Thus, if residual monomer were a cause for denture-sore mouth, its effect might be expected to appear comparatively rapidly but the majority of clinical cases reporting irritation under the denture occur months, or even years, after insertion. Careful clinical evaluation of large numbers of so-called allergy to acrylic resins show that the causative factor is either unhygienic conditions under the denture,[64] or an ill-fitting denture which is traumatizing the tissue. A true allergy to acrylic resin can be recognized by a patch test.

## Literature

1. Sweeney, W. T.: *Acrylic Resins in Prosthetic Dentistry.* D. Clin. North America, November 1958, pp. 593–602.
2. Skinner, E. W., and Cooper, E. N.: *Physical Properties of Denture Resins: Part I, Curing Shrinkage and Water Sorption.* J.A.D.A., *30:*1845–1852 (Dec.), 1943.
3. Schroeder, A.: *Die Eignung der Methakrylate als Prothesenstoffe im Lichte neuer Untersuchungen.* Schweiz. Mschr. Zahnheilk., *63:*971 (Oct.), 1953.
4. Sweeney, W. T.: *Denture Base Materials: Acrylic Resins.* J.A.D.A., *26:*1863–1873 (Nov.), 1939.
5. Peyton, F. A., and Mann, W. R.: *Acrylic and Acrylic-styrene Resins: Their Properties in Relation to Their Uses as Restorative Materials.* J.A.D.A., *29:*1852–1864 (Oct.), 1942.
6. Sweeney, W. T., Paffenbarger, G. C., and Beall, J. R.: *Acrylic Resins for Dentures.* J.A.D.A., *29:*7–33 (Jan.), 1942.
7. Osborne, J.: *Acrylic Resins in Prosthetic Dentistry.* Internat. D. J., *4:*299–310 (March), 1954.
8. Skinner, E. W., and Jones, P. M.: *Dimensional Stability of Self-curing Denture Base Acrylic Resins.* J.A.D.A., *51:*426–431 (Oct.), 1955.
9. Steck, N. S.: *Making the Denture Dimensionally Accurate.* J. D. Res., *27:*751 (Dec.), 1948. Abstract.
10. Jørgensen, K. D.: *Investigations on the Expansion Properties of Some Dental Model Plasters.* Acta Odont. Scandinavica, *12:*24–38 (Oct.), 1954.
11. Vieira, D. F.: *Influencia de Materiais e Tecnicas Sobre a Posiçao Relativa dos Dentes, na Construçao de uma Base de Dentadura.* Thesis—Universidade de São Paulo, Brazil, 1958, p. 112.
12. Brauer, G. M., White, E. E., Burns, C. L., and Woelfel, J. B.: *Denture Reliners— Direct, Hard, Self-curing Resins.* J.A.D.A., *59:*270–283 (Aug.), 1959.
13. Kline, G. M., Martin, A. R., and Crouse, W. A.: *Proceedings: American Society for Testing Materials.* 40:1273, 1940.
14. Brauer, G. M., and Sweeney, W. T.: *Sorption of Water by Polymethyl Methacrylate.* Modern Plastics, *32:*138–143 (May), 1955.
15. Vernonite Work Bench: Vol. 6, No. 3 (March), 1947.
16. Caul, H. J., Stanford, J. W., and Serio, A. F.: *Properties of Self-curing Denture Base Resins.* J.A.D.A., *44:*295–298 (March), 1952.
17. Stanford, J. W., Burns, C. L., and Paffenbarger, G. C.: *Self-curing Resins for Repairing Dentures: Some Physical Properties.* J.A.D.A., *51:*307–315 (Sept.), 1955.
18. Grunewald, A. H., Paffenbarger, G. C., and Dickson, G.: *The Effect of Molding Processes on Some Properties of Denture Resins.* J.A.D.A., *44:*269–284 (March), 1952.
19. Tuckfield, W. J., Worner, H. K., and Guerin, B. D.: *Acrylic Resins in Dentistry, Part II.* Austral. D. J., *47:*1–25 (March), 1942.
20. Pryor, W. J.: *Internal Strains in Denture Base Materials.* J.A.D.A., *30:*1382–1389 (Sept.), 1943.
21. Woelfel, J. B., and Paffenbarger, G. C.: *Method of Evaluating the Clinical Effect of Warping a Denture: Report of a Case.* J.A.D.A., *59:*250–260 (Aug.), 1959.
22. Horton, E.: *An Experimental Investigation of Internal Strains in Polymerized*

*Methyl Methacrylate as Revealed by Polarized Light.* Brit. D. J., *86:*133–142 (March 18); 176–180 (April 1), 1949.

23. Matthews, E., and Wain, E. A.: *Stresses in Denture Bases.* Brit. D. J., *100:*167–171 (April), 1956.

24. Taylor, P. B.: *Acrylic Resins: Their Manipulation.* J.A.D.A., *28:*373–387 (March), 1941.

25. Osborne, J.: *Internal Strains in Acrylic Denture Base Materials.* Brit. D. J., *82:* 204–212 (May 16), 1947.

26. Atiyyah, A. R.: *Dimensional Changes of the Acrylic Denture Base.* Northwest. Univ. Bul., Den. Res. and Grad. Study, *47:*9–15 (Autumn) 1946.

27. Smith, E. H.: *Dimensional Stability of Acrylic Resin Dentures.* Thesis, Northwestern University Dental School, 1947.

28. Darley, H. P.: *Strain Release in Acrylic Resin Dentures Molded by Injection.* Thesis, Northwestern University Dental School, 1948.

29. Hsiao, C. C., and Sauer, J. A.: *On Crazing of High Polymers.* J. App. Phys., *21:* 1071–1083 (Nov.), 1950.

30. Sweeney, W. T., Brauer, G. M., and Schoonover, I. C.: *Crazing of Acrylic Resins.* J. D. Res., *34:*306–312 (June), 1955.

31. Furguson, G. W., Paffenbarger, G. C., and Schoonover, I. C.: *Deficiencies of Tin-foil Substitutes in the Processing of Acrylic Resin.* J.A.D.A., *38:*573–586 (May), 1949.

32. Skinner, E. W., Cooper, E. N., and Molnar, E. J.: *An Estimate of the Fit of One Hundred Acrylic Denture Bases.* J. D. Res., *30:*496 (Aug.), 1951. Abstract.

33. Fairhurst, C. W., and Ryge, G.: *Tin-foil Substitute: Warpage and Crazing of Acrylic Resin.* J. Pros. Den., *4:*274–287 (March), 1954.

34. Fairhurst, C. W., and Ryge, G.: *Effect of Tin-Foil Substitutes on the Strength of Denture Base Resins.* J. Pros. Den., *5:*508–513 (July), 1955.

35. Mowery, W. E., Burns, C. L., Dickson, G., and Sweeney, W. T.: *Dimensional Stability of Denture Base Resins.* J.A.D.A., *57:*345–353 (Sept.), 1958.

36. Dolder, E.: *Physikalische Workstoffprüfungen an Zahnprothesen im Laboratorium und am Patienten.* Schweiz. Mschr. Zahnheilk., *53:*435 (May), 1943; *53:*597 (June), 1943.

37. Rupp, N. W., Dickson, G., Lawson, M. E., and Sweeney, W. T.: *A Method for Measuring the Mucosal Contours of Impressions, Casts and Dentures.* J.A.D.A., *54:*24–32 (Jan.), 1957.

38. Ryge, G., and Fairhurst, C. W.: *An Evaluation of Denture Adaptation on the Basis of Contour Meter Recordings.* J. Pros. Den., *9:*755–760 (Sept.), 1959.

39. Anthony, D. H., and Peyton, F. A.: *Evaluating Dimensional Accuracy of Denture Bases with a Modified Comparator.* J. Pros. Den., *9:*683–692 (July), 1959.

40. Tylman, S. D., and Peyton, F. A.: *Acrylic and Other Dental Resins.* Philadelphia, J. B. Lippincott Co., 1946, pp. 377–385.

41. Gehl, D. H., and Dresen, O. M.: *Complete Denture Prosthesis,* 4th ed. Philadelphia, W. B. Saunders Co., 1958, pp. 416–422.

42. Caul, H. J., and Schoonover, I. C.: *A Method for Determining the Extent of Polymerization of Acrylic Resins and Its Applications for Dentures.* J.A.D.A., *39:*1–9 (July), 1949.

43. Ware, A. L., and Docking, A. R.: *The Strength of Acrylic Repairs.* Austral. D. J., *54:*27–32 (Feb.), 1950.

44. Jeffreys, F. E.: *Use of Self-curing Resins in Repairing and Relining Dentures.* J.A.D.A., *44:*298–301 (March), 1952.

45. Tylman, S. D., and Peyton, F. A.: *loc. cit.,* pp. 387–390.

46. Cornell, J. A., Jordan, J. S., Ellis, S., and Rose, E. E.: *A Method of Comparing the Wear Resistance of Various Material Used for Artificial Teeth.* J.A.D.A., *54:* 608–614 (May), 1957.

47. Dirksen, L. C.: *Plastic Teeth: Their Advantages, Disadvantages and Limitations.* J.A.D.A., *44:*265–268 (March), 1952.

48. Leader, S. A.: *Acrylic Crazing: Its Significance, Prevention and Treatment.* Brit. D. J., *87:*205–207 (Oct. 21), 1949.

49. Sweeney, W. T., Yost, E. L., and Fee, J. G.: *Physical Properties of Plastic Teeth.* J.A.D.A., *56:*833–841 (June), 1958.

50. Schoonover, I. C., Fischer, T. E., Serio, A. F., and Sweeney, W. T.: *Bonding of Plastic Teeth to Heat-cured Denture Base Resins.* J.A.D.A., *44:*285–287 (March), 1952.
51. Gabel, G. B., and Smith, E. N.: *Flow of Methyl Methacrylates.* J. D. Res., *22:*237–241 (Aug.), 1943.
52. Harman, I. M.: *Effects of Time and Temperature on the Polymerization of a Methacrylate Resin Denture Base.* J.A.D.A., *38:*188–203 (Feb.), 1949.
53. Swaney, A. C., Paffenbarger, G. C., Caul, H. J., and Sweeney, W. T.: *American Dental Association Specification No. 12 for Denture Base Resin: Second Revision.* J.A.D.A., *46:*54–66 (Jan.), 1953.
54. Sweeney, W. T., and Schoonover, I. C.: *A Progress Report on Denture Base Material.* J.A.D.A., *23:*1498–1512 (Aug.), 1936.
55. Koivumaa, K. K.: *On the Properties of Flexible Dentures.* Acta Odont. Scandinavica, *16:*159–175 (Nov.), 1958.
56. Matthews, E., and Smith, D. C.: *Nylon as a Denture Base Material.* Brit. D. J., *98:*231–237 (April 5), 1955.
57. Anthony, D. H., and Gibbons, P.: *The Nature and Behavior of Denture Cleansers.* J. Pros. Den., *8:*796–810 (Sept.-Oct.), 1958.
58. Sexson, J. C., and Phillips, R. W.: *Studies on the Effects of Abrasives on Acrylic Resins.* J. Pros. Den., *4:*454–471 (July), 1951.
59. Morden, J. F. C., Lammie, G. A., and Osborne, J.: *Effect of Various Denture Cleansing Agents on Chrome-cobalt Alloys.* D. Practitioner and D. Record, *6:*304–310 (June), 1956.
60. Nyquist, G.: *Study of Denture Sore Mouth. An Investigation of Traumatic, Allergic and Toxic Lesions of the Oral Mucosa Arising from the Use of Full Dentures.* Acta Odont. Scandinavica, 10, suppl., *9:*11–154, 1952.
61. Van Huysen, G., Fly, W., and Leonard, L.: *Artificial Dentures and the Oral Mucosa.* J. Pros. Den., *4:*446–460 (July), 1954.
62. Smith, D. C., and Bains, M. E. D.: *Residual Methyl Methacrylate in the Denture Base and Its Relation to Denture Sore Mouth.* Brit. D. J., *98:*55–58 (Jan.), 1955.
63. Smith, D. C.: *The Acrylic Denture Base—Some Effects of Residual Monomer and Peroxide.* Brit. D. J., *106:*331–336 (May), 1959.
64. Nyquist, G.: *Influence of Denture Hygiene and the Bacterial Flora on the Condition of the Oral Mucosa in Full Denture Cases.* Acta Odont. Scandinavica, *11:*24–60, 1953.

# CHAPTER 13

# Tooth Restorations

# with Acrylic Resin

Acrylic resin has been developed as a material for restorations in teeth because of its esthetic properties. The use of acrylic resin as a denture base material has been discussed in Chapters 10, 11, and 12. Further development of the previous discussion will be made in the present chapter, in relation to the use of acrylic resin in dental operative procedures.

The early resin restorations were made by cementation of heat-cured acrylic inlays or crowns in the prepared cavity. However, the low modulus of elasticity and a lack of dimensional stability invariably resulted in a fracture of the cement with a subsequent leakage and failure of the restoration. The use of this type of resin in operative procedures is now confined to the self-curing acrylic resin.

Its use has been, and still is, the subject of much controversy. Certain properties, such as its esthetic quality and insolubility, make it superior to the silicate cement restoration, to be described in a subsequent chapter. On the other hand, inherent weaknesses discussed later have cast doubt on its suitability as a restorative material. In all fairness it should be recognized that improved compositions and technics have eliminated some of the faults found in the earlier materials and procedures. If the self-curing acrylic resin is employed as tooth restorative material, it should be used in only selected types of cases. It is only by a knowledge of its basic chemical and physical properties that one can intelligently evaluate its proper role in the restoration of the carious tooth.

**Polymer.** The chemical composition of the polymer used in the self-curing resins is essentially poly(methyl methacrylate). The polymer may also contain an initiator, usually benzoyl peroxide (0.5 to 2.0 per cent).[1, 2]

The production of the proper shade and hue is accomplished in essentially the same manner as described for dental porcelain (p. 273). The polymer particles are generally pigmented by a ball-mill process in which the pigment is ground into the surface of the polymer particle, the same procedure used for many denture base resins.[3]

The size of the polymer particles may be of considerable importance in relation to the total surface presented for the monomer-polymer reaction. All other factors being equal, the attack on the polymer by the monomer will be more rapid, the smaller the particle size. As a result, the solution rate of the polymer and thus the hardening time will be more rapid with the ultra-fine polymers. Materials which have this type of polymer in the main may be mixed on a glass slab. If, however, the powder is composed of larger polymer particles (100–200 mesh) the solution rate will be too slow for slab mixing and a Dappen dish is employed.[1]

The particle size and shape of three acrylic resin polymers used for direct tooth restoration are shown in Figures 13–1, 13–2 and 13–3. Although none of the particles shown in the figures is as large as those generally used in a denture base material, there is a significant difference in their size and shape when they are compared with each other. It should be noted that the shape of the particles shown in Figure 13–3 is different from that of the other particles. Apparently, these particles are grindings obtained from a solid polymer.

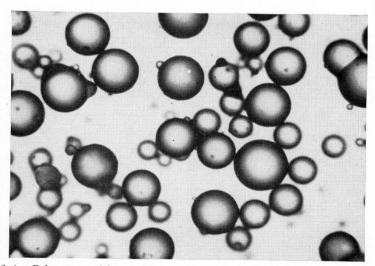

Fig. 13–1.   Polymer particles used in a self-curing acrylic resin for tooth restoration. Note that the polymer pearls are of graded sizes. ×100.

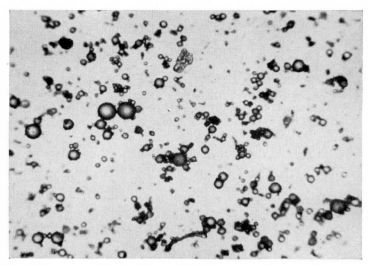

Fig. 13–2. Polymer particles used in a different brand of direct filling acrylic resin for tooth restoration. ×100.

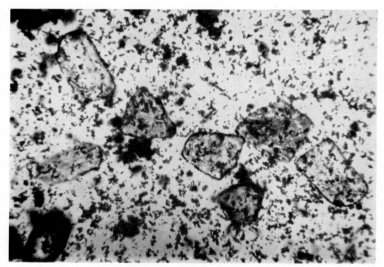

Fig. 13–3. A third type of polymer particle employed in a direct filling acrylic resin for tooth restoration. The particles are ground from a solid polymer. Their size varied so widely that it was necessary to photograph them compositely. ×100.

The molecular weight distribution of the polymer should be adjusted to control the initial reaction between the polymer and the monomer, as with the denture base polymers (p. 161). The polymer may contain a limited amount of plasticizer to enhance this reaction.

**Monomer.** The composition of the monomer is mainly methyl methacrylate, although some manufacturers claim the presence of a cross-linking agent as well, probably in a minor amount. In addition, the monomer contains a minute amount of inhibitor (*e.g.*, hydroquinone, 0.006 per cent). If an initiator is included in the resin by the manufacturer, it is incorporated in the monomer. A cross-linking agent may also be present.

**Chemistry.** In contrast to the reaction in the case of the denture base self-curing resins, it is highly desirable that the polymerization of a direct restorative resin be completed in a comparatively short time. The resin is usually polymerized directly in the prepared cavity, and the chair time should be as short as possible. Also, the more rapid the polymerization, the less apt is the adaptation to the cavity walls to be disturbed during the finishing of the restoration. Consequently, a short initiation period is desirable.

A number of factors which influence the polymerization time of acrylic resins regardless of the method of activation, such as the possible effects of particle size, molecular weight distribution, and composition of the polymer, have already been enumerated in the previous chapters. In the last analysis, the total time of hardening will depend upon the monomer-polymer reaction and, most important, upon the rate at which the activated radicals of the initiator are supplied. The higher the rate of production of free radicals, the shorter will be the initiation period. Any increase in temperature will facilitate the production of free radicals in the presence of a chemical activator by virtue of the increase in kinetic energy, and consequently the initiation period will be shortened.

Actually, there are two general methods by which the active radicals can be supplied at mouth temperatures. The first is the method already described wherein two chemicals are used. For example, dimethyl-*p*-toluidine is incorporated in the monomer as an activator and benzoyl peroxide in the polymer as the initiator. When the two are mixed, the molecules of benzoyl peroxide react with the dimethyl-*p*-toluidine to liberate free radicals which in turn act as the initiators and the polymerization reaction proceeds. All other factors being equal, the rate at which the activated molecules will be supplied will depend upon the initiator-activator ratio. Regardless of all factors involved, there will always be an initiation period.

A slight modification of this mode of polymerization is the addition of a methacrylic acid additive to the conventional amine containing monomer,[4] added mainly for the purpose of reducing any subsequent discoloration.

The other method entails the use of some type of chemical which can act to supply free radicals without the presence of a second chemical. Dimethyl-*p*-toluidine can effect a polymerization without the presence of benzoyl peroxide, but the process is too slow.

It has been shown that *p*-toluene sulfinic acid[5] ($CH_3 \cdot C_6H_4 \cdot SO_2H$), among other chemicals, can initiate the polymerization of methyl methacrylate. The *p*-toluene sulfinic acid is dissolved in the monomer and the reaction starts immediately, without a measurable induction period. Initially, free radicals are produced at a more rapid rate than in the reaction which occurs between dimethyl-*p*-toluidine and benzoyl peroxide under the same conditions.[1] Methyl methacrylate polymerizes more rapidly at 20° C. (68° F.) with *p*-toluene sulfinic acid than at 60° C. (140° F.) with benzoyl peroxide.

One objection to the use of *p*-toluene sulfinic acid is that this chemical is unstable. It readily oxidizes to *p*-toluene sulfonic acid ($CH_3 \cdot C_6H_4 \cdot SO_3OH$), which does not activate polymerization. Commercially, this difficulty has been partially overcome by an immersion of the *p*-toluene sulfinic acid in an inert silicone oil, in order to keep it away from the air. Under these conditions, its shelf life is approximately six months.

In practice, the dentist squeezes a measured amount of the silicone-sulfinic acid paste from a flexible tube onto a blotting paper. The paste is then pressed against the blotting paper in order to remove the oil, and the powder remaining is dissolved in the monomer. The polymerization begins immediately.

**Pressure Technic.**     A number of different technics for the insertion of direct acrylic resin restorations have been reported in the dental literature. There are at least three methods for the insertion of the material in the prepared cavity which are in general use. They are (1) the bulk pack or compression technic, (2) the non-pressure or brush technic, and (3) the combination non-pressure and pressure technic. All of the individually employed procedures are basically variations of these three.

In the pressure technic, the polymer and monomer are mixed in much the same manner as that described for the denture resins. The mixture is prepared either on a mixing slab or in a Dappen dish. One objection to this method of mixing is the danger of the incorporation of air bubbles which may affect the final restoration deleteriously.

One method for the mixing procedure which entails the least possible risk of the incorporation of air is to add the polymer to the monomer without any stirring or mixing.[6] Sufficient monomer is placed in a Dappen dish, and the polymer is added gradually. The dish is rapped sharply on the top of the table to allow all the polymer to be saturated. This process is continued until all of the monomer has been absorbed. The mass is now ready for insertion into the cavity.

After the monomer and polymer have been mixed, the mass is inserted into the prepared cavity at once. A contoured matrix strip of some material which is not attacked by the monomer is applied so that the monomer-polymer mixture can be held under pressure. The matrix strip is clamped tightly in position until the polymerization has been virtually completed. Any disturbance of the matrix during the polymerization is apt to cause a subsequent leakage of the restoration.

The functions of the matrix are (1) to prevent the evaporation of the monomer during the period of polymerization, (2) to consolidate the material into the cavity and reduce the size of any air bubbles which may be present, and (3) supposedly to direct the polymerization shrinkage to areas where it will not be a cause for the leakage of the restoration.

The bulk pack or pressure technic[7, 8] is no doubt one of the most practical methods and, when properly executed, it gives reasonably good results. Its basic principle is supposedly the exertion of pressure on the already inserted polymerizing resin by means of the matrix and, thereby, to force excess resin into the cavity. Unfortunately in practice this action does not take place. Actually, any excess resin not confined in the cavity is flowed over the tooth surface outside the cavity by the pressure of the matrix strip and a flash is formed. Finally, therefore, the pressure of the matrix is exerted on the tooth surface surrounding the prepared cavity and not on the polymerizing resin in the cavity itself. Apparently the basis for the satisfactory results possible with the pressure technic are not due to pressure but, at least in part, to other factors such as the pattern of the contraction, a mechanical locking of the material to the cavity walls, and the presence of excess material from which the contracting resin may draw.

It is important, regardless of the technic employed, to prevent the evaporation of monomer during the early periods of the polymerization. Otherwise, the polymer pearls are not surrounded by a polymer matrix after polymerization, and the surface exhibits a sandy appearance. As previously stated, the matrix protects the surface from evaporation. However, for other technics where the matrix may not be employed, evaporation can be prevented by immediately coating the restoration with a layer of tin foil or cocoa butter.

***Non-pressure (Brush) Technic.*** The non-pressure or brush technic[9, 10] is accomplished by the application of the monomer-polymer mixture in increments, rather than all at one time. The polymer is placed in one Dappen dish and the monomer in another. The prepared cavity is saturated with monomer. The tip of a small sable-hair brush is dipped into the monomer, and then into the polymer so that a few pearls cling to it (Fig. 13–4). The "bead" so formed is placed in the prepared cavity in contact with the monomer already present. The process is repeated again and again. The period between application of the "beads" may vary from ten to sixty seconds depending upon the temperature, the size of polymer powder, and the experience of the operator. When the prepared cavity has been properly filled, the surface of the restoration is then covered with some type of inert material, such as tin foil, until the initial polymerization is complete, in order to

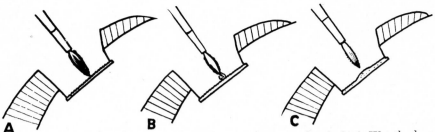

Fig. 13–4.    Filling a prepared cavity by the non-pressure method. *A.* Wet the base of the cavity with monomer. *B.* Place a "bead" of polymer on the wet surface. *C.* Withdraw the brush and allow the monomer-saturated polymer to flow over the surface. Wait 10–15 seconds. Repeat until the cavity is overfilled. (Simon, *Clinical Operative Dentistry.*)

prevent the evaporation of monomer. In this case, no pressure is necessary.

When the non-pressure technic is used, special care should be taken not to allow any polymer to drop into the Dappen dish containing the monomer, or to drop any of the monomer into the dish containing the polymer. Any premature contact of the powder and liquid will destroy the effectiveness of the reactions involved, and the restoration will be weakened thereby.

Another precaution to be observed is to insure that the fresh increments of monomer and polymer are always added to a monomer-saturated surface. If the monomer is allowed to evaporate so that the resin already present in the prepared cavity exhibits a dull surface, a good union with the added resin may not be possible.

Because of the difficulties involved with pressure technics, such as movement of the matrix during polymerization, the brush technic is more generally employed and it appears to produce somewhat better adaptation to the cavity walls.[11] The reasons are probably that there is less chance for error and the thinner mass of resin, having a lower viscosity and surface tension, tends to flow better into the minute crevices of the cavity walls. The resin is thus held in close apposition during polymerization.

Another aid in increasing adaptation is by the use of certain cavity liners supplied by the resin manufacturer. Although the exact compositions of these liners are not known, an analysis[12] of one indicated that it contained 5 to 10 parts of phosphoric ester, 5 to 10 parts of methacrylic acid and 80 to 90 parts of methyl methacrylate. If such a liner is painted on the cavity walls before the insertion of the resin, these solutions improve the adaptation.[12–14] Another suggested method for the improvement of the adaptation of the resin restoration is to etch the enamel or dentin and thus roughen the cavity walls.[15]

There are other modifications of the brush technic. It is not possible to use the bead procedure with the sulfinic acid type of resin so "flow" technics are better suited for that type of material.[16] In this method a thin or medium-thin mix is prepared and carried to the cavity on a small sable brush. This increment is touched to the base of the preparation and allowed to flow into the retention until the cavity is approximately one-third filled (Fig. 13–5). At subsequent intervals additional slightly thicker mixes are flowed into the cavity until it is filled and a slight excess is humped in the center surface area. The surface is then covered as previously described.

**Combination Non-pressure and Pressure Technic.**   The non-pressure procedures are easily managed in class V restorations and open areas where the excess resin may be controlled. However, in certain cases, the pull of gravity on large amounts of resin while it is fluid makes it difficult to control the material in order to secure desired contour. A combination technic using both non-pressure and a bulk pack application may be preferred.

A non-pressure application of resin is used to secure maximum retention on the first third of the preparation. A bulk pack-strip matrix procedure is used for the remainder of the restoration. Thus the non-pressure phase of the technic assures adaptation to the retentive areas and cavity walls while the bulk pack, if properly done with a contoured and confining matrix, assures proper contour and contact.

Whatever the technic employed, the final finishing of the restoration should take place not less than 24 hours after its insertion, in order to insure that the polymerization is complete and that the maximum strength and hardness of the resin have been attained.

**Evolution of Heat.**   The temperature attained on the interior of the resin will depend, among other factors, upon (1) the temperature of the environment in which the resin polymerizes, (2) the rate of polymerization, and (3) the bulk of the restoration.

The temperatures attained in the interior of resin specimens of various commercially available self-curing resins, two cubic centimeters in volume, are shown graphically[17] in Figure 13–6. Curve 8 in the figure represents the temperature rise of a typical silicate cement during setting, in contrast to the heat evolved in the resins. It is obvious that the

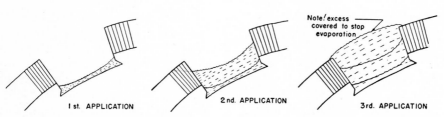

Fig. 13–5.   "Flow" technic. 1. Flow a mixture of monomer and polymer to fill approximately one-third of the cavity. 2. Add a second mix somewhat thicker. 3. Overfill the cavity as shown. (Boyd, *D. Clin. North America*, March, 1957.)

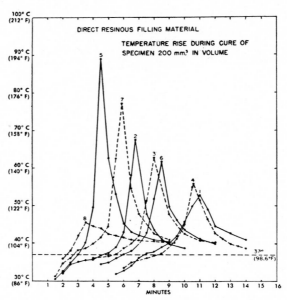

Fig. 13–6.   Temperature of seven commercial self-curing resin products for tooth restoration and one silicate cement (curve 8), plotted as a function of the time after mixing. (Wolcott, Paffenbarger and Schoonover, *J.A.D.A.*, March, 1951.)

increase in temperature for the silicate cement is much less than that for the self-polymerizing resin of the same volume.

As can be noted, the maximum temperatures obtained, and the times at which the maxima occur, vary with different brands of resin. The greatest polymerization rate occurs before and at the peak temperature. Since most of the polymerization has taken place when the peak temperature has been attained, the time period measured from the time the polymer and monomer are combined until the peak temperature is reached can be defined as the *hardening* or *setting time* of the resin.

The time at which the maximum temperature is attained can be determined readily by the heat sense if a small piece of the material is held between the thumb and forefinger during polymerization. Such a determination of the hardening time is particularly practical when the pressure technic is used. After the resin begins to cool as sensed by the fingers, the matrix can be removed, and the initial finishing of the restoration can be started, when the pressure technic is employed.

It is of interest to note the effect of the particle size on the rate of polymerization as evidenced by the curves in Figure 13–6. The larger polymer particles shown in Figure 13–1 produced a comparatively low temperature rise (curve 4, Fig. 13–6). On the other hand, the higher temperature rise of the products with the smaller pearls shown in Figures 13–2 and 13–3 is represented by curves 7 and 5, respectively, in Figure 13–6.

**Effect of Temperature.** As previously noted, the higher the environmental temperature of the heat-curing resins, the greater is the rate of polymerization, and, consequently, the higher is the temperature rise above the initial temperature. This factor is of considerable importance in connection with the resins used for tooth restorative purposes.

For example, the temperature rise during the polymerization of the commercial resins used in connection with Figure 13–6 will be greater at body temperature than at room temperature, even though the same amount of resin is employed in each case. Furthermore, it has been shown that the exothermic heat as indicated by the change in temperature during polymerization varies greatly with different commercial brands of resin in its relation to the environmental temperature.[18] In other words, a determination of the temperature change at room temperature of a given amount of self-curing resin is not necessarily an indication of the temperature change which may occur at mouth temperature.

The same considerations apply in connection with the time of occurrence of the peak temperature (*i.e.*, the setting time). The setting times at body temperature of the different commercial resins cannot be predicted from their setting times at room temperature.[18] The greater the bulk of the self-curing resin, the higher the peak temperature will be. However, differences in bulk do not affect the time of the peak temperature (*i.e.*, the setting time).[17]

It should be noted that the peak temperature is of practical importance only to the extent that it indicates the proper time at which the matrix strip can be removed. The temperature rise during polymerization is not likely to be of sufficient magnitude that the pulp will be harmed.

**Effect of Water.** Water incorporated in the resin before or during its polymerization definitely increases the maximum temperature rise and decreases the initiation period.[19] The incorporation of water is generally to be avoided, however, since the shade of the restoration may be affected. In the case of those resins which contain *p*-toluene sulfinic acid, the incorporation of water should be completely avoided. The *p*-toluene sulfinic acid is unstable in water. If the resin becomes contaminated by saliva, for example, during its polymerization in the tooth, the *p*-toluene sulfinic acid decomposes and the material will not set properly.[1]

**Polymerization Shrinkage.** As noted in Chapter 12, it can be calculated that a volume shrinkage of approximately 7 per cent can be expected when an acrylic resin is polymerized according to dental procedures. Such a calculation is based on the assumption that one-third of the monomer-polymer mixture is monomer. If more monomer than this is present, a greater shrinkage can be expected.

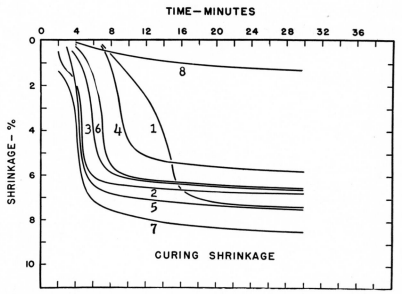

Fig. 13–7. Effective volumetric shrinkage of various commercial direct filling resins during polymerization. (Smith and Schoonover, *J.A.D.A.*, May, 1953.)

The volume shrinkage of the commercial products tested for heat evolution (Fig. 13–6) and other similar products has been determined.[18, 20] Some of the results are shown graphically in Figure 13–7. The numbers on the curves correspond to the similar numbers in Figure 13–6.

It should be noted that all of the resins shrink more than the silicate cement (curve No. 8). It is also of interest that the materials in which the most shrinkage occurred are materials number 5 and 7 in Figure 13–6 which exhibited the greatest temperature rise during polymerization. Furthermore, the material which exhibited the least shrinkage (curve No. 4, Fig. 13–7) also produced one of the lowest peak temperatures (Fig. 13–6). Such a qualitative correlation between the amount of shrinkage and the heat of reaction can be generalized for the conditions described. The relation possibly can be accounted for by the differences in the completeness of the polymerization attained by the various resins, since it is logical that the more complete the polymerization, the greater will be the polymerization shrinkage and the greater the heat of reaction, other factors being equal.

The magnitude of the shrinkages, ranging from 5 to 8 per cent (Fig. 13–7), is perhaps less than might be expected on the basis of the theoretical calculation of 7 per cent or above, if more monomer is used. At least two reasons can be given for these apparently lower shrinkage values: (1) part of the polymerization probably occurred before the measurements began, and (2) the polymerization is not completed when this type of self-polymerizing resin is employed within the time indicated in the figure.

Although various brands of direct restorative resins exhibit different amounts of polymerization shrinkage, it is doubtful that the differences are of practical significance. If a restorative material shrinks as much as 5 per cent by volume during its hardening in the mouth, it is doubtful that an additional shrinkage of 3 per cent will be significant clinically, so far as a possible leakage of the restoration is concerned.

**Shrinkage Compensation.** If a shrinkage of the magnitude of 5 to 8 per cent actually occurred in dental practice, the restoration would exhibit such a great leakage in practice that the material could not be used. Since it is used with a certain measure of success, it is reasonable to assume that the leakage can be prevented to some extent.

In connection with the pressure technic, the importance of holding the resin under pressure with a matrix during polymerization was discussed. As previously stated, one possible purpose of the matrix is to direct the shrinkage into areas which will not be of consequence so far as the leakage of the filling is concerned. For example, some experimental "fillings" in cylindrical holes in a brass die are shown in Figure 13–8. The holes were filled according to the pressure technic, and the resin was allowed to polymerize under pressure at 37° C. (98.6° F.). As can be noted, a shrinkage occurred on the surface of each specimen, but the margins were held tightly closed by the flash.

Since the surface of the resin pulled away from the matrix as it shrank, the pressure exerted by the matrix on the bulk of the resin became zero soon after the polymerization started. However, the flash

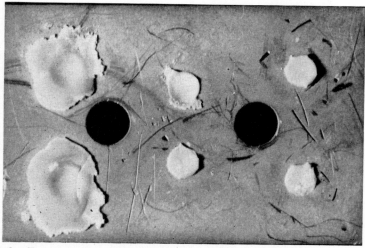

Fig. 13–8. Experimental "fillings" prepared in a brass die according to the pressure technic.

was so thin that there was probably very little shrinkage because of its small bulk. Consequently, it can be assumed that the pressure of the matrix on the flash was positive at all times. As a result, it is conceivable that the flash may have aided in the prevention of shrinkage at the margin of the restoration, since its resultant action under pressure was to hold the resin tightly to the margin of the prepared cavity.

If a close adaptation of the resin to the surface of the tooth is attained during the insertion of the monomer-polymer mixture, a mechanical adhesion to the surface of the dentin can be obtained.[20] Such an adhesion is effective only during the early stages of polymerization, and it is lost as soon as the restoration is exposed to moisture.[1, 13, 14, 20] This loss of adhesive characteristics is, of course, common to other dental materials, particularly the dental cements. However, this initial close adaptation may be effective in the prevention of polymerization shrinkage at the margins of the restorations.

In the case of the non-pressure technic, the shrinkage is directed toward the walls of the prepared cavity. When the monomer-polymer mixture is added gradually, there is sufficient mechanical adhesion to the dry walls of the prepared cavity during the initial stages of the polymerization so that the resin tends to shrink toward the walls. As more material is added, it tends to shrink against the material already added, and so on.

**Water Sorption.**    The weight increase due to water sorption of the autopolymer resins is not essentially different from that of the resins cured by heat activation.

As in the case of the heat-cured acrylic resin denture bases (p. 184), the dimensional change which occurs during the water sorption is not necessarily an increase in volume, as might be expected. When it is measured linearly, the result is often similar to the changes shown in Figure 12–5 (p. 185). However, the changes in volume which accompany the water sorption of a small cylindrical bulk of resin polymerized by heat activation indicate an initial expansion, a contraction, and then a gradual expansion[21] as indicated in Figure 13–9. On the other hand, self-cured acrylic resin specimens of the same size exhibited little or no change in volume when they were treated in the same manner.[22]

The reason for such erratic changes in dimension during water sorption is related to the release of processing stresses as described in the case of the acrylic resin denture bases. If the autopolymer resin is first annealed, the linear change in water sorption is manifested as an expansion of 0.3 to 0.5 per cent, which is virtually completed after an immersion in water for 24 hours.[18]

Water sorption probably has little clinical significance in the resin restoration. It does not seriously alter the physical properties, neither is the resulting expansion produced by the water sorption to be relied upon to assure better adaptation to the cavity walls.

**Surface Hardness and Strength.** The acrylic resin is undoubtedly the weakest and softest of the existing restorative materials. A comparison of the Knoop hardness numbers of tooth structure and various types of restorative materials is given in Table 13–1. As can be noted, the acrylic resin is softer than any of the materials or hard tissues listed. Such data are a definite indication that the tooth restorations with this material should be confined to regions where they are not subjected to the forces of mastication.

This limitation of their use is further evidenced by examination of other mechanical properties.[23] The average yield strength under compression is only 450 kilograms per square centimeter (6,400 pounds per square inch). As biting forces above 45 kilograms (100 pounds) are common in the oral cavity, stresses above 450 kilograms per square centimeter can easily occur on the occlusal surfaces of resin restorations and plastic flow would occur on the resin placed in that area.

The modulus of elasticity of poly(methyl methacrylate) is 21,800 kilograms per square centimeter (310,000 pounds per square inch), as compared to that of gold alloys used for inlays which have a modulus of 1,000,000 kilograms per square centimeter (14,000,000 pounds per square inch). In short, equal forces on similar specimens of resin and gold will produce approximately fifty times as much deformation in the resin as in the gold. Thus, stresses of mastication will likely result in a deformation of the resin restoration with resultant movement at the marginal areas.

Addition of filler agents, such as aluminum oxide or fiberglass, has been made by some manufacturers with a view to increasing these

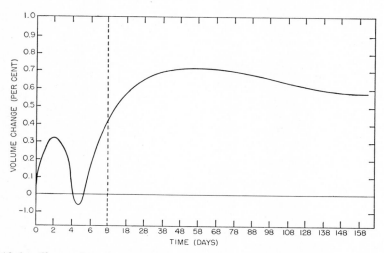

Fig. 13–9. Change in volume of small cylinders of heat cured poly(methyl methacrylate) after immersion in water.

properties. Although these inert agents may appear to give a harder, stronger resin, they do not measurably alter the properties.

It is readily evident from the foregoing that intelligent consideration of the basic properties of the present resins contraindicate their use except where they are not subject to stress. This consideration, then, limits their use primarily to the class V restoration and, where there is access, to the class III. As a temporary measure, reinforced with wire,[7] they have been used with some effectiveness in the class IV cavity. As a rule, they should never be employed on the two or three surface restoration.

**Germicidal Properties.**     The ability of the filling material to resist caries is an important consideration that will often be mentioned in relation to tooth restorative materials. Many materials of this type, especially silicate cement (Chapter 15), possess some bacteriostatic or germicidal characteristics. Unfortunately the current resin restorative materials are totally inert in this respect.

Addition of antibacterial agents has been attempted[24, 25] with little success. The more soluble agents produce good marginal protection at first but due to their high solubility they soon leach out and lose potency. Less soluble compounds seem to have little effect. One promising approach, however, is the possibility of adding small concentrations (2 per cent) of sodium fluoride.[26] The mechanism in this case is essen-

*Table 13–1.*     *Comparative Hardness of Tooth Restorative Materials*

| MATERIAL | K.H.N. |
|---|---|
| Tooth enamel | 300 |
| Tooth dentin | 65 |
| Silicate cement | 70 |
| Acrylic resin (heat-curing) | 16 |
| Acrylic resin (self-curing) | 16 |
| Pure gold | 32 |
| Soft inlay gold alloy | 55 |
| Amalgam | 90 |

*Table 13–2.*     *Differential Thermal Dimensional Change between Tooth Structure and Various Restorative Materials*

| MATERIAL | FACTOR* $\left(\dfrac{\alpha \text{ for material}}{\alpha \text{ for tooth}}\right)$ |
|---|---|
| Acrylic resin (dry) | 7.1 |
| Amalgam | 2.2 |
| Gold inlay | 1.9 |
| Gold foil | 1.3 |
| Silicate cement | 0.8 |

* $\alpha$ = linear coefficient of expansion.

tially that of the silicate cement, namely, a reduction in the acid solubility of the adjoining tooth structure. It is because of this total lack of antibacterial qualities of the current resin products that marginal leakage is so acute with this type of restorative material.

**Percolation.**    As can be noted from Table 2–1 (page 28), the linear coefficient of expansion of a tooth across its crown is $11.4 \times 10^{-6}$ per degree centigrade, whereas that of dry acrylic resin is $81 \times 10^{-6}$ per degree centigrade. When the resin is wet, its thermal expansion may be 40 to 65 per cent greater.[27] It follows that an acrylic resin will, therefore, shrink or expand seven or more times as much as the tooth structure for every degree change in temperature. Similar calculations for other restorative materials given in Table 2–1 are presented in Table 13–2 for purposes of comparison. As can be noted, the differential expansion of the acrylic resin and the tooth is definitely greater than that of any of the other restorative materials.

That this phenomenon may be of clinical interest is shown in Figure 13–10. An acrylic restoration was inserted in an extracted tooth. The tooth was immersed in ice water for 30 seconds, removed and dried. As the tooth was warmed with the fingers, small droplets of liquid exuded from the margin as shown in the figure.[28]

Studies in the mouth showed a similar effect when the acrylic filling was chilled to 9° C. (48° F.) while the patient drank ice water and when heated to 52° C. (125° F.) with hot coffee. The restoration is, therefore, assumed to be chilled and warmed according to the foods

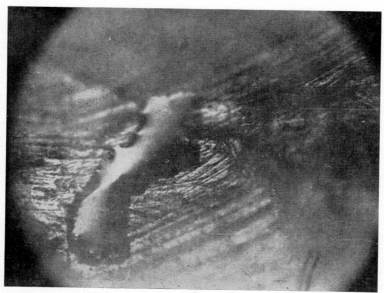

Fig. 13–10.    Marginal percolation of a direct filling acrylic resin. (Nelsen, Wolcott, Paffenbarger, *J.A.D.A.*, March, 1952.)

taken in, and, at the same time, the margin is imagined as opening at lower temperatures, imbibing fluids and then exuding them as the temperature rises. This pumping action of alternately imbibing and exuding fluids has been termed *percolation.*

**Marginal Leakage.**    It is possible that the temperature changes in the dental restoration are not as extreme as previously quoted,[29] but it is difficult to imagine that the teeth, and particularly the restorations, do not change temperature to some extent, at least, when hot and cold food and liquids are taken into the mouth. Whatever the change, the facts indicate that the effect of percolation in the acrylic resin restoration is much greater than for the other filling materials.

There appears to be some difference of opinion as to its clinical importance. Certain experiments *in vitro* indicated that the marginal leakage of the acrylic resin restorations is no worse than with other restorative materials,[30-33] but other investigators found that percolation causes definite marginal leakage of these restorations.[34, 35]

One clinical investigation,[34] extending over a two-year period, indicated that a significant number of the 412 acrylic resin restorations examined were found to have caries in the dentin beneath the restoration when it was removed. Unfortunately, removal of the restoration is the only method by which the caries can be detected in this area. Since in most cases faulty margins of the fillings were observed also, it is difficult to pinpoint the exact cause of the leakage. Percolation may have been one of the causes, but marginal failure due to masticatory stresses could also be the reason.

Another clinical investigation in which only marginal adaptation was measured, showed a relatively good marginal seal was still present in the acrylic restorations at the end of nine months.[36]

Regardless of its clinical significance, percolation is not a desirable characteristic for a restorative material such as a resin. Numerous ideas have been advanced[37-39] for its minimization but none is sufficiently successful. The best method yet found for minimizing this disadvantage is the use of a proper technic intelligently applied.

**Discoloration.**    Any impurities incorporated in the resin during its manufacture or manipulation are apt to result in a subsequent discoloration of the restoration. Clean utensils should be employed by the dentist and at no time should the resin be touched with the fingers before or during the polymerization.

General discoloration of the resin restoration was a common occurrence with the early products. It was not unusual to find the resin changing to a yellow or orange color after a short period of time in the oral cavity. Most of this discoloration could probably be attributed to chemical changes in the initiator. For example, if a drop of amine is added to benzoyl peroxide,[1] oxygen is liberated and the residue is amine anhydrobenzoic acid and colored products of decomposition.

This type of reaction, on a smaller scale, occurs in the resin restoration. Although not totally stable, such discoloration has been practically eliminated by the addition of stabilizers, such as cross-linking agents, or by the use of different initiator systems, such as *p*-toluene sulfinic acid.

The exact relationship of ultra-violet light to color change is not known but it has long been considered a contributing factor.[40] For this reason it is well to expose as little of the restoration to the labial as possible and whenever possible to place it below or above the lip line.

In any event, under the ideal conditions of formulation and technic, it can be expected that the acrylic resin restoration will not change color perceptibly in service, and that the material will maintain its esthetic properties indefinitely. Furthermore, it is virtually insoluble in the mouth fluids; consequently, no deterioration from solubility need be expected.

**Finishing.** Preferably, the finishing should not be completed for at least 24 hours after the restoration has been inserted, until the polymerization reaction is completed. During the finishing, the operator should remove the flash or overhang by cutting or abrading it *away* from the margins. If the flash is pulled toward the margins, it will likely tear and leave an opening for subsequent leakage.

The trimming can be effected with a thin-bladed, sharp knife, a sandpaper disk, or a bur held lightly against the surface. The surfaces can then be smoothed effectively with a dull bur or wet disks and sandpaper strips. The final finish can be enhanced by the use of wet chalk on a buff wheel,[41] or with wet flour of pumice in a rubber cup. Excessive glazing of the surface should be avoided since it will destroy the esthetic qualities of the resin.

**Pulp Reaction.** All materials used for restoring the carious tooth produce some pulpal reaction. The resin in particular has often been blamed for pulp injury and resulting death of the tooth. Although the resin restorations have been condemned from this standpoint,[42, 43] it is generally agreed that the pulp reaction is reversible and that any injury is not permanent.[44-46]

The fact that early use of the resin apparently resulted in greater incidence of pulpal reaction probably may be attributed to the fact that severe leakage routinely occurred with the technics being employed. As has been mentioned, the bulk pack technic is easily abused. In the beginning, this technic was the only one available. Improper use of this method, premature finishing of the resin, and inferior products unquestionably lead to poor adaptation. If leakage is severe and deleterious agents enter between the tooth structure and filling material, pulp reaction is inevitable regardless of the restorative used. Because of the lack of any bactericidal characteristics in the resin, one must again emphasize the importance of securing proper adaptation with this material.

## Literature

1. McLean, J. W., and Kramer, I. R. H.: *A Clinical and Pathological Evaluation of a Sulphinic Acid Activated Resin for Use in Restorative Dentistry.* Brit. D. J., *93:*255–269 (Nov. 18); 291–293 (Dec. 2), 1952.
2. Blumenthal, L. M.: *Recent German Developments of Dental Resins.* Final Report No. 1185, May 27, 1947, Washington, D. C.
3. McLean, J. W.: *A Review of Current Acrylic Filling Materials and Techniques.* D. Practitioner, *1:*176–182 (Feb.), 1951.
4. Morrant, G. A.: *Acrylic Resin Activator Systems and Associated Clinical Techniques.* D. Record, *73:*725–736 (Dec.), 1953.
5. Hagger, V.: *New Catalyst for the Polymerization of Ethenes at Room Temperature.* Helv. Chem. Acta, *31:*1624–1630, 1948.
6. Skinner, E. W.: *An Appraisal of Self Hardening Resins in Operative Dentistry.* W. Virginia D. J., *26:*4–11 (Oct.), 1951.
7. Simon, W. J.: *Clinical Operative Dentistry.* Philadelphia, W. B. Saunders Co., 1956, pp. 244–274.
8. Boyd, D. A.: *Symposium on Dental Materials.* D. Clin. North America, November, 1958, pp. 603–614.
9. Nealon, F. H.: *Acrylic Restorations: Operative Non-pressure Procedure.* New York J. D., *22:*201–206 (May), 1952.
10. Nealon, F. H.: *Acrylic Restorations by the Operative Non-pressure Procedure.* J. Pros. Den., *2:*513–527 (July), 1952.
11. Sausen, R. E., Armstrong, W. D., and Simon, W. J.: *Penetration of Radiocalcium at Margins of Acrylic Restorations made by Compression and Non-compression Technics.* J.A.D.A., *47:*636–638 (Dec.), 1953.
12. Buonocore, M., Wileman, W., and Brudevold, F.: *A Report on a Resin Composition Capable of Bonding to Human Dentin Surfaces.* J. D. Res., *35:*846–851 (Dec.), 1956.
13. Swartz, M. L., and Phillips, R. W.: *Method of Measuring the Adhesive Characteristics of Dental Cement.* J.A.D.A., *50:*172–177 (Feb.), 1955.
14. Swartz, M. L., Phillips, R. W., Day, R., and Johnston, J. F.: *A Laboratory and Clinical Investigation of Certain Resin Restorative and Cementing Materials.* J. Pros. Den., *5:*698–710 (Sept.), 1955.
15. Buonocore, M. G.: *A Simple Method of Increasing the Adhesion of Acrylic Filling Materials to Enamel Surfaces.* J. D. Res., *34:*849–853 (Dec.), 1955.
16. Boyd, D. A.: *The Direct Self-curing Resin Restoration.* D. Clin. North America, March, 1957, pp. 107–122.
17. Wolcott, R. B., Paffenbarger, G. C., and Schoonover, I. C.: *Direct Resinous Filling Materials: Temperature Rise During Polymerization.* J.A.D.A., *42:*253–263 (March), 1951.
18. Smith, D. L., and Schoonover, I. C.: *Direct Filling Resins: Dimensional Changes Resulting from Polymerization Shrinkage and Water Sorption.* J.A.D.A., *46:*540–544 (May), 1953.
19. Schoonover, I. C., Brauer, G. M., and Sweeney, W. T.: *Effect of Water on the Induction Period of the Polymerization of Methyl Methacrylate.* J. Res. Nat'l. Bur. Standards, *49:*359–364 (Dec.), 1952.
20. Christie, D. R.: *Acrylic Fillings—General Comments and Some Experimental Data.* J. Canad. D. A., *17:*427–434 (Aug.), 1951.
21. Dahl, G. S. A.: *Dimensional Stability of Small Cylinders of Acrylic Resin.* Thesis, Northwestern University Dental School, 1946.
22. Emmerson, J. H.: *A Physical, Clinical and Histo-pathological Investigation of the Self-hardening Resins Designed for Restoring Natural Teeth.* Thesis, Northwestern University Dental School, 1950.
23. Sweeney, W. T., Sheehan, W. D., and Yost, E. L.: *Mechanical Properties of Direct Filling Resins.* J.A.D.A., *49:*513–521 (Nov.), 1954.
24. Harris, N. O., and Fischer, J. E.: *A Study of the Antibacterial Properties of Plastic Filling Materials.* J. D. Res., *34:*742 (Oct.), 1955. Abstract.
25. Colton, M. B., and Ehrlich, E.: *Bactericidal Effect Obtained by Addition of Anti-*

biotics to Dental Cements and Direct Filling Resins. J.A.D.A., 47:524–531 (Nov.), 1953.

26. Phillips, R. W., and Swartz, M. L.: *Effect of Certain Restorative Materials on Solubility of Enamel.* J.A.D.A., 54:623–636 (May), 1957.

27. Spreter von Kreudenstein, Th.: *Thermal Volume Changes and Marginal Adaptation of Self-curing Resin Fillings.* Dent. zahnartztl. Zschr. 8:143 (July), 1953.

28. Nelsen, R. J., Wolcott, R. B., and Paffenbarger, G. C.: *Fluid Exchange at the Margins of Dental Restorations.* J.A.D.A., 44:288–295 (March), 1952.

29. Docking, A. R.: *The Present Status of Self-hardening Resins in Conservative Dentistry.* Bul. Alabama D. A., 41:6–19 (Jan.), 1957.

30. Fusayama, T., Ishibashi, M., and Kitazaki, T.: *Comparison of the Technics for Direct Acrylic Fillings.* Tokyo Med. & Dent. Bull., 2:235–242, 1956.

31. Swartz, M. L.: *In Vitro Studies on Marginal Leakage of Restorative Materials as Assessed by* $Ca^{45}$. Thesis, Indiana University School of Dentistry, September, 1959.

32. Buchanan, G. A.: *Resistance of Self-curing Acrylic Resin to the Passage of Dye Between Filling and Cavity Wall.* J. Canad. D. A., 17:131–138 (March), 1951.

33. Seltzer, S.: *The Penetration of Microorganisms between the Tooth and Direct Resin Fillings.* J.A.D.A., 51:560–566 (Nov.), 1955.

34. Hedegård, B.: *Cold-polymerizing Resins as Restorative Materials.* Sartryck ur. Odont. Tidsk., 65:173–212 (March), 1957.

35. Hirsch, L., and Weinreb, M. M.: *Marginal Fit of Direct Acrylic Restorations.* J.A.D.A., 56:13–21 (Jan.), 1958.

36. Phillips, R. W., Gilmore, H. W., Swartz, M. L., and Schenker, S. I.: *Adaptation of in vivo Restorations as Assessed by* $Ca^{45}$. Paper presented at 37th Annual Meeting of the International Association for Dental Research, San Francisco, California, March 21, 1959.

37. Rose, E. E., Lal, J., Green, R., and Cornell, J.: *Direct Resin Filling Materials: Coefficient of Thermal Expansion and Water Absorption of Polymethyl Methacrylate.* J. D. Res., 34:489–496 (Aug.), 1955.

38. Bowen, R. L.: *Use of Epoxy Resins in Restorative Materials.* J. D. Res., 35:360–369 (June), 1956.

39. Rose, E. E., Lal, J., Williams, N. B., and Falcetti, J. P.: *The Screening of Materials for Adhesion to Human Tooth Structure.* J. D. Res., 34:577–588 (Aug.), 1955.

40. Fischer, T. E., Butt, B. G., Sartose, J., and Eichel, B.: *Spectrophotometric Characterization of Light-induced Changes in Direct-filling Resins.* J. D. Res., 34:741 (Oct.), 1955. Abstract.

41. Coy, H. D.: *Auto-polymerizing Resin Fillings.* J.A.D.A., 44:251–260 (March), 1952.

42. Nygaard-Ostby, B.: *Pulp Reactions to Direct Filling Resins.* J.A.D.A., 50:7–13 (Jan.), 1955.

43. Langeland, K.: *Pulp Reactions to Resin Cements.* Acta Odont. Scandinavica, 13:230–256, 1956.

44. Councils on Research and on Dental Therapeutics: *Status Report on the Reactions of the Pulp to Self-curing Resinous Filling Materials.* J.A.D.A., 42:449–450 (April), 1951.

45. Massler, M.: *Effects of Filling Materials on the Pulp.* J. Tennessee D. A., 35:353–374 (Oct.), 1955.

46. Kramer, I. R. H., and McLean, J. W.: *The Response of the Human Pulp to Self-polymerizing Acrylic Restorations.* Brit. D. J., 92:255–261 (May 20); 281–287 (June 3); 311–314 (June 17), 1952.

# CHAPTER 14

# Dental Cements for

# Luting and Thermal

# Insulation. Cavity Liners

Dental cements are materials of comparatively low strength but they are used extensively in dentistry where strength is not a prime consideration. Unfortunately, they are not truly adhesive to enamel and dentin and they dissolve and erode in the oral fluids. These defects are likely to make them impermanent. However, regardless of certain inferior properties they do possess so many desirable characteristics that they are used in from 40 to 60 per cent of all restorations.[1] They are used as luting agents for fixed cast restorations or orthodontic bands, as thermal insulators under metallic restorations, as temporary or permanent restorations, as root canal fillings, and for pulp capping. It should be emphasized that as a group their chemical and physical properties leave much to be desired and the manipulative technics should be designed to provide the optimum behavior.

**Classification of Dental Cements.** Dental cements can be classified according to their composition, as presented in Table 14–1. The zinc phosphate cements are used principally for the cementation of inlays and other restorations fabricated outside of the mouth. Occasionally, silicate cement or a combination of silicate and zinc phosphate cement may be used for this purpose, particularly when a translucent filling material, such as porcelain or resin, is used.

Copper, silver, and mercury salts are sometimes added to the cements

*Table 14–1.* *Classification of Dental Cements*

| CEMENT | USES | |
|--------|----------|----------|
| | PRINCIPAL | SECONDARY |
| Zinc phosphate | Luting agent for fabricated restorations | Temporary restorations<br>Thermal insulating base |
| Zinc phosphate with copper or silver salts added | Temporary restorations<br>Root canal restorations | Thermal insulating base |
| Copper phosphate (red and black) | Temporary restorations | |
| Zinc oxide-eugenol | Temporary restorations<br>Thermal insulating base<br>Pulp capping | Root canal restorations |
| Calcium hydroxide | Pulp capping | |
| Silicate | Tooth restorations | Luting agent for restorations |
| Zinc phosphate-silicate | Luting agent for fabricated restorations | Posterior tooth restoration |
| Acrylic resin (cements) | Luting agent for fabricated restorations | Temporary restorations |

for the purpose of rendering them bacteriostatic or bactericidal. Copper oxide may also be used in place of zinc oxide for this reason. Although many investigations have been concerned with the antibacterial properties of all dental materials, the exact influence of each is not yet known. While some investigations have shown definite antibacterial effects from certain types of dental cements,[2, 3] other research[4, 5] has cast doubt on these findings. Thus the germicidal influence of added metallic ions must still be considered controversial. The same situation also exists in respect to adding polyantibiotics to the cement for dentin sterilization.[6, 7]

When the prepared cavity approaches the pulp, a cement base is employed as a protection to the pulp against both mechanical and thermal shock. Any of the cements can be used for this purpose except the silicate cements, which are generally considered to be too irritating. The zinc phosphate cements are the strongest of the cements used as bases, and probably afford the best protection against mechanical shock to the pulp. They, as well as most of the other commonly used cavity base materials, are excellent thermal insulators.[8] It can be seen from Table 14–2 that these values are in the same general range as other recognized insulators, such as asbestos and cork. Dentin itself is, of course, a very poor heat conductor and therefore a good insulator from temperature changes in the mouth and from heat evolved during cavity preparation or setting of restorative materials.

The zinc oxide-eugenol cements are increasing in their popularity as a base material. They apparently have a palliative, non-irritating

*Table 14–2.    Thermal Conductivity of Various Cement Base Materials and Dentin as Compared to Two Commonly Recognized Insulators*

| MATERIAL | THERMAL CONDUCTIVITY [cal. sec.$^{-1}$ cm.$^{-2}$($^{\circ}$C./cm.)$^{-1}$] $\times 10^{-4}$ |
|---|---|
| Dentin | 2.57 |
| Zinc phosphate cement (dry) | 3.11 |
| Zinc phosphate cement (wet) | 3.88 |
| Resin cement | 3.25 |
| Gutta-percha | 3.53 |
| Zinc oxide-eugenol | 3.98 |
| Silicate cement | 4.58 |
| Asbestos fiber | 1.90 |
| Cork | 7.00 |

action[9, 10] on the pulp as well as being good thermal insulators. Their effect on the pulp is most mild.

The silicate cements are used almost exclusively as permanent filling materials. They possess excellent esthetic properties when they are first inserted in the tooth. Unfortunately, they gradually disintegrate in the mouth fluids, and they may stain and craze; thus they should not be called permanent in comparison with the metallic filling materials, for example.

So far as is known, all of the cements shrink during setting. They are all soft and weak in comparison to metals, and they all slowly disintegrate in the mouth fluids. Research has not as yet provided a solution to these inherent weaknesses and they must be taken into consideration whenever these materials are used.

## ZINC PHOSPHATE CEMENTS

**Composition.**    The compositions of 16 zinc phosphate cement powders and liquids are presented in Tables 14–3 and 14–4, respectively.[11] The compositions given do not necessarily represent those of the modern zinc phosphate cements, but they are sufficiently typical for all practical purposes.

The chief difference between the various cements appears to be in the composition of the powders. According to Table 14–3, the first four cement powders contain zinc oxide almost exclusively. The next seven powders (E, F, G, H, I, J and K) contain one principal modifier in the form of magnesium oxide in the approximate ratio of nine parts of zinc oxide to one of magnesium oxide. The last five powders (L, M, N, O and P) contain modifiers in addition to magnesium oxide, such as silica, rubidium trioxide and bismuth trioxide. Powder N contains an appreciable amount of barium sulfate.

The chemical analyses of the liquids given in Table 14–4 for the corresponding powders in Table 14–3 show that the liquids are essentially aluminum phosphate, phosphoric acid, and, in some cases, zinc phosphate. The metallic salts are added as buffers to reduce the reaction rate of the liquid with the powder.

The average water content of the liquids is $33 \pm 5$ per cent. The

*Table 14–3.*   *Composition of Zinc Phosphate Cement Powders**
(PERCENTAGE BY WEIGHT)

| SAMPLE | ZnO | MgO | SiO$_2$ | R$_2$O$_3$ | Bi$_2$O$_3$ | MISCELLANEOUS |
|---|---|---|---|---|---|---|
| A . . . . . . . . . . . | 100.0 | . . . . | 0.05 | 0.05 | . . . . | |
| B . . . . . . . . . . | 99.7 | . . . . | 0.1 | 0.1 | . . . . | CaO, 0.1 |
| C . . . . . . . . . . | 98.0 | . . . . | . . . . | . . . . | 1.9 | |
| D . . . . . . . . . . | 99.4 | . . . . | 0.6 | 0.1 | 0.04 | |
| E . . . . . . . . . . | 92.4 | 7.5 | 0.1 | 0.06 | . . . . | CuO, 0.1 |
| F . . . . . . . . . . | 90.3 | 8.2 | 1.4 | 0.1 | . . . . | |
| G . . . . . . . . . . | 90.2 | 9.4 | 0.4 | 0.07 | . . . . | |
| H . . . . . . . . . . | 89.9 | 9.1 | 0.4 | 0.5 | . . . . | |
| I . . . . . . . . . . | 89.5 | 9.4 | 0.3 | . . . . | . . . . | BaCrO$_4$, 0.8 |
| J . . . . . . . . . . | 89.3 | 9.4 | 0.3 | 0.1 | . . . . | CuO, 0.02; BaCrO$_4$, 1.0 |
| K . . . . . . . . . . | 88.0 | 9.4 | 0.8 | . . . . | 1.8 | |
| L . . . . . . . . . . | 89.1 | 4.0 | 1.8 | 0.5 | 4.5 | |
| M . . . . . . . . . . | 82.2 | 9.0 | 3.0 | 0.9 | 4.1 | CuO, 0.8 |
| N . . . . . . . . . . | 83.1 | 7.2 | 0.1 | 0.04 | . . . . | BaSO$_4$, 8.2; CaO, 1.3 |
| O . . . . . . . . . . | 84.0 | 7.2 | 4.9 | 1.0 | . . . . | CaF$_2$, 2.7 |
| P . . . . . . . . . . | 74.9 | 13.0 | 1.3 | 2.6 | . . . . | BaO, 2.2; B$_2$O$_3$, 5.1 |

\* Paffenbarger, Sweeney and Isaacs, *J.A.D.A.*, Nov., 1933.

*Table 14–4.*   *Composition of Zinc Phosphate Cement Liquids**
(PERCENTAGE BY WEIGHT)

| COLUMN | ANALYSIS | | | | CALCULATIONS | | | | |
| | 1 | 2 | 3 | 4 | 5 | 6 | 7 | 8 | 9 |
| SAMPLE | PO$_4$ | Al | Zn | Mg | FREE H$_3$PO$_4$ | COM-BINED H$_3$PO$_4$ | TOTAL H$_3$PO$_4$ | PHOS-PHATE | WATER |
|---|---|---|---|---|---|---|---|---|---|
| A . . . . . . | 57.4 | 1.8 | 10.0 | . . . : | 42.8 | 16.6 | 59.4 | 27.8 | 28.8 |
| B . . . . . . | 55.2 | 3.4 | 3.1 | . . . . | 41.6 | 15.5 | 57.1 | 21.5 | 36.4 |
| C . . . . . . | 64.3 | 2.7 | . . . . | . . . | 56.8 | 9.8 | 66.6 | 12.2 | 30.7 |
| D . . . . . . | 57.3 | 2.1 | 10.0 | . . . | 41.7 | 17.6 | 59.3 | 29.2 | 28.6 |
| E . . . . . . | 64.6 | 2.7 | 1.6 | . . . | 55.5 | 11.4 | 66.9 | 15.4 | 28.8 |
| F . . . . . . | 52.6 | 2.5 | 7.1 | . . . | 38.2 | 16.2 | 54.4 | 25.3 | 36.0 |
| G . . . . . . | 59.9 | 2.9 | 2.0 | . . . | 49.4 | 12.6 | 62.0 | 17.0 | 33.1 |
| H . . . . . . | 59.7 | 2.1 | 4.1 | . . . | 50.1 | 11.7 | 61.8 | 17.6 | 32.0 |
| I . . . . . . | 57.9 | 2.8 | . . . . | 0.3 | 48.9 | 11.0 | 59.9 | 13.7 | 37.0 |
| J . . . . . . | 61.1 | 2.8 | . . . . | . . . | 53.1 | 10.2 | 63.3 | 12.7 | 33.9 |
| K . . . . . . | 64.0 | 3.2 | . . . . | . . . | 54.7 | 11.6 | 66.3 | 14.5 | 20.5 |
| L . . . . . . | 64.2 | 2.7 | 0.9 | . . . | 55.8 | 10.7 | 66.5 | 14.0 | 29.9 |
| M . . . . . . | 67.2 | 3.0 | . . . . | . . . | 58.7 | 10.9 | 69.6 | 13.6 | 27.4 |
| N . . . . . . | 64.9 | 2.9 | . . . . | . . . | 56.6 | 10.6 | 67.2 | 13.1 | 29.9 |
| O . . . . . . | 54.6 | 2.3 | 10.3 | . . . | 37.8 | 18.7 | 56.5 | 30.7 | 30.9 |
| P . . . . . . | 53.4 | 2.7 | . . . . | . . . | 45.5 | 9.8 | 55.3 | 12.2 | 42.0 |

\* Paffenbarger, Sweeney and Isaacs, *J.A.D.A.*, Nov., 1933.

amount of water present is a factor in the control of the ionization of the liquid, and it is a critical ingredient in the rate and type of the liquid-powder reaction.

In spite of the fact that the compositions of the liquids are similar, generally the liquids cannot be interchanged for use with the various powders. The composition of the liquid is quite critical, and the manufacturer is compelled to take special care in compounding it.

**Chemistry of Setting.** When a zinc oxide powder is mixed with phosphoric acid, a solid substance is formed very rapidly with a considerable evolution of heat. The exact nature of the product of the reaction is not known, but it is thought that tertiary zinc phosphate $[Zn_3(PO_4)_2 \cdot 4H_2O]$ is finally formed.[12] The reaction probably consists of a solution of the surface of the powder particles in the phosphoric acid to saturation. A reaction then possibly takes place to form primary zinc phosphate:

$$Zn O + 2H_3PO_4 \rightarrow Zn(H_2PO_4)_2 + H_2O$$

The available evidence indicates that the mixture at the time it is placed in the mouth may be composed of undissolved powder particles and a solution of phosphoric acid and primary zinc phosphate.[13] The solidification or setting process consists of a further reaction to form the stable water-insoluble tertiary zinc phosphate which precipitates in a crystalline form from a supersaturated solution.

Any magnesium oxide present in the dental cement powder (Table 14–3) probably reacts in a similar manner to form a tertiary magnesium phosphate $[Mg_3(PO_4)_2 \cdot 4H_2O]$. This product is quite insoluble in water, although it is not as insoluble as is the tertiary zinc phosphate.

In the dental cement, the reaction is retarded by the addition of the buffers to the liquid as already described. Also, the reactivity of the powder is reduced by a sintering of the ingredients at temperatures in the neighborhood of 1000° to 1400° C. (1830° to 2550° F.) into a cake which is ground and sifted to a fine powder.[12]

The reaction does not go to completion, since all of the powder is not attacked by the liquid. The surface layer of the powder particles is first dissolved by the liquid, and then the above reactions take place. As the crystals of the final product precipitate, the density of the crystalline deposition is greatest at the surface of the particle. Consequently, subsequent attack by the phosphoric acid becomes more difficult owing to the protective action of the dense, crystalline sheath around the particle.

The final product is crystalline in structure,[13] with undissolved powder particles suspended in the crystals of the zinc phosphate and other reaction products. Such a condition is typical of the *cored structure* which is found in many dental materials of this type. The undissolved powder particles are called the *core*, and the crystalline phase in which they are suspended is called the *matrix*. Thus, the set cement is essentially powder particles cemented together with the phosphate compounds.

**Control of the Setting Time.** The setting time of the cement must be controlled accurately. If the cement sets too rapidly, the crystal formation will be disturbed and broken up during the mixing of the cement, or upon insertion of the inlay or crown into the prepared cavity, and the set product may, therefore, be weak and lack cohesion. If the setting time is prolonged, the dental operation will be delayed unduly. A reasonable setting time at mouth temperature for a zinc phosphate cement would be between four and ten minutes.

The setting time is usually measured with a 1 pound Gillmore needle at a temperature of 37° C. (99° F.) and a relative humidity of 100 per cent. It is defined as the time elapsing from the start of mixing until the point of the needle no longer penetrates the surface of the cement when the needle is gently lowered onto it.

The control of the setting time as influenced by the manufacturing process is affected by the following factors:

1. The composition and the sintering temperature of the powder undoubtedly are factors in control of the setting time.

2. The composition of the liquid, as already described, is a factor since the presence of the buffering salts and the water definitely influences the setting time.

3. The larger the particle size of the powder, the less rapid will be the reaction because of the decreased surface contact of the powder with the liquid.

In a sense, when the dentist mixes the powder and liquid, he continues the manufacturing process. The factors under the control of the dentist are as follows:

1. The lower the temperature during mixing the longer will be the setting time. The temperature can be controlled by cooling the mixing slab.

2. In some cases, the rate at which the powder is added to the liquid may influence the setting time markedly. Generally, the more slowly the powder is added, the longer is the setting time.

3. The more liquid employed in ratio to the powder, the slower will be the setting rate.

4. The longer the mixing time, within practical limits, the longer will be the setting time.

The best method for the control of the setting time by the dentist is to regulate the temperature of the mixing slab. Generally, it is desirable to increase the setting time in order to be certain that sufficient time will be available for the manipulation of the cement, and so that the maximum amount of powder can be incorporated at the desired consistency. For this reason, the mixing slab is cooled. It should not be cooled below the dew point of the environment, otherwise moisture will collect on the slab and an accelerated setting time will result.

The rate of addition of the powder to the liquid may also be an effective means by which the dentist can control the setting time. The powder is usually added in uniform and small increments in order to control this factor. A prolonging of the setting time by the use of a higher liquid-powder ratio and by the prolongation of the mixing is usually to be avoided because of the adverse effect on the strength and solubility.

**Water Content of the Liquid.**   As previously noted, the water content of the liquid is established by the manufacturer, and the dentist should maintain it; otherwise the chemical equilibrium may be disturbed. Erratic behavior of the cement may often be traced to improper care of the liquid.

If the bottle of liquid is left unstoppered, the water content of the liquid will be altered according to the vapor pressure of the atmosphere in relation to the vapor pressure of the liquid. The change in weight of a cement liquid when stored in air and over water[14] is shown in Table 14–5. When the liquid is stored in air, it generally loses water, as shown in the table. However, if the humidity is sufficiently high, so that the vapor pressure of the air is higher than that of the liquid, water will be absorbed by the liquid. Such a condition is evident in Table 14–5 when the liquid is stored over water. It follows that the bottle of liquid should be left unstoppered for as short a time as possible. Also, the liquid should not be left on the mixing slap in contact with the air for any length of time before it is mixed with the powder.

The effect of the change in the water content of the liquid on the setting time may be quite marked. A dilution produces a decrease in setting time. The general effect of the water combined with the cement which was mixed on a slab which was chilled to a temperature below the dew point would, therefore, be to decrease the setting time.

*Table 14–5.*   *Effect of Water Vapor Pressure on the Change in Weight of a Zinc Phosphate Cement Liquid**

| TIME | LIQUID IN AIR † (CHANGE IN WEIGHT, PER CENT) | LIQUID OVER WATER (CHANGE IN WEIGHT, PER CENT) |
|---|---|---|
| 15 minutes | −0.3 | . . . . . . |
| 1 hour | −0.7 | . . . . . . |
| 3.5 hours | . . . . . . | +1.2 |
| 5 hours | . . . . . . | +2.0 |
| 1 day | −7.5 | +6.9 |
| 1 week | −17.7 | +23.7 |
| 1 month | −24.6 | +76.0 |

* Souder and Paffenbarger, *Nat'l. Bur. Standards Circular C433.*
† Temperature 21°–26° C. (70°–80° F.); relative humidity 25–50 per cent.

If water evaporates from the liquid, the setting time will be prolonged. Insufficient water in the liquid is often evidenced by the formation of crystals on the walls of the bottle, or a general cloudiness of the liquid. Such a condition is the result of the precipitation of the buffering salts. Unfortunately, if water is absorbed by the liquid, no change in appearance can be observed. Repeated opening of the bottle over a long period of time undoubtedly alters the water-acid ratio of the remaining liquid. Therefore, approximately the last one-fifth of the liquid should be discarded. Most manufacturers provide a slight excess in proportion to the powder for this reason.

The neck of the bottle should be kept clean and free of débris. Agitation of the liquid is not necessary.

**Acidity.** As might be expected from the presence of the phosphoric acid, the acidity of the cements is quite high at the time they are inserted in the tooth. Measurement of acidity in the setting or set cement is difficult and the exact $pH$ changes are probably not well known. According to one researcher, the hydrogen ion concentration of the mixture during this period[13] is approximately $pH$ 1.6. As the reaction proceeds, the $pH$ increases. The ultimate $pH$ of the cement may be in the neighborhood of 7 (neutrality).[15] It is probable that any damage occurring to the pulp occurs during the first few hours after insertion of the cement.

**Standard Consistency.** The consistency of the initial mixture of powder and liquid is often of considerable importance. From the standpoint of the physical properties of the cement, a mix of thick consistency is the best. However, in the seating of an inlay in a prepared cavity an extremely thick mix might not be indicated, since the mix might not flow from beneath the inlay readily, and thus the casting would not seat in the tooth properly.

The consistency of a cement is definitely related to the liquid-powder ratio used. The more powder incorporated in the liquid, the thicker will be its consistency.[16] Owing to the difference between various brands of cement, the liquid-powder ratio to produce the proper consistency usually varies from one cement to another.

The manufacturer should specify the proper liquid-powder ratio to provide the desired consistency.

The *standard consistency* as defined by the American Dental Association Specification No. 8 is determined with a modified slump test. It is the consistency obtained when the proper amount of powder is mixed with 0.5 cubic centimeter of liquid so that a disk, 30 millimeters (1.18 inches) in diameter, will be formed from 0.5 cubic centimeter of the mixed, unset cement when it is pressed between two glass plates under a load of 120 grams (4.2 ounces). The average properties of modern certified cements are shown at the bottom of Table 14–6, as determined with a standard consistency.

*Table 14-6.    Detail Requirements of A.D.A. Specification No. 8 for Dental Zinc Phosphate Cement, and Range of Values for Zinc Phosphate Cements on the List of Certified Dental Materials**

| | STANDARD CONSISTENCY OF MIX | TIME OF SETTING AT 37° C. (99° F.) | | COMPRESSIVE STRENGTH | FILM THICKNESS | SOLUBILITY AND DISINTEGRATION | ARSENIC CONTENT |
|---|---|---|---|---|---|---|---|
| | | Minimum (minutes) | Maximum (minutes) | | | | |
| Detail requirements of A.D.A. Specification No. 8 for Dental Zinc Phosphate Cement | To produce disk 30 ± 1 mm. in diameter | 4 | 10 | Minimum (7 days) kg./cm.$^2$ 840 $\left[\begin{array}{c}\text{lb./in.}^2\\12{,}000\end{array}\right]$ | Maximum (microns) 40 | Maximum (percentage by weight) 0.30 | Maximum (percentage by weight) 0.0002 (1 part in 500,000) |
| Range of values for Zinc Phosphate Cements on List of Certified Dental Materials | (Grams of powder in 0.5 ml. of liquid) 1.3 ± 0.3 | (Minutes) 7 ± 1 | | (lb./in.$^2$) 16,800 ±4,000 | (Microns) 30 ± 10 | (Percentage) 0.1 ± 0.1 | (Percentage) < 0.0002 |

* Paffenbarger, and Stanford, *D. Clin. North America*, November, 1958.

**Film Thickness.** In order for an inlay or crown to be seated properly, the film of cement should be sufficiently thin so that it will not interfere with the fit of the restoration.

The minimum thickness of the film is logically related to the particle size of the powder employed. However, the actual film thickness can be less than that of the maximum particle dimension. Undoubtedly the size of the original particle is reduced by its solution in the liquid during mixing, and it may be crushed during mixing and by the pressure exerted on the inlay when it is seated. For instance, it has been determined that a cement made from a powder having one or more particles 75 microns in one dimension possessed a film thickness as low as 35 microns.[17]

The test employed for film thickness is that described in the American Dental Association Specification No. 8. A cement mix of standard consistency is placed between two glass plates of 2 square centimeters (0.31 square inch) in area, under a load of 15 kilograms (33 pounds) for 10 minutes. According to the Specification, the increase in thickness of the two plates caused by the cement film should not be greater than 40 microns. The average film thickness range of a number of commercial products determined in this manner is presented in Table 14–6.

**Contact with Moisture.** In the light of the previous discussion of the critical nature of the water content of the cement, it is evident that the area in the vicinity of the cement must be kept dry while the powder-liquid mixture is being mixed and inserted in the tooth, and during hardening. If the cement is allowed to harden under a film of saliva, some of the phosphoric acid will be leached out, and the surface of the cement will be dull, soft and easily dissolved by the mouth fluids.

Such a statement does not indicate, however, that a condition of complete desiccation need exist. For example, if the walls of a prepared cavity are desiccated with alcohol and hot air, it is possible that more phosphoric acid may be absorbed from the cement liquid into the dentinal tubules and the pulp may be injured.

Once the cement has set, it should not be allowed to dry out. A drying of the set cement results in a shrinkage and a crazing of the surface, which will inevitably result in its disintegration.

**Adhesion.** Strictly speaking, adhesion refers to a molecular attraction between unlike molecules. It has been clearly established that adhesion in a physical sense does not exist between the cement and the tooth structure.[18, 19] Ideally, such an adhesion would be desirable and its attainment should be the objective of future development of superior cementing mediums.

In a broader sense, however, adhesion can refer to a mechanical interlocking, such as a gluing action in paper or wood joints. For example, when two pieces of wood are joined by an ordinary glue, the liquid glue penetrates into minute openings and crevices. When the glue sets, these many tiny finger-like extensions act as a bond and hold the two parts tightly in contact. It is then necessary to shear these extensions in separating the parts.

Whenever an inlay is seated in the prepared cavity, the surfaces of both the inlay and the tooth structure present slight roughnesses and scratches into which the plastic cement is forced. After the cement hardens, such extensions, many of which are undercut, assist in providing retention of the inlay. It has been shown that highly polished surfaces do not exhibit as great retention when they are bonded with dental cement as do slightly roughened surfaces.[20]

The thickness of the film between the inlay and the tooth also is a factor in the bonding strength. The thinner the film, the better is the bonding action. This effect is probably the result of a number of factors, one of which is the fact that the cement itself is subject to internal flaws such as air spaces and structural defects in bulk which are minimized in a thin film. Other factors which may be responsible for the difference are connected with surface chemistry, surface tension, atmospheric pressure, and similar phenomena.

There are, however, other inherent properties that influence the cement bond beside film thickness. For example, the compressive and shear strength of the cement affect the ease with which the small extensions, or locks, can be fractured. The mechanical retention is also dependent upon the dimensional changes occurring in the cement during setting, by the water gain or loss, and by the differences in the thermal coefficient of expansion of the tooth, of the structure luted, and of the cement itself.

**Dimensional Stability.** The zinc phosphate cements shrink during setting. The shrinkage of cement F, the composition of which is given in Tables 14–3 and 14–4, is presented[11] in Figure 14–1. As can be noted, the cement shrinks much more when it is in contact with air than when it is under water. It is evident that the cement should not be allowed to dry out. If the cement is in contact with water, its shrinkage is negligible as related to cementation. For example, if the film under an inlay is 0.1 millimeter in thickness, and if the cement shrinks 0.08 per cent linearly, the actual shrinkage of the film would be 0.00008 millimeter or 0.08 micron. Such a minute change is not of practical consequence.

**Strength.** The strength of dental cements is generally determined under compressive stress. The range of compressive strength of certified zinc phosphate cements is shown in Table 14–6. According to the American Dental Association Specification No. 8 the compressive strength of a zinc phosphate cement should not be less than 840 kilograms per square centimeter (12,000 pounds per square inch) seven days after it has been mixed.

As previously stated, the strength of the cement is dependent upon the liquid-powder ratio. The nature of this dependence is illustrated by the curve in Figure 14–2. As can be noted, the compressive strength increases rapidly as the amount of powder used for mixing with 0.5 milliliter of liquid is increased. The mixture for a standard consistency for this particular cement was 1.4 grams of powder to 0.5 milliliter of liquid. It can be noted from the curve that the strength obtained by increasing the powder above this amount is relatively small, particularly when compared to the decrease in strength when less powder is used.

As can be noted from Table 14–7, the set cement gains its maximum strength, for all practical purposes, within the first day.[11] As a matter of fact, it attains approximately 75 per cent of its maximum strength during the first hour.

When zinc phosphate cements are placed in contact with water for long periods of time, there is a gradual decrease in strength, probably due to the slow dissolution of the material similar to that which takes place in the mouth.

The strength of a zinc phosphate cement is probably sufficient when it is placed under an inlay or crown, but when it is exposed to the mouth forces, as a temporary filling material, for example, it exhibits brittleness and a definite lack of strength. Under such conditions of stress and erosion, it fractures and disintegrates relatively soon.

**Solubility and Disintegration.** Probably the one property of greatest clinical significance is the solubility and disintegration of the cement. In fact, this property is one of the most important considera-

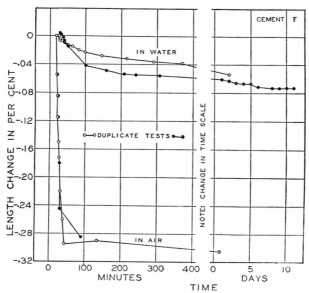

Fig. 14–1. Dimensional change of a zinc phosphate cement on setting. (Paffenbarger, Sweeney and Isaacs, *J.A.D.A.*, Nov., 1933.)

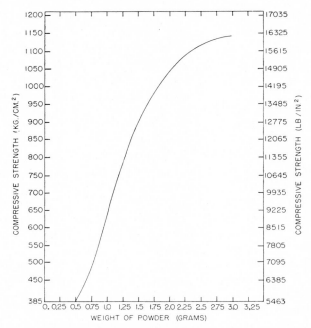

Fig. 14–2. Effect on the compressive strength of the amount of powder added to 0.5 milliliter of cement liquid. (Data from Paffenbarger, Sweeney and Isaacs, *J.A.D.A.*, Nov., 1933.)

*Table 14–7.*    *Change in Compressive Strength with Time**

| TIME | COMPRESSIVE STRENGTH (KG./CM.²) | (LB./IN.²) |
|------|------|------|
| 1 Hour | 770 | 11,000 |
| 3 Hours | 910 | 13,000 |
| 1 Day | 1010 | 14,500 |
| 1 Week | 1080 | 15,500 |
| 4 Weeks | 1050 | 15,000 |

* Paffenbarger, Sweeney and Isaacs, *J.A.D.A.*, June, 1937.

tions in the use and selection of any dental material. In the case of the cemented cast restoration, solubility of the cement is of utmost significance. There is always a thin line of cement exposed to oral fluids at the margins even though this cement line may not be readily visible to the naked eye. It must be remembered that visual acuity under oral conditions is approximately 50 microns.[21] Thus whenever any cement line is visible in the mouth it must be thicker than 50 microns. This exposed layer gradually dissolves so that the inlay becomes loose and caries develops.

Other than errors in cavity preparation, probably cement solubility is the main factor contributing to recurrent caries around the inlay or fixed bridge. Every precaution must be taken to produce an accurately fitting restoration that will minimize the layer of exposed cement and then to handle the material in such a manner that its solubility will be as low as possible.

The solubility is usually measured by immersion in distilled water for seven days (American Dental Association Specification No. 8). As shown in Table 14–6, the maximum solubility should not exceed 0.30 per cent and the better products show considerably lower values.

However, when the cement is immersed in dilute organic acids the solubility is much greater.[22] This fact is evident in Figure 14–3 where solubility has been measured in lactic, acetic, and citric acids as well as in ammonium hydroxide and distilled water. It is obvious that the solubility in all other solutions is greater than in distilled water. Likewise the solubility increases when the solution is changed daily and when the *p*H of the media is lowered.

In the oral cavity, deleterious agents such as organic acids and ammonia are present in varying concentrations, depending upon the flora and nutrients available. The data in Figure 14–3 suggest that durability of the cement is basically related to the type and *p*H of the acids to which it is exposed. Thus, the solubility in such media is indicative of the dangers inherent when the zinc phosphate cements are exposed to oral fluids.

Since no single *in vitro* test can duplicate all the oral conditions, immersion in distilled water is accepted as a standard laboratory test method. Experience has shown that there is some correlation with this

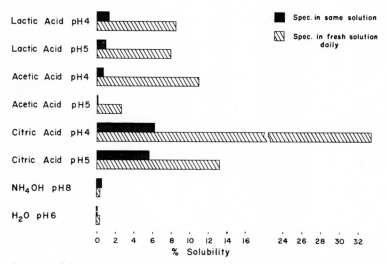

Fig. 14–3. Solubility of a typical zinc phosphate cement when immersed in solutions of varying *p*H for 1 week with solutions changed daily as compared with immersion in the same solution.

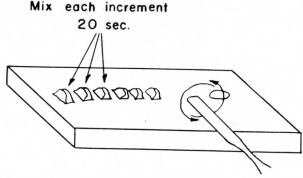

**Mix each increment**
**20 sec.**

Fig. 14–4. Diagrammatic sketch showing the proper mixing procedure for zinc phosphate cement. (Peterson, *Clinical Dental Hygiene.*)

test and durability in the mouth. However, such a correlation should be confined to cements of a single type and not between different types.

The exact mechanism of this solubility is unknown. Analyses[22] of the material leached from the cements show zinc in greater quantity than any other element with phosphorus, magnesium, aluminum and traces of calcium also present. Probably the matrix is attacked first and then erosion results as the cement crumbles and disintegrates. On this basis, it is obvious that the greater the amount of powder incorporated into the liquid, the less will be the disintegration. Thus, the use of a cool slab is essential in order to provide ample time for the incorporation of the maximum amount of powder within the limit of the proper cementing consistency.

**Technical Considerations.** In summary, the following points should be observed in the manipulation of dental cements.

1. It is probably not necessary to use a measuring device for proportioning the powder and liquid, as the consistency may vary for the purpose used. However, the maximum amount of powder possible for the operation at hand should be used in order to reduce the solubility and to increase the strength of the cement.

2. A cool mixing slab should be employed. The temperature of the slab should not be below the dew point of the room, however. The cool slab delays the setting and allows the operator to incorporate the maximum amount of powder before the crystallization proceeds to a point where the mixture stiffens.

3. Mixing is initiated as shown in Figure 14–4, by the addition of a small amount of powder at the start. This procedure assists in neutralizing the acid and thus the buffering action of the salts present in the acid is complemented. Small quantities are incorporated at a time, using a brisk, rotary motion of the spatula. A considerable portion of the mixing slab is used. A good rule to follow is to spatulate for about 20 seconds after adding each increment. The mixing time is not unduly

critical and completion of the mix will usually require approximately one and a half minutes. The actual consistency will vary with the purpose for which the cement is to be used and for the individual operator. The desired consistency is always attained by the addition of more powder and *never* by allowing a thin mix to stiffen.

4. Because of the increased rate of set of the cement at body temperature in comparison to that at room temperature, the cavity side of the inlay should be coated with cement first and then the surface of the prepared cavity should be coated. The inlay should be seated immediately, before any crystallization of the cement occurs.[23] A premature crystallization will definitely weaken the cement. After the inlay has been seated, it should be held under pressure until the cement sets, in order to minimize the effect of any air spaces which may have been inadvertently included. The field of operation should be kept dry during the entire procedure.

5. The cement liquid should be stored away from the air in a stoppered bottle. It should be exposed to the air as little as possible. If the liquid becomes cloudy, it should not be used. Such liquid may eventually become chemically unbalanced during the time the bottle is unstoppered, even though the minimum time is observed for this operation. As previously noted, the bottle of cement liquid should be discarded before the liquid is completely used.

## COPPER CEMENTS

Silver salts or copper oxides are sometimes added to the powders of the zinc phosphate cements supposedly in order to increase their antiseptic properties. The cement is black when cupric oxide ($CuO$) is used; it is red if cuprous oxide ($Cu_2O$) is employed, and it is white or green if cuprous iodide ($Cu_2I_2$) or the silicate ($CuSiO_3$), respectively, is added to the zinc phosphate cement powder. The two copper oxides are mostly used. They can be combined directly in powdered form with the phosphoric acid to produce a cement.

The chemistry of the copper cements is very similar to that of the zinc phosphate cements, and they should be manipulated in the same manner. They have been used primarily as temporary restorative materials, particularly in children's dentistry. They are seldom used any more since their clinical behavior does not seem to be superior to any other temporary restorative material and their toxic reaction to the pulp is generally recognized. They rank high on the list of pulp irritating materials.[9, 10]

Very little information on the physical properties of these cements has been published. One publication[24] lists the compressive strength of a red copper cement as 1470 kilograms per square centimeter (21,000 pounds per square inch) and its disintegration as 0.05 per cent. On the other hand, the compressive strength of a black copper cement was

*Table 14–8.*     *Composition of a Zinc Oxide-Eugenol Cement\**

| INGREDIENT | COMPOSITION (PER CENT) |
|---|---|
| Powder | |
| Zinc oxide | 70.2 |
| Hydrogenated rosin | 29.4 |
| Zinc acetate | 0.4 |
| Liquid | |
| Eugenol | 85 |
| Olive oil | 15 |

\* Accepted Dental Remedies, American Dental Association, 1959.

found to be 630 kilograms per square centimeter (9000 pounds per square inch) and its disintegration was 3.7 per cent. It is not known whether or not these values are typical for the cements of this type.

## ZINC OXIDE-EUGENOL CEMENTS

These cements are dispensed in the form of a powder and a liquid, which are mixed together in much the same manner as the zinc phosphate cements. They can be used as temporary fillings, as thermal insulating bases, and as root canal fillings. Their hydrogen ion concentration is $pH$ 7–8, even at the time when they are inserted in the tooth.[13] This is one of the reasons why they are the least irritating of any of the dental cements. In addition, they may act as an obtundent, and they also possess certain antiseptic properties by virtue of the eugenol; however, the clinical significance of the latter characteristic is unknown.

**Composition.**     Their composition is essentially the same as that of the impression pastes discussed in Chapter 6, with the exception that no fillers or plasticizers are normally introduced. The composition of a reasonably successful cement of this type[25] is presented in Table 14–8.

As in the case of the impression pastes, different types of zinc oxide produce different rates of reaction with the eugenol. Zinc oxide powders which have been decomposed from zinc hydroxide, zinc carbonate and similar salts at temperatures in the neighborhood of 300° C. (570° F.) appear to be the most active in their reaction with eugenol.[26, 27] Such zinc oxide is also the type which exhibits a catalytic action in certain organic reactions, and it may be that this catalytic activity is important in connection with the setting of the zinc oxide-eugenol cements.

Magnesium oxide (MgO), prepared from the carbonate at temperatures of 300° to 500° C. (570° to 930° F.), will also set to a hard mass when it is mixed with eugenol.

Although a satisfactory zinc oxide-eugenol cement can only be made with a zinc oxide of the proper type, and eugenol, the strength and mixing properties of the cement are greatly improved by the addition of rosin. For example, the crushing strength of a set cement containing only zinc oxide and eugenol is approximately 140 kilograms per square centimeter (2000 pounds per square inch) whereas that of the cement with the composition given in Table 14–8, with the rosin added, is 385 kilograms per square centimeter (5500 pounds per square inch).[24] Other agents have been suggested for increasing the strength. The addition of dicalcium phosphate to the powder[28] increased the strength as much as 300 per cent. Likewise the use of o-ethoxybenzoic acid in the eugenol showed promise as a strengthening agent.[29]

Most salts will accelerate the setting reaction but zinc compounds, such as zinc acetate, are especially effective. Many other chemicals, such as water, alcohol, and glacial acetic acid, are also commonly used accelerators.[29-31] As in the case of the zinc oxide-eugenol impression paste, the set can be retarded with glycol or glycerine.

Clove oil, which is approximately 85 per cent eugenol, oil of bay, and guaiacol may be substituted for the eugenol.

**Setting Time.** As previously noted, the type of zinc oxide used is of considerable importance in the production of a proper setting time. Furthermore, the smaller the particle size of the zinc oxide, the faster is the setting time. The most effective means for the control of the setting time is the addition of an accelerator to either the powder or the liquid, or to both.

The greater the amount of zinc oxide incorporated in the eugenol, the faster the material will set. The lower the temperature of the mixing slab, the longer the setting time, provided that the temperature is above the dew point.

Water is essential and is an accelerator for the setting reactions. Under conditions of a high relative humidity, it is sometimes difficult or even impossible to obtain an adequate mixture before the material sets. Control of the water content in the liquid is a critical problem for the manufacturer.

**Strength and Consistency.** As noted earlier, a compressive strength as high as 385 kilograms per square centimeter (5500 pounds per square inch) has been reported.[24] In order to obtain a mix of testing consistency, as for zinc phosphate cement in American Dental Association Specification No. 8, much more powder must be incorporated into the eugenol. In this study[24] 8.5 grams of powder were mixed with 0.4 ml. of eugenol.

Very likely, such a stiff consistency is not often employed with the zinc oxide-eugenol cements. For example, when 0.5 to 1.5 grams of powder were mixed with 0.25 cubic centimeter of eugenol using various compositions and types of powder, compressive strengths of 100 to 240 kilograms per square centimeter (1440 to 3400 pounds per square inch) were obtained after 1 to 3 days.[26] In any event, it is evident that these cements are weaker than the zinc phosphate cements.

This lack of strength is unquestionably one of their weaknesses. Although the exact strength necessary for a cement base is not known, it is generally thought that values in this range may not be adequate to resist the condensation force used in the insertion of an amalgam restoration, for example, or even to resist the biting force transmitted to it through any type of restoration. Thus, it is a common precaution in most instances to place a layer of zinc phosphate cement over the zinc oxide-eugenol cement base. Future research designed to improve the strength of these materials may amplify their use.

The solubility of zinc oxide-eugenol mixtures in distilled water has been reported as approximately the same as that of zinc phosphate cements.[32] Solubility in dilute organic acids generally shows the same trend.[33] The eugenol is not markedly affected by aqueous solutions, being immiscible with water, whereas the zinc oxide is quite soluble in solutions of relatively low $p$H. The range of solubility for these materials does not indicate this to be a serious disadvantage if they are exposed to most oral fluids.

**Uses.** The zinc oxide-eugenol cements are probably the most effective materials known for a temporary filling, before a permanent restoration is placed in the mouth. The eugenol exerts a palliative effect on the pulp of the tooth. The use of radioactive tracer elements to measure adaptation of various materials to tooth structure has shown that zinc oxide-eugenol is excellent from the standpoint of minimizing leakage, at least during the first few days or weeks. It is quite possible that its mild effect on the pulp is related to its ability to prevent ingress of fluids and organisms which might produce pulp pathology during that time when the pulp is injured.

The cementation of fixed bridges with zinc oxide-eugenol cements is a frequently used procedure.[34] This technic is usually considered as a temporary measure to make the tooth more comfortable while the pulp is healing. The bridge later is cemented permanently with zinc phosphate cement. Recently, however, its use as a permanent cement has increased. Although its low strength and the possible increase in film thickness might contraindicate its use for this purpose, the clinical behavior of the material when used in this way should be followed with interest.

## CALCIUM HYDROXIDE

Another cement type material which is used for capping the pulp of a tooth unavoidably exposed during a dental operation is calcium hydroxide. Abundant research,[35–37] substantiated by clinical experience, indicates that calcium hydroxide tends to accelerate the formation of secondary dentin over the exposed pulp. Secondary dentin is a most effective barrier to further irritants. Usually the thicker the dentin, primary and/or secondary, between the surface of the cavity and the pulp, the better is the protection from chemical and physical trauma. It is considered by some as superior to zinc oxide-eugenol cement for this purpose and is often used as a base in the deep cavity even if there is no obvious pulp exposure.

In practice, aqueous or non-aqueous suspensions of calcium hydroxide are flowed over the prepared area. The thickness of this layer is usually approximately two millimeters. This layer of calcium hydroxide does not gain sufficient hardness or strength to recommend its use alone as a base so it is usually overlaid with zinc phosphate cement.

The compositions of the commercial products vary.[38] Some are merely suspensions of calcium hydroxide in distilled water. One product contains 6 per cent calcium hydroxide and 6 per cent zinc oxide suspended in a chloroform solution of a resinous material.[39] Aqueous methyl cellulose is also a common solvent for some products, while one such paste contains salts of human serum, calcium chloride, and sodium bicarbonate.

### CAVITY LINERS

The use of cavity varnishes or liners, in conjunction with certain restorative materials, has been advocated for a number of reasons. These varnishes are painted in the prepared cavity, leaving a thin film. They are employed in an effort to seal the dentinal tubules and thus prevent the penetration of constituents in the restorative or cementing material. Research seems to indicate that while certain of these varnishes, acting as semi-permeable membranes, do not prevent pulp damage from the acids of the cementing mediums, they may reduce it.[40, 41] Their penetration by phosphoric acid has been studied[42] and they have been shown to be poor electrical but good thermal insulators.[8] Their exact merit in regard to reducing postoperative sensitivity thus remains unanswered.

These varnishes are usually natural gums, such as copal and rosin, dissolved in chloroform, acetone or ether.[43] Another recently introduced product makes use of a synthetic resin rather than a natural gum while nitrocellulose is sometimes used as a part of the base. In any event, the liner should be kept in a tightly stoppered bottle to prevent evaporation of the solvent.

Other than the research on permeability there is little information on the physical and chemical properties of these products. Their solubility is low. They are virtually insoluble in distilled water. Two commercial products show an average solubility of only 1.3 per cent after one week storage in citric acid.

It is possible one of their merits is that they may assist in preventing leakage around certain restorative materials. Radioactive tracers may be used to measure infiltration between the walls of the cavity preparation

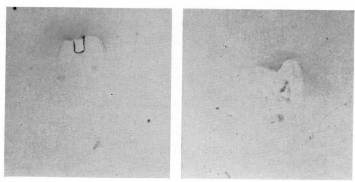

Fig. 14–5.  Radioautographs showing leakage around amalgam restorations. Ca[45] was used as the tracer. The dark line surrounding the restoration at left shows severe penetration of the 48-hour old *in vivo* restoration. No leakage can be seen on the restoration at the right where a cavity liner was first applied before inserting restoration.

and the filling material. Using this technic it can be shown that the penetration of fluids is less, particularly during the first few weeks or months, around an amalgam restoration when a cavity liner is used as indicated in Figure 14–5.

Amalgam restorations were placed, both with and without a cavity liner. The teeth were extracted 48 hours after placement of the restoration. All surfaces of the teeth were sealed except for the marginal areas of the amalgam restoration. The teeth were then immersed in a solution of Ca[45] for two hours, washed and sectioned through the restoration. The ground section was then placed on x-ray film and developed. The dark line indicates the penetration of the tracer around the restoration.

These typical results indicate markedly less leakage when the cavity liner was used. This observation suggests that if they actually do reduce tooth sensitivity it may well be due to the reduced infiltration of irritating fluids.

## ACRYLIC RESIN

Acrylic resin cement is dispensed in the usual powder and liquid form of a self-curing resin. The powder contains fine particles of poly (methyl methacrylate) and the usual initiator, together with a filler and plasticizer. The filler agents, added to enhance certain properties such as the thermal coefficient of expansion, include quartz, calcium carbonate, and barium carbonate.[44] The filler and plasticizer also aid in increasing the smoothness of the mix. The liquid is essentially methyl methacrylate with the typical quantity of activator and inhibitor.

The powder and liquid can be mixed in the same manner as any other cement, with the advantage that the rate of addition of the powder to the liquid is not important. A cool slab is desirable in order to prolong the initiation period, but the slab temperature should not be below the dew point. As with any self-curing acrylic resin, the incorporation of water at any stage of the technic reduces the length of the initiation period. For this reason, the area of operation should be kept dry. The technic of seating the inlay is the same as for any other cement.

Acrylic resin cement can be used over a base of zinc phosphate cement, but its use in connection with eugenol in any manner is not indicated. The eugenol is an inhibitor for the polymerization of the resin, and it also attacks the polymer. In fact, a phenolic compound of any type will act as an inhibitor. The practice of treating the prepared cavity with phenol is definitely not indicated if a self-curing acrylic resin of any type is to be placed in contact with a surface so treated.

According to the available experimental evidence,[44, 45] the film thickness of the acrylic resin cements is satisfactory. It may be as low as ten microns. Although poly(methyl methacrylate) is virtually insoluble in the mouth fluids, the solubility of the acrylic resin cements may be somewhat greater, because of the effect of the filler and plasticizer.[44] Its compressive strength is comparable to that of zinc phosphate cement.

The lack of dimensional stability of the acrylic resin is possibly not a great factor in its use as a cementing medium, provided that the cement film is very thin. However, the dentist should take into consideration the changes in dimension which are brought about by curing shrinkage, water sorption, relaxation and thermal expansion and contraction. The acrylic resin cement cannot be expected to function properly as a cement when it is used primarily as a filling material to compensate for the errors in an ill-fitting inlay.

Although the adaptation of the resin cements to tooth structure is superior initially to zinc phosphate cement, this bond is lost rapidly as the resin cement becomes saturated with water.[18, 46] Moisture has a deleterious effect on adhesion of any present cementing material but apparently the resin cements are inferior in this respect.

Just as with the resin filling materials, the effect of these cements on the pulp remains controversial. One study[47] showed rather severe reaction to three resin cements while other research on the resin restorative materials indicated their effect is mild.[48]

The interest in this type of cement has waned. Although one clinical evaluation[18] showed satisfactory behavior after a 28-month observation period in the oral cavity, there was no evidence that they were superior to the other type cements. The lack of any germicidal or bacteriostatic characteristics warrants further clinical observations over a longer period of time.

## Literature

1. Paffenbarger, G. C., Sweeney, W. T., and Schouboe, P. J.: *Dental Cements.* Internat. D. J., *5:*484–496 (Dec.), 1955.
2. McCue, R. W., McDougal, F. G., and Shay, D. E.: *The Antibacterial Properties of Some Dental Restorative Materials.* Oral Surg., Oral Med. & Oral Path., *4:* 1180–1184 (Sept.), 1951.
3. Kinnear, J. S.: *Germicidal Actions of Dental Filling Materials.* New Zealand D. J., *31:*5–18 (Jan.), 1935.
4. Turkheim, H. J.: *In Vitro Experiments on the Bactericidal Effect of Zinc Oxide-Eugenol Cement on Bacteria-containing Dentin.* J. D. Res., *34:*295–301 (April), 1955.
5. Shay, D. E., Allen, T. J., and Mantz, R. F.: *The Antibacterial Effects of Some Dental Restorative Materials.* J. D. Res., *35:*25–32 (Feb.), 1956.
6. Colton, M. B., and Ehrlich, C.: *Polyantibiotic Dental Cement as a Cavity Sterilant. In Vitro and in Vivo Report.* N. Y. J. Den., *23:*23–30 (Jan.), 1957.
7. Frisbie, H. E., and Nuckolls, J.: *Caries of the Enamel.* J. Am. Col. Den., *13:*84–100 (June), 1946.
8. Phillips, R. W., Johnson, R. J., and Phillips, L. J.: *An Improved Method for Measuring the Coefficient of Thermal Conductivity of Dental Cement.* J.A.D.A., *53:*577–583 (Nov.), 1956.
9. Massler, M.: *Effects of Filling Materials on the Pulp.* J. Tennessee D. A., *35:*353–374 (Oct.), 1955.
10. Massler, M.: *Pulp Protection and Preservation.* Practical Dental Monographs, Year Book Publishers, Chicago, Ill., January, 1958.
11. Paffenbarger, G. C., Sweeney, W. T., and Isaacs, A.: *A Preliminary Report on the Zinc Phosphate Cements.* J.A.D.A., *20:*1960–1982 (Nov.), 1933.
12. Crowell, W. S.: *Physical Chemistry of Dental Cements.* J.A.D.A., *14:*1030–1048 (June), 1927.
13. Harvey, W., Le Brocq, L. F., and Rakowski, L.: *The Acidity of Dental Cements.* Brit. D. J., *77:*61–69 (Aug. 4); 89–99 (Aug. 18), 1944.
14. Souder, W., and Paffenbarger, G. C.: *Physical Properties of Dental Materials.* National Bureau of Standards Circular C433, Washington, U. S. Government Printing Office, 1942, p. 105.
15. Eberly, J. A.: *Development of a Silicate Cement Tending to Eliminate Pulp Irritation.* Dent. Cos., *76:*419–424 (April), 1934.
16. Souder, W., and Paffenbarger, G. C.: *loc. cit.,* pp. 97–98.
17. *Ibid.,* p. 108.
18. Swartz, M. L., Phillips, R. W., Day, R. A., and Johnston, J. F.: *A Laboratory and Clinical Investigation of Certain Resin Restorative and Cementing Materials.* J. Pros. Den., *5:*698–704, 705–710 (Sept.), 1955.
19. Rose, E. E., Lal, J., Williams, N. B., and Falcetti, J. P.: *The Screening of Materials for Adhesion to Human Tooth Structure.* J. D. Res., *34:*577–588 (Aug.), 1955.
20. Berkson, R.: *Dental Cement: A Study of Its Property of Adhesion.* Am. J. Orthodont., *36:*701–710 (Sept.), 1950.
21. Nelsen, R. J., Wolcott, R. B., and Paffenbarger, G. C.: *Fluid Exchange at the Margins of Dental Restorations.* J.A.D.A., *44:*288–295 (March), 1952.
22. Norman, R. D., Swartz, M. L., and Phillips, R. W.: *Studies on the Solubility of Certain Dental Materials.* J. D. Res., *36:*977–985 (Dec.), 1957.
23. Henschel, C. J.: *The Effect of Mixing Surface Temperature upon Dental Cementation.* J.A.D.A., *30:*1583–1589 (Oct. 1), 1943.
24. Paffenbarger, G. C., and Caul, H. J.: *Dental Cements.* Proc. Dent. Cent. Celebration, March, 1940, pp. 232–237.
25. Wallace, D. A., and Hansen, H. L.: *Zinc Oxide-Eugenol Cements.* J.A.D.A., *26:* 1536–1540 (Sept.), 1939.
26. Harvey, W., and Petch, N. J.: *Acceleration of the Setting of Zinc Oxide Cements.* Brit. D. J., *80:*1–8 (Jan. 4); 35–42 (Jan. 18), 1946.
27. Smith, D. C.: *The Setting of Zinc Oxide-Eugenol Mixtures.* Brit. D. J., *105:*313–321 (Nov.), 1958.

28. Roland, N., Kutscher, A. H., and Ayers, H. D.: *Effect of Dicalcium Phosphate on the Crushing Strength of Zinc Oxide and Eugenol Cement. Preliminary Report.* N. Y. State D. J., *25:*84–86 (Feb.), 1959.
29. Brauer, G. M., White, E. E., and Moshonas, M. G.: *The Reaction of Metal Oxides with o-Ethoxybenzoic Acid and Other Chelating Agents.* J. D. Res., 37:547–560 (June), 1958.
30. Copeland, H. I., Brauer, G. M., Sweeney, W. T., and Forziati, A. F.: *Setting Reactions of Zinc Oxide and Eugenol.* J. Research N. B. S., *55:*134–138 (Sept.), 1955.
31. Molnar, E. J., and Skinner, E. W.: *A Study of Zinc Oxide-Rosin Cements.* J.A.D.A., *29:*744–751 (May), 1942.
32. Souder, W., and Paffenbarger, G. C.: *loc. cit.*, p. 96.
33. Norman, R. D., Swartz, M. L., and Phillips, R. W.: *Additional Studies on the Solubility of Certain Dental Materials.* J. D. Res., 30:1028–1037 (Sept.), 1959.
34. Baraban, D. J.: *Cementation of Fixed Bridge Prosthesis with Zinc Oxide-Rosin-Eugenol Cements.* J. Pros. Den., *8:*988–991 (Nov.), 1958.
35. Glass, R. L., and Zander, H. A.: *Pulp Healing.* J. D. Res., *28:*97–107 (April), 1949.
36. Berman, D. S., and Massler, M.: *Experimental Pulpotomies in Root Molars.* J. D. Res., *37:*229–242 (April), 1958.
37. Stewart, D. J., and Kramer, I. R. H.: *Effects of Calcium Hydroxide on the Unexposed Pulp.* J. D. Res., *37:*758 (Aug.), 1958. Abstract.
38. Zawawi, H. A. M.: *Rat Connective Tissue Reactions to Implants of Certain Pulp Capping and Cavity Lining Materials.* Thesis for M. S. degree, Indiana University School of Dentistry, Sept., 1958.
39. Council on Dental Therapeutics: *Accepted Dental Remedies*, Chicago, American Dental Association, 1959, p. 145.
40. Zander, H. A., Glenn, J. F., and Nelson, C. A.: *Pulp Protection in Restorative Dentistry.* J.A.D.A., *41:*563–573 (Nov.), 1950.
41. Paynter, K., Nikiforuk, G., and Wood, A. W. S.: *Pulp Protective Effect of Silicone under Silicate Fillings.* J. D. Res., *34:*718–719 (Oct.), 1955. Abstract.
42. Newcomer, C. E.: *Penetration of Cavity Varnishes by Phosphoric Acid.* J. D. Res., *37:*43 (Feb.), 1958. Abstract.
43. Council on Dental Therapeutics: *Accepted Dental Remedies, loc. cit.* p. 186.
44. Schouboe, P. J., Paffenbarger, G. C., and Sweeney, W. T.: *Resin Cements and Posterior-type Direct Filling Resins.* J.A.D.A., *52:*584–600 (May), 1956.
45. Anonymous: *Cementing Inlays with Self-hardening Resin.* D. J. Australia, *25:* 25–27 (Jan.-Feb.), 1953.
46. Stüben, J., and Lockowandt, P.: *Experimentelle Untersuchungen über die Haftintensität des Schnellhärtenden Kunststoffs.* Zahnärztliche Welt, *7:*298 (July), 1952.
47. Langeland, K.: *Pulp Reaction to Resin Cements.* Acta Odont. Scandinavica, *13:* 239–256 (Feb.), 1956.
48. Council on Dental Research: *Status Report on the Reactions of the Pulp to Self-curing Resinous Filling Materials.* J.A.D.A., *42:*449–450 (April), 1951.

# CHAPTER 15

# Silicate Cement

As noted in the previous chapter, the silicate cements are used chiefly as materials for the restoration of tooth structure which has been removed in the preparation of a carious cavity.

As in the case of the zinc phosphate cements, the silicate cements are in the form of a powder which is mixed with a liquid containing phosphoric acid. The mixture sets to a relatively hard, translucent substance which resembles dental porcelain, although it should not be classified as a porcelain.

The cements are supplied in a variety of shades so that the tooth color can be imitated very closely. Unfortunately such a restoration may, after a few months, discolor and gradually disintegrate in the mouth fluids. For this reason such a restoration is not considered permanent. Although the average lifetime has been estimated at four years,[1] some restorations may last 25 years while others fail in six months. As will be seen, the reason for this erratic behavior is probably due both to variations in technic and in oral environments.

**Composition.** The powders are finely ground ceramic compositions. They are essentially acid-soluble glasses.

The powders consist primarily of silica ($SiO_2$), alumina ($Al_2O_3$), lime (CaO), and sodium fluoride (NaF), calcium fluoride ($CaF_2$), cryolite ($Na_3AlF_6$) or combinations. It has been found[2] that there is only a very narrow range of compositions containing CaO, $SiO_2$ and $Al_2O_3$ which can be fused to give clear glasses which, when powdered, would set within a suitable time with the usual cement liquids. The reaction is essentially a function of these compounds.[3] The ingredients are fused together at a temperature of approximately 1400° C. (2550° F.). The fluorides melt at a lower temperature than the other ingredients, and act as a fusing agent. Such substances are known as *fluxes* in ceramics. Beryllium silicate ($Be_2SiO_4$) was formerly used as a flux, but the fluorides apparently produce better cements. It is possible to obtain a ceramic product which will set in combination with phosphoric acid which contains no flux,[2] but so far as is known, such compositions are not used to a great extent.

While the mass is in a fused condition, it may be plunged into water. The sudden cooling produces a cracking and crazing which facilitates the later grinding of the powder. Except for the fluxes employed, the manufacturing process is not unlike that of dental porcelain, described in the next chapter.

The compositions[4] of twelve powders for silicate cements are shown in Table 15–1. These compositions may not be representative of modern silicate cement powders even though silicate cement compositions have been fairly well standardized for many years. They are presented as possible combinations of ingredients which can be used.

So far as can be interpreted from Table 15–1, all of the powders contain one or more fluxes. Probably sodium carbonate ($Na_2CO_3$) was used as a flux in powders A, B and H. The remaining powders were fluxed with sodium or calcium fluoride or cryolite. The cements made from these latter powders generally possessed the best physical properties. The use of a fluoride flux usually reduces the solubility of the cement in water, for example.

The setting time of the cement is related to the ratio of the silica present to the alumina and lime incorporated. In other words, the more alumina or lime added, the shorter will be the setting time of the cement, other factors being equal. Very likely, the alumina and lime may be substituted for each other to a certain extent.[2] The ratio of the silica to the alumina-lime combination in Table 15–1 varies from 1.02 (powder H) to 1.44 (powder D).

Cement H differs from the other powders in that a considerable amount of phosphate was used as a flux. As can be noted from column 8 in Table 15–1, most of the powders contained a phosphate flux, probably incorporated as calcium or aluminum phosphates. A phosphate flux decreases the setting time of the cement, but it may affect the other properties deleteriously.

The compositions of the liquids used for the powders in Table 15–1 are given in Table 15–2. The compositions of the liquids for the silicate cements are not greatly different from those of the liquids for the zinc phosphate cements (Table 14–4), except that zinc and magnesium phosphate have been used in more cases as buffering agents in the silicate cement liquids in addition to the usual aluminum phosphate; also, the silicate cement liquids generally contain more water than do the liquids for the zinc phosphate cements. It is possible that the combina-

*Table 15-1.*     Composition of Silicate Cement Powders (Percentage by Weight)*

| COLUMN | 1 | 2 | 3 | 4 | 5 | 6 | 7 | 8 | 9 | |
|---|---|---|---|---|---|---|---|---|---|---|
| CEMENT POWDER | SILICA (SiO$_2$) (PER CENT) | ALUMINA (Al$_2$O$_3$) (PER CENT) | CALCIUM OXIDE (CaO) (PER CENT) | CALCIUM (Ca) (PER CENT) | FLUORINE (F) (PER CENT) | SODIUM OXIDE (Na$_2$O) (PER CENT) | SODIUM (Na) (PER CENT) | PHOSPHORUS PENTOXIDE (P$_2$O$_5$) (PER CENT) | LOSS ON IGNITION† (PER CENT) | (°C.) |
| A | 47.2 | 33.1 | 10.4 | ... | .... | 8.7 | ... | .... | 0.7 | 900 |
| B‡ | 44.0 | 21.4 | 13.6 | ... | ... | 2.6 | ... | 7.6 | 0.8 | 120 |
| C§ | 32.0 | 29.5 | .... | 8.6 | 14.3 | ... | 7.3 | 5.8 | 2.4 | 850 |
| D | 39.9 | 27.7 | .... | 5.9 | 15.4 | ... | 6.6 | 4.0 | 0.8 | 110 |
| E‖ | 35.1 | 29.9 | .... | 7.9 | 14.2 | ... | 7.3 | 5.4 | 0.1 | 120 |
| F¶ | 14.6 | 15.6 | .... | 3.2 | 5.9 | ... | 2.9 | 2.1 | 0.1 | 120 |
| G | 37.7 | 31.7 | .... | 6.2 | 12.9 | ... | 7.4 | 3.3 | 0.9 | 900 |
| H** | 29.7 | 23.1 | 5.8 | ... | ... | 7.6 | ... | 24.0 | 2.7 | 900 |
| I†† | 41.7 | 28.1 | .... | 6.7 | 12.2 | ... | 7.6 | 2.2 | 1.0 | 900 |
| J | 39.7 | 35.8 | .... | 3.2 | 11.0 | ... | 6.5 | 3.9 | 0.0 | 110 |
| K | 40.1 | 29.8 | .... | 6.6 | 14.3 | ... | 6.3 | 3.2 | 1.1 | 900 |
| L‡‡ | 36.5 | 26.3 | .... | 5.9 | 12.0 | ... | 4.6 | 3.2 | 6.9 | 900 |

* Paffenbarger, Schoonover and Souder, *J.A.D.A.*, Jan., 1938.

† Ignition losses at 900° C. on these cements containing fluorides may be in error because of the volatilization of some silicon tetrafluoride (SiF$_4$).

‡ Contained 4.8 per cent of beryllium oxide (BeO) and 0.3 per cent of nickel oxide (NiO).

§ Contained 0.3 per cent of strontium.

‖ Contained 0.2 per cent of ferric oxide (Fe$_2$O$_3$).

¶ Contained 53.2 per cent of zinc oxide (ZnO); 2.3 per cent of magnesia (MgO), and 0.1 per cent of ferric oxide (FeO$_3$).

** Contained 4.1 per cent of zinc oxide (ZnO); 2.9 per cent of beryllium oxide (BeO), and 0.2 per cent of magnesia (MgO).

†† Contained 0.5 per cent of lithium oxide (Li$_2$O).

‡‡ Contained 9.4 per cent of zinc oxide (ZnO) and 0.5 per cent of magnesia (MgO).

*Table 15–2.* *Composition of Silicate Cement Liquids\**
*(Percentage by Weight)*

| COLUMN.... | ANALYSES | | | | CALCULATIONS | | | |
|---|---|---|---|---|---|---|---|---|
| | 1 | 2 | 3 | 4 | 5 | 6 | 7 | 8 |
| CEMENT LIQUID † | $PO_4$ (PER CENT) | Al (PER CENT) | Zn (PER CENT) | Mg (PER CENT) | FREE $H_3PO_4$ (PER CENT) | COM-BINED $H_3PO_4$ (PER CENT) | TOTAL $H_3PO_4$ (PER CENT) | WATER ‡ (PER CENT) |
| A......... | 60.1 | 1.9 | 7.7 | ... | 47.6 | 14.5 | 62.1 | 28.3 |
| B......... | 52.3 | 2.1 | 6.2 | 0.1 | 39.8 | 14.2 | 54.0 | 37.6 |
| C§....... | 56.8 | 2.1 | 2.5 | 0.7 | 46.5 | 12.1 | 58.6 | 36.1 |
| D......... | 47.8 | 2.3 | 5.6 | ... | 35.0 | 13.8 | 48.8 | 43.3 |
| E‖ ....... | 56.1 | 2.4 | 3.1 | 0.8 | 44.1 | 13.8 | 57.9 | 35.8 |
| F‖ ....... | 55.7 | 2.4 | 3.1 | 0.7 | 43.6 | 13.9 | 57.5 | 36.3 |
| G......... | 48.6 | ... | 9.1 | ... | 41.1 | 9.1 | 50.2 | 40.7 |
| H¶...... | 51.9 | 3.3 | ... | ... | 41.7 | 11.8 | 53.5 | 43.2 |
| I......... | 51.7 | 2.5 | 5.8 | ... | 37.6 | 15.7 | 53.3 | 38.4 |
| J......... | 48.6 | ... | 8.9 | ... | 41.3 | 8.9 | 50.2 | 40.9 |
| K....... | 48.1 | 1.9 | 4.4 | ... | 38.3 | 11.3 | 49.6 | 44.1 |
| L........ | 48.1 | 1.9 | 4.4 | ... | 38.3 | 11.3 | 49.6 | 44.1 |

\* Paffenbarger, Schoonover and Souder, *J.A.D.A.*, Jan., 1938.
† Unless otherwise noted, arsenic content was less than 0.0002 per cent.
‡ Water content calculated by difference.
§ Contained 0.0002 per cent of arsenic.
‖ Contained 0.0005 per cent of arsenic.
¶ Contained 0.3 per cent of calcium.

tion of aluminum and zinc together as a modifier aids in the prevention of precipitation of the modifiers during the storage of the liquid.[2] When the two modifiers are combined, the saturation point of neither metal is likely to be reached.

Traces of arsenic are often found in cement powders and liquids as it is very difficult to remove this impurity from some of the ingredients. It imposes no deleterious effect if it is present in amounts less than 1 part in 500,000, the maximum limit established in American Dental Association Specification No. 9.

Although innumerable powder and liquid modifications have been attempted,[2] none has as yet been found to be appreciably superior to the representative compositions shown in Tables 15–1 and 15–2. For example, the addition of silicones[5] to the cement reduced the solubility slightly but at the same time the compressive strength was sometimes lowered.

Recently several products have appeared which contain small amounts of fiberglass added to the powder. Although claims are made for reduced solubility and higher strength, they have not been substantiated by unbiased tests. One might not expect significant improvements since the addition of fiberglass particles less than ½ inch in length does not re-inforce the cement but acts simply as a filler.[6]

**Clinical Significance of the Fluoride.** As can be noted from Table 15–1, most commercial silicate cement powders contain fluorine up to 15 per cent. The exact fluoride compound in the final restoration is unknown. However, the clinical significance of this fluorine is tremendously important.

It is commonly recognized that the incidence of recurrent caries is markedly less around the silicate restoration as compared to all other filling materials.[7–9] Although the silicate cement has many weaknesses, it is superior from this standpoint. This protective mechanism has been attributed to the fluorine present in the cement. Since the silicate cement restoration is quite soluble in the oral fluids, it has been believed that a sufficient amount of fluoride is continually leached from the restoration and thus acts in some manner as a germicidal or anti-enzyme agent. However, only approximately 14 parts per million fluoride[10] is dissolved from the silicate at the end of the fifth day and the amount continues to diminish with time. It is doubtful that such small concentrations of fluorine could have any inhibitory effect.[11, 12] Any bacterial inhibition occurs only during the first 24 or 48 hours and is probably due to the phosphoric acid present.[13]

The more logical explanation for this unique anticariogenic property seems to be a reduction in enamel solubility,[8, 14, 15] similar to the effect of fluoride solutions which are applied topically. The reduction in solubility and fluoride uptake for two fluoride containing cements, A and B, may be seen in Table 15–3.

Silicate C is one of the very few available silicates which contains no fluoride, a beryllium flux being used. Apparently this material actually removes fluorine from the tooth and increases enamel solubility. The same results can be shown with most non-fluoride materials such as zinc phosphate cements and resins. Thus, it is quite possible that certain commonly used filling materials differ in their effect on the adjacent tooth; some increase its resistance to caries and others lower it.

*Table 15–3.* *Effect of Three Silicates on Solubility of Adjacent Enamel and the Uptake of Fluorine by the Tooth as Compared to Normal Fluorine Content of Enamel*

| SILICATE | AVERAGE CHANGE IN CALCIUM SOLUBILITY (PER CENT) | FLUORINE CONTENT OF ADJACENT ENAMEL (P.P.M.) |
|---|---|---|
| A | −27.5 | 713 |
| B | −22.8 | 700 |
| C (no fluoride) | +20.4 | 88 |
| Untreated enamel | | 120 |

**Setting Reactions and Structure.** A cored structure results from the setting of a silicate cement, as shown in Figure 15–1. The core is composed of undissolved powder particles, and the matrix is essentially a silicic acid gel. The formation and structure of the gel is of interest.

The reactions between the powder and liquid are complex and not entirely understood, but based on the knowledge of the simpler process of the formation of a silicic acid gel from sodium silicate (water glass), a tentative theory can be given.

Presumably, the acid attacks the surface of the powder particles and silicic acid is formed. When the proper $p$H is attained, the gel structure forms according to the following reactions:[16]

$$
\begin{array}{ccc}
\text{OH} & \text{OH} & \text{OH} \quad \text{OH} \\
| & | & | \quad\quad | \\
\text{HO—Si—OH} + \text{HO—Si—OH} \rightarrow & \text{HO—Si—O—Si—OH} + \text{H}_2\text{O} \\
| & | & | \quad\quad | \\
\text{OH} & \text{OH} & \text{OH} \quad \text{OH}
\end{array}
$$

$$
\begin{array}{cc}
\text{OH} \quad \text{OH} & \text{OH} \\
| \quad\quad | & | \\
\text{HO—Si—O—Si—OH} + \text{HO—Si—OH} \rightarrow \\
| \quad\quad | & | \\
\text{OH} \quad \text{OH} & \text{OH}
\end{array}
$$

$$
\begin{array}{ccc}
\text{OH} & \text{OH} & \text{OH} \\
| & | & | \\
\text{HO—Si—O—Si—O—Si—OH} + \text{H}_2\text{O}, \text{ etc.} \\
| & | & | \\
\text{OH} & \text{OH} & \text{OH}
\end{array}
$$

The reaction can be recognized as a process of polymerization by condensation. Not only can the polymerization continue in chain formation, but also cross-linkages can occur in three dimensions. A schematic structural formula for the gel in two dimensions would be as follows:

$$
\begin{array}{ccc}
\vdots & \vdots & \vdots \\
| & | & | \\
\text{O} & \text{O} & \text{O} \\
| & | & | \\
\cdots\text{—O—Si—O—Si—O—Si—O—}\cdots \\
| & | & | \\
\text{O} & \text{O} & \text{O} \\
| & | & | \\
\cdots\text{—O—Si—O—Si—O—Si—O—}\cdots \\
| & | & | \\
\text{O} & \text{O} & \text{O} \\
| & | & | \\
\cdots\text{—O—Si—O—Si—O—Si—O—}\cdots \\
| & | & | \\
\text{O} & \text{O} & \text{O} \\
| & | & | \\
\vdots & \vdots & \vdots
\end{array}
$$

The fibril structure of the gel is apparently the framework of the —Si—O— combination, linked together by primary valences. The gel is, therefore, of the irreversible type. Furthermore, although dimensional changes can be expected during syneresis and imbibition, the

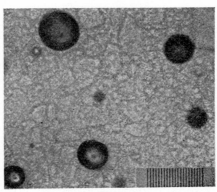

Fig. 15–1.   Photomicrograph of a silicate cement after it has set. The core is undissolved powder particles, and the matrix is a silicic acid gel. The dark circles are air bubbles. × 200. (Paffenbarger, Schoonover and Souder, *J.A.D.A.*, Jan., 1938.)

changes cannot be as marked as in the case of the agar gels discussed in Chapter 7. Also, because of this molecular network, the gel possesses considerable strength and rigidity.

The final disposition of the water of condensation and the metal and phosphate ions is not clear. Very likely, they are contained in the capillary network formed by the polymerized silicic acid. Whatever the final products are, their insolubility in the mouth fluids will be a potent influence on the final success of the restoration. Thus the nature and relative amounts of the metallic ions will have an important bearing on the properties of the cement.

As in the case of the zinc phosphate cements, the density of the matrix is greatest in the vicinity of the powder particle. The sheath formed around the particles effectively reduces the rate of the reaction. As a result, free phosphoric acid may be present in the silicate restoration for a considerable time before it is entirely reacted.

The proportion of the gel to the undissolved particles will depend upon the amount of powder incorporated into the liquid during the mixing. Generally, for reasons of increased strength and insolubility, it is advisable to incorporate as much powder as is consistently possible. In a properly mixed cement it is estimated[17] that 10 per cent of the mass of solid particles is dissolved before the gel forms. The final structure of the set cement consists of 20 to 30 per cent gel matrix, with the undissolved powder particles occupying the remainder of the mass.

**Standard Consistency.**    As can be noted in Table 15–4, a standard consistency for silicate cement is prescribed in the American Dental Association Specification No. 9 for Dental Silicate Cement. The powder-liquid ratio to produce a standard consistency is the amount of powder which can be combined with 0.4 milliliter of liquid so that a disk 25 millimeters (0.985 inch) in diameter is formed from 0.5 milliliter of the mixed, unset cement, when it is pressed between two glass plates under a load of 2500 grams (5.51 pounds). For cements certified to meet this specification, the range of weight of powder required for a standard consistency mixture was 1.25 to 1.55 grams (Table 15–4)[18] with 0.4 milliliter of liquid.

The standard consistency is not necessarily the optimum consistency so far as the physical properties of the cement are concerned. Usually a thicker mixture of powder and liquid is used in order to increase the strength and the insolubility in the mouth fluids. For comparative testing purposes, however, the standard consistency is satisfactory.

**Setting Time.** The setting time of these cements should be controlled. If the setting time is too short, the gel may start to form before the insertion of the cement in the prepared cavity has been completed. As with any substance of this type, any fracture or disturbance of the gel will be permanent, and the structure will be weak and soluble in the mouth fluids. According to the American Dental Association Specification No. 9, the setting time at 37° C. (98.6° F.) should be between three and eight minutes when it is tested with the 1 pound Gillmore needle. The range of setting times of certified commercial silicate cements at 37° C. (98.6° F.) was found to be four to six minutes (Table 15–4).

The setting time is definitely influenced by the composition of the powder and liquid, as already described. The finer the powder, the faster the cement will set, as in the case of the zinc phosphate cements. The factors that are under the control of the dentist are as follows:

1. In general, the longer the mixing time, the longer is the setting time.

2. The less liquid used with the same amount of powder, the shorter is the setting time.

3. Addition of small amounts of water will decrease the setting time. Conversely, a loss of water from the liquid will increase the setting time.

4. The temperature during mixing affects the setting time in that the lower the temperature of the mixing slab, the longer will be the setting time of the cement.

Generally, the rate of addition of the powder to the liquid has little practical effect on the setting time, although the tendency is for the setting time to be reduced if the powder is added more rapidly.

The reason for the first factor is probably connected with the production of the gel. When the mixing is prolonged the gel is broken up, and the acquirement of sufficient strength to withstand the weight of the Gillmore needle is delayed. The second factor is likely related to the number of reactive powder particles present. The less the liquid-powder ratio, the more reactive powder particles there will be per unit volume, and consequently the gelation will be completed sooner.

The influence of the concentration of the liquid can be accounted for

*Table 15–4.*    Detail Requirements of American Dental Association Specification No. 9 for Dental Silicate Cement and Range of Values for Certified Silicate Cements*

| | STANDARD CONSISTENCY OF MIX | TIME OF SETTING AT 37° C. (99° F.) | | COMPRESSIVE STRENGTH | OPACITY | | SOLUBILITY AND DISINTEGRATION | ARSENIC CONTENT |
|---|---|---|---|---|---|---|---|---|
| | | Minimum (minutes) | Maximum (minutes) | | Minimum $C_{0.70}$ | Maximum | | |
| Detail requirements of A.D.A. Specification No. 9 for Dental Silicate Cement | To produce disk 25 ± 1 mm. in diameter | 3 | 8 | Minimum 24 hours kg./cm.² 1,620 $\left[\begin{array}{c}\text{lb./in.}^2\\23,000\end{array}\right]$ | 0.35 | 0.55 | Maximum 24 hours percentage by weight 1.4 | Maximum percentage by weight 0.0002 (1 part in 500,000) |
| Range of values for Silicate Cements on List of Certified Dental Materials | Grams of powder in 0.4 ml. of liquid 1.40 ± 0.15 | Minutes 5 ± 1 | | lb./in.² 25,200 ± 2,000 | $C_{0.70}$ all within 0.35–0.55 | | Percentage 1.0 ± 0.3 | Percentage <0.0002 |

* Paffenbarger and Stanford, *D. Clin. North America,* November, 1959.

on the basis of the ionization of the phosphoric acid, and its effect on the chemical activity.

Unfortunately, if the mixing time is altered, if the liquid-powder ratio is increased, or if the water content of the liquid is changed, a decreased strength and an increased solubility of the set cement in water are observed, and a greater shrinkage of the cement during hardening occurs. The best method for the dentist to control the setting time is to change the temperature of the slab. As in the case of the zinc phosphate cements, a cool mixing slab is usually indicated.

**Dimensional Stability.**    Once the cement has acquired a sufficient rigidity, a shrinkage occurs during hardening, as shown in Figure 15–2. "Durosim" was an oily substance added to the cements at one time in the hope that their acidity could be reduced.

Clinically, the seemingly small shrinkages, indicated in Figure 15–2 for short intervals of time, are important. Even the slightest opening of the silicate cement restoration at the margins may result in a leakage. Such leakage may then result in discoloration and possible recurrence of caries.

A swelling of the surface layers of the silicate has been demonstrated, if water is allowed to contact the cement during its early stages of hardening.[19] It appears that the swelling is greater if the water contacts the cement early during its gelation period. Unfortunately, such an imbibition cannot be taken advantage of in practice, since a premature contact with water causes the cement to lose most of its desirable properties, as will be described in a subsequent section. The proper procedure is to cover the restoration with a water-impervious film as

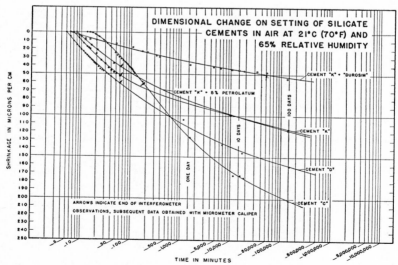

Fig. 15–2.   Dimensional change of silicate cements during setting in air. (Paffenbarger, Schoonover and Souder, *J.A.D.A.*, Jan., 1938.)

soon after the cement initially hardens as possible, in order to prevent its contact with the saliva for several hours. During this period, a shrinkage occurs. When the saliva is finally allowed to contact the cement, the gel has been so completely formed that only a small expansion results from any imbibition of water.

If the restoration is exposed to the air at any time subsequent to its hardening, a syneresis will occur with a consequent shrinkage. The surface of the cement is damaged by such a drying, and it loses its translucence. Although an imbibition of water may follow when it is again exposed to the saliva, the restoration never completely recovers its original volume.[20] Consequently, the use of silicate cement restorations is not indicated for use in the mouths of mouth-breathers, for example.

From the standpoint of thermal dimensional change, the silicate restoration is excellent. The thermal coefficient of expansion for the human tooth[21] is approximately $8.0 \times 10^{-6}$ per degree centigrade, depending on the area measured. Silicate cement has been measured at almost the same value, $7.6 \times 10^{-6}$ per degree centigrade. Thus, even severe thermal change should have little effect on the differential dimensional stability between the restoration and the tooth. Silicate cement is superior to all other restorative materials from this standpoint while acrylic resin is the poorest (Chapter 13).

**Solubility and Disintegration.**    Although the silicate cement restorations exhibit good esthetic qualities for a short time after they have been inserted, probably their greatest disadvantage is the fact that too often they gradually erode in the mouth fluids, and their esthetic qualities are apt to be soon lost.

According to American Dental Association Specification No. 9, the solubility and disintegration should not be greater than 1.4 per cent after immersion in distilled water for 24 hours at 37° C. (99° F.). Typical range of values for certified products may be seen in Table 15–4.

If one compares this weight loss to that of zinc phosphate cement, Table 14–6, it would indicate that the solubility of silicate cements is greater. Such a relationship, however, is not borne out by clinical observations since zinc phosphate cement disintegrates more rapidly in the mouth than does silicate cement. The explanation possibly lies in the data shown in Figure 15–3, where the solubility of various types of dental cements has been determined in different media.[22, 23] As can be noted, silicate cement is less soluble in both lactic and acetic acids than is the zinc phosphate cement, but it is more soluble in water. As discussed in the previous chapter, although the water solubility test is accepted as a standard test, it does not necessarily represent the true conditions if one type of cement is compared with another.

Since both acetic and lactic acid are present in plaque material and in oral fluids, it can be expected that the zinc phosphate cement will be attacked more rapidly than the silicate cement as observed clinically. Another possible factor might be the lower compressive strength of the zinc phosphate cements compared with that of the silicate cements.

This relationship of the oral environment to disintegration of the cement has been demonstrated clinically. Clinical surveys[7, 24] have noted that the lingual and labial areas of silicate restorations, which are exposed to the greatest washing action of the saliva and to mechanical wear, remain relatively intact. Most disintegration occurs adjacent to gingival areas where débris and food plaques collect.

These observations suggest that although the durability of the clinical silicate restoration is dependent on many factors, such as diet and bacterial flora of the mouth, basically it is related to the type and $pH$ of the acids to which it is exposed. For example, a mouth that normally may have areas of low $pH$ from degradation of foodstuffs, or where citric acid is prevalent, will invariably contribute to the disintegration of the silicate cement restoration regardless of its type or manipulation.

The solubility of a silicate cement, plotted against time, is of interest as indicated in Figure 15–4. Even though the solutions indicated were

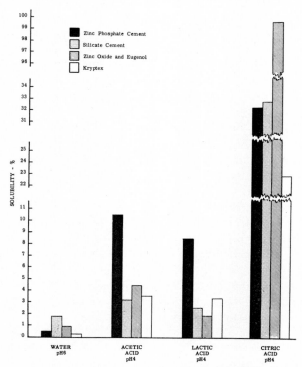

Fig. 15–3. Comparison of various cementing mediums in different solutions after immersion for seven days. The solutions were changed each day. "Kryptex" is the trade name for a combination silicate-zinc phosphate cement.

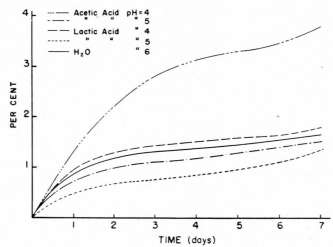

Fig. 15–4. Solubility of a typical silicate cement in various solutions which were changed each day.

changed daily, there was a decrease in the rate of solution at the end of the second or third day.[4, 22] However, with zinc phosphate cement, the solubility in acid increased almost in direct proportion to the time under similar conditions. Likewise, the *p*H of the storage environment increased more rapidly for zinc phosphate cement. The *p*H of distilled water in which silicate cement was stored for one week is between 5.5 and 5.8.

It should not be inferred that this decrease in solubility with time will result in an arrest of further clinical disintegration. It is a progressive erosion that, even though slight, leads to continual destruction of the restoration. The breakdown will, however, be governed by the concentration, *p*H, and type of fluids present.

The products of disintegration, as determined from solutions in which silicate cement has been stored, were relatively large quantities of silica, as well as smaller amounts of phosphorus, aluminum, calcium, magnesium, zinc, and fluorine. The last was discussed previously.

The solubility of the silicate cement is generally decreased by the presence of the fluoride flux. Possibly the substitution of the soluble phosphate flux (*e.g.*, Cement H, Table 15–1) is more responsible for the increased solubility than is the absence of the fluoride flux.

It is interesting to compare solubilities of cements of previous years with the modern products. A review[4] of the properties obtained in a survey of 13 silicate cements in 1938 showed solubilities, at one week in distilled water, ranging from 0.13 to 5.0 per cent. As seen in Table 15–4, the solubilities of present materials in 24 hours is generally less than 1.0 per cent. Since there is no significant difference between the 24 hour and 7 day data, the improvement, following the publication of the first American Dental Association Specification for silicate cement, is evident.

The solubility of the cement is undoubtedly related to the gel matrix and not to the core of undissolved particles. It has been shown[4] that the solubility of the cement powder itself is not greater than 0.4 per cent in distilled water. This solubility is less than that of powdered tooth enamel, which is 0.8 per cent.[4] Consequently, it is hardly conceivable that the core is the component which is being dissolved by the mouth fluids. It follows, therefore, that the less the amount of the gel matrix present in the set cement, the less will be its solubility.

The disintegration is probably better described as an erosion by solution than strictly as a solution process. The gel probably dissolves, and the particles are washed away.

**Strength.**      The ultimate strength of silicate cement is generally measured under compressive stress. The compressive strength of the certified commercial products is given in Table 15–4. According to the American Dental Association Specification No. 9, the compressive strength of a silicate cement should be not less than 1620 kilograms per square centimeter (23,000 pounds per square inch) 24 hours after mixing. Although the strength of these cements is greater than that of any other type of cement, they are the weakest of the tooth restorative materials with the exception of the acrylic resins.

The greater the amount of powder incorporated in a given amount of liquid, within practical limits, the greater the compressive strength will be. The more powder particles present in the hardened cement, the greater will be the binding action of the matrix or gel, since the binding action is dependent upon the surface area of the core. However, all of the particles must react with the liquid; if an excessive amount of powder is used, so that all of the particles are not chemically attached, the cement will be weak. This relationship between powder-liquid ratio and strength is evident in Figure 15–5 in that the greater the amount of powder added to 0.4 cubic centimeter of liquid, the higher is the compressive strength until a critical ratio is attained, beyond which the strength decreased.

It is interesting to note (Fig. 15–5) that the solubility decreases with an increase in the incorporated powder and that it reaches a minimum beyond which the cement becomes more soluble. This observation is in line with the previous conclusion as to the effect of the gel matrix on the solubility. It follows that the greater the amount of powder employed, the less will be the amount of matrix formed. However, each undissolved particle should be surrounded by gel, otherwise the mouth fluids will penetrate the voids formed by the absence of silica gel, and the exposed surface of the cement will be considerably increased.

Another fact implied in Figure 15–5 is that maximum strength and

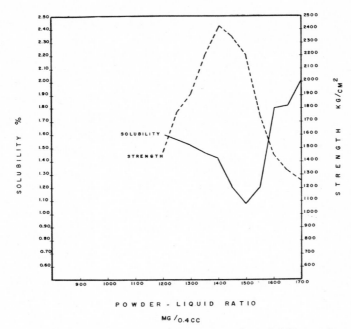

Fig. 15–5.   Influence of the powder-liquid ratio on the solubility and compressive strength of a silicate cement. (Corrêa, Thesis, University of São Paulo, 1955.)

minimum solubility do not coincide at the same powder-liquid ratio. However, it is not likely that the difference is of practical interest.

The strength increases somewhat slowly after the initial hardening has taken place, a fact which indicates that the rate of reaction between the powder and liquid is slow. For example, in 15 minutes one cement developed a strength approximately 40 per cent of its strength attained in 14 months.[4] In three hours its strength was 60 per cent of the 14 month value, and in 1 week it had developed only 80 per cent of the strength at 14 months, which was approximately 1750 kilograms per square centimeter (25,000 pounds per square inch).

The strength of some silicate cements decreases with time when they are stored in distilled water. Such an observation indicates a possible relation between the solubility and erosion of the cement and its strength.

*Hardness.*     The surface hardness of the silicate cements ranges from K.H.N. 65 to 80. This value for surface hardness is essentially the same as that of the human tooth dentin. The surface hardness of tooth enamel is in the neighborhood of K.H.N. 300. The surface hardness of the silicate cement is more than twice as great as that of any other type of cement.

*Optical Properties.*     The color and shade of the silicate cement should be comparable to that of the tooth. The color and shading is incorporated in the powder. During the process of manufacture, highly colored powders are prepared, as well as the colorless or white powder. The colored powders are blended with the white powder to provide the proper shade. The dentist, in turn, can blend the powders supplied to produce new shades.

In order for the silicate cement restoration to match that of the tooth, the index of refraction of the two should be the same. The index of refraction[25] of enamel is approximately 1.60 and that of dentin is in the neighborhood of 1.56. The index of refraction of the silicate cement powders varies between 1.47 and 1.60, and that of the gel matrix is approximately 1.46.

The translucence of the cement restoration should also approximate that of the enamel. The *opacity of a substance,* which is actually the reciprocal of its translucence, is more easily measured. The opacity of specimens of enamel one millimeter in thickness is 21 to 67 per cent.[25] In other words, the enamel will absorb from 21 to 67 per cent of the light passing through it. On the same basis, the opacity of the dentin was found to be 50 to 91 per cent, and that of the silicate cements ranged from 23 to 57 per cent.

In practical testing the opacity of a specimen of a cement is compared with that of certain specified glass standards, placed over a black and white background[4] according to the instructions given in the American Dental Association Specification No. 9.

The opacity of the cement is represented by the contrast ratio $C_{0.70}$. This value is the ratio between the daylight apparent reflectance ($R_o$) of the part of a cement specimen one millimeter in thickness which is placed over a black background and the daylight apparent reflectance ($R_{0.70}$) of the part of the specimen which is placed over a white backing which has a reflectance value of 70 per cent relative to that of magnesium oxide. When the reflectances are equal, the $C_{0.70}$ value would be 1.00 and the cement would be 100 per cent opaque. If the $C_{0.70}$ is equal to 0.50, the cement would be 50 per cent opaque.

In the specification test, two opal glass standards with $C_{0.70}$ values of 0.35 and 0.55 are used and the cement opacity should fall within those limits (Table 15–4).

It is possible that the use of a color difference meter might eventually prove to be more suitable for standardizing color in these materials.[26]

**Discoloration.**     Any impurities in the cement powders or liquids may cause a subsequent discoloration of the restoration in service, particularly if the impurities form colored sulfides in the presence of hydrogen sulfide. The manufacturer should accept only the purest ingredients to be incorporated into the powders and liquids. The dentist should be on guard constantly not to contaminate the cement during its manipulation.

In some instances the observed change in the optical properties of a

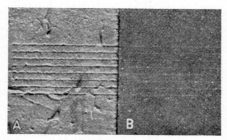

Fig. 15–6.   Effect of premature exposure to water. *A.* Immersed in water two minutes prior to setting. *B.* Immersed in water four minutes after setting. (Paffenbarger, Schoonover and Souder, *J.A.D.A.*, Jan., 1938.)

silicate cement restoration may actually be a change in the translucence or opacity. As the restoration erodes, the margins dissolve and a black line may appear, owing to the staining of the crevice between the restoration and the cavity margin. Stain of this nature, as with metallic restorations, may probably be related primarily to the formation of sulfides. Also, more light may be reflected from the eroded surface which renders it more opaque in appearance.

The restoration may become particularly objectionable in appearance if it is allowed to dry out in the mouth. The surface becomes soft and chalky in appearance, and its former translucence is not restored when it becomes wet again. Such a restoration may erode quite rapidly as a result.

**Effect of Water.**      Like the zinc phosphate cements, the silicate cements will not set properly in the presence of water. The operating area must be kept dry and the restoration should not be exposed to water for several hours after it has set.

A premature exposure of the cement during or immediately after setting results in a soft surface, totally lacking in translucence. The specimen[4] in Figure 15–6 is an illustration of the effect of premature exposure to water. Half of the surface of the specimen was covered with a water impervious film. The specimen was then placed in water two minutes before setting as determined with the Gillmore needle. Four minutes after it had set, the film was removed, and this surface was also exposed to water. Lines were then drawn across the two surfaces with the same tool and under the same pressure. As can be observed, the lines on the side *A*, which was exposed to water prematurely, are wider and deeper than those on side *B*. Side *A* was soft and totally lacking in translucence, whereas side *B* was reasonably normal. Side *A* will stain readily, and it will disintegrate rapidly in comparison to side *B*.

When the silicate cement is prematurely exposed to water, the phosphoric acid is leached out, and the water replaces it in the weak gel framework which has partially formed. A swelling takes place, and the surface of the restoration is irreparably ruined.

Very likely, a prolonged exposure of the surface of the restoration to water, even four minutes after the gel has set, is too soon for the best results. As soon as the initial finishing of the restoration has been completed, its surface should be coated with a varnish, or a wax before the patient is dismissed. The restoration should not be exposed to the saliva for several hours after it has been inserted.

On the other hand, as already noted, the surface of the restoration should never be exposed to the air. When the dentist operates on teeth adjacent to a silicate restoration, its surface should always be protected from the air.

**Care of the Liquid.**     All of the precautions in the care of the liquid listed for the zinc phosphate cements in the preceding chapter apply equally well for the liquids used for the silicate cements. A lack of water in the liquid will delay the setting of the cement, and an excess of water will accelerate the set unduly. In either case, the physical properties of the set cement will be changed undesirably. For example, it has been shown that either loss or gain in water will increase the solubility of the set cement.[27]

The changes in weight of the liquids used with the silicate cements when they are exposed to the atmosphere are of the same nature as those described for the zinc phosphate cement liquids. The change in weight of a silicate cement liquid is shown graphically[20] in Figure 15–7. As can be noted, only at a relative humidity of 80 per cent were the vapor pressures of the cement liquid and the atmosphere in balance so that no exchange of water took place across the interface.

It has been suggested[28] that the unstoppered bottle of cement liquid might be kept in a closed container in which the relative humidity is controlled so that the vapor pressure of the enclosed air is in equilibrium with that of the cement liquid.

Another method is to cover the liquid in the bottle with a thin layer of light liquid petrolatum, U.S.P.[28] The layer of liquid petrolatum will provide a barrier to the exchange of water vapor. In practice, a glass pipette or dropper is inserted through the cover of the bottle, which is always kept tightly closed unless it is in use. The opening of the dropper is placed beneath the oil film, and sufficient liquid is drawn in. The dropper is withdrawn, any oil clinging to it is wiped off, and the required amount of liquid is deposited on the mixing slab. The dropper is then returned to the bottle and the top is securely fastened in place.

It has been estimated[4] that a bottle of cement liquid may be open a total of 30 minutes during repeated withdrawals of liquid for the individual mixes with a single bottle of powder, even though it is assumed that the stopper is replaced immediately after each withdrawal. Such a length of time is sufficient to affect the liquid deleteriously. As with the zinc phosphate cement liquids, when approximately three-fourths of a bottle of cement liquid has been used, it should be discarded and a new bottle opened.

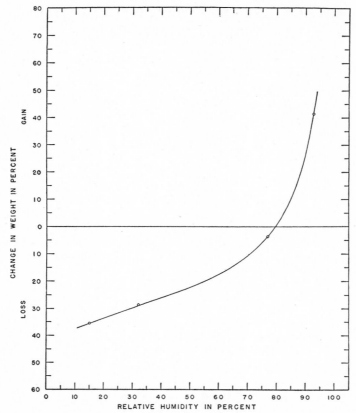

Fig. 15–7.   Effect on a silicate cement liquid as shown by its loss or gain in weight when it was exposed to different relative humidities for 200 days. (Paffenbarger, *North-West Den.*, Jan., 1948.)

**Temperature of the Mixing Slab.**     Possibly the most important consideration in the mixing of a silicate cement is the temperature of the glass mixing slab. As previously noted, the lower the temperature, the more slowly the material sets. A cool slab is important in the prevention of a premature gel formation before the mixed cement has been inserted into the prepared cavity.

As previously noted, a cool slab is important with the silicate cements for still another reason: the more powder that can be incorporated into the liquid, the less will be the volume of the gel matrix in the set cement, and consequently the less will be its solubility and disintegration in the mouth. The lower the temperature of the slab, the more powder can be incorporated before the reaction begins and causes a thickening of the mass.

On the other hand, the cooling of the slab will be limited by the relative humidity. Under no conditions should the temperature of the slab be lower than the dew point of the atmosphere. If moisture collects on the slab, the silicate cement restoration will possess poor physical properties regardless of the amount of powder added. When a silicate cement is mixed on a warm, humid day at a temperature above the dew point, the service-life of the resulting restoration will probably not be very long. It has been suggested that the operation should be postponed until better atmospheric conditions prevail,[29] unless the dental office is air-conditioned.[30]

**Mixing.** When a mixing slab is used, the cement powder and liquid should be placed on the cool slab just before they are to be mixed. For the reasons previously discussed, the liquid should not be in contact with the air any longer than is necessary.

The proper amount of powder and liquid to be used should be proportioned. Many manufacturers supply dispensers that are quite adequate for the powder, and a syringe may be used for the liquid. However, if the mixing temperature is somewhat variable, it is difficult to determine exactly the amount of powder that can be incorporated in a given amount of liquid. For this reason, a slight excess of powder should be provided. Once the mixing process has begun, it is inadvisable to stop it in order to obtain a fresh supply of powder. Any excess powder should be discarded since it is likely to be contaminated.

Unlike the zinc phosphate cements, the rate at which the powder is added to the liquid is relatively unimportant. Probably one-half of the entire mass can be added at once, and then smaller increments as the mixture becomes thicker (Fig. 15–8). The mixing procedure consists of rapidly "folding" the powder into the liquid, so that every particle of powder is coated with liquid. The area of mixing should be confined to a narrow limit on the mixing slab in order to minimize the exposure of the hygroscopic unset cement to the atmosphere. The time

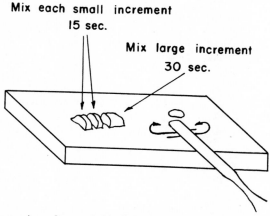

Fig. 15–8. Approximately one-half of the silicate cement powder is "folded" into the liquid at once for 30 seconds. Smaller units should be mixed about 15 seconds. (Peterson, *Clinical Dental Hygiene.*)

of mixing should never exceed one minute. At completion of the mixing it should have a heavy, putty-like consistency.

A novel method has been suggested for mixing the powder and liquid by which the air is virtually excluded and a cool temperature can be used regardless of the climatic conditions.[31] A thin-walled, paddle-shaped toy balloon (uncolored) is used as the mixing container. The balloon is cut off approximately one inch from the bottom, and a weighed amount of powder is sealed inside. The liquid is stored in a small serum bottle with a self-sealing rubber stopper. The proper amount of liquid is removed from the bottle with a tuberculin syringe fitted with a hypodermic needle. The needle is inserted into the balloon, and the liquid is expelled. The balloon is then kneaded between the thumbs and fingers of both hands under cool water. The proper mixture is thus obtained regardless of the dew point. The balloon is cut open and the mixed cement is used at once. More powder can be incorporated into the liquid in this manner than can be accomplished in mixing in the usual manner on a cool mixing slab.

Other methods of mixing have also been employed, such as by the attachment of the balloon to the dental handpiece and whirling it in a bowl of ice water,[32] and by the use of a gelatin capsule in a mechanical amalgamator.[33] The results indicate no significant improvement in the physical properties of the cement with these devices.

In short then, one should make a thick mix on a cool slab as fast as possible.

**Insertion and Finishing.**    A textbook on operative dentistry should be consulted for the details of this procedure. In brief, a strip of cellulose acetate or similar material is fashioned so that it can be drawn around the tooth. As soon as the mixing of the cement is completed, the material is inserted into the prepared cavity, and the cellulose strip is drawn tightly against it so that it is held under pressure. It is imperative that the strip be held tightly and rigidly until the set is completed. Otherwise, the gel may be fractured, and the restoration will be ruined irreparably. As discussed in previous sections, it is also imperative that the field of operation be completely dry. The time of hardening should never be left to guess work but should be judged by the feel of a piece of the excess cement left on the slab.

The strip can be removed after the set has occurred, but the cement should be immediately protected with cocoa butter or a similar material, in order to allow the hardening to progress further out of contact with air or water. Some dentists allow as much as a half hour to elapse before further work is completed. The restoration should be finished only roughly at the first sitting. Under no circumstances should the surface of the restoration be finished flush with the enamel at this time.[34] Such a procedure encourages fracture of the weak margins and the production of a V-shaped crevice. The final finishing should not be done for

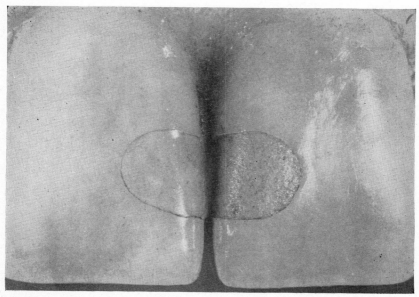

Fig. 15–9. Two silicate restorations made with the same brand of silicate cement. Restoration on left was properly manipulated and the one on the right was over-spatulated on a warm slab and finished immediately. (Paffenbarger and Stanford, *D. Clin. North America*, Nov., 1958.)

several days, preferably for at least one week, in order to allow the cement time to approach its maximum strength.

The restoration should be contoured as much as possible by the cellulose strip at the time it initially hardens in the tooth in order to provide the smoothest surface possible. Later abrading and polishing will not produce as smooth a surface as that left by the strip. If the restoration is subsequently contoured by grinding or trimming, the undissolved particles are apt to be displaced from the gel matrix. Since the gel is mainly responsible for the subsequent dissolution of the restoration, any undue exposure of the gel at the surface of the restoration tends to reduce the useful life of the filling. In finishing, only the finest grit disks should be used, at low speeds and covered with grease to minimize heat.

All of these manipulative variables markedly affect the clinical behavior of the material, as shown in Figure 15–9. Both of the restorations in the photograph[34] were made with the same brand of silicate cement. The good restoration at the left was made from a mix spatulated for 30 seconds on a slab at 16° C. (60° F.). Petrolatum was placed on the restoration just after the matrix strip was removed. The restoration was finished a week later.

The poor restoration on the right was made from a mix spatulated on a slab at 37° C. (98.6° F.) for two minutes. Saliva was allowed to contact the restoration immediately after the matrix strip was removed. The restoration was immediately dressed down flush with the enamel.

The photograph of the two restorations was obtained only a few weeks after their insertion. It is obvious that the laboratory evidence previously presented is borne out by clinical experience.

**Acidity.** The acidity of the silicate cement is considerable ($p$H 1.6) when it is placed in contact with the tooth.[35] However, when measurements were made with the cement in distilled water, the acidity decreased rapidly in most cases as the cement hardened. It approached neutrality in 24 hours under such conditions of testing.

**Pulp Injury.** Considerable experimental work seems to indicate that the silicate cements, without some truly protective base, irritate the pulp if placed in a freshly cut cavity.[36, 37] The reaction is usually attributed to the phosphoric acid, not to the fluoride flux.[2] These investigations suggest that the reaction in the pulp may often be irreversible and more severe, therefore, than that incurred with zinc phosphate cement. On the other hand, other research has not supported this thesis.[38] One experienced worker in this field strongly suggests that more pulp infection can be attributed to undetected pulp exposures during the preparation of the cavity than from the materials themselves.[39]

More recent work involving the tissue reaction to subdermal implants in rats indicates that the relative irritational characteristics of a silicate cement are moderate; some filling materials cause more severe responses.[40] Suffice to say, though, that it is sound procedure to take special precaution in protecting the pulp against possible injury from silicate cement. As mentioned in Chapter 14, zinc oxide and eugenol cement or calcium hydroxide, either alone or with other agents,[41] are effective barriers against the phosphoric acid. Cavity varnishes are not totally effective,[42] as discussed in the previous chapter.

**Combination Cements.** Powders F and L in Table 15–1 contain zinc oxide and magnesium oxide in considerable amount, in addition to the usual constituents of the silicate cements. In the case of powder F, the ingredients were fused together, but the fusion was incomplete. With powder L, the silicate powder was mixed mechanically with the zinc and magnesium oxides after the latter had been sintered.[4] These cements are hybrid combinations of zinc phosphate cement with silicate cement and are commonly employed by many dentists. They are often referred to as "silico-phosphate" cement.

The strength of these cements is comparable to that of the conventional silicate cements. The solubility is of the same order, although it may be lower in certain mediums (Fig. 15–3).[23, 43] As could be expected, the translucence of this type of cement is definitely less than that of silicate cement.[44] They are generally manipulated in a manner similar to silicate.

These products are occasionally used as cements for cast restorations. Their manipulative characteristics, such as working time and film thickness, are somewhat inferior to those of a zinc phosphate cement, but in terms of strength and solubility (Fig. 15–3) they are probably superior. Likewise the fact that they contain a fluoride offers protection against recurrent caries. If the manipulation can provide adequate working time and a sufficiently thin film thickness, their use as a cement may possibly be indicated.

**Causes of Failure.** The two most common causes for difficulty are: (1) use of liquid which has either changed through exposure to the atmosphere or by contamination, and (2) improper mixing technique.

If the cement sets too slowly, the probable cause is (a) the mix is too thin (insufficient powder incorporated in the mix), or (b) prolonged spatulation (increased spatulation time increases setting time), or (c) an unbalancing of the liquid by loss of water.

If the cement sets too fast, the probable cause is (a) mixing on a warm slab, or (b) insufficient spatulation time, or (c) the liquid has gained water.

Precipitation or cloudiness in the liquid denotes contamination or evaporation of water and it should be discarded. Surplus powder that has been on the mixing slab should never be returned to the bottle. The powder may have come in contact with the liquid and when returned to the bottle it will affect the properties of subsequent mixes.

Addition of liquid to the mix is contraindicated once the spatulation has begun. If the mix is too viscous or has started to set, it should be discarded. By the same token, additional powder should not be added to a mix which is too thin after the completion of spatulation. As previously stated, the mixing should be completed promptly. Once the powder and liquid have come into intimate contact, the silica gel begins to form. Further radical disturbance of the mix will disperse the gel and the restoration will be unserviceable.

## Literature

1. Paffenbarger, G. C.: *An Investigation by a Group of Practicing Dentists under the Direction of the A.D.A., Research Fellowship at the National Bureau of Standards.* J.A.D.A., 27:1611–1622 (Oct.), 1940.
2. Manly, R. S., Baker, C. F., Miller, P. N., and Welch, F. E.: *The Effect of Composition of Liquid and Powder on the Physical Properties of Silicate Cements.* J. D. Res., 30:145–156 (Feb.), 1951.
3. Crepaz, E.: *Constitution and Reactivity of Dental Cements.* Chimica e Industria (Milan), 33:137–140, 1951.
4. Paffenbarger, G. C., Schoonover, I. C., and Souder, W.: *Dental Silicate Cements: Physical and Chemical Properties and a Specification.* J.A.D.A., 25:32–87 (Jan.), 1938.
5. Brauer, F. J., White, E. E., and Burns, C. L.: *Investigations to Reduce the Solubility of Silicate Cements.* J. D. Res., 37:89–90 (Feb.), 1958.
6. Crowell, W. S.: Personal communication.

7. Henschel, C. J.: *Observations Concerning in Vivo Disintegration of Silicate Cement Restorations.* J. D. Res., *28:*528 (Oct.), 1949.
8. Volker, J., Bekaris, B., and Melillo, S.: *Some Observations on the Relationship between Plastic Filling Materials and Dental Caries.* Tufts D. Outlook, *18:*4–8 (May), 1944.
9. Paffenbarger, G. C., Nelsen, R. J., and Sweeney, W. T.: *Direct and Indirect Filling Resins: a Review of Some Physical and Chemical Properties.* J.A.D.A., *47:*516–524 (Nov.), 1953.
10. Norman, R. D., Phillips, R. W., and Swartz, M. L.: *Fluoride Uptake by Enamel from Certain Dental Materials.* J. D. Res., *39:*11–16 (Jan.-Feb.), 1960.
11. Lilienthal, B., and Martin, W. D.: *Investigation of the Anti-enzymatic Action of Fluoride at the Enamel Surface.* J. D. Res., *35:*189–196 (April), 1956.
12. Lilienthal, B.: *The Effect of Fluoride on Acid Formation by Salivary Sediment.* J. D. Res., *35:*197–204 (April), 1956.
13. Mangi, S. L., Summers, W. A., Phillips, R. W., and Swartz, M. L.: *Antibacterial Action of Certain Fluoride-containing Dental Restorative Materials.* J. D. Res., *43:*88–95 (Jan.), 1959.
14. Phillips, R. W., and Swartz, M. L.: *Effect of Certain Restorative Materials on Solubility of Enamel.* J.A.D.A., *54:*623–636 (May), 1957.
15. Swartz, M. L., and Phillips, R. W.: *Effect of Certain Restorative Materials on Solubility of Dentin.* J. D. Res., *37:*811–815 (Sept.), 1958.
16. Alexander, A. E., and Johnson, P.: *Colloid Science.* London, Oxford University Press, 1949, Vol. II, p. 608.
17. Souder, W., and Schoonover, I. C.: *Probable Chemical Reactions in Silicate Cements.* J. D. Res., *18:*250 (June), 1939.
18. Paffenbarger, G. C., and Stanford, J.: *Zinc Phosphate and Silicate Cement.* D. Clin. North America, November, 1958, p. 566.
19. Souder, W., and Paffenbarger, G. C.: *Physical Properties of Dental Materials.* National Bureau of Standards Circular C433, Washington, U. S. Government Printing Office, 1942, pp. 125–127.
20. Paffenbarger, G. C.: *Silicate Cements, How to Select and Use Them.* North-West Den., *27:*29–35 (Jan.), 1948.
21. Souder, W., and Paffenbarger, G. C.: *loc. cit.,* p. 13.
22. Norman, R. D., Swartz, M. L., and Phillips, R. W.: *Studies on the Solubility of Certain Dental Materials.* J. D. Res., *36:*977–985 (Dec.), 1957.
23. Norman, R. D., Swartz, M. L., and Phillips, R. W.: *Additional Studies on the Solubility of Certain Dental Materials.* J. D. Res., *30:*1028–1037 (Sept.), 1959.
24. Voelker, C. C.: *Dental Silicate Cements in Theory and Practice.* D. Cosmos, *58:* 1098–1111 (Oct.), 1916.
25. Souder, W., and Paffenbarger, G. C.: *loc. cit.,* p. 121.
26. Oglesby, P. L., and Dickson, G.: *Standardization of the Colors of Silicate Cements.* J. D. Res., *37:*89 (Feb.), 1958. Abstract.
27. Docking, A. R.: *Recent Advances in the Non-resinous Filling Materials.* Internat. D. J., *4:*482–494 (June), 1954.
28. Souder, W., and Paffenbarger, G. C.: *loc. cit.,* p. 132.
29. Tingley, H. E.: *A Code for Silicate Cements.* J.A.D.A., *26:*183–192 (Feb.), 1939.
30. Ringsdorf, W. M.: *Temperature and Humidity Control with Silicate Cement Restorations.* J.A.D.A., *38:*715–721 (June), 1949.
31. Grunewald, A. H., Dickson, G., Paffenbarger, G. C., and Schoonover, I. C.: *Silicate Cement: Method of Mixing in a Closed Container to Prevent Effects of Exposure to Atmosphere.* J.A.D.A., *46:*184–187 (Feb.), 1953.
32. Brauer, F. J.: *Mechanical Manipulation of Silicate Cements.* J.A.D.A., *51:*713–717 (Dec.), 1955.
33. Brauer, F. J., and Dickson, G.: *Effect of Mechanical Mixing on Silicate Cement.* J. D. Res., *35:*111–112, 1957. Abstract.
34. Paffenbarger, G. C., and Stanford, J.: *loc. cit.,* p. 567.
35. Harvey, W., Le Brocq, L. F., and Rakowski, L.: *The Acidity of Dental Cements.* Brit. D. J., *77:*61–69 (Aug. 4), 1944.
36. Massler, M.: *Effects of Filling Materials on the Pulp.* J. Tennessee D. A., *35:*353–374 (Oct.), 1955.

37. Manley, E. B.: *Investigations into the Early Effects of Various Filling Materials on the Human Pulp.* D. Record, *62:*1–16 (Jan.), 1942.
38. Barker, J. N.: *Reactions of the Pulp to Various Filling Materials and Clinical Procedures.* Austral. J. Den., *46:*226–232 (Dec.), 1942.
39. Van Huysen, G.: *Conservation of Pulp Vitality.* New York D. J., *21:*185–191 (May), 1955.
40. Mitchell, D. F.: *The Irritational Qualities of Dental Materials.* J.A.D.A., *59:*954–966 (Nov.), 1959.
41. Zander, H. A., Glenn, J. F., and Nelson, C. A.: *Pulp Protection in Restorative Dentistry.* J.A.D.A., *41:*563–573 (Nov.), 1950.
42. Zander, H. A., and Pejko, I.: *Protection of the Pulp under Silicate Cements with Cavity Varnishes and Cement Linings.* J.A.D.A., *34:*811–819 (June 15), 1947.
43. Ross, J. H.: *The Silico-phosphate Cement as a Permanent Filling Material.* D. Practitioner, *2:*370–374 (Aug.), 1952.
44. Paffenbarger, G. C., and Caul, H. J.: *Dental Cements.* Proc. Dent. Cent. Celebration, March, 1940, pp. 232–237.

CHAPTER 16

# Dental Porcelain

Dental porcelain may be divided into two types, depending upon its use. One type, which is of the greatest importance so far as the actual quantity used, is employed for the construction of artificial teeth. The second type is used by the dentist in powdered form for the construction of porcelain jacket crowns and inlays. Although the basic principles of composition, chemistry, and technic are essentially the same for both types, more attention will be given to the second type which is fired by the dentist or technician in the laboratory.

Regardless of the type of dental porcelain, basically a fine ceramic powder, pigmented to produce the color and shade of a human tooth, is mixed with water to form a paste. The paste is then formed into the shape desired and fused at a high temperature to form a ceramic body which exhibits excellent esthetic qualities in the mouth.

**Uses of Dental Porcelain.** Before the advent of the synthetic resins, porcelain was employed for the construction of denture bases. The "all-porcelain" denture was considered to be the ultimate in denture construction. Although these denture bases were excellent from an esthetic standpoint, there were many technical difficulties involved in their construction. Furthermore, the porcelain was easily fractured upon accidental impact, and the service life of such dentures was apt to be short.

A general technic for the construction of a porcelain jacket crown is briefly as follows: an impression is taken of the crown preparation on the tooth. A die is prepared in the impression. A thin sheet of platinum, called the matrix, is burnished over the preparation as it is reproduced on the die. A porcelain powder of the desired shade is then mixed with water to form a paste, which is applied to the platinum matrix by

**Page 270**

methods to be described in a subsequent section. The paste is applied in such a manner that the form of the finished crown is attained. The matrix with the porcelain is removed from the die to a fire-clay slab, and fired in an electric furnace to the desired condition. Actually the crown may be fired several times before the final form is attained. For the details of this procedure, a textbook on the subject should be consulted.[1]

During the firing, the porcelain shrinks as much as 40 per cent by volume. Although the shrinkage can be directed in such a manner that the actual shrinkage of the finished restoration may not be as much as might be expected, such a shrinkage is definitely disadvantageous in the use of the material.

**Composition.** Dental porcelain for crowns and bridges may be classified according to its fusion temperature, *i.e.*, the temperature to which the porcelain must be subjected to complete the firing reactions, or "maturing." There are three types of dental porcelain generally recognized:

High fusing 1300°–1370° C. (2350°–2500° F.)
Medium fusing 1090°–1260° C. (2000°–2300° F.)
Low fusing 870°–1065° C. (1600°–1950° F.)

Porcelain A in Table 16–1 is probably used for the manufacture of porcelain teeth. The clay, or kaolin, is added to provide body or strength for the molded tooth before firing. As previously noted, the fine powder is mixed with water and formed to the desired shape. The clay acts as a binder to hold the form together before it is fired.

The clay also contributes to the strength of the fired product, but it tends to reduce the translucence and consequently its use in dental porcelains has been virtually discontinued.[2]

Very likely, porcelains B and C are of a lower fusing type than A, since the addition of borax lowers the fusion temperature. Feldspar is a mineral with the chemical formulas of $KAlSi_3O_8$ (microline), or $NaAlSi_3O_8$ (albite). When it is fused it does not exhibit a sharp melting point, but rather gradually begins to melt at approximately 1100° C. (2000° F.). It becomes a viscous liquid at about 1300° C. (2370° F.)

*Table 16–1.* *Composition of Dental Porcelain*

| PORCELAIN | KAOLIN | SILICA | FELDSPAR | SODIUM CARBONATE | BORAX | CALCIUM CARBONATE | POTASSIUM CARBONATE |
|---|---|---|---|---|---|---|---|
| | (Per Cent) | (Per Cent) | (Per Cent) | (Per Cent) | (Per Cent) | (Per Cent) | (Per Cent) |
| A | 4 | 15 | 81 | .. | .. | .. | .. |
| B | .. | 29 | 61 | 2 | 1 | 5 | 2 |
| C | .. | 12 | 60 | 8 | 11 | 1 | 8 |

*Table 16–2.* *Constituents of Dental Porcelain Powders for Crowns and Inlays\**

| PORCELAIN | TYPED BY FUSING TEMP. | PREDOMINANT PHASE | PRINCIPAL MINERAL PHASE |
|:---:|:---:|:---:|:---:|
| A | Low | Glass | Feldspar |
| B | Low | Glass | Feldspar |
| C | Low | ½ Glass ½ Mineral | Feldspar |
| D | Medium | Glass | Feldspar |
| E | Medium | Glass | Feldspar |
| F | Medium | Glass | |
| G | High | Glass | Feldspar |
| H | High | Glass | Feldspar |
| I | High | Mineral | Feldspar \*\* |
| J | High | Mineral | Feldspar † |
| K | High | Mineral | Feldspar |
| L | High | ½ Glass ½ Mineral | Feldspar |

\* Hodson, *J. D. Res.*, May-June, 1959.
\*\* Some Quartz.
† Some Glass.

with a very high viscosity, approximately 1,000,000 times that of fused glass.[3]

The quartz is present in the usual form of $SiO_2$.

The results of petrographic analyses of 12 crown and inlay porcelains in use at the present time are presented in Table 16–2. With the exception of porcelains H and L, the high fusing types contain feldspar as the predominant constituent with little or no glass. As can be noted from the Table, most of the porcelains contain glass as the principal constituent. These dental porcelains should actually be classified as glasses. Quartz was identified only in porcelain I, and no kaolin was found.[3]

**Manufacture.** Very few of the modern dental porcelain powders used in the dental office contain the original raw products. However, in the case of the manufacture of porcelain teeth, the raw ingredients are employed. As the powders are received by the dentist, the raw ingredients have been fired together to form a fused mass which is plunged into water while hot. As a result, the hot mass is stressed to the extent that considerable cracking and fracturing occur. Such a ceramic body is known as a *frit*. The frit is then ground to a fine powder.[4]

The thermochemical reactions which occur during this fritting process are extremely complex. The feldspar separates into a glass and a feldspathic crystalline form known as *leucite* ($KAlSi_2O_6$) at about 1100° C. (2000° F.). As the temperature rises the glass dissolves the leucite. When the fusion is complete, the porcelain is said to have *matured*. At this stage, approximately 1300° C. (2356° F.), the glass has dissolved all of the leucite. If a dental structure is being constructed, the firing is stopped at this stage since a further temperature rise only reduces the viscosity and causes a loss of shape.

Any silica or kaolin which may be present does not enter into the thermochemical reactions, but rather remains an inert filler. The ingredients added to reduce the fusion temperature of the feldspar (porcelains B and C, Table 16–1), are first pre-fused to form an insoluble glass in order to prevent their dissolution during subsequent firings.

The frit can be completed at any desired stage of the above reactions. As can be noted from the petrographic analyses in Table 16–2, the lower fusing porcelains contain more glass than mineral or crystalline phase, whereas the reverse is true for the high fusing porcelains. In other words, the farther advanced the thermochemical reactions before fritting, the lower is the fusing temperature of the porcelain as received by the dentist. In addition, as noted previously, the lower fusing porcelains are of a different composition so as to provide a lower fusing temperature.

It is possible that no fritting was employed in the case of porcelains J and L.

The coloring and shading of dental porcelain are produced by the addition of colored pigments to the base powder. The porcelain can be colored either by the fusing of certain metallic oxides into the porcelain body, or by the dispersion of colloidal particles into the fused mass. The vitreous substances so obtained are generally brilliant in hue. After they have been ground, the colored powders are blended in the proper amount with the uncolored base to give the desired shade and color.

**Glazes.** A *glaze* is a ceramic veneer which may be added to a porcelain restoration after it has been fired. A glaze for dental purposes is generally a transparent glass, with a fusing temperature lower than that of the porcelain body. A jacket crown, for example, can be fired; then a glaze is applied as a paste and the crown is again fired to the fusion temperature of the glaze. The result is a glossy or semi-glossy surface which is completely non-porous.

The thermal coefficient of expansion of the glaze ideally should be equal to that of the porcelain body to which it is applied. If the glaze has a higher thermal coefficient of expansion than the body, it will cool under tension. The stresses resulting may cause a crazing of the surface. The greater the stressed condition, the finer will be the crazing network produced.

On the other hand, if the thermal coefficient of expansion of the glaze is considerably less than that of the body, compressive stresses may develop cracks in the glaze known as "peeling." In either case, an erosion of the glaze may gradually occur in the mouth. A smooth surface on the porcelain is always necessary, particularly where the porcelain contacts the soft tissues. If the glaze is removed, the rough and sometimes porous surface of the body becomes exposed.

Glasses in general are more capable of withstanding compressive stresses than they can tensile stress or shear. Since it is virtually impossible to match the thermal coefficients of expansion of the body and the glaze precisely, a desirable glaze probably should exhibit a thermal coefficient of expansion slightly less than that of the body.[4]

**Stains.**    Often slight markings or defects are placed in porcelain restorations in imitation of a similar dental condition. Colored minerals known as *spinels* may be used for staining purposes, although in dentistry ordinary colored, low-fusing porcelain is usually employed. In any event, the stain should fuse into the body or the glaze, and it should be sufficiently stable not to react with either the glaze or the body during the firing.

The stain is used in finely powdered form, suspended in a vehicle such as water, glycerin and water, or similar liquids which will completely volatilize during firing. The suspension is applied with a brush to the porcelain body, usually before it is glazed.

**Condensation.**    The porcelain jacket crown or inlay must first be formed before it is fired. The porcelain powder is mixed with water to form a thick paste, which is applied to the platinum matrix with a brush or a porcelain carver.

The added water by virtue of its surface tension serves as a binder for the porcelain powder so that the crown or inlay can be shaped before firing. Some powders contain an organic binder in addition, such as sugar or starch. Whatever the binder, it does not react chemically with the powder. During the subsequent firing it is driven off, and as the particles of porcelain fill in the space formerly occupied by the binder, a shrinkage occurs. It follows, therefore, that the smaller the amount of water present at the time the firing is begun, the more closely the powder particles will have been packed before firing and the less should be the shrinkage during firing. The process of packing the particles together and of removing the water is known as *condensation.*

There are many variations in the methods employed for condensation, but the methods can be fairly well classified into five groups, the *brush application* method, the *gravitation* method, the *spatulation* method, the *whipping* method, and the *vibration* method. The spatulation and vibration methods, separately or in combination, are employed to a much greater extent than are the other three methods.

The brush application method consists of adding the paste to the matrix, and then dry powder is sprinkled onto the wet surface. The dry powder removes the excess water by capillary action from the mixture already applied. The particles move closer together as the water is withdrawn.

In the gravitation method, water is added to the wet porcelain after it has been applied to the matrix. The sudden addition of water is thought to agitate the particles so that they will settle again in a compact manner. The water is then drawn off with a linen cloth or a clean blotting paper. This method is open to the objection that only the coarser particles will settle during the time allowed. Many porcelain powders are so fine that they may remain suspended in water for hours.

In the spatulation method, the wet porcelain is applied with the blade of a porcelain carver or a small spatula, and then the surface is smoothed with the instrument. Such an action disturbs the particles and causes them to become more closely packed. The water rises to the surface, and it is removed as described before with a linen cloth or a piece of blotting paper.

After the paste has been applied to the matrix, it may be whipped with the brush. The water is thus brought to the surface and it is removed as before.

In the vibration method, the paste on the matrix is vibrated slightly to give the particles a chance to settle and to pack together, and the excess water is removed as usual. A slight vibration is indicated, since a heavy vibration may cause the particles to vibrate upwards, and the purpose of the condensation would be defeated.

Whatever the method employed, a bit of porcelain paste is carried to the matrix with a small brush or porcelain carver, and treated to remove as much water as possible. The crown or inlay is built up in this manner, piece by piece. Different shades of porcelain may be added. For example, a darker shade may be used toward the base of the crown than toward the incisal surface. The proper shade is determined by a comparison of the natural teeth present in the mouth with a prepared shade guide.

In the manufacture of teeth, the condensation is accomplished in flexible rubber molds of the proper size. A thinner paste, or slurry, is used than in the dental office. The molds are then vibrated automatically for an extended period of time until a much better condensation is effected than by the usual dental technic. The formed teeth are then extruded from the mold and fired in a specially designed furnace.

**Theory of Condensation.** One of the factors which determines the effectiveness of the condensation in the prevention of firing shrinkage is the shape and size of the porcelain powder particles.[5] Since the object of the condensation is to produce the most compact arrangement or greatest density of the particles before firing, the size distribution of the powder becomes important.

This fact is demonstrated diagrammatically in Figure 16–1. In Figure 16–1*A*, when only one size of particle is used, it can be calculated that the greatest condensation will leave a void space between the

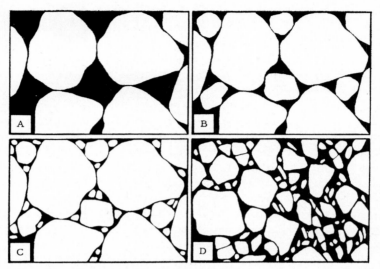

Fig. 16–1. The effect of particle size on condensation. *A.* One particle size, void space of 45 per cent. *B.* Two sizes, void space of 25 per cent. *C.* Three or more sizes, void space of 22 per cent. *D.* Many sizes, dental porcelains shrink 30 to 40 per cent. (Hodson, *J. Pros. Den.,* March-April, 1959.)

particles of 45 per cent. It follows that if this space is filled during firing, the body of porcelain will likely shrink this amount.

If two sizes of porcelain particles are used, as in Figure 16–1*B,* the void space can be reduced to 25 per cent. If three or more sizes are employed (Fig. 16–1*C* and *D*), a void space of as low as 22 per cent can be obtained. However, such calculations are theoretical limits of contraction, and they can only be approached with the best available condensation technic.

It can be noted that all of the condensation methods previously described have one procedure in common, and that is the removal of the water from the paste after it has been applied to the matrix or to the partially built crown. The water should be removed by a blotting action, and not by a simple drying. The less the amount of the water in the paste, the less is the amount that will need to be removed, but there must be sufficient water originally so that the particles can settle and pack.

The sudden removal of the water is an important factor in the condensation. Bernoulli's theorem states that the greater the velocity of a fluid, the less is its pressure. It is conceivable that when the water is withdrawn from the paste, it rushes between the particles with a variable velocity, depending upon the spacing of the particles, their surface roughness, etc. In such a case, the particles will move toward the areas where the water is moving with the greatest velocity.

The most important factor in condensation is the effect of surface tension. As the water is withdrawn, surface tension causes the powder particles to pack more closely together. The same effect can be seen if a camel's-hair brush is dipped in water; while the bristles are in the water, they may move apart in all directions, but if the brush is removed from the water, the bristles move toward each other, because of the action of the surface tension of the water remaining in the brush. If the brush is now touched with a blotter, for example, the bristles will pack even closer together.

It should be noted, however, that sufficient water must remain in the brush to wet all of the bristles. As the brush dries, for example, the bristles spring apart again. As previously noted, a binder is sometimes added to the porcelain powder to prevent the disintegration of the crown or inlay after it is dried before firing.

**The Porcelain Furnace.**[6]      One type of porcelain furnace is shown in Figure 16–2. The *muffle* containing the heating unit is shown on top of the box containing the rheostat or variable transformer for the control of the current. After the work has been placed inside the muffle, the door can be closed, as shown in the insert.

The instrument shown to the rear and above the muffle is a *pyrometer* which registers the electric potential produced in the thermocouple. The *hot junction* of the thermocouple is placed toward the top of the muffle, halfway between the back and the front. The *cold junction* is completed through the pyrometer.

The thermocouple circuit is diagrammed in Figure 16–3. The principle of the thermocouple is dependent upon the electromotive force

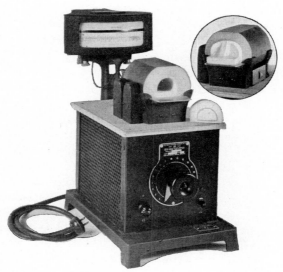

Fig. 16–2.   An electric furnace for the firing of dental porcelain. (Courtesy of S. S. White Dental Manufacturing Co.)

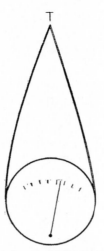

Fig. 16–3.  A typical thermocouple circuit with a pyrometer.

generated between the junctions of two dissimilar metals when they are held at different temperatures. In Figure 16–3, the hot junction at $T$ is placed in the furnace as described and the temperature of the cold junction is that of the pyrometer. A platinum wire is joined with a wire composed of 90 per cent platinum and 10 per cent rhodium to form the thermocouple for high fusing porcelains. If the furnace is to operate at temperatures less than 1100° C. (2000° F.), alloys of chromium may be used for the thermocouple more economically.

The heating element usually consists of platinum wire, coiled around the interior of the muffle and embedded in a refractory cement. If only low fusing porcelain is to be fired, an ordinary type of nickel-chromium resistance wire can be substituted for the platinum.

Some type of variable transformer is superior to a rheostat for the regulation of the current, but a heavy duty rheostat is often provided in the units for the dental office.

The pyrometer is usually a millivoltmeter, calibrated to read in degrees of temperature. The connection of the thermocouple through the instrument constitutes the cold junction. Since the difference in potential between the hot junction in the furnace and the cold junction is proportional to the difference in temperature between the two, the temperature of the pyrometer itself should be constant throughout the firing procedure. In practice, this temperature is that of the room. It is possible to compensate automatically for small variations in room temperature, but if the pyrometer is not sufficiently insulated thermally from the muffle during firing, it is possible that it may read low as its temperature increases above that of the room. Such a consideration should be taken into account in the original design of the unit.

Other types of furnaces are available. For example, some furnaces are equipped for vacuum firing as described in a subsequent section.

**Firing Procedure.**     After the condensation has been completed, the article is placed on a fire-clay slab or tray, and inserted in the muffle, directly under the hot junction of the thermocouple. The porcelain should never be allowed to come directly into contact with the muffle walls or floor. At high temperatures, the porcelain will melt and some of the ingredients may fuse into the heating element. Such a contamination renders the heating element extremely brittle, and it may fracture during cooling or a subsequent heating. Such a precaution is particularly important when a platinum-wound muffle is used.

Since the thermochemical reactions between the ingredients have been virtually completed in most cases during the original fritting process the purpose of the firing by the dentist is simply to fuse the particles of powder together properly.

At the time the firing begins, the interstices between the particles are filled with either water or air. In any event, the thermal conductivity of the mass is very low at this stage, and the temperature of the muffle should be raised slowly so that the condensed porcelain will be heated as uniformly as possible.

During the initial heating, the door of the muffle should be left ajar in order to allow any water vapor or products of combustion to escape. If such products are confined in the furnace, the heating element may become contaminated. Usually all such reactions are completed below 870° C. (1600° F.), at which temperature the muffle door can be closed.

Not only does the size of the powder particles influence the degree of condensation of the porcelain but it also influences the soundness or apparent density of the final product. The progressive changes which occur during the firing of porcelain powders of coarse and fine particle sizes respectively are shown[7] in Figure 16–4. The upper row of photomicrographs represents the structure during firing at the temperatures indicated of a porcelain with particles greater than 125 microns in diameter, and the lower row the same vitrification changes for particles 44 microns or less in diameter.

Regardless of the particle size, the white areas at 2150° F. (1177° C.) are the powder particles. The areas between are the voids shown diagrammatically in Figure 16–1, which at this temperature would be occupied by the atmosphere of the furnace. As fusion begins, the particles unite at their points of contact (Fig. 16–4, 2200° F.). As the temperature is raised the fused glass gradually flows to fill up the air spaces, but the air becomes trapped in the form of bubbles since the fused mass is too viscous to allow all of it to escape.

**Stages in Firing.**     There are at least three stages generally recognized in the firing of dental porcelain. The temperature at which each occurs will depend upon the type of porcelain employed. The lower the fusing temperature of the porcelain, the lower will be the temperature of each firing stage.

A *low bisque* firing is recognized as the stage when the fluxes have softened and have started to flow between the particles. The fired article exhibits rigidity, but it is very porous. The powder particles lack complete cohesion. A negligible amount of firing shrinkage can be noted.

A *medium bisque* firing is characterized by the fact that the fluxes have flowed to the extent that the powder particles exhibit complete cohesion; the article is still porous and this stage is accompanied by a definite shrinkage in size.

After a *high bisque* firing, the shrinkage is complete, and the mass exhibits a smoother surface. A very slight amount of porosity may be visible, but the body does not exhibit a glazed appearance.

The work can be removed from the furnace and cooled at any of these stages, so that additions can be made.

**Glazing.**     The surface of the crown or inlay should be completely smooth when the restoration is placed in the mouth. Otherwise food and other débris may cling to it.

Only if the condensation has been complete can the fired porcelain be polished. As a rule, the condensation procedure employed in the dental office is seldom effective in the complete elimination of blebs and surface porosity. Such surface defects are removed by a glazing of the body.

A glaze can be applied to the surface as described in a preceding section, or the body itself can be glazed by a separate firing. If the body, previously fired to a high bisque, is heated rapidly (10 to 15 minutes) to its fusion temperature, and maintained at that temperature for approximately five minutes before it is cooled, the fluxes will flow over the surface to form a vitreous layer, which will act as a glaze. Owing to the surface tension of the fluid flux at the firing temperature, any sharp edges and angles are likely to be rounded slightly by such a procedure.

**Cooling.**     The method of cooling the jacket crown after it has been fired may affect its subsequent strength considerably. If the crown is cooled too rapidly, the premature cooling of the outer layers before the inner part has cooled to the same extent will result in an introduction of stresses. Such stresses may decrease the strength of the porcelain considerably.

For example, it has been shown[8] that the modulus of rupture of dental porcelain may be increased as much as 25 per cent by a proper cooling, or by an annealing of the porcelain at a temperature slightly below its fusing point for a specified time after an initial cooling. The safest method is to allow the work to cool in the muffle of the furnace after the current has been shut off.

**Shrinkage.**     The principal cause of the shrinkage during the firing of the dental porcelain is a lack of condensation. When dry porcelain powder was condensed into an experimental specimen under a load of 150 tons, very little firing shrinkage was noted.[9]

Authorities appear to differ as to the volume shrinkage which occurs in different types of porcelain. According to one study,[10] the volume shrinkage did not vary with the fusion temperature of the porcelain, but the results of a more recent research[11] indicate that the high fusing porcelains shrink approximately 29 per cent by volume, medium fusing about 31 per cent, and low fusing in the neighborhood of 36 per cent. Such differences are not of practical importance, however, and are likely related to differences in technic.

The usual methods of condensation do not appear to be a considerable factor in the control of the firing shrinkage, however. As can be noted from Table 16–3, the differences in firing shrinkage observed with the different methods of condensation, or with no condensation of any kind are negligible from a practical standpoint.[12]

The immediate cause for the shrinkage is the contraction of the body as the powder particles melt and fuse together as indicated in Figure 16–4. There is a surface tension action by the fused mass which acts to draw any unfused portions toward the center and into the voids or interstices. The final structure may be cored (Fig. 16–5) with the crystalline phases, the glass phase forming the matrix.

The effect of the firing temperature on the shrinkage is demonstrated by the data in Table 16–4. Small specimens of a high fusing porcelain were fired to the temperatures indicated in 15 minutes, and held at those temperatures for 30 minutes before cooling. As can be noted, the volume shrinkage did not change to any extent once the high bisque firing temperature (1175° C.) was attained.[13]

**Specific Gravity.** When the specific gravity or the density of a dental porcelain is discussed, a distinction must be made between the *apparent specific gravity* and the *true specific gravity*. The values for the specific gravity given in Tables 16–3 and 16–4 were obtained from fired specimens of dental porcelain. Any blebs or other internal voids in the porcelain would reduce the specific gravity. Consequently, the fig-

*Table 16–3.*    *Influence of Condensation Method on the Physical Properties of Dental Porcelain*

| METHOD OF CONDENSATION | FIRING SHRINKAGE, VOLUMETRIC (PER CENT) | APPARENT SPECIFIC GRAVITY | MODULUS OF RUPTURE | |
|---|---|---|---|---|
| | | | (KG./CM.²) | (LB./IN.²) |
| Vibration | 38.1 | 2.35 | 490 | 7000 |
| Spatulation | 38.4 | 2.34 | 500 | 7200 |
| Brush application | 40.5 | 2.36 | 370 | 5300 |
| No condensation | 41.5 | 2.36 | 340 | 4900 |

*Table 16–4.     Effect of the Firing Temperature on the Physical Properties of a High Fusing Porcelain*

| TEMPERATURE | | APPARENT SPECIFIC | FIRING SHRINKAGE BY VOLUME | MODULUS OF RUPTURE | |
|---|---|---|---|---|---|
| (°C.) | (°F.) | GRAVITY | (PER CENT) | (KG./CM²) | (LB./IN.²) |
| 1040 | 1900 | 1.73 | 16.0 | 130 | 1870 |
| 1100 | 2000 | 2.14 | .... | 335 | 4800 |
| 1150 | 2100 | 2.35 | 27.7 | 560 | 8000 |
| 1175 | 2150 | 2.37 | 35.4 | 670 | 9560 |
| 1200 | 2200 | 2.33 | 24.5 | 590 | 8430 |

ures represent the specific gravity of the specimens and not necessarily that of the porcelain itself.

On the other hand, if the porcelain specimens were ground to a fine powder so that the effect of the flaws was eliminated, the specific gravity of the powder would indicate the true or actual specific gravity of the porcelain. The true specific gravity of the porcelain used to obtain the data in Tables 16–3 and 16–4 was 2.42. Consequently, since none of the values for specific gravity in either table was as high as the true specific gravity, it can be concluded that the fired porcelain is not free from internal voids and similar flaws, regardless of the method of condensation or firing.

It is apparent that the specific gravity of the porcelain is not greatly affected by the method of condensation (Table 16–3).

**Strength.**     The strength of dental porcelain is generally measured in terms of its flexure strength or modulus of rupture.

Like the values for the firing shrinkage, the strengths of the various types of dental porcelain are approximately the same.[10] The strength is, however, greatly affected by the method of condensation and the firing temperature. It is evident from Table 16–3 that the vibration and spatulation methods of condensation are superior to the brush method or to no condensation whatever, so far as their effect on strength is concerned. Such a conclusion implies that the packing of the porcelain particles is definitely important in the production of the strength, even though it apparently exerts little influence on the volume shrinkage so far as the method of condensation is concerned.

The strength increases as the firing temperature increases, but it reaches a maximum at the high bisque firing (Table 16–4). A decrease in strength occurs if the porcelain is fired beyond the high bisque temperature,[13] at which the porcelain normally matures. A separate glaze applied to the porcelain usually results in greater strength than if the body itself is glazed by a glaze firing.[8] As previously noted, however, the glaze material must possess a coefficient of thermal expansion identical with, or slightly less than, that of the body. Otherwise, a stressed condition in both the glaze and the body will occur during cooling, and the strength may be reduced below that of either the glaze or body.

The method of firing also affects the strength. Although the same high fusing porcelain was used to obtain the data in Tables 16–3 and 16–4, the method of firing employed in the latter case resulted in the production of a higher strength. These studies indicate that a firing schedule which employs a lower temperature and a longer time is superior, so far as strength is concerned, to a shorter firing period at a higher temperature. It was also observed that the contours of the sharp edges and angles were better preserved at the lower firing temperatures.[13]

Evidently, sufficient time at the proper temperature should be allotted for the viscous melt to flow completely through the unmelted parts to weld them together. As the temperature rises, the viscosity of the molten phase decreases and it flows more easily, but perhaps too much of the material is fused at the higher temperature, with the result that the strength is decreased. As with other similar materials, an optimum ratio between the matrix and the core should be maintained for the maximum strength.

**Bubbles.** As previously described, the bubbles, or voids, in the photomicrographs on the right in Figure 16–4 are due to the inclusion of air during fusion, although there is evidence that in the case of some of the high fusing porcelains they may appear as a by-product of the vitrification of the feldspar.[3]

As might be expected, the bubbles reduce the translucence and strength of the dental porcelain. As can be noted from Figure 16–4, the bubbles formed with the larger size porcelain powders, although larger

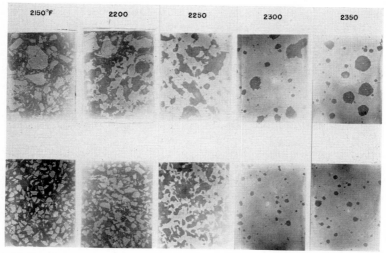

Fig. 16–4. Progressive vitrification of coarse- and fine-grained porcelain. Top row: diameter of powder particles greater than 125 microns. Bottom row: diameter of particles less than 44 microns. Cross sections of porcelain teeth fired on a 15-minute cycle to the temperatures indicated. Orig. mag. ×200. (Vines and Semmelman, *J. D. Res.*, December, 1957.)

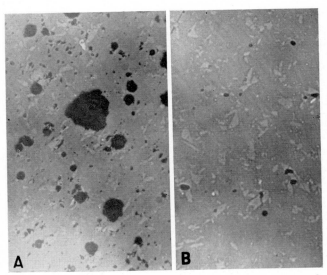

Fig. 16–5.   A. Air-fired porcelain. B. Vacuum-fired porcelain. The cored structure is crystalline quartz. (Vines and Semmelman, *J. D. Res.*, December, 1957.)

in size, are not as numerous as are the smaller bubbles formed with the smaller size particles. Because of the difference in indices of refraction between the porcelain body and the entrapped gas, the porcelain with the larger particle sizes with fewer bubbles is more translucent than that fired with the smaller particle size. When the bubbles are reduced in number or are eliminated, the finer size porcelain produces the more translucent body.[14]

These bubbles seldom appear on the surface of a ceramic tooth or crown, since the entrapped gases can be released because of the decreased pressure in this area. By the same token, gas bubbles are not as numerous in low fusing porcelains as in high fusing ones. The viscosity of the glass phase in low fusing porcelains is sufficiently low to allow the escape of the air during vitrification.[11]

Three methods for the reduction or elimination of such voids have been suggested.[7]

1. The porcelain is fired in a vacuum so that the air will be removed before it is entrapped.

2. A diffusible gas is substituted for the ordinary furnace atmosphere. The air will then be driven out of the interstices during the firing and the diffusible gas will be substituted. During fusion such entrapped gases diffuse outward through the porcelain or are dissolved in the porcelain.

3. If the fused porcelain is cooled under pressure during cooling, the air bubbles can be compressed in size so that their effect will be negligible.

The vacuum firing of porcelain is used for crowns and inlays as well as porcelain teeth. According to one authority,[15] the impact strength of porcelain fired in this manner is increased 48.8 per cent, and its compressive strength is increased 29.2 per cent. Since one of the disadvantages of a dental porcelain crown is its lack of strength, the increased strength obtained by this method of firing is important.

The reduction in number and size of the air bubbles by vacuum firing is shown in Figure 16–5. Since not all of the air can be evacuated from the furnace, a few bubbles are present in Figure 16–5B but they are quite in contrast to the bubbles obtained with the usual air firing method shown in Figure 16–5A.

The diffusible gases which can be introduced into the furnace during vitrification are helium, hydrogen, or steam.[14] As previously noted, when these gases are trapped in the voids they diffuse into the porcelain body. The structure of the final product resembles that of the vacuum fired porcelain shown in Figure 16–5B.

The structure shown in Figure 16–5 was obtained with a high bisque firing. When the porcelain is self-glazed by reheating, the diffusible gas method is somewhat superior to the others, since further gas diffusion takes place and the bubbles virtually disappear. When the vacuum-fired porcelain is reheated, the bubbles remain virtually unchanged.

If the porcelain is fired in air, the bubbles can be reduced by increasing the air pressure to 10 atmospheres, for example; the bubbles will be reduced to a size comparable to that obtained with the other two methods. The pressure is, of course, maintained until the porcelain has cooled to rigidity.

The pressure method offers a disadvantage in that the porcelain cannot be refired or glazed at atmospheric pressure without the bubbles being restored to their original size by the entrapped gas previously compressed.

**Fusion to Metal.** Porcelain can be fired against a gold alloy casting to provide a veneer. For example, instead of constructing a crown entirely of porcelain, a casting can be made with a gold alloy as will be described in Chapter 28, and the porcelain is then fused to the labial or buccal side so as to provide the same esthetic quality of the porcelain jacket crown. Such a veneer crown provides superior strength in comparison to the porcelain jacket crown.

A slight modification is made in the composition of the porcelains for this technic. The crystalline phases are increased in order to increase the thermal expansion more nearly to match that of the metal. Such a modification, however, increases the opacity of the porcelain.[2] As a matter of fact, *opaque porcelains* are available in which the crystalline phase is so predominant that very little translucence is evident. In some instances, however, the porcelain is rendered opaque by pigmentation. The porcelains of this variety which are fused to the average type of gold alloy must be low fusing so that the gold will not be softened or melted during the firing of the porcelain. An opaque porcelain is first fused to the gold and then the tooth contour is reproduced using a translucent porcelain of the proper shade.[16]

The exact nature of the bond between the porcelain and the metal is not known, but it probably is effected by a union of oxides between the two substances. A green line always appears between the porcelain and a gold alloy which contains copper. The green color is probably due to a copper oxide. Unless the green line is present, a bond is not effected.[17] The design of the cast crown and the application of the porcelain is accomplished so that the green line is inconspicuous in the finished restoration.

Whatever is the value of the bond between the porcelain and the gold, it is stronger than is the porcelain itself, when tested in tension.[17] The modulus of rupture of the porcelain employed compares favorably with that of the crown and inlay porcelain previously studied (Table 16–3).

The linear coefficient of expansion of the opaque porcelain is slightly less than that of the gold alloy, and that of the translucent body is less than that of the opaque material.[18] Thus, the porcelains are subjected to compressive stress during cooling as previously discussed.

The gold casting surface to be veneered is carefully cleaned with a bur and chloroform to remove any oil or grease that would interfere with the bonding of the opaque to the metal.[17] An opaque porcelain is now applied, sufficiently thick to mask out the gold. After fusing this at the proper temperature, a somewhat translucent or iridescent porcelain of proper shade is mixed, applied and baked. Although proper technic may provide excellent contour with only one application and bake, porcelain may be added to deficient areas and baked as before.

In order to eliminate the green line at the junction between the porcelain and the gold alloy, a gold alloy or a palladium alloy without copper can be employed. In this case, a higher fusing porcelain can be used since such alloys usually have a higher melting temperature than the gold alloy containing copper. In this case, the union between the porcelain and the metal is not visible.

**Physical Properties.** The modulus of rupture of dental porcelain varies from 260 kilograms per square centimeter (3700 pounds per square inch)[10] to as high as 700 kilograms per square centimeter (10,000 pounds per square inch)[11] depending upon its composition and the technic employed in condensation and firing. As previously noted, the presence of bubbles weakens the porcelain, but they are not necessarily the determining factor in this respect.[11]

The compressive strength of dental porcelain is approximately 3,360 kilograms per square centimeter (48,000 pounds per square inch). Its coefficient of thermal expansion is 6.4 to 7.8 $\times$ 10⁻⁶ per degree Centigrade, a value which is close to that of the human tooth[19] (Table 2–1, page 28).

The solubility of the porcelain after it has been powdered is 0.1 to 0.3 per cent in a 4 per cent solution of acetic acid.[19] The high fusing porcelain tested was slightly less soluble than the low fusing type. Such values are of academic interest only. No case of a dental porcelain *per se* being affected by the mouth fluids has ever been reported.

So far as the optical properties of the porcelains are concerned, strength is sacrificed in order to obtain the translucence and color shade so necessary in order to approach the similar properties of the tooth itself. The strength of porcelain can be increased by the inclusion of kaolin, for example, but the translucence is reduced. The glass present with the minerals provides the proper translucence.

The optical properties of the porcelain are the result of many reflections, transmissions, refractions, and scattering of the incident light ray. It will be recalled from the study of physics that whenever a light ray passes from one medium to another, a reflection and refraction occur. If the transmitting substance is birefringent, a polarization of the light occurs in addition.

As previously indicated, the dental porcelain is heterogeneous in structure. The glass phase is not always continuous, the mineral phase is usually birefringent with a different index of refraction,[3] the air bubbles provide a different transmission medium, and the coloring pigment will produce selective reflection. All of these factors are combined to provide the proper translucence. It is for this reason that the condensation and firing procedures are as important to the color and shade of the ceramic product as is its composition. Underfiring results in too much opacity and overfiring may produce a glass transparency which is equally undesirable. For this reason, the manufacture and practice of dental ceramics often involves more art than it does science.

**General Considerations.** The construction of a porcelain restoration which will function properly requires considerable skill and knowledge on the part of the dentist. The shear strength of the fired porcelain is so low that the slightest imperfection in the preparation of the cavity in the tooth may cause the jacket crown to fracture in service.

On the other hand, the porcelain restoration possesses excellent esthetic qualities, it is completely insoluble in the mouth fluids, and it is dimensionally stable after it has been fired. It is doubtful, however, that a porcelain inlay or crown can be constructed with sufficient accuracy so that the margins are completely sealed, owing to the unavoidable errors caused by the firing shrinkage.

The restoration is usually cemented in position with a luting cement. As noted in Chapter 14, such cements eventually erode in the mouth fluids. A porcelain inlay in time may exhibit a bluish line at its margins; the cement has eroded, and the crevice left becomes stained from the deposit of débris. If the cement erodes from beneath the jacket crown, it may take on a bluish hue. The use of an opaque porcelain base can prevent such a change in color, however.

The porcelain restoration is compatible with the soft tissues, and it is resistant to abrasion. When all factors are considered, dental porcelain is probably the most serviceable of the tooth restorative materials which possess good esthetic qualities.

### Literature

1. Johnson, J. F., Phillips, R. W., and Dykema, R. W.: *Modern Practice in Crown and Bridge Prosthodontics.* Philadelphia, W. B. Saunders Co., 1960, pp. 307–344.
2. Semmelman, J. O.: Personal communication.
3. Hodson, J. T.: *Phase Compositions of Crown and Inlay Porcelains.* J. D. Res., *38:* 483–490 (May-June), 1959.
4. Hodson, J. T.: *A Preliminary Study of Dental Porcelains.* J. South. California D. A., *26:*334–338 (Sept.), 1958.
5. Norton, F. N.: *Elements of Ceramics.* Cambridge, Addison-Wesley Press, 1952.
6. Maier, M., and Heiliman, H.: *Porcelain Furnace Specifications and Construction.* Dent. Items Int., *61:*868–880 (Sept.), 1939.
7. Vines, R. F., and Semmelman, J. O.: *Densification of Dental Porcelain.* J. D. Res., *16:*950–956 (Dec.), 1957.
8. Sartori, J. C.: *Influence of Different Firing Methods upon the Physical Properties of Dental Porcelains.* Northwest. Univ. Bul., *39:*8–12 (Autumn Quarter), 1939.
9. Clark, E. B.: *Manipulation of Dental Porcelain.* J.A.D.A., *22:*33–40 (Jan.), 1935.
10. Skinner, E. W., and Fitzgerald, P. A.: *Physical Properties of Dental Porcelains.* J.A.D.A., *25:*861–865 (June), 1938.
11. Hodson, J. T.: *Some Physical Properties of Three Dental Porcelains.* J. Pros. Den., *9:*325–335 (March-April), 1959.
12. Sayre, L. D.: *Effect of Varying Manipulation upon Certain Physical Properties of Dental Porcelain.* Northwest. Univ. Bul., *38:*3–11 (May), 1938.
13. Moldal, O. H.: *Physical Properties of Opaque Porcelain.* Northwest. Univ. Bul., *39:*7–11 (April), 1939.
14. Vines, R. F., Semmelman, J. O., Lee, P. W., and Fonvielle, F. D.: *Mechanisms Involved in Securing Dense, Vitrified Ceramics from Preshaped Partly Crystalline Bodies.* J. Am. Cer. Soc., *41:*304–309 (Aug.), 1958.
15. Klaffenback, A. O.: *Vacuum Fired Porcelain.* Iowa D. J., *41:*247–249 (Oct.), 1955.
16. Cohn, L. A.: *The Acrylic Faced Cast Gold Crown.* J. Pros. Den., *1:*112–134 (Jan.), 1951.
17. Dykema, R. W., Johnston, J. F., and Cunningham, D. M.: *The Veneered Gold Crown.* D. Clin. North America, November, 1958, pp. 663–669.
18. Smith, D. L., Coleman, R. S., and Wain, R.: *Porcelain Fused to Gold.* J. D. Res., *38:*759 (July-Aug.), 1959. Abstract.
19. Sacchi, H., and Paffenbarger, G. C.: *A Simple Technic for Making Dental Porcelain Jacket Crowns.* J.A.D.A., *65:*366–367 (March), 1957.

CHAPTER 17

# Metals: Solidification

# and Structure

The next few chapters will be devoted to an introduction to the theory of physical metallurgy. Only those principles of value to the dentist will be discussed.

**Metals.** Although metals are very common elements in human experience, it is difficult to give a concise, all-inclusive definition. Ordinarily, a metal is thought of as a solid, but such a conception is narrow indeed. For example, mercury is a metal which is a liquid at normal room temperature. Hydrogen, a very active metal, is a gas at room temperature. If the normal temperature for the human environment were 1000° C. (1800° F.), most of the ordinary solid metals would be liquids and some of them would be gases.

There are some properties of a metal which are characteristic of it in the solid state, however. A clean, metallic surface exhibits a luster which is difficult to duplicate in other types of solid matter. A metal exhibits a certain metallic ring when it is struck, although certain silica compounds can emit a similar sound. Generally all metals are good thermal and electrical conductors, and they possess a relatively high hardness, strength and density. They also generally exhibit a high ductility and malleability in comparison to the nonmetals.

One definition which is possibly unique for a metal can be derived from its chemical properties. *Any chemical element which ionizes positively in solution is a metal.*

There are at least three chemical elements which behave like metals under certain circumstances, but which do not ionize positively in solution. These elements are carbon, silicon and boron. They are fairly good conductors of heat and electricity, but they are almost totally lacking in plasticity at ordinary temperatures. However, they can be alloyed with metals to provide important combinations. They are known as *metalloids*.

**Alloys.**    The use of pure metals for dental purposes is quite limited. Most of the "metals" commonly used are mixtures of two or more pure metals. Although such mixtures can be effected in a number of ways, they are generally produced by a fusion of the metals above their melting points. Such a solid mixture of two or more metals or metalloids is called an *alloy*. The metals most useful to civilization can be alloyed. A list of such metals, together with some of their physical constants, is presented in Table 17–1.

An *amalgam* is a type of alloy which contains mercury as one of its elements. Amalgams of silver, tin and mercury are used quite extensively in dentistry. They will be discussed in Chapters 22 to 24.

The term "metal" is often used all-inclusively, to include alloys as

*Table 17–1.*    *Physical Constants of the Alloy-forming Elements**

| ELEMENT | SYMBOL | ATOMIC WEIGHT | MELTING POINT (°C.) | BOILING POINT (°C.) | DENSITY (GM./CC.) | LINEAR CO-EFFICIENT OF THERMAL EX-PANSION (PER °C. $\times 10^{-4}$) |
|---|---|---|---|---|---|---|
| Aluminum | Al | 26.97 | 660.2 | 2060 | 2.70 | 0.239 |
| Antimony | Sb | 121.76 | 630.5 | 1440 | 6.62 | 0.108 |
| Bismuth | Bi | 209.00 | 271.3 | 1420 | 9.80 | 0.133 |
| Cadmium | Cd | 112.41 | 320.9 | 765 | 8.37 | 0.298 |
| Carbon | C | 12.01 | 3700.0 | 4830 | 2.22 | 0.06 |
| Chromium | Cr | 52.01 | 1890.0 | 2500 | 7.19 | 0.068 |
| Cobalt | Co | 58.94 | 1495.0 | 2900 | 8.90 | 0.123 |
| Copper | Cu | 63.54 | 1083.0 | 2600 | 8.96 | 0.165 |
| Gold | Au | 197.20 | 1063.0 | 2970 | 19.32 | 0.142 |
| Indium | In | 114.8 | 156.4 | 1450 | 7.31 | 0.33 |
| Iridium | Ir | 193.1 | 2454.0 | 5300 | 22.5 | 0.068 |
| Iron | Fe | 55.85 | 1539.0 | 2740 | 7.87 | 0.117 |
| Lead | Pb | 207.21 | 327.4 | 1740 | 11.34 | 0.293 |
| Magnesium | Mg | 24.32 | 650.0 | 1110 | 1.74 | 0.26 |
| Mercury | Hg | 200.61 | −38.87 | 357 | 13.55 | 1.8182† |
| Molybdenum | Mo | 95.95 | 2625.0 | 4800 | 10.2 | 0.049 |
| Nickel | Ni | 58.69 | 1455.0 | 2730 | 8.9 | 0.133 |
| Palladium | Pd | 106.7 | 1554.0 | 4000 | 12.0 | 0.118 |
| Platinum | Pt | 195.23 | 1773.5 | 4410 | 21.45 | 0.089 |
| Rhondium | Rh | 102.91 | 1966.0 | 4500 | 12.44 | 0.083 |
| Silicon | Si | 28.06 | 1430.0 | 2300 | 2.33 | 0.073 |
| Silver | Ag | 107.88 | 960.5 | 2210 | 10.49 | 0.197 |
| Tantalum | Ta | 180.88 | 2996.0 | .... | 16.6 | 0.065 |
| Tin | Sn | 118.70 | 231.9 | 2270 | 7.298 | 0.23 |
| Titanium | Ti | 47.90 | 1820.0 | .... | 4.54 | 0.085 |
| Tungsten | W | 183.92 | 3410.0 | 5930 | 19.3 | 0.043 |
| Zinc | Zn | 65.38 | 419.46 | 906 | 7.133 | 0.397 |

* Compiled from the Metals Handbook (1948).
† Volume coefficient of thermal expansion.

well as pure metals. If the phenomenon discussed does not apply to both alloys and pure metals, a distinction should be made as to which is meant.

**Solidification of Metals.** All metals are crystalline in character, and those metals which are useful in dentistry generally belong to the cubic system. The metals exhibit characteristic melting and freezing temperatures; a pure metal, and often an alloy, can be identified by its melting temperature.

The solidification phenomena which occur during the freezing of a pure metal will be considered first. The solidification of alloys will be discussed in a subsequent chapter.

If a metal is melted, and then allowed to cool, and if its temperature during cooling is plotted as a function of the time, a graph similar to that in Figure 17–1 will result. As can be noted, the temperature decreases regularly from $A$ to $B'$. An increase in temperature then occurs to $B$ when the temperature becomes constant until the time indicated by $C$. After $C$ time has elapsed, the temperature decreases normally to the temperature of the room.

The temperature $T_f$, as indicated by the straight or "plateau" portion

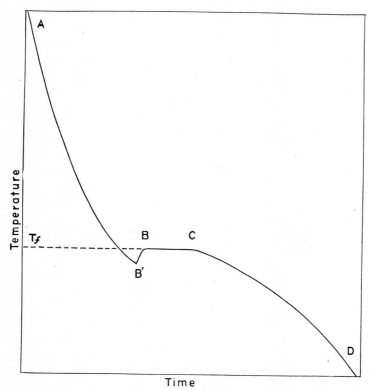

Fig. 17–1. A time-temperature cooling curve for a pure metal showing supercooling.

of the curve at *BC*, is the fusion or melting temperature. As can be noted, during melting or freezing the temperature remains constant. During freezing or solidification, heat is evolved as the metal changes from the liquid to the solid state. This heat is the familiar *latent heat of fusion*, studied in the course in physics. It is defined as the *number of calories of heat liberated from 1 gram of a substance when it changes from the liquid to the solid state.*

The interpretation of the curve in Figure 17–1 is that at all temperatures above $T_f$, as indicated by the plateau *BC*, the metal will be molten, and at all temperatures below this temperature, it will be a solid. The initial cooling to *B'* is called *supercooling*. During the period of supercooling, the crystallization begins. Once the crystals begin to form, the latent heat of fusion causes the temperature to rise to the temperature $T_f$, where it remains until the crystallization is completed.

The fusion temperature of metals and alloys is of considerable interest to the dentist. Many metallic dental structures are *cast*. A *pattern* is prepared which is an exact duplication of the dental appliance or restoration to be cast. A mold is prepared from the pattern, into which a molten alloy can be forced under pressure. When the alloy solidifies, the original pattern has been reproduced in a metallic form, known as a *casting*. The procedures and materials involved will be discussed at some length in subsequent chapters.

**High Temperature Measurement.**     There are a number of ways to measure high temperatures. Specially designed mercury thermometers made of quartz can be used to gauge temperatures as high as 525° C. (977° F.). In such high temperature measurements, an inert gas such as nitrogen is introduced into the thermometer under pressure, in order to increase the boiling point of the mercury.

In dentistry, the thermocouple is usually used, with the circuit shown in Figure 16–3. Usually the temperatures involved are sufficiently low that a platinum, platinum-rhodium thermocouple is not necessary. Commercial alloys of aluminum and chromium are often used. Such thermocouples will withstand temperatures as high as 1100° C. (2000° F.).

After a certain amount of experience, the temperature of a body can be gauged with reasonable accuracy by its color. As a body is heated it begins to emit radiant energy in the form of electromagnetic waves. As the temperature increases, the wave length of the radiation becomes smaller. When the temperature reaches a certain value, the electromagnetic waves are of a length to affect the retina of the eye with a sensation of a faint red color. The shade becomes lighter and the intensity becomes greater as the temperature increases; gradually, with further increase in temperature, the color changes from a red to an orange, then to a yellow, and finally to a white light, such as can be observed in a lamp filament.

### Table 17–2. *Howe's Color Scale*

| | TEMPERATURE | |
|---|---|---|
| COLOR | (°C.) | (°F.) |
| Lowest visible red | 475 | 890 |
| Dull red | 550–625 | 1020–1150 |
| Cherry red | 700 | 1300 |
| Light red | 850 | 1560 |
| Orange | 900 | 1650 |
| Full yellow | 950–1000 | 1740–1830 |
| Light yellow | 1050 | 1920 |
| White | 1150 or above | 2100 or above |

The colors associated with each temperature are given in Table 17–2. The environment of the heated object influences the perception of the color considerably. For example, in a bright sunlight, a red color would actually indicate a temperature close to that of the yellow color, whereas in total darkness, the temperature might be gauged too high because of the contrasting brilliance of the color emitted. Actually, a shadowed environment with a black background is the most reliable for the observation of temperature colors.

**Mechanism of Solidification.** The metals crystallize from the molten state on nuclei of crystallization. Any nuclei not already present at the solidification temperature form during the period of super-cooling.

Once a nucleus of the proper size is present, the crystals begin to grow and to branch outward. In dental structures, the growth may produce treelike formations called *dendrites*. The process, in three dimensions, is not unlike that of the two-dimensional formation of beautiful frost crystals on a window pane in the winter.

A schematic representation of such a crystallization in two dimensions is shown in Figure 17–2. As can be observed, the growth starts from the nuclei of crystallization, and the crystals grow toward each other. When two or more crystals collide in their growth, the growth is stopped. Finally, as diagrammed in Figure 17–2*f*, the entire space is filled with crystals. However, each crystal remains a unit in itself. It is differently oriented from its neighbors. The metal is, therefore, made up of thousands of tiny crystals. Such a metal is said to be *polycrystalline* in nature, and each crystal is known technically as a *grain*.

If any metal is highly polished, and if the polished surface is etched with an appropriate reagent, the grain structure can be made visible in a microscope. The *photomicrograph* of the grain structure of a gold ingot prepared in this manner is shown in Figure 17–3. The resemblance between the grain structure in Figure 17–3 and that of the diagram in Figure 17–2 is evident. The lines in Figure 17–3, somewhat

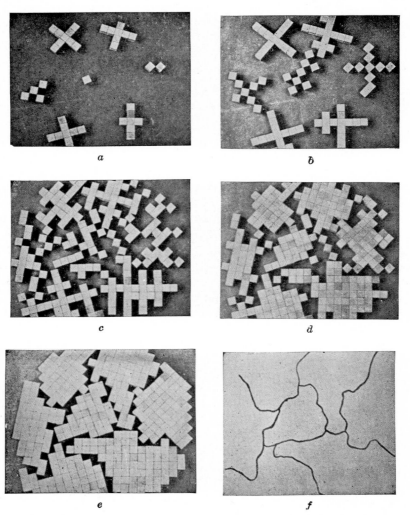

*a*          *b*

*c*          *d*

*e*          *f*

Fig. 17–2.  Stages in the formation of metallic grains during the solidification of a molten metal. (Rosenhain, *Introduction to Physical Metallurgy*, Constable and Co., Ltd.)

indistinct at times, represent the periphery of the grains, or the boundaries where the grains met during their original growth.

**Grain Size.**   The size of the grains will depend upon the number and location of the nuclei at the time of the solidification. If the nuclei are equally spaced with reference to each other, the grains will be approximately equal in size.

The solidification can be pictured as proceeding from the nuclei in all directions at the same time in the form of a sphere, which is constantly increasing in diameter. When these spheres meet, they will be flattened along various surfaces. The tendency for each grain to remain spherical still exists, however, and the grain tends, therefore, to be the same diameter in all dimensions. Such a grain is said to be *equiaxed.* Dental castings generally tend to exhibit an equiaxed grain structure, and such a structure is of considerable dental importance.

**Control of Grain Size.** In general, the smaller the grain size of the metal, the better will be its physical properties. Consequently, the obtaining of a small grain size during casting is an advantage.

The size of the equiaxed grain when a pure metal freezes will depend primarily upon the number of nuclei present at the time of solidification. The more nuclei present, the smaller will be the grain size.

Another factor of equal importance is the rate of crystallization. If the crystals form faster than do the nuclei of crystallization, the grains will be larger than if the reverse condition prevails. Consequently, if the nuclear formation can occur faster than the crystallization, a small grain size can be obtained.

Nuclei of crystallization are formed rapidly during the period of supercooling, and the greater the degree of supercooling, the faster will be the rate of formation of the nuclei. It is an observed fact that the faster the cooling rate from the liquid to the solid state, the greater will be the number of nuclei formed, and, consequently, the smaller will be the grain size. Therefore, a rapid cooling rate immediately before and during solidification aids in the production of small grains.

Conversely, a slow cooling results in large grains. For example, some

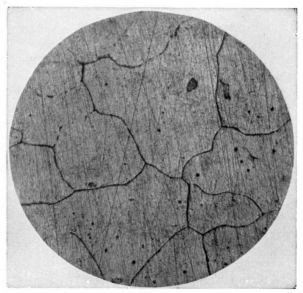

Fig. 17–3. Microstructure of an ingot of gold. × 100. (Courtesy of S. D. Tylman, University of Illinois.)

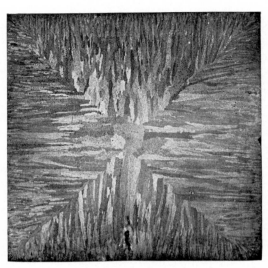

Fig. 17–4.   Metallic grains formed by the solidification of a metal in a square mold. (Williams and Homerberg, *Principles of Metallography*, McGraw-Hill Book Co., Inc.)

metals can be held at their fusion temperatures and caused to crystallize in contact with a crystal or "seed" of the metal. If the crystal is withdrawn at a constant speed as the crystallization proceeds, a rod or bar made up of a single grain can be formed. Such a metal is known as a *single crystal* in contrast to the polycrystalline form usually present.

In a polycrystalline metal, the shape of the grains may be influenced by the shape of the mold in which the metal solidifies. For example, if a metal solidifies in a square mold which is at a temperature considerably below the melting temperature of the metal, the crystal growth may proceed from the edges to the center as shown in Figure 17–4. The grains are called *columnar grains*. If the mold had been cylindrical, the grains would have radiated from the center to the edge. Such grains are called *radial grains*.

**Grain Boundaries.**     As previously noted, the orientation of the space lattice of the various grains is different, although each grain may possess the same space lattice as its neighbor. The probability is very small for two neighboring grains to grow from different nuclei and to meet so that the planes of their space lattices would join in exact continuity. Consequently, there must be a discontinuity of lattice structure at the *grain boundaries,* as this area is designated.

The structural nature of the grain boundaries has been under discussion by metallurgists for many years. That the lattice structure at the boundaries must be different from that of the grains themselves is evidenced by the fact that they are etched more by a reagent than are the grains themselves. Otherwise, the boundaries would not be visible under the microscope as in Figure 17–3.

The grain boundaries are actually under a condition of permanent stress. As indicated in Figure 17–2, crystal growth of the grains is interrupted when they meet at the grain boundaries. In the similar case described for the gypsum products (page 41), the entire mass expanded due to the outward thrust of the crystals to produce a setting expansion. No expansion necessarily occurs in this case, and the stresses incurred by the outward thrust of the crystals remain to a great extent. Thus a condition of a permanent stress exists.

As described in Chapter 2, a condition of stress is accompanied by a strain or, in other words, a localized distortion of the space lattice. The lattice structure in the grain boundaries, therefore, can be imagined as a gradual change in regularity from one grain to the other. The greatest irregularity (or condition of stress and strain), approaching that of random arrangement, will occur approximately midway between the grains themselves. One can imagine the irregularity to be caused either by the resultant atomic forces between the two grains as the orientation of the crystalline planes is changed from one grain to the other, or it might be the result of atomic displacement occasioned by the collision of the two grains during growth. Either conception is adequate.

The irregular lattice structure of the grain boundaries results in certain properties which are different from those of the grains. As already mentioned, the boundaries are less resistant to chemical attack than the grains. Owing to the lack of regularity in arrangement, they tend to be brittle at room temperature. However, as the metal is heated to a higher temperature, the grain boundaries appear to soften, much in the same manner as an amorphous thermoplast such as glass. Such a phenomenon is also related to the lack of regularity in the lattice formation in this region. These properties of the grain boundaries will be dealt with further in the next chapter.

Another condition which often accentuates the brittleness and susceptibility to chemical attack at the grain boundaries is the fact that impurities in the metal may be expelled from the grain to the grain boundaries during solidification. Such a condition may often be responsible for a serious corrosion of the metal or alloy during its use.

# CHAPTER 18

# Wrought Metal: Strain Hardening, Recrystallization and Grain Growth

In the preceding chapter, the discussion was limited to cast metal. Most of the dental structures placed in the mouth are castings. However, wires are used by the orthodontist and are sometimes used for clasps in connection with partial dentures. Wires are not castings. Rather, wires are made from castings by drawing a cast metal through a die. Many of the accessory dental materials and tools have been rolled to form plate metal, or forged or ground to form knives, burs and many other dental instruments.

Whenever a casting is worked in any manner to form any type of structure of a different type or shape, it is no longer a cast metal, but rather it becomes a *wrought metal*, and it will exhibit certain metallurgical phenomena not generally associated with a cast structure. The differences are so marked that the dentist should always analyze any situation presented in terms of whether he is concerned with cast metal or wrought metal before he proceeds with any dental operation or procedure.

Although, as stated, most dental appliances are of cast metal, the proper treatment of the many wrought metal tools employed in the preparation of the mouth structures for the reception of the cast dental appliance is of equal importance to the success of the operation as is the fabrication of the appliance itself. Actually, if one considers the many useful metallic articles that he encounters in everyday life, most of them are wrought metal and are not castings, although all wrought metal structures originated from cast metal.

**Deformation of Metals.** In Chapter 2 (page 27), it was pointed out that stresses and strains were manifested in the space lattice by distortions and irregularities. If these distortions disappeared when the load was removed, the structure was described as having been deformed under elastic deformation. If the distortions did not disappear, the structure suffered permanent deformation, with the stresses and strains becoming inherent in the structure. The important observation to be noted is that in any type of deformation, or whenever stresses or strains are present, an irregularity of the space lattice exists.

In permanent deformation, it is generally thought that the planes of the space lattice slip over one another, without change in either atomic spacing or type of space lattice. A diagram of such a slip is shown in Figure 18–1. The small circles indicate the position of the atoms before the slip occurred. The black dots indicate their position after slip.

In the diagram, the upper four rows of atoms have slipped three atomic spacings, but they could as well have slipped one or a thousand atomic spacings. The slip generally occurs along a principal plane, as shown. It can occur in any principal plane in three dimensions, theoretically any number of times until fracture occurs. Each slip takes place through one or more integral atomic spacings. A twisting of the

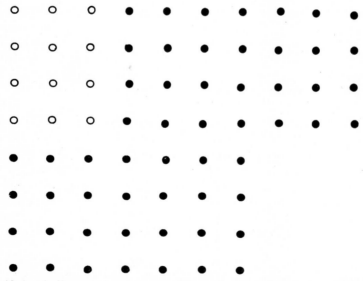

Fig. 18–1. A diagram showing a possible mechanism of translational slip in two dimensions. The circles show the positions of the atoms before slip occurred. The relation of the atoms after slip is indicated by the black dots.

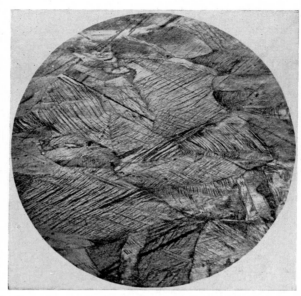

Fig. 18–2.   A photomicrograph of gold, showing slip bands. ×100. (Courtesy of S. D. Tylman, University of Illinois.)

lattice may also take place to produce a *twinning* of the crystal, in which one part of the crystal becomes a mirror image of the other part. However, the amount of twinning which occurs is normally much less than the movement by translation.

The result of slip can be seen in the grains pictured in the photomicrograph shown in Figure 18–2. The "lines" across the grains are *slip bands*. They are steps on the surface of the polished metal which have resulted from slip which caused certain blocks or fragments of the grain to be elevated and others to be depressed. The slip planes themselves are, of course, much too small to be visible under a microscope.

By means of slip, a structure can be deformed permanently with a resulting change in shape. When this change in shape is accomplished at normal temperatures, the process is known as *cold work.* Any structure which is bent, twisted, rolled, drawn or similarly cold worked becomes a wrought metal.

**Slip Interference.**     The stresses and strains during slip can be recognized as shear. The deformation can be the result of any type of loading, but the resultant stress in the metal during slip will be a shear stress.

So far as the diagrammatic representation in Figure 18–1 is concerned, after the slip has occurred, a regular space lattice remains, and no stress is evident after the loading has ceased. Unfortunately, the situation is not so simple as this, particularly in the case of the polycrystalline metal. In a polycrystalline metal, if slip occurs in a single grain, all of the grains will need to slip in equal amount, or else a lattice distortion must occur at some position.

It was shown in the previous chapter that the atoms in the grain boundaries tend to form discontinuities in the space lattice. The grain boundary should not be conceived as a discontinuity of structure beginning abruptly, however. The irregularity of the lattice in these regions is presumably caused by the difference in orientation in the space lattice of adjacent grains. Not only will the atoms in the grain boundaries tend to be irregularly spaced, but they in turn will produce certain displacements in the space lattice of the grain proper, at the edges of the grain.

In other words, as the boundary of the grain is approached, the structure of the lattice becomes irregular. A careful study of Figure 18–1 will indicate that for easy slip, the space lattice should be regular. If the space lattice is irregular, the slip becomes more difficult because of the internal friction developed in the irregularity. The principle is much the same as the difference in the ease with which two glass plates slide over one another in contrast to the friction developed with the same movement when two pieces of coarse sandpaper are substituted for the glass.

Owing, therefore, to the irregularities of the space lattice near and in the grain boundaries, slip between grains becomes difficult. It can be assumed that the slip on the interior of the grain occurs as shown in Figure 18–1, but as it approaches the grain boundary, the slip is interrupted. Such a condition is known as *slip interference.*

**Strain Hardening.** If the loading of the metal is continued, the amount of slip must increase, and, because of slip interference, a distortion of the space lattice occurs. For example, the slip in a given plane may not be completed, and the atoms may be out of line with the rest of the atoms in the lattice. Slip interference will result in this area. As the slip continues, the grains may be fractured along certain planes; they may break off, and fragments may be wedged in the grain boundaries, or in disoriented areas in the grain itself. The system finally becomes so disrupted that no further slip can occur, and the structure fractures by a complete separation of the atoms across an entire area.

Such a situation has been encountered by everyone. For example, one way to "cut" a wire is to bend it back and forth rapidly between the fingers. When all the slip possible has occurred, the wire fractures. When a nail is flattened with a hammer, the first few blows are quite effective. However, as the blows are continued, it is noted that they are not so effective, until finally no further deformation occurs. Instead, the metal fractures. Furthermore, one senses that the metal has become stiffer and harder during the deformation. Such a hardening of the structure under cold work is known as *strain hardening.*

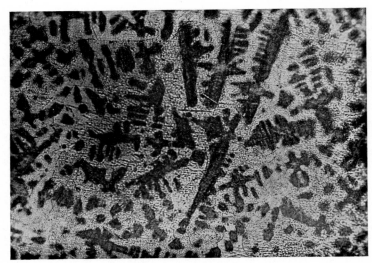

Fig. 18–3.   Grain structure of a gold alloy casting to be drawn into a wire. (Courtesy of R. L. Coleman, J. M. Ney Co.)

The surface hardness, strength and proportional limit of the metal are increased with strain hardening, whereas the ductility and resistance to corrosion are decreased. Sometimes the color of the metal may be changed by strain hardening. For example, certain alloys of gold, copper and silver which contain sufficient silver to render them white under conditions approaching equilibrium, may first become a pale yellow upon strain hardening, with a gradual deepening in the color to a greenish-yellow as the deformation continues.[1]

The change in physical properties of a metal effected by strain hardening is often a practical method in dentistry for the control of such properties. For example, it will be shown in the next chapter that a strain hardening of a gold foil restoration is necessary to provide its proper strength and hardness.

The resultant deformation of the grain is usually in the direction of the working. For example, a photomicrograph of a gold alloy casting is shown in Figure 18–3. When this casting is drawn through dies to fabricate a wire, the grains become elongated, as shown in Figure 18–4. The grain structure in Figure 18–4 is characteristic of this type of wire, and any change in its form would definitely affect the physical properties of the wire.

An illustration of the effect on the grain structure of the flattening of a metal between rollers is shown in the first row of photomicrographs at the top of Figure 18–5. The rolling took place in a direction perpendicular to the photomicrographs, and it can be observed that the less the thickness of the specimen, as designated above each photomicrograph, the flatter or thinner the grains appear to be. If the specimens were observed in a plane 90 degrees to that shown (*i.e.*, parallel to the direction of rolling), the area of the grains would, of course, appear to be greater. Although brass was used, the same effect would be present with wrought gold alloys.

**Annealing.** There are conditions of cold working, such as the contouring of a clasp wire to the surface of a tooth, for example, where the necessary cold work may be considerable. In such a case, the question arises as to how the operation can be continued without the occurrence of a fracture. In other words, once a structure has been cold worked, how can the inherent stresses be relieved?

Metals exhibit a property of atomic diffusion in the solid state. In the case of metals used in dentistry, the ability of the atoms to diffuse through the space lattice at room temperature is negligible, but if the temperature is raised sufficiently, a diffusion can take place quite readily owing to the increased internal energy.

After a strain hardening has taken place, the metal is obviously not in equilibrium, and, therefore, if a diffusion of the atoms is allowed to occur, the tendency is for the atoms to reform into a regular space lattice. The heating of a metal after strain hardening to allow atomic diffusion is known as *annealing*. After an annealing, the properties which were increased by strain hardening are decreased, and the properties that were decreased in strain hardening are increased by the anneal. The important consideration is that the regular space lattice

Fig. 18–4. Grain structure of a wire drawn from the cast ingot shown in Figure 18–3. ×500. (Courtesy of R. L. Coleman, J. M. Ney Co.)

ORIGINAL
ANNEALED METAL
THICKNESS                    COLD ROLLED TO THICKNESS
  0.110″          0.100″          0.090″          0.080″          0.070″          0.060″
NO. 9 B. & S. GA.  NO. 10 B. & S. GA.  NO. 11 B. & S. GA.  NO. 12 B. & S. GA.  NO. 13 B. & S. GA.  NO. 14 B. & S. GA.

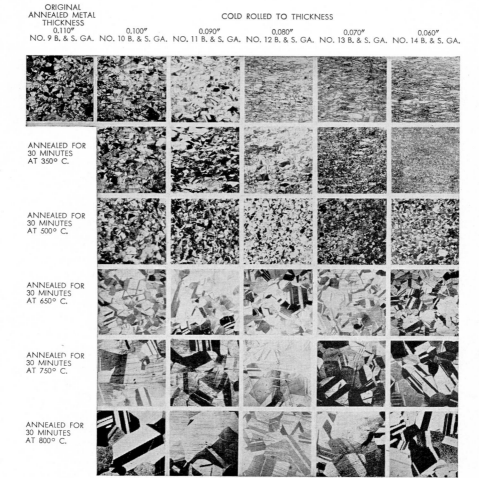

ANNEALED FOR
30 MINUTES
AT 350° C.

ANNEALED FOR
30 MINUTES
AT 500° C.

ANNEALED FOR
30 MINUTES
AT 650° C.

ANNEALED FOR
30 MINUTES
AT 750° C.

ANNEALED FOR
30 MINUTES
AT 800° C.

Fig. 18–5.   Grain size of brass (copper 66 per cent, zinc 34 per cent) after cold working and annealing. ×40. (Prepared by L. H. DeWald.)

has been reformed, the ductility has been restored, and the cold work can proceed.

The rearrangement by diffusion is a special type of crystallization. Nuclei form in the area with the greatest amount of strain, such as the slip planes, the grain boundaries, and similar irregular lattice points. As the annealing proceeds, the new crystals grow. The annealing can be stopped at any stage by cooling the structure. If the cooling is accomplished by plunging the heated structure into water or oil, the process is called *quenching.*

**Recrystallization.**     If the annealing is allowed to proceed far enough, new equiaxed grains can be seen under the microscope. Such an annealing process is called *recrystallization.* Once the structure has been recrystallized, it generally possesses its maximum ductility. The temperature at which the recrystallization occurs is known as the *recrystallization temperature.*

There are several factors which affect the recrystallization. Time is important, in that the higher the temperature, the less time is required for the recrystallization. However, the lower the temperature employed for a given time, the smaller the recrystallized grains will be. Also, the smaller the grains before recrystallization, the lower will be the recrystallization temperature. The composition of an alloy is also a factor; this factor will be discussed in a subsequent chapter.

In regard to the temperature, there is a minimum temperature below which recrystallization will not take place regardless of other factors. Such a temperature is characteristic of the particular metal or alloy.

Probably the greatest single factor in recrystallization is the amount of strain hardening present prior to annealing. The greater the amount of previous strain hardening, the lower the recrystallization temperature will be.

Many of these factors are illustrated in the photomicrographs in Figure 18–5.

As previously noted, the top row of photomicrographs in Figure 18–5 represent the grain structure of various pieces of brass which have been rolled into progressively thinner pieces. As can be noted, the thickness of each piece has been reduced by 0.01 inch (0.25 millimeter) by each successive rolling. As a result, the strain hardening of each specimen increases progressively as the specimen is rolled thinner.

After the rolled specimens were annealed at 350° C. (660° F.) for 30 minutes, the grain structure obtained for each rolling is shown in the second row of photomicrographs. Only when the thickness was reduced to 0.070 inch (1.8 millimeters) is there any evidence of recrystallization. Apparently, a certain amount of strain hardening must originally be present if a recrystallization is to be effected. Careful observation indicates, however, that the recrystallization is not complete. Only when the thickness was reduced another 0.01 inch (0.25 millimeter) was a condition of complete recrystallization attained, as indicated by the grain structure of the specimen at the extreme right of the second row. Also, the extremely fine grain structure of this specimen should be noted.

When the annealing temperature was raised to 500° C. (930° F.) for thirty minutes, the first three specimens, which were not previously recrystallized at the lower temperatures, were recrystallized, but the recrystallized grains are larger than those of the recrystallized specimens in the second row. Evidently, the previous statement is true that the higher the recrystallization temperature, the greater is the size of the recrystallized grain.

A few metals such as tin, zinc and lead will not strain harden readily because of the fact that their recrystallization temperatures are close to or below normal room temperature. However, if they are worked at lower temperatures, they exhibit a strain hardening similar to that of any other metal.

**Grain Growth.** If the annealing at a high temperature is prolonged, the grains get larger as shown in Figure 18–5, rows four, five and six. This phenomenon is called *grain growth*. It occurs as a type of boundary migration by diffusion, where one grain absorbs others.

The cause of grain growth may be related to the surface energy of the grains, which always tends to become a minimum. Consequently, any decrease in the number of grains will result in a decrease in surface energy. The ultimate growth would be the formation of one huge grain, or a single crystal, but grain growth does not progress to this extent under practical conditions.

The ultimate size of the grains after grain growth will be larger, the greater the amount of strain hardening originally present. It is possible that grain growth may not accompany an over-annealing at a low temperature, even though a recrystallization occurs, if the metal has not been sufficiently worked. Like recrystallization, however, grain growth is dependent on time as well as temperature, and it may be that a lack of grain growth at low annealing temperatures is the result of the impractically long period that may be required for the proper atomic diffusion.

Grain growth results in a general weakening of the structure. Since there are fewer grains, there is less chance for slip, and as a result the strength, hardness and ductility are all reduced. Once grain growth occurs, the only remedy is to re-work-harden the structure, and then to recrystallize it to form small equiaxed grains.

**Practical Application.** Under no circumstances should a dental wrought structure be subjected to sufficient heating so that grain growth occurs. During the cold working of a plate metal, it may be necessary to recrystallize it occasionally to prevent a fracture. Should a grain growth be inadvertently introduced, the metal can be strain hardened and recrystallized.

The dentist, particularly the orthodontist, uses wires much more than plate metal. If the wire exhibits an elongated or a *banded* grain structure, similar to that shown in Figure 18–4, it may exhibit mechanical properties superior to that of an equiaxed grain structure. Consequently, even the recrystallization of a wire during an annealing or heating is to be avoided. Also, once a recrystallization is effected, it is sometimes difficult to prevent grain growth at the same time, since the degree of strain hardening of the metal cannot be controlled exactly under the varying conditions of dental manipulation.

The wire is, therefore, partially annealed only, to relieve a certain amount of the strain hardening without a recrystallization.

**Hot Work.** The dentist does not ordinarily work any metal at a high temperature, but a limited discussion of hot work or *forging* may be valuable, since further information of interest regarding grain structure can be presented.

Hot work, as distinguished from cold work, may be defined as the mechanical working of a structure at or above its recrystallization temperature. Generally, under such conditions, the grains may be somewhat refined, but the room-temperature mechanical properties remain unchanged, provided that the working temperature is not sufficient to cause grain growth. When it is properly done, hot working may produce the same effect as cold working followed by a recrystallization.

It is interesting to note, in this connection, that fractures which occur at a high temperature are different in nature from those which occur below the recrystallization temperature. As previously noted, a strain hardening may result in slip until no further movement of the planes can occur. Further loading results in a fracture, caused by the separation of the atoms in the grain. It should be noted that the fracture takes place across the grain, and never along the grain boundaries.

On the other hand, when fracture occurs at a high temperature, it usually takes place along the grain boundaries and not through the grains themselves. It is thought that the lack of regularity in the atomic spacings in the grain boundaries results in a plasticity or a softening at a high temperature. A similar effect occurs in amorphous materials, owing to a lack of regularity in their molecular spacing.

At lower temperatures, then, the grain boundaries can be considered to be stronger than the grains, but at higher temperatures, the grains are the stronger. The temperature at which the strength of the grains is equal to that of the boundaries is called the *equicohesive temperature*.

## Literature

1. Boas, W.: *An Introduction to the Physics of Metals and Alloys.* New York, John Wiley & Sons, Inc., 1947, p. 126.

## CHAPTER 19

# Gold Foil and Its Manipulation

Very few metals are used in the pure condition for dental restorative purposes, gold being the outstanding exception. Because of its extreme softness, pure gold is not indicated for use in the mouth except in the form of *gold foil*. Since gold is the most malleable of metals, it may be rolled into extremely thin sheets, and then beaten until it is so thin that it will transmit light. Gold foil appears yellow by reflected light, but it is green by transmitted light.

Pure gold is the most noble of metals; it neither tarnishes nor corrodes in the mouth. When used in the form of foil, it is an ideal dental restorative material from the standpoint of permanently preserving tooth structure. Its chief disadvantages are its color, high thermal conductivity, and difficulty of manipulation.

If the surface of the foil is free from adsorbed gases and other impurities, it can be welded at room temperature, that is, complete cohesion can be established between the space lattices of two different pieces of foil, a phenomenon which is usually exhibited by metals and alloys only at higher temperatures. This property of the foil is taken advantage of in the construction of a gold foil restoration by driving pieces of foil together in the prepared cavity, thus gradually building up a coherent mass by welding. The gold foil condenser is a rodlike instrument approximately 6 inches long, with a small flat surface at one end, which is called the face or working point. The point is placed on the foil to be condensed, and the other end of the instrument is struck with a small mallet.

The gold foil is generally supplied in sheets 4 inches square and of varying thicknesses. If the sheet weighs 4 grains, it is called "No. 4"; if it weighs 6 grains, it is called "No. 6"; etc. The sheets may be made into pellets by cutting them into eighths, sixteenths, sixty-fourths, etc., and then by compressing the sections into cubes. The foil also may be made into ropes, or corrugated, by placing it between sheets of paper, which are ignited in a closed container. This latter form of gold foil is of historical interest since it was an outcome of the great Chicago fire of 1871. A dental depot had some books of gold foil in a safe. After the fire, the safe was opened, and it was found that the paper had charred, but the gold leaf itself was unharmed, except that it had become corrugated because of the shriveling of the paper while oxidizing in the air-tight safe. After the carbon was removed, it was found that the gold exhibited a superior welding property.

A form of pure gold known as *mat gold* is often used in certain types of prepared cavities. The base of the cavity may be covered with mat gold and then overlaid with cohesive foil.[1] The mat gold is not actually a foil in the sense that it is a thin sheet formed by rolling and beating. Rather it is composed of very thin flake-like crystals of gold formed by electrodeposition.

A sheet of pure platinum may be sandwiched between two sheets of pure gold and so-called *platinum foil* can be formed. The platinum content of the foil may vary from 10 to 40 per cent.

**Cohesive and Noncohesive Gold Foil.**   Cohesive gold foil, as previously noted, will cohere or weld at room temperature under pressure because of its clean surface free from impurities. Most metals attract gases to their surfaces, particularly oxygen, and the gas film prevents coherence of the surface atoms. Only when the metals are heated sufficiently to drive off the adhering gas molecules will the surface cohere or weld.

There are gases which will contaminate the surface of the gold foil to the extent that the foil must be heated to restore its welding property. For example, ammonia vapor and chlorine gas are of this type.[2] Gas containing sulfur and phosphorus groups is said to render the foil permanently noncohesive.[2]

Noncohesive gold foil is sometimes used as a base for cohesive foil as described for mat gold. It is driven into the prepared cavity in rolls so that retention is attained solely by wedging the rolls between the cavity walls. It is then veneered with cohesive foil.

**Annealing of Gold Foil.**   So far as is known, the gold foil is no longer rendered noncohesive by the manufacturer. It is supposedly received by the dentist in so-called "annealed" condition.

Nevertheless, it is customary to anneal the rope of foil before it is condensed into the tooth. The annealing of the foil as a precautionary measure is probably good practice. Even though the foil as received from the manufacturer may be pure, annealing will drive off any contaminating gases inadvertently acquired during storage. Apropos of such a possibility of contamination, it is important that the foil be

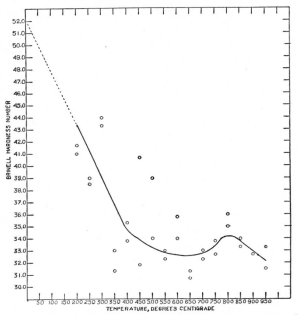

Fig. 19–1.    Relation between the Brinell hardness number of condensed gold foil and the annealing temperature of the foil before condensation.

stored in a stoppered bottle and exposed to the air as little as possible before use.

Aside from the surface purification of the foil, the total result obtained by annealing is not entirely known. On the basis of previous discussions concerning the annealing of polycrystalline wrought metals, the temperature and time of annealing gold foil should be an important factor. Although the gold is frequently annealed during the forming of the foil, it is reasonable to assume that the grain structure of the foil should be subject to recrystallization and grain growth at comparatively low temperatures because of the intense strain hardening the metal has undergone.

In an attempt to determine the proper annealing temperature of gold foil, pieces of cohesive gold foil were condensed after annealing at various temperatures for a uniform time.[3] The Brinell hardness numbers of the foils so condensed are shown in Figure 19–1 as a function of the annealing temperature. As can be noted, the lower the annealing temperature, the harder was the condensed foil. When even lower annealing temperatures were employed than shown in Figure 19–1, the hardness of the condensed foil continued to increase as the annealing temperature decreased. With the particular foil employed, the greatest hardness was found when the foil was condensed at room temperature with no temperature annealing whatever.[4] It is not known whether such a finding is typical for all of the dental gold foils commercially available, since annealing may be necessary in some instances to remove surface contamination.

It is not possible to evaluate the clinical importance of these findings without further research. However, these observations indicate strongly that the annealing temperature and time may be important to the grain structure and physical properties of the gold foil restoration.

In practice, the ropes of foil are cut into convenient lengths and placed on a mica annealing tray. Care should be taken to handle the pieces only with stainless steel tweezers and similar instruments. The foil should never be touched with the hands because of the danger of contamination.

Electrical heat is probably best for annealing. Not only is the heat more uniform and easier to control than gas heat, but also there is less chance of contamination by possible contact with illuminating gas.

If gas heat is used, a hood may be placed over the mica tray as a precautionary measure for the prevention of contamination.

It is doubtful whether the foil should ever be annealed directly in the gas flame under any circumstances. Not only is the danger of contamination increased, but also a uniform annealing is virtually impossible.

**Condensation of Cohesive Gold Foil.**    Originally, each piece of foil was malleted into place with a condenser, the point of which was placed against the foil, and the other end struck sharply with a small mallet. A complete account of the insertion of a gold foil restoration is not within the scope of the present discussion.

In brief, starting points are cut in the prepared cavity into which the first pieces of foil are wedged. Subsequent pieces of foil are welded to the pieces already present and condensed in such a manner that the prepared cavity is gradually filled.

The operation with the hand condenser and mallet is tedious for both dentist and patient. Each piece of foil is "stepped" by placing the condenser point against the piece of foil in successive adjacent positions as it is struck with the mallet.

The modern gold foil condensers consist of points activated by comparatively light blows repeated with a frequency of 360 to 3600 per minute.[1] In other words, a vibratory motion is employed. The vibrations are produced either pneumatically or electrically. With these devices, it is not necessary to raise the condenser point each time during the stepping procedure. The condensation is quite rapid with much greater comfort for the patient and less danger from traumatic injury than with the earlier methods.

Whatever the condensation method employed, each piece of foil should be condensed over its entire length so that no voids will be bridged. Photomicrographs of a condensed gold foil are shown in

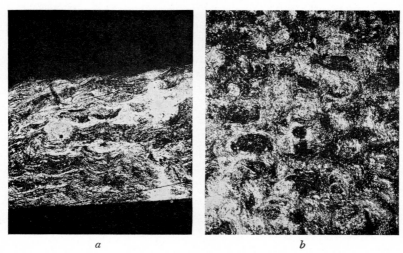

*a*    *b*

Fig. 19–2.  Photomicrographs of condensed gold foil. *a*. Section parallel to the direction of condensation. *b*. Section perpendicular to the direction of condensation. ×50.

Figure 19–2, *a*, parallel to the direction of the condensing force and *b*, perpendicular to the condensing force. The laminated structure shown in Figure 19–2*a* is the result of the welding procedure, one piece of foil being welded to the one below and so on.

**Voids.**    Voids caused by insufficient condensation are evident in the photomicrographs, particularly in Figure 19–2*a*. Apparently such voids are unavoidable, but they should be kept to a minimum, a factor which depends upon the skill of the operator. In a poor foil restoration, the voids may be present to the extent that a recurrence of caries can occur due to leakage.[5] With a properly condensed gold foil restoration, however, any leakage is minimal.[6]

The number of voids in a condensed gold foil restoration can be estimated by the specific gravity of the condensed foil. It can be assumed that the specific gravity of a gold foil restoration should be approximately the same as that for pure gold (19.32). A survey[7] of the specific gravity of a number of restorations condensed by gold foil operators indicated that the values varied from 17 to 19.

Specific gravities of the specimens used for the hardness tests in Figure 19–1 were also obtained.[3] It was found that the same type of curve was obtained as in Figure 19–1 when the specific gravity values were plotted as a function of the annealing temperature. Consequently, it is usually assumed that the hardness number is also a measure of the soundness of the condensed foil.

**Energy Considerations.**    The direction of the force applied during condensation should always be perpendicular to the surface of the foil that is being welded. Otherwise, one of the stress components will be a shear, and the foil will be more likely to be dislodged than to be welded.

Whatever the method of the condensation, the applied force is an impact or blow and, therefore, its magnitude cannot be measured directly, but some interesting conclusions can be reached if the energy involved is considered.

For example, the energy of the blow with a mallet on a hand condenser can be given by the familiar equation:

$$\text{Kinetic Energy} = \tfrac{1}{2}\, mv^2 \tag{1}$$

where m = mass of the mallet.

     v = velocity of the mallet at the instant of impact.

Since the mass of the mallet and its velocity at impact are both under the control of the operator, he can control the energy of the blow.

Unfortunately, there is a limit to the amount of energy which the operator can exert on the delicate dental structures. Whatever the magnitude of the blow, the energy of the impact is dissipated in some manner by the foil and the dental structures. Certainly, the energy transmitted to the dental structures through the foil should be absorbed by these structures without permanent deformation. It will be recalled that the ability of a structure to resist impact depends upon a design factor, its volume and its modulus of resilience.*

In other words, the energy of the blow is limited according to the ability of the oral structures to resist the impact. A large tooth can withstand a greater impact force than a small one because of its greater volume. A heavy bone structure of the face will be conducive to a greater impact resistance than a small, light structure, and so on.

Although the energy considerations in connection with the mouth structures involved are important, they are not the prime consideration. Any energy dissipated by the surrounding structures represents energy lost from the prime purpose, namely, the condensation of the gold foil. Energy absorbed by the foil results in the welding process plus the deformation of the space lattice of the foil. Both of these considerations are important to the success of the gold foil restoration. The welding, of course, provides cohesion and density, and the deformation of the foil provides a surface hardness and strength by virtue of the strain hardening involved.

The Brinell hardness number of pure gold is in the neighborhood of 27, whereas the hardness number of a condensed gold foil may be as high as 70 or 80. By virtue of the strain hardening during condensation, the hardness and strength of a gold foil restoration may be as high as that of a medium hard inlay gold alloy, for example.

In the case of the modern automatic gold foil condensers, the total energy applied to the foil per unit of time will be much greater than that transmitted by the single blow method. Furthermore, the magnitude of the impact force can be reduced with the automatic condenser.

* Formula (4), page 18.

For example, as can be noted from equation (1) above, the kinetic energy at impact can be reduced either by a reduction of the mass or of the velocity. If this energy is reduced but applied more frequently, the end result should be the same as that obtained with a single blow of greater energy. This fact is taken advantage of in the automatic condensation equipment, with the result that the operation is faster, more efficient and completed with much less discomfort to the patient.

**Size of the Condenser Point.** The diameter of the condenser point is an important factor in determining the effectiveness of the welding. Assuming the condenser point to be circular, its surface area will be directly proportional to the square of its diameter. The energy distribution of the impact onto the foil will depend upon the area of the condenser point. For example, a given amount of energy will be distributed over four times as much area of foil with a condenser point 2 millimeters in diameter than with a similar point 1 millimeter in diameter. In other words, the *concentration* of the energy, and consequently the strain hardening of the foil, should be four times as great with the 1-millimeter condenser as with the larger condenser.

It follows, therefore, that small condenser points are indicated for use with gold foil in order to provide effective energy distribution without increasing the impact energy to an extent that the oral structures will be damaged. The surface area of the points in use may vary between equivalent circular areas with diameters 0.5 to 1 millimeter. It should be understood that the points can be of any contour desired provided their surface areas are within the limits specified.

The lower limit for the point diameter is established on the basis of a possible penetration of the foil by the point. For example, a piece of steel will likely not be indented by a piece of ⅛-inch drill rod if one attempts to drive it into the steel. However, if the end of the drill rod is pointed to form a center punch, the surface of the steel can easily be indented with the sharp point. In the same manner, the condenser point should not be so small in area that it will penetrate and chop the foil during condensation.

**Physical Properties of Condensed Foils.** Extensive tests have been made on the mechanical properties of gold foil and gold-platinum foil.[8] The results of these tests are summarized in Tables 19–1 and 19–2.

As can be noted in Table 19–1, the tensile strength of the condensed foil was determined as a measure of the cohesion obtained during condensation. It was later demonstrated from the data that the Brinell hardness number was directly proportional to the tensile strength of the condensed foil. In fact, the tensile strength of the foil can be computed in pounds per square inch within the limits of experimental error by multiplying the Brinell hardness number by 550.

As can be noted from Table 19–1, the cohesion is less with the larger

*Table 19–1.* *Influence of the Method of Condensation and Composition of Gold Foil on the Surface Hardness and Tensile Strength\**

| METHOD AND COMPOSITION † | B.H.N. | TENSILE STRENGTH (KG./CM.²) | (LB./IN.²) |
|---|---|---|---|
| Hand malleted (average) | 54 | 2520 | 36,000 |
| Hand malleted (nib area 0.36 mm.²) | .. | 2790 | 38,500 |
| Hand malleted (nib area 1 mm.²) | .. | 2020 | 28,800 |
| Pneumatic condenser | 64 | 2940 | 42,000 |
| Condensed in resin teeth | 59 | 2170 | 31,000 |
| Condensed in steel die | 65 | 3150 | 45,000 |
| Condensed with ¼-gr. pellets (Au-Pt) | .. | 3710 | 53,000 |
| Condensed with ½-gr. pellets (Au-Pt) | .. | 2100 | 30,000 |
| Gold 85–90%, platinum 10–15% | 78 | 3150 | 45,000 |
| Gold 60–70%, platinum 30–40% | 96 | 3500 | 50,000 |

\* Rule, *J.A.D.A.*, April, 1937.

† Unless otherwise stated, the composition is 100 per cent gold.

*Table 19–2.* *Effect of Thickness of Gold-Platinum Foil on Hardness\**

| NO. OF FOIL | PLATINUM (%) | B.H.N. |
|---|---|---|
| 4 | 30 | 98 |
| 8 | 30 | 88 |
| 8 | 16 | 74 |
| 12 | 30 | 72 |
| 40 | 30 | 70 |

\* Rule, *J.A.D.A.*, April, 1937.

condenser, as predicted in a previous section. Also as might be expected from resilience considerations, both the Brinell hardness and the strength are greater when the foil is condensed in a steel die than in a plastic tooth. The same properties of the foil condensed with ½-grain pellets are lower in value than those of the specimens condensed with ¼-grain pellets, since the smaller pellets are strain hardened more than the larger pellets with the same energy of condensation. Such a result is also to be expected on the basis of theory.

According to Table 19–1, the greater the platinum content of the foil, the greater is its hardness and cohesion. The platinum strain hardens more than the gold, and therefore its presence causes an increase in the hardness number.

According to Table 19–2, the greater the thickness of the foil for a given composition, the less is its Brinell hardness number. This condition may also be accounted for on the basis of the amount of strain hardening, if it is assumed that the condensation factor is constant as before. In all such cases, it should be evident that the thickness or bulk will affect the degree of strain hardening under a given stress.

Obviously, the greater the thickness or bulk, the greater will be its resilience in the absorption of the impact energy, as previously described.

**The Gold Foil Restoration.** There can be no doubt that a gold foil restoration, properly inserted, is unsurpassed in operative dentistry from the standpoint of service. With modern equipment, the time factor objected to by many dentists has been reduced.

As previously noted, the adaptation of a good foil restoration is excellent. Radioactive tracer experiments indicate that although leakage may occur into the condensed foil itself, it does not usually penetrate around the restoration.[6] Retention is initially obtained by wedging the foil between the dentin cavity walls which are actually distended by the process. This wedged retention is lost, however, within a few months by a relaxation of the stresses in the dentin.[9] Nevertheless, sufficient retention remains so far as service is concerned.

It should be emphasized, however, that the skill of the dentist is of paramount importance in the success of a gold foil restoration. A gold foil restoration of poor quality can rate as one of the poorest restorations so far as service is concerned.

The proper insertion of a gold foil restoration challenges the skill of the dentist as does no other type of restoration.[10] If he is not ready or cannot meet this challenge, then he should employ some other type of restoration.

## Literature

1. Koser, J. R. and Ingraham, R.: *Mat Gold Foil with a Veneer Cohesive Gold Foil Surface for Class V Restorations.* J.A.D.A. 52:714–727 (June), 1956.
2. Black, G. V.: *Operative Dentistry,* ed. 6, Chicago, Medico-Dental Publishing Co., 1924, Vol. II, p. 229.
3. Peterson, H. W.: *A Study of the Annealing Temperature of Gold Foil.* Northwestern Univ. Bull. Dent. Res., 41:9–15 (Oct.), 1941.
4. Spencer, P. N., Romnes, A. F. and Skinner, E. W.: *Effect of the Annealing Temperature on the Hardness of Condensed Gold Foil.* Paper read at the Annual Meeting of the Dental Materials Group, I.A.D.R., March, 1960.
5. Black, G. V.: *Practical Utility of Accurate Studies of the Physical Properties of the Teeth and of Filling Materials,* Dent. Cos., 38:302–310 (April), 1896.
6. Taylor, J. B., Stowell, E. C., Murphy, J. F. and Wainwright, W. W.: *Microleakage of Gold Foil Fillings.* J. D. Res., 38:748 (July-Aug.), 1959. Abstract.
7. Souder, W. and Paffenbarger, G. C.: *Physical Properties of Dental Materials.* Washington, U. S. Government Printing Office, 1942, p. 35.
8. Rule, R. W.: *A Further Report on Physical Properties and Clinical Values of Platinum-Centered Gold Foil as Compared to Pure Gold Filling Materials.* J.A.D.A., 24:583–595 (April), 1937; *Gold Foil and Platinum-Centered Foil; Methods of Condensation.* J.A.D.A., 24:1783–1792 (Nov.), 1937.
9. Heussel, E.: *Die Elastischen Eigenschaften von Stahl-un Gold-Klammern.* Deutsche Zahnärz. Woch., 37:507–511, 1934.
10. Kramer, W. S., Trandall, T. R. and Diefendorf, W. L.: *A Comparative Study of the Physical Properties of Variously Manipulated Gold Foil Materials.* J. Am. Acad. Gold Foil Operators, 3:8–24 (May), 1960.

CHAPTER 20

# Constitution of Alloys.
# Heat Treatment

An alloy is defined for dental purposes as a combination of two or more metals which are mutually soluble in the molten condition. So far as the general principles of cast and wrought structure are concerned, the reactions of alloys are not essentially different from those of the pure metals already described. However, the presence of other metals in addition to the pure metal complicates the picture in relation to certain fundamental aspects not yet considered.

For example, most alloys solidify over a range in temperature rather than at a single temperature as does a pure metal. The range of the solidification temperature is as typical for any one particular alloy composition as is the single fusion temperature for the pure metal.

The presence of more than one metal may also bring about certain reactions in the solid state which cannot occur in the presence of a single metal, and which directly affect the properties of the alloy. These and other alloy phenomena will now be discussed.

**Classification of Alloys.** Alloys can be classified according to the number of alloying elements. For example, if two metals are present, a *binary* alloy is formed; if three metals are present, a *ternary* alloy is said to result, and so on. As the number of elements increases above two, the structure becomes increasingly complex. Consequently, only binary alloys will be studied in detail.

For dental purposes, the alloys can also be classified on the basis of the miscibility of the atoms in the solid state. The simplest alloy is one in which the atoms of the two metals intermingle randomly in a common space lattice. Under the microscope the grains of such alloys

**Page 317**

may resemble those of pure metals; the structure is entirely homogeneous. The metals are said to be *soluble* in each other in the solid state, and the alloys are called *solid solutions*.

If the metals are only partially soluble in one another, an *intermediate compound* may appear. One of the alloys of this type is the *intermetallic compound*. The intermetallic compound alloy also exhibits a homogeneous grain structure, but the atoms do not intermingle randomly in all proportions. Instead, they combine in stoichiometric proportions, without regard to valence, in a somewhat complex space lattice. They are characterized by an extreme brittleness and hardness. An example is the alloy $Ag_3Sn$ which is an essential constituent in the hardening of a dental amalgam and which will be discussed in a subsequent chapter.

If the metals are completely insoluble in each other in the solid state, a *eutectic alloy* is formed. The system is characterized by the fact that the melting limits of the alloy are less than the melting points of the components. The alloy composition with the lowest melting point is called the *eutectic*. In a eutectic alloy, each grain will be composed solely of one metal, and there will be as many different grain compositions as there are metals in the alloy. This situation occurs when an ordinary liquid solution is frozen. For example, when a liquid solution of sugar and water is frozen, the solid is composed of crystals of sugar and of water.

A fourth type of alloy may be classified as a *mixed type*. For example, the maximum solid solubility of copper in silver is 8.8 per cent. When more copper than this amount is present, a eutectic is formed with two types of grains, each composed of a different solid solution. Also, an intermetallic compound can be formed in combination with a eutectic alloy. In other words, the mixed type alloy may be a combination of the other three types, under different conditions of limited solid solubility.

**Definitions.**    There are a few terms which are used in metallurgy, which are also familiar in connection with other branches of science. Some of these terms have already been used in previous discussions. Before the technical discussion proceeds further, these terms will be explained to insure that a common ground of understanding is reached.

An alloy *system* is an aggregate of two or more metals in all their possible combinations which are being considered as a whole. For example, the "gold-silver system" means that all of the possible alloys of gold and silver are being considered in their various relations to one another.

From a metallurgical standpoint, a *phase* is any physically distinct, homogeneous, and mechanically separable portion of a system. Everyone is familiar with the fact that matter can exist in three different states or phases, liquid, solid or gas. However, in metallurgy it is not uncommon to find that more than one phase is present in the solid state. For example, a binary eutectic alloy can be termed a two-phase system. There are grains of two different compositions present which are mechanically separable.

Actually, the system must be in *equilibrium* before a true phase can exist. Polycrystalline metals and alloys never reach true equilibrium conditions in the solid state. There are at least three reasons for this condition: (1) The rigidity of the metal prevents the ready diffusion of the atoms to attain equilibrium. (2) At room temperature, the diffusion may be entirely arrested. If the alloy has been quenched in water from a high temperature where the rate of atomic diffusion is considerable, an unstable structure at the high temperature may be made permanent and apparently stable at room temperature. (3) The stresses at the grain boundaries described in Chapter 17 are not relieved as long as any grain boundaries persist, and, therefore, complete equilibrium is never attained in this area.

Nevertheless, equilibrium conditions must be assumed in the subsequent discussions. The conditions to be described are approached as a limit only under conditions of slow cooling and prolonged annealing, with ample opportunity for atomic diffusion.

**Solid Solutions.** By far the greatest number of alloys which are useful as dental restorations are solid solutions. Therefore special attention should be given to this type of alloy.

The term "solution" as applied to liquids is familiar to everyone. For example, a solution of sugar and water connotes a homogeneous system in which molecules of sugar diffuse through and intermingle with those of the water. The same is true of a molten solution of silver in palladium. However, if the sugar and water are frozen, each component will crystallize separately, but a palladium-silver alloy, low in silver content, will crystallize in such a manner that the atoms of the silver will be scattered randomly through the space lattice of the palladium, replacing the palladium atoms in a manner analogous to the molecular arrangement of the solute in the liquid solution. Such an alloy is called a solid solution. Since the atoms of silver enter directly into the space lattice of the palladium, the system is not mechanically separable and it has only one phase. Furthermore, if the atoms of silver are segregated for any reason, and are not scattered randomly throughout the palladium space lattice, they may be made to diffuse in a manner quite analogous to that of undissolved sugar in water.

**Solute and Solvent.** When the sugar is dissolved in water, the water is known as the solvent and the sugar as the solute. When two metals are soluble in one another in the solid state, the solvent is that metal whose space lattice persists, and the solute is the other metal. In the case of the palladium-silver alloys, the two metals are completely soluble in all proportions, and the same type of space lattice persists

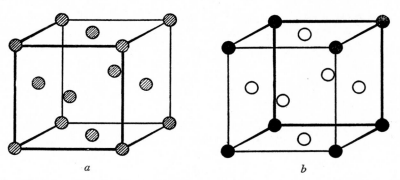

*a*                    *b*

Fig. 20–1.  *a.* A unit cell of a face-centered cubic space lattice of a copper-gold substitutional space lattice. The positions of the copper atoms cannot be distinguished from the gold atoms. *b.* The superlattice or ordered arrangement. The gold atoms are situated at the corners and the copper atoms on the faces of the cube. (Barrett, *Metals and Alloys,* Sept., 1937.)

throughout the entire system. In such a case, the solvent may be defined as the metal whose atoms occupy more than one-half the total number in the space lattice.

The configuration of the space lattice of solid solutions may be of several types: in the *substitutional* type, the atoms of the solute occupy the space lattice positions which normally are occupied by the solvent atoms in the pure metal. For example, in a palladium-silver alloy in which the palladium is the solvent, the silver atoms will replace the palladium atoms randomly in certain space lattice positions.

The presence of unlike atoms in the space lattice appears to allow the atoms to diffuse within the lattice more readily than in the case of the pure metal. Therefore, under certain conditions, a diffusion may take place so as to produce an *ordered* arrangement.

For example, the gold-copper alloys exhibit a random or substitutional solid solution structure of the face-centered type at high temperatures (Fig. 20–1*a*), but if an alloy of composition 50.2 per cent gold and 49.8 per cent copper by weight is allowed to cool slowly to below 400°C. (840°F.), the gold atoms will be found at the corners of the cube of the unit lattice cell, and the copper atoms on the faces (Fig. 20–1*b*).

When the unit cells are combined to form the space lattice, it can be noted that there are three times as many copper atoms as there are gold atoms, and as a result such a structure is represented as $AuCu_3$. The structure is called a *superlattice.*

**Conditions for Solid Solubility.**     In any substitutional type of solid solution, the distance between the atoms changes according to the size of the solute atom. The entire lattice may be expanded or contracted, sometimes non-uniformly, according to the size of the solute atom in relation to the solvent atom. Generally, however, such changes in atom distances are not great, since one of the primary requisites for two or more metals to form solid solutions is that their sizes be approximately the same.

For extensive solid solubility between the metals, the diameters of their atoms should not differ more than 10 to 15 per cent. Within this range, the *size factor* is said to be favorable for solid solubility. If the difference between their diameters is greater than this, the solid solubility becomes limited, or it may not exist.

A second factor is the valency of the metals. Metals of the same valence and size are more apt to form extensive solid solutions than are metals of different valence with a favorable size factor. In the case of a difference in valence, the metal with the higher valence often exhibits a greater solubility in a metal of lower valence, than does the metal with a lower valence in one with a higher valence.

A third requisite for solid solubility is that the metals be closely associated in the electromotive series (see Table 21–1). If the metals are widely separated in this regard, there is a strong tendency for the formation of stable intermediate compounds, such as intermetallic compounds, instead of solid solutions.

Although it is not necessary that the two metals possess the same crystal structure to form a solid solution, when they are of the same lattice structure with a favorable size factor and with the same valence, a continuous series of solid solutions is nearly always formed.

**Examples of Solid Solutions.** Some of the atomic properties of metals used in dental alloys are given[1] in Table 20–1. The first five metals are commonly used in dental gold alloys. All of these metals belong to the face-centered cubic system, and this factor, at least, is favorable for the formation of solid solutions. As might be expected from both the size and valence factors, silver and gold form a continuous series of solid solutions with each other, with very little disturbance of the lattice dimensions. Silver and palladium also form a continuous series of solid solutions.

*Table 20–1.* *Atomic Diameters of Metals of Dental Interest**

| METAL | ATOMIC DIAMETER (ÅNGSTROMS) | CRYSTAL STRUCTURE |
|---|---|---|
| Gold | 2.878 | Face-centered cubic |
| Platinum | 2.769 | Face-centered cubic |
| Palladium | 2.745 | Face-centered cubic |
| Silver | 2.882 | Face-centered cubic |
| Copper | 2.551 | Face-centered cubic |
| Tin | 3.016 | Body-centered tetragonal |
| Zinc | 2.659 | Close-packed hexagonal |
| Silicon | 2.346 | Diamond cubic |

* Metals Handbook (1948).

Although the diameter of the copper atom differs as much as 10 to 12 per cent from that of the other four metals under consideration, it is an important alloy component. As will be discussed later, it forms a limited series of solid solutions with silver. Solid solutions of copper in gold, platinum and palladium are continuous at high temperatures, but upon cooling, superlattice changes take place, as already discussed in connection with the formation of the $AuCu_3$ superlattice, for example.

According to Table 20–1, the difference between the silver and the tin atomic diameters is in the neighborhood of 4 per cent. However, the two metals are different in valence, and they are not closely associated in the electromotive series. It will be shown in a subsequent chapter that silver is a limited solvent for tin. As the tin content increases, an intermetallic compound forms, which is an important factor in the hardening of dental amalgams.

**Physical Properties of Solid Solutions.**    It was previously noted that the lattice structure of a solvent metal is expanded or contracted by the introduction of solute atoms by substitution. Such a statement is true only if the situation is considered as an average condition over the entire space lattice. Actually, wherever a solute atom displaces or substitutes for a solvent atom, the difference in size of the solute atom results in a localized distortion or strained condition of the lattice. As noted in Chapter 18, whenever a lattice distortion occurs, slip becomes more difficult, and the strength, proportional limit and surface hardness are increased, whereas the ductility is decreased.

Consequently, the alloying of metals may be a means of strengthening the metal. The general theory of slip interference in alloys is the same as in strain hardening, except that a different type of lattice distortion is present initially to inhibit slip before the structure is stressed or worked.

There are a number of useful alloys in dentistry which are examples of this. Gold itself cannot be used as a restorative material unless it is strain hardened, as in the condensation of gold foil. Gold in the cast condition is too weak and ductile. However, if as little as 5 per cent by weight of copper is alloyed with the gold, the latter loses practically none of its ability to resist tarnish and corrosion, yet a strength and hardness is imparted to it so that it can be used for the casting of inlays.

In general, the hardness and strength of any metallic solvent are increased by the atoms of a solute. The more nearly the atoms are of the same size, the less the effect of the solute atoms will be, but some increase in strength can be expected nevertheless.

Generally, the more of the solute metal added to the solvent, the greater is the strength and hardness of the alloy. In the case of two metals which form a continuous series of solid solutions with one another, the maximum hardness will be reached at approximately 50 atomic per cent* of each metal. As might be expected from the theory, the ductility usually decreases progressively as the strength and hardness increase.

The density of a solid solution under conditions of complete solubility can be calculated from the composition. In the cases of limited solubility, however, the calculated density is apt to be lower than the density determined by experiment.

**Constitution Diagrams.** Alloys can often be distinguished from pure metals by means of their time-temperature cooling curves. As noted previously, most alloys solidify over a range in temperature. Solidification under these conditions may result in a grain structure characteristic of a given alloy composition. If the type of grain structure can be predicted, as well as the range of solidification of a particular alloy composition, valuable information is available as to the probable behavior of the alloy in the mouth as a dental appliance. Such information can be obtained from a *constitution diagram*, which will now be described. An explanation of the diagram will be given, with no attempt to justify the statements with theoretical considerations. A reference book on this subject[2] should be consulted, if further information is desired.

Let Figure 20–2 represent the time-temperature cooling curves for alloy combinations of 0 per cent palladium and 100 per cent silver, 10 per cent palladium and 90 per cent silver, 20 per cent palladium and 80 per cent silver, and so on, up to 100 per cent palladium and 0 per cent silver. At either end of the graph, where the pure metals are indicated, a constant freezing temperature is present, but for all the alloys, a range of freezing temperatures occurs.

For example, consider the time-temperature cooling curve for the alloy composition 20 per cent palladium and 80 per cent silver. At the temperature designated by *B*, the solidification commences and the alloy will be partly liquid and partly solid until the temperature falls to *C*, when it will be completely solidified. In other words, at all temperatures above *B*, the alloy will be wholly molten, and it will be entirely solid at temperatures below *C*, whereas between *B* and *C* it will be partially liquid and partially solid. This is true for all of the alloys given in the illustration.

Now if the temperatures corresponding to the points *B* and *C* of all the cases illustrated are plotted against their corresponding compositions, and if a smooth curve is drawn through the points thus plotted, Figure 20–3 will result. For example, in Figure 20–2, if the temperature at which 0 per cent palladium and 100 per cent silver solidify is plotted, only one point in Figure 20–3 will result, namely at 960°C.

---

* *Atomic per cent* is calculated on the basis of the atomic weight of each metal, rather than the gravity weight. When the latter is employed, the percentage is known as *weight per cent.*

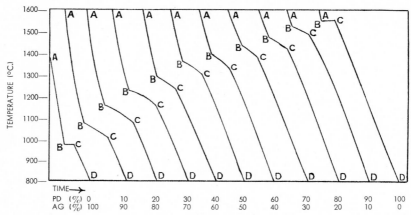

Fig. 20–2. A diagrammatic representation of the time-temperature cooling curves for the palladium-silver system.

(1762°F.), which is the melting point of silver. In Figure 20–2, *B* occurs at approximately 1060°C. (1942°F.), and *C* at 1000°C. (1832°F.) for the alloy of composition 10 per cent palladium and 90 per cent silver. Both of these temperatures are plotted in Figure 20–3 for the composition 10 per cent palladium and 90 per cent silver. Each alloy composition in Figure 20–2 is treated similarly until the pure metal palladium is reached, when the temperatures *B* and *C* again coincide in one point in Figure 20–3, at the melting point of palladium.

Considering the diagrams as a whole, the line *ABC* in Figure 20–3 is evidently a curve passing through all the points *B* of Figure 20–2, and the lower curve *ADC* represents the locations of the points *C* in the other figure. Since in Figure 20–2 the alloys are molten above all temperatures *B*, the alloy must be liquid at all temperatures above the line *ABC* in Figure 20–3. For this reason, the curve *ABC* is called the *liquidus*. By similar reasoning, the alloy must be solid at all temperatures below the curve *ADC*, which is therefore called the *solidus*. In the area between the curves, the alloy is partially liquid and partially solid.

***Interpretation of the Constitution Diagram.*** As an illustration of how the constitution diagram is used practically, consider an alloy of composition 65 per cent palladium and 35 per cent silver, which cools from the liquid state along the dotted line *PO* in Figure 20–3. At any temperature above the point of intersection *R* of the line *PO* with the liquidus, the alloy will be molten. When the temperature falls to approximately 1400°C. (2552°F.) at *R*, the first solidification begins. The composition of the alloy first solidifying may be found by drawing the line *RM* through *R*, parallel to the base line such that it intersects both the liquidus and solidus; the point of intersection with the solidus (*M*) gives the composition of the solid as determined by projecting *M* onto the base line, and the composition of the remaining liquid is determined by projecting the point $R$ to the base line in the same manner. In the case just cited, the solid phase will be approximately 77 per cent palladium and 23 per cent silver, whereas the composition of the remaining liquid will be 65 per cent palladium and 35 per cent silver.

Now assume that the temperature decreases to approximately 1370°C. (2497° F.) as denoted by the point $S$. At this temperature, the material will be partially solid and partially liquid. As before, the composition of the solid and liquid at this stage may be determined by drawing the line $YW$, and locating its point of intersection with the liquidus and solidus respectively in terms of composition as before. Hence, the approximate composition of the liquid will be 58 per cent palladium and 42 per cent silver, as given by the projection of the point $Y$ on the base line, whereas that of the solid will be about 71 per cent palladium and 29 per cent silver, determined by projecting the point $W$ to the base line. At the temperature corresponding to the point $T$ on the graph (approximately 1340° C., or 2442° F.), the last liquid to solidify will have the composition of 52 per cent palladium, and the solid phase will be 65 per cent palladium. No further change occurs as the temperature falls to that of the room. In a similar manner, any alloy composition of the entire system can be analyzed.

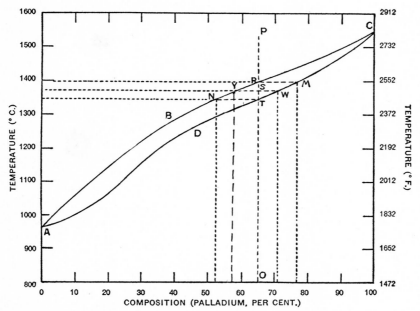

Fig. 20–3. Constitution diagram for the palladium-silver system. Only the percentage composition for the palladium is given; the percentage composition for the silver is determined by subtracting the palladium composition from 100.

*Table 20–2.    Compositions of the Alloy Palladium 65 Per Cent and Silver 35 Per Cent, Which Can Occur During Solidification*

| TEMPERATURE | | COMPOSITION (BY WEIGHT) | | | |
| | | LIQUID | | SOLID | |
| °C. | °F. | Pd (%) | Ag (%) | Pd (%) | Ag (%) |
|---|---|---|---|---|---|
| >1400 | >2552 | 65 | 35 | 0 | 0 |
| 1400 | 2552 | 65 | 35 | 77 | 23 |
| 1370 | 2497 | 58 | 42 | 71 | 29 |
| 1340 | 2442 | 52 | 48 | 65 | 35 |
| <1340 | <2442 | 0 | 0 | 65 | 35 |

It should be noted that the composition line *PO* must intersect the horizontal line at or between the liquidus and solidus for the proper interpretation of the diagram. For example, a line drawn parallel to the base line at the temperature 1450° C. will intersect the liquidus and the solidus but not the original composition line *PO* at/or between these points of intersection. In this case, it would be meaningless to draw perpendiculars to the base line since the alloy is known to be molten at 1450° C. The same argument can be applied to any temperature below point *T*.

A summary of the compositions of the solid and liquid as determined at the various temperatures is given in Table 20–2.

**Coring.**    The situation depicted in Table 20–2 is highly theoretical, and it exists only if it is assumed that the alloys can be cooled instantaneously from their liquidus temperatures. On the basis of such an assumption, the composition of the first minute grain or nucleus of crystallization to form would be palladium 77 per cent and silver 23 per cent. As more solid forms, its content will be lower in palladium and higher in silver. The solid can be pictured as forming dendrites, each succeeding "layer" of which contains less of the component with the higher melting temperature (palladium, in this case).

The outermost "layer" of the dendrites will have a composition of palladium 65 per cent and silver 35 per cent at the solidus temperature, but the last liquid to solidify will have a composition high in silver and low in palladium. The grain structure of the alloy will be cored. The core will consist of the dendrites with the higher melting compositions, and the matrix will be composed of the last liquid metal to solidify at the solidus temperature of the alloy. The matrix will, therefore, be composed mainly of the lower melting constituents.

Generally, the greater the solidification temperature range of the alloy, the greater is the extent of the coring, since a large solidification range is generally accompanied by a considerable composition range between the liquidus and solidus at a given temperature. Consequently, a small solidification range in temperature is generally advantageous in dental alloys.

An excellent example of a cored structure can be observed in the photomicrographs presented in Figures 18–3 and 20–4. The dark dendritic structure represents the core composed of the high melting alloys. The matrix which solidified last between the dendrites is lighter in shade.

**Homogenization.** In the previous discussion, an instantaneous cooling was assumed, a condition which is impossible of attainment. Actually, the atoms tend to diffuse to relieve the segregation as much as possible. Under conditions of complete equilibrium, the composition of the palladium-silver alloy should be palladium 65 per cent and silver 35 per cent throughout, and the atomic diffusion during cooling tends to produce such a situation. However, the faster the alloy is cooled from its liquidus temperature, the more nearly the compositions in Table 20–2 are approached. On the other hand, during a slow cooling, the greater will be the amount of atomic diffusion toward equilibrium conditions.

Atomic diffusion does not take place in a cast structure as rapidly as it does in a wrought metal structure. If a cored structure can be cold worked and then annealed at its recrystallization temperature, a homogeneous structure can be obtained in a short time. If the casting cannot be cold worked, it can be recrystallized or *homogenized* either by cooling it slowly from its liquidus temperature, or by annealing it at a temperature just below its solidus temperature for a considerable time, often many hours. The cored structure in Figure 20–4*a* is shown in Figure 20–4*b* after such a homogenizing treatment.

It will be shown in the next chapter that an inhomogeneous dental gold alloy is more subject to tarnish and corrosion than the same alloy after it has been homogenized. Not only does such tarnish cause

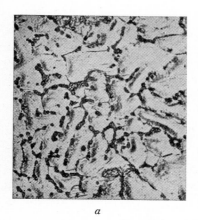 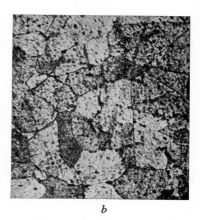

*a* *b*

Fig. 20–4. *a.* Copper-silver alloy (1 per cent silver) as cast. *b.* Same structure after homogenization. ×100. (Van Wert, *An Introduction to Physical Metallurgy*, McGraw-Hill Book Co., Inc.)

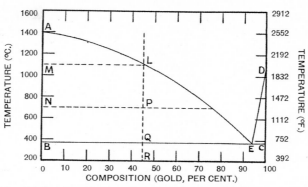

Fig. 20–5. Constitution diagram of the gold-silicon system.

an undesirable discoloration of the dental structure, but also it may be a factor in the production of pathologic changes in the surrounding soft tissue.[3]

As might be expected, the inhomogeneous grain structure offers more resistance to slip than does the homogenized structure because of the heterogeneous grain structure of the former. Consequently, although the difference is not great, the ductility of the alloy is greater after homogenization.

**Eutectic Alloys.**  Although they are mutually soluble in the molten state, the components of a eutectic alloy are insoluble in the solid state.

A typical example of such an alloy would be any composition of the gold-silicon system. According to Table 20–1, the diameters of the gold and silicon atoms are much different. The two elements are far apart in the electrochemical series; in fact, silicon is a metalloid, and not a true metal. Their space lattices are different (Table 20–1), as are their valences. Consequently, none of the conditions exist for solid solubility.

The constitution diagram for the gold-silicon eutectic alloy system is shown in Figure 20–5. The line *ABECD* is the solidus and the line *AED* is the liquidus, both of which are obtained from a series of time-temperature cooling curves, as previously described for the palladium-silver alloys. The points *A* and *D* represent the melting points of silicon and gold, which are 1430° C. (2610° F.) and 1063° C. (1945° F.), respectively. Whereas the addition of palladium to silver raised the melting temperature of the solid solution, if approximately 40 per cent or less silicon is added to gold, the liquidus temperature of the alloy will be lowered below the fusion temperature of gold, in spite of the fact that the fusion temperature of silicon is much greater than that of gold. On the other hand, the addition of gold to silicon in any proportion will lower the melting temperature of the alloy below that of silicon.

In order to clarify this point, let us consider the cooling of an alloy composition of 45 per cent gold and 55 per cent silicon, as represented by the dotted line *LR* in the figure. As the alloy cools from the molten state, it starts to solidify at the temperature represented by *L*. As before, the composition of the first solid phase is found by drawing the line *LM*, which intersects the solidus at *M;* hence, the composition of the solid is 100 per cent silicon. As the temperature falls to *P*, the silicon is still the only solid phase. Furthermore, as the temperature decreases, the liquid gradually becomes richer in gold until the solidus is reached, when the entire mass freezes with the composition *E*, 94 per cent gold and 6 per cent silicon, which solidifies as a mechanical mixture at 370° C. (698° F.) and is called the *eutectic.*

The compositions which form during the solidification as described are summarized in Table 20–3. It is interesting to note that the composition of the solid at all temperatures from the liquidus to the solidus is pure silicon. It is evident that a cored structure results wherein the core is pure silicon, and the matrix has a composition of silicon 6 per cent, and gold 94 per cent. The grain structure of a similar alloy is pictured in Figure 20–6.

The matrix merits special attention. Its grain structure at a higher magnification is shown in Figure 20–7. It is composed of minute grains of gold and silicon. Presumably the dark grains are pure silicon, and the light grains are pure gold. A study of the constitution diagram in Figure 20–5 reveals further characteristics of this particular alloy composition.

1. Regardless of the composition of the molten alloy, an alloy of this composition is always the last to solidify. In other words, regardless of the total composition, the matrix is always of the same composition.

2. If the alloy is of this particular composition (gold, 94 per cent, and silicon, 6 per cent), it will melt and freeze at a constant temperature, similar to the solidification of a pure metal. This point is proven by the fact that the liquidus and solidus coincide at this particular composition.

3. The lowest melting temperature of the entire system occurs with

*Table 20–3.    Compositions of the Alloy Silicon 55 Per Cent and Gold 45 Per Cent, Which Can Occur During Solidification*

| TEMPERATURE | | COMPOSITION | | | |
| | | LIQUID | | SOLID | |
| °C. | °F. | Si (%) | Au (%) | Si (%) | Au (%) |
| --- | --- | --- | --- | --- | --- |
| >1100 | >2012 | 55 | 45 | 0 | 0 |
| 1100 | 2012 | 55 | 45 | 100 | 0 |
| 700 | 1292 | 23 | 77 | 100 | 0 |
| 370 | 698 | 6 | 94 | 100 | 0 |
| <370 | <698 | 0 | 0 | 55 | 45 |

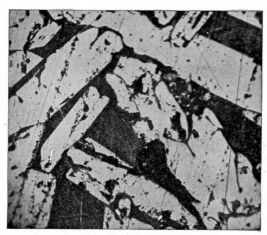

Fig. 20–6.   Microstructure of an alloy of composition silicon 50 per cent and gold 50 per cent. The core is silicon. ×75. (Ray, *Metallurgy for Dental Students*, P. Blakiston's Son & Co.)

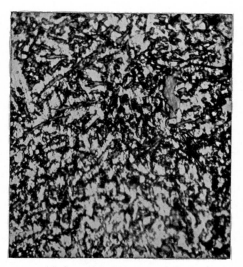

Fig. 20–7.   Microstructure of the gold-silicon eutectic. ×300. (Ray, *Metallurgy for Dental Students*, P. Blakiston's Son & Co.)

this composition. For this reason, it is called the *eutectic* (meaning "lowest melting"). A eutectic alloy is, then, any combination of metals containing a eutectic.

Since the eutectic is always the last composition to solidify, it is evident why the core is always a pure metal. If the silicon content is greater than 6 per cent, the silicon will solidify as the temperature decreases until 6 per cent of this metal remains, at which composition the eutectic will solidify at 370° C. (698° F.). If more than 94 per cent of gold is present, the core will be gold as shown in Figure 20–8, but when the gold content is reduced to 94 per cent, the eutectic will solidify as the matrix.

Owing to their inhomogeneous grain structure, the eutectic alloys are apt to be brittle. They are used chiefly in dental solders, where a low melting point is desirable. Usually, such a structure is avoided in dental alloys if possible because of its tendency to tarnish and corrode in the mouth fluids.

**Silver-Copper System.** Copper is a very important component of dental alloys. It forms a continuous series of solid solutions with many of the precious metals.

The solubility of copper in silver, as well as silver in copper, is limited as previously discussed. The constitution diagram for the silver-copper system is shown in Figure 20–9. The liquidus can be identified as the line *AED*, and the solidus connects the points *ABEGD*.

The line *BC* extends below the solidus, and it indicates the solid solubility of copper in silver at the various temperatures. For example, copper can exist as a solute in silver at any temperature and composition in the area between the vertical ordinate and the boundary line *ABC*. The alloys in this area are designated as *α-solid solutions*. The line *GF* provides a similar boundary for the *β-solid solutions* of silver in copper.

The alloy is a mixed type. A eutectic is formed if the copper is present in combination with the silver to an extent greater than 8.8 per cent or if the silver is present in combination with the copper to an extent

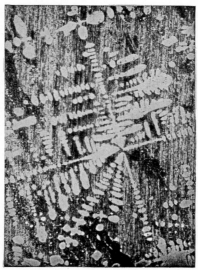

Fig. 20–8. Microstructure of an alloy composition gold, 96 per cent and silicon, 4 per cent. The core is gold. ×75. (Ray, *Metallurgy for Dental Students,* P. Blakiston's Son & Co.)

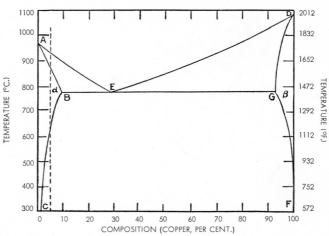

Fig. 20–9.  Constitution diagram for the silver-copper system.

greater than 8.0 per cent. The composition of the eutectic is silver, 71.9 per cent, and copper, 28.1 per cent. Its melting temperature is 779.4° C. (1434.9° F.). Its grain components will be the α- and β-solid solutions. If the copper content is greater than 28.1 per cent, the core will be the β-solid solution, and if it is less than this it will be the α-solid solution.

Owing to the susceptibility of most of the high copper alloys to tarnish and corrosion, in dentistry only the α-solid solution is of interest. Consequently, special attention will be given this type of alloy.

Let it be assumed that an alloy of composition 5 per cent copper and 95 per cent silver cools slowly, as shown by the dotted line in Figure 20–9, from the molten state to room temperature. It will begin to solidify at a temperature slightly above 900° C. (1650° F.), and it will freeze completely as an α-solid solution at approximately 860° C. (1580° F.). As the temperature falls, the solid solution phase will remain intact until a temperature of 630° C. (1166° F.) is reached, when the copper will appear in a mixture with the α-solid solution as a precipitated phase. The reason for this change is related to the solid solubility of copper in silver. Just as the line *AB* represents the solubility limit of the copper in the silver at the respective solidification temperatures, so does the line *BC* represent the solubility limit of the two metals in the solid state. As previously noted, if more than 8.8 per cent copper is added to the melt, the eutectic appears upon solidification. But the solubility of the copper in the silver becomes less as the temperature decreases below the eutectic solidification temperature, as indicated by the line *BC*. Consequently, when the above-mentioned alloy is slowly cooled below 630° C., the solid solution becomes *supersaturated* with copper, and the excess phase is *precipitated*. The process is analogous to similar phenomena in supersaturated liquid solutions.

Although silver-copper alloys are used in dentistry only in pedodontics, the significance of the phenomenon described is of practical importance by analogy. When this process is compared with the more complicated heat treatments of dental gold alloys, this complex phenomena will be more easily comprehended.

This precipitation of copper from a solid solution of silver and copper is a typical example of a method for controlling the physical properties of an alloy by a reversible heat treatment. For example, if the alloy described above is quenched in water at a temperature above 630° C. (1166° F.) but below the temperature of the solidus, the solid solution condition is preserved intact with no precipitation of copper at room temperature. As has been previously discussed, the rate of atomic diffusion of a metal or alloy is greater at the higher temperatures. In the case of the alloy under discussion, the rate of diffusion at room temperature approaches zero. Consequently if the temperature change during the quenching of the alloy is sufficiently rapid, any precipitation of copper will be negligible. As a result, the solid solution is, for all practical purposes, seemingly stable at room temperature.

This precipitation reaction is reversible. For example, if the slowly cooled alloy with the precipitated copper lattice as described above is again heated above 630° C. (1166° F.) to 700° C. (1292° F.), the copper atoms will diffuse randomly, or dissolve, into the space lattice of the solid solution.

As might be predicted from previous theory, these changes in lattice structure result in a change in the physical properties of the alloy. When the copper lattice is precipitated in the space lattice of the $\alpha$-solid solution, a distortion results, and a condition for slip interference is produced. As in other cases of slip interference, after the precipitation an increase in hardness, strength and proportional limit can be observed, with a decrease in ductility. This method of heat treatment is called *age hardening.* If it is desired, the ductility can be restored by heating the alloy to a temperature at which the copper is soluble in the silver. If the alloy is then quenched in water, the solid solution condition will remain at room temperature. Such a heat treatment is known as a *solution heat treatment.*

Age hardening is the third method available to the dentist for increasing the strength and hardness of a metal structure. Other examples of age hardening will be outlined in subsequent sections, and it will be shown that this method of heat treatment is very important in the proper manipulation of partial denture and orthodontic appliances, for example.

Silver-copper alloys are sometimes used for the filling of deciduous teeth. One particular composition is especially adaptable to such use because of its tarnish resistance. The composition is copper, 7.5 per cent and silver, 92.5 per cent. The alloy is called *sterling silver.*

*Table 20–4.*     *Heat Treatment of Sterling Silver*

| PHYSICAL PROPERTY | SOLUTION HEAT TREATMENT | AGE HARDENING TREATMENT |
|---|---|---|
| Ultimate Tensile Strength | | |
| (Kg./Cm.$^2$) | 2,620 | 3,040 |
| (Lb./In.$^2$) | 37,400 | 43,400 |
| Yield Point | | |
| (Kg./Cm.$^2$) | 1,370 | 2,100 |
| (Lb./In.$^2$) | 19,680 | 30,000 |
| Elongation (%) | 42 | 26 |

It is of interest to note that sterling silver is susceptible to heat treatment as shown in Table 20–4. For a solution heat treatment, the alloy was held at 650° C. (1200° F.) for 30 minutes and then quenched. It was age hardened at 325° C. (617° F.) for thirty minutes. As predicted by theory, the yield point and strength were increased by age hardening whereas the ductility decreased.

**Gold-Copper System.** The gold-copper alloys were probably the first to be used for cast dental restorations, and, in a sense, they can be considered basic to most dental gold alloys.

The constitution diagram for these alloys is shown in Figure 20–10. Above approximately 400° C. (750° F.) all of these alloys form a continuous series of solid solutions. The system is characterized by the fact that the liquidus and solidus are almost identical. At a composition of gold 75.6 per cent (by weight) the liquidus and solidus join (*A*, Fig. 20–10). None of the alloys exhibit much coring, since their temperature range of solidification is so small.

Another interesting characteristic of the system is that all of the alloys possess melting ranges at temperatures less than the fusion points of either copper or gold. Such a depression of the freezing point is more characteristic of a eutectic system than it is of a solid solution.

In the case of gold-copper alloys, with compositions between 39 and 88 per cent gold by weight, superlattice transformations take place as the alloy is cooled slowly from above 400° C. (750° F.). Three superlattices have been identified, as shown by the enclosed areas toward the bottom of Figure 20–10. They are the $\beta$-superlattice with the formula $AuCu_3$, the $\gamma$-superlattice with the formula $AuCu_2$, and the $\delta$-superlattice with the formula $AuCu$. The effects of such solid-solid transformations are similar to those described for the silver-copper system in the preceding section.

The $AuCu_3$ superlattice has already been discussed (page 320). Since the dimensions of this superlattice are the same as those of the parent lattice from which it was formed, there is little distortion of the parent lattice. Consequently, no appreciable age hardening occurs after such a transformation, as happens in the case of the precipitation of copper.

Owing to the fact that the conditions in the mouth require a relatively high gold content in the alloy in order to prevent tarnish and corrosion, only the AuCu superlattice is of dental interest. When the alloys of composition 65 to 85 per cent gold are age hardened below 400° C., a tetragonal face-centered superlattice may appear in the face-centered cubic space lattice of the substitutional solid solution. The ordered arrangement in the tetragonal lattice consists of five copper atoms on each of two opposite sides (one at each corner, and one face-centered on each side), and one gold atom, face-centered, on each of the remaining four sides. A unit cell of such a lattice is diagrammed in Figure 20–11.

Since the tetragonal lattice has one dimension longer than the other two, a definite distortion of the parent face-centered cubic lattice occurs after age hardening. Consequently, a condition of slip interference is produced. The usual properties are increased and the ductility is decreased by such an age hardening. The age hardening can be relieved by heating the alloy at a temperature above 400° C., followed by a quenching, so that the substitutional solid solution condition will be restored.

**Other Systems.** The platinum-gold system exhibits a considerable spread in temperature between the liquidus and solidus, and an undesirable cored structure results. The alloys may be age hardened between 350° C. (660° F.) and 650° C. (1200° F.); the temperature and time of aging for the best results depend on the composition. The transforma-

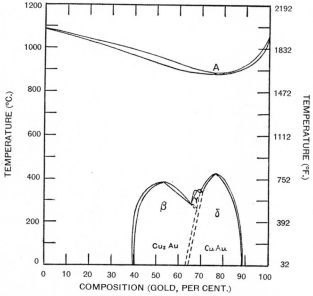

Fig. 20–10. Constitution diagram for the gold-copper system.

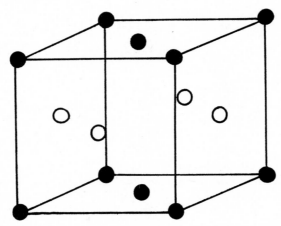

Fig. 20–11. A unit cell of the face-centered tetragonal superlattice corresponding to AuCu. The circles represent the gold atoms.

tions involved are thought to be a breaking down of the solid solution near the solidus into two solid solutions, one being rich in gold, and the other rich in platinum. At 400° C. (750° F.), this heterogeneous structure may be spread over compositions which range from 4 to 90 per cent gold.

The palladium-copper system is characterized by a relatively short melting range, particularly in comparison to that of the platinum-gold system. Although the melting range is never less than the melting temperatures of the constituents, the copper effectively reduces the liquidus and solidus temperatures over a considerable range of composition. In some respects, this system resembles that of the gold-copper system. Transformations which correspond to the compositions PdCu (62.6 per cent palladium) and PdCu₃ (36 per cent palladium) occur on age hardening below 600° C. The range of the PdCu transformation is approximately from 48 to 63 per cent palladium, and it involves an atomic diffusion to an ordered face-centered cubic structure of the same dimensions as the parent lattice. As might be expected, the increase in hardness on age hardening is not great.

The platinum-copper system resembles the palladium-copper system somewhat. Age hardening may be brought about with the compositions corresponding to PtCu (75.5 per cent platinum) and PtCu₃ (50.6 per cent platinum). The hardening in the region of PtCu is the more efficient.

There are a number of other transformations which are known to occur in ternary and quaternary systems of the precious metals, but their consideration involves the use of three or more dimensional constitution diagrams, and they are not within the scope of the present discussion. It will be noted in a subsequent chapter that some dental alloys may contain as many as six component metals: gold, platinum, palladium, silver, copper and zinc. There are very likely superlattice combinations present in the age hardening of such complex alloys that are not known at present. It is not possible, therefore, to predict with surety from the composition of such a complex alloy that it will age harden. When age hardening occurs, however, the phenomena involved are basically the same as those described for the binary alloys.

**Theory of Age Hardening.**      In practice, the alloy is first given a solution heat treatment at a temperature above any transformation limits in order to obtain the substitutional solid solution. In the case of dental alloys, the solution heat-treatment temperature is 700 to 800° C. (1292 to 1472° F.). The optimum time for this treatment has never been determined, but it is usually given arbitrarily as ten minutes. After this treatment, the alloy is quenched rapidly, in order to maintain the substitutional solid-solution condition at room temperature. Equilibrium conditions do not exist under such a treatment, but the atomic diffusion is so sluggish at the lower temperatures that the metastable condition is rendered permanent. The ductility of the alloy is increased by this treatment, but the other tensile properties and surface hardness are reduced, since the solid solution space lattice presents the more favorable conditions for slip.

If the alloy is cooled slowly, or if it is held at a temperature below the transformation limits, an age hardening may occur, owing to the precipitation of some new phase or component. For example, in the case of the silver-copper alloys, copper is precipitated from a solid solution supersaturated with respect to copper; in the gold-copper system, $AuCu$ and/or $AuCu_3$ are formed, and so on, as described for each combination of metals. Regardless of the complexity of the precipitated lattice, a new phase of some type appears. In any event, the new phase may produce a decrease in ductility and an increase in hardness and in the other tensile properties, provided that the precipitated phase produces a region of interruption or discontinuity in the original solid solution space lattice. In other words, the essential conception is the same as in strain hardening or alloying, *i.e.*, the space lattice of the parent lattice is distorted by the precipitated phase, and slip is rendered more difficult.

The actual mechanism by which the slip interference is accomplished can be illustrated by the diagrams in Figure 20–12. Figure 20–12*a* represents a series of "slip planes," in which there is no interruption. The planes can slip over each other easily, with little internal friction. If hard spheres or blocks of some nature are inserted in the planes, as shown in Figure 20–12*b*, the ability to slip will be prevented by the new phase; only those few planes in which no block is present will be able to slip as before. The planes are said to be "keyed," in such a case, and the blocks are sometimes called "keys."

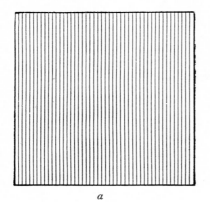
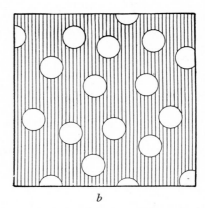

*a*                                                  *b*

Fig. 20–12.   *a.* Set of planes with easy slip, no interruptions. *b.* Slip planes "keyed" by space lattice discontinuities and distortions represented by circles. (Jeffries and Archer, *The Science of Metals*, McGraw-Hill Book Co., Inc.)

The analogy is evident. The condition represented in Figure 20–12*a* is that of the substitutional solid solution. During age hardening, "keys" are produced by the distortions in the space lattice occasioned by the formation of a new phase. It should be emphasized, however, that the "keys" formed by the superlattices are not necessarily hard or brittle. The slip is inhibited by the lattice distortions, and not by the hardness of the particles.

From a practical standpoint, the control of the formation of the dispersed phase is a matter of importance, and it forms the basis for the optimum conditions of age hardening. For example, if too much of the precipitated phase is allowed to form, the alloy may become too brittle. The proper control will depend not only upon the composition of the alloy, but also upon its previous history; for example, a strain hardened alloy will age harden more readily than will a cast structure.

The dispersed phases are localized in such small regions that it is often impossible to see them under a microscope unless the age hardening is prolonged beyond practical limits. For example, an alloy[4] of palladium 8.2 per cent, gold 60.6 per cent, silver 16.6 per cent, copper 14.1 per cent, and zinc 0.5 per cent was age hardened at 450° C. (840° F.) for 100 hours after a solution heat treatment at 700° C. (1292° F.), with the result shown in Figure 20–13. The light part is the solid solution phase and the dark is the precipitated phase. Evidently, the precipitation occurred at the grain boundaries.

It is apparent that the rate of atomic diffusion in age hardening is slow, at least soon after the initial precipitation has occurred. In dental practice, the usual time for age hardening is 15 minutes. If the time is prolonged beyond this limit, many alloys become too brittle.

An inspection of Figure 20–12*b* will indicate that many small areas of discontinuity might be more effective in interrupting slip than a few large areas. As a matter of fact, if too much of the new phase is pre-cipitated in particles of relatively large size, it is conceivable that the slip might take place in the new phase in preference to the old, and that the ductility might be increased. Such a condition is not likely to occur in dental alloys, however, because of the impractically long time required for such a precipitation.

**Conditions for Precipitation.** Whether or not a precipitation will occur in an alloy system during age hardening is in part dependent upon the size factor of the alloy components. For example, as previously noted, the size factor is not favorable for a complete solubility of copper in silver. The parent space lattice (silver) is so distorted by the solute atoms of copper, that the latter tend to be precipitated in order to re-lieve the induced stresses.

The same theory can be applied to the ordering of the atoms to produce the superlattlice. It can be noted from Table 20–1 that the diameters of the copper and gold atoms are almost as different as are those of copper and silver. Although the copper and the gold form a continuous series of substitutional solid solutions at high temperatures, it follows from the theory there must be strained areas wherever the copper atoms are randomly situated in the gold lattice. It is evident that a regularity of the spacing of the copper atoms in the gold lattice would reduce (but not completely eliminate) the strained condition below that of the random arrangement. The AuCu superlattice pre-

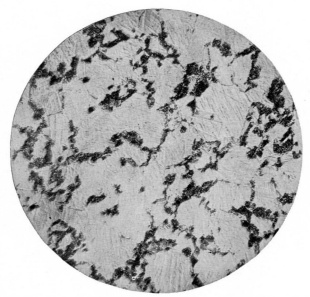

Fig. 20–13. A photomicrograph of a dental alloy which has been age hardened at 450° C. for 100 hours. ×250. (Courtesy of E. M. Wise, International Nickel Co.)

viously described is one of the possible results of such an ordered rearrangement. In essence, then, the precipitation of the superlattice is an attempt to attain equilibrium in the space lattice, or a reduction in the internal energy.

## Literature

1. *Metals Handbook*, 1948 edition, Cleveland, American Society for Metals, 1948, pp. 20–21.
2. Committee on Solids, Division of Physical Sciences, National Research Council: *Phase Transformations in Solids*. New York, John Wiley & Sons, Inc., 1951.
3. Hedegård, B.: *Homogenization*. Dept. Pros., Royal Sch. Dent., Stockholm, 1958.
4. Wise, E. M. and Eash, J. T.: *The Role of the Platinum Metals in Dental Alloys, III*. Trans. A.I.M.E. Inst. Met. Div., *104:*276–203, 1933.

*CHAPTER 21*

# Tarnish and Corrosion

One of the primary requisites of any metal or alloy which is to be placed in the mouth is that it should not tarnish or corrode in the oral fluids. If not too marked, tarnish and corrosion are often overlooked as they have no deleterious effect. However, when they are present in a more noticeable form, they not only lead to loss of esthetic qualities but they may even alter the physical properties of an alloy to such an extent that the applicance may be weakened or it may fail.

Unfortunately, the oral environment is very conducive to corrosion. The mouth is warm and moist. The foods and liquids ingested have wide ranges of $p$H, as do the acids liberated during the breakdown of foodstuffs. This food débris often adheres tenaciously to the metallic restoration, thus providing a localized condition that is extremely conducive to corrosion.

Since gold resists chemical attack very well, it was natural that this "noblest of the metals" was early employed for the construction of dental appliances.

**Tarnish and Corrosion.**     A differentiation should be made between *tarnish and corrosion*. Even though there is a definite technical difference, it is difficult clinically to differentiate between the two phenomena and the terms are often used interchangeably in the dental literature. *Tarnish* is a surface discoloration on a metal[1] or even a slight loss or alteration of the surface finish or luster. In the oral cavity tarnish usually occurs from the formation of hard and soft deposits on the surface of the restoration. Calculus is the principal hard deposit and its color varies from light yellow to brown. The longer it remains on the surface, the darker it becomes. Its color varies also with the mouth hygiene of the patient and is especially dark in the mouths of heavy smokers.[2] The soft deposits are plaques and films composed mainly of microorganisms and mucin. Stain or discoloration arises from pigment-producing bacteria,[2] drugs containing such chemicals as iron or mercury[3] and adsorbed food débris. These hard and soft deposits, and thus tarnish, may be found anywhere in the mouth but are more apt to be on surfaces that are protected from the abrasive action of foods and the toothbrush.

Although such deposits are the main cause for tarnish in the oral cavity, surface discoloration may also arise on a metal from the formation of thin films, such as oxides, sulfides, or chlorides.[1] This phenomenon may then be only a simple deposition on the surface or it may be the first step of the more serious condition of corrosion.

*Corrosion* is not merely a surface deposit but is an actual attack on the surface by some medium in contact with it.[1] This disintegration of a metal may occur through the action of moisture, atmosphere, acid or alkaline solutions and certain chemicals. Tarnish is often the forerunner of the more serious condition of corrosion. The film which is deposited and produces tarnish may in time form, or accumulate, elements or compounds which chemically attack the metallic surface. For example, eggs and certain other foods contain significant amounts of sulfur. Various sulfides, such as hydrogen or ammonium sulfide, corrode silver, copper, mercury and similar metals which are present in dental alloys and amalgam.[4] Oxygen, chlorine and acids such as phosphoric, acetic and lactic are also present at times. If they are at the optimum concentration and $pH$, corrosion can occur.

Of all these elements and compounds, sulfur is probably the most important consideration in the usual dental metallic restoration. For example, x-ray diffraction patterns of clinically tarnished amalgam restorations indicate a sulfide, with a tentative formula of $(Hg, Ag)S_x$, to be the dominant factor in discoloration with only trace amounts of chlorides and other compounds present.[4] Thus, the sulfur content of ingested foods and saliva may account for the marked corrosion often noted in the mouths of patients even where good mouth hygiene is practiced.

**Classification of Corrosion.** The exact phenomenon of corrosion is often complex and not completely understood. The less homogeneous the metal or alloy and the more complex the environment, the more complicated is the corrosion process. The composition, physical state and surface condition of the metallic material, as well as the chemical components of the surrounding medium—their phases and concentrations—determine the nature of the corrosion reactions. Other important variables affecting corrosion processes are the temperature, temperature fluctuation, movement or circulation of the medium in contact with the metal surface, and the nature and solubility of the corrosion products.[5] In spite of all these complexities, if the general mechanism of corrosion is understood, it is usually possible to recognize the controlling variables in a given instance of corrosion.

There are two general classifications of corrosion reactions. One type is so-called *chemical corrosion* in which there is a direct combination of metal and non-metallic elements. This type is exemplified by oxidation, halogenation or sulfurization reactions. A good example is the rusting of iron in the presence of oxygen, particularly if water and carbon dioxide are present.

As pointed out, in the oral cavity, sulfides, in some form are the most common cause of chemical corrosion. A direct chemical attack by acid or alkaline media is rare unless the structure is grossly inhomogeneous or certain types of surface deposits are already present.

Chemical corrosion is seldom isolated and almost invariably is accompanied by the second type of corrosion known as *electrolytic corrosion*. This type is caused by a flow of electrical current. In this reaction the corroding metal usually involves the replacement of hydrogen from water or acids.

The basis for any discussion of electrolytic corrosion is, of necessity, the *electromotive force series*. This classification is an arrangement of the elements in the order of their dissolution tendencies. The values for potential are calculated for the elements in solutions containing one atomic weight, in grams, of ions in 1000 grams of water at 25° C.[5] These standard potentials may be considered as the voltage of electrolytic cells in which one pole is the hydrogen electrode, designated arbitrarily as zero, and the other is the electrode of the element designated. The sign of the electrode potential indicates the polarity in such a cell. The series for the elements which might be useful to the dentist is seen in Table 21–1.

According to this theory, if two metals are immersed in an electrolyte and are connected by an electrical conductor, an electric couple is formed and the metal with the lowest solution potential will go into solution. The strength of the current and the direction in which it passes depend primarily upon the electrode potentials of the individual metals. A familiar example of this phenomenon is the dissolving of the zinc electrode in a voltaic cell when it is in electric contact with copper or some metal with a greater electrode potential than itself. Thus, the solution of the zinc and the corresponding disintegration of the surface is an example of the process of corrosion.

It should be empasized that the relative position of any of the elements in the series is dependent not only on the inherent solution tendencies, but also upon the effective concentration of ions of that element which are present in the environment. As the ionic concentration of the element increases in the environment, the tendency of that element to dissolve decreases. The significance of the concentration factor in determining the position of a metal in the electromotive series

*Table 21–1.*      *Electromotive Series of the Metals*

| METAL | ION | ELECTRODE POTENTIAL (VOLTS) |
|---|---|---|
| Gold | $Au^+$ | +1.50 |
| Gold | $Au^{+++}$ | +1.36 |
| Platinum | $Pt^{++}$ | +0.86 |
| Palladium | $Pd^{++}$ | +0.82 |
| Mercury | $Hg^{++}$ | +0.80 |
| Silver | $Ag^+$ | +0.80 |
| Copper | $Cu^+$ | +0.47 |
| Bismuth | $Bi^{+++}$ | +0.23 |
| Antimony | $Sb^{+++}$ | +0.10 |
| Hydrogen | $H^+$ | 0.00 |
| Lead | $Pb^{++}$ | −0.12 |
| Tin | $Sn^{++}$ | −0.14 |
| Nickel | $Ni^{++}$ | −0.23 |
| Cadmium | $Cd^{++}$ | −0.40 |
| Iron | $Fe^{++}$ | −0.44 |
| Chromium | $Cr^{++}$ | −0.56 |
| Zinc | $Zn^{++}$ | −0.76 |
| Aluminum | $Al^{+++}$ | −1.70 |
| Sodium | $Na^+$ | −2.71 |
| Calcium | $Ca^{++}$ | −2.87 |
| Potassium | $K^+$ | −2.92 |

is well illustrated again by zinc and copper. In a zinc cyanide solution, under certain circumstances, the copper actually dissolves and corrodes more readily than the zinc and it displaces zinc from the solution.

This increase in metal content in the environment may finally prevent further corrosion. Metals usually cease corroding merely because their immediate environments have become saturated with ions of the metals. Such a situation does not usually occur in dental restorations since the dissolving ions are removed by fluids and the toothbrush. Thus the corrosion continues.

**Electrolytic Corrosion.**      Since electrolytic corrosion is of the greater significance and is usually associated also with chemical corrosion, it will be discussed in greater detail and with special reference to the oral cavity.

Provided an electrolyte is present, there are four general types of electrolytic corrosion possible and all may occur to some extent in the oral cavity since saliva, with the salts which it contains, is a weak electrolyte. The electrochemical properties of saliva depend upon its composition, concentration of its components, $p$H, surface tension and buffering capacity.[6] All of these factors may influence the strength of any electrolyte and thus the magnitude of the resulting corrosion.

The first type of electrolytic corrosion is that found with combinations of *dissimilar metals*. The metallic combinations which may produce "galvanic currents" may or may not be in intermittent contact.

The effect of "galvanic shock" is well known in dentistry. For example, assume that an amalgam restoration, as discussed in the following chapters, is placed on the occlusal surface of a lower tooth directly opposing a gold inlay in an upper tooth. Since both restorations are wet with saliva, potentially an electric couple exists, with a difference in potential between them. When the two fillings are brought into contact, the potential is suddenly short-circuited through the two alloys. The result is sharp pain. A similar effect may be observed by touching the tine of a silver fork to a gold foil or inlay restoration, and at the same time allowing some other portion of the fork to come in contact with the tongue.

When the teeth are not in contact, the difference in electrical potential or electromotive force between the two fillings still exists. A circuit also exists. The saliva forms the electrolyte, and the hard and soft tissues can constitute the external circuit. The resistance of the external circuit is considerable in comparison to that which exists when the two fillings are brought into contact. The electric currents measured under these conditions between a gold and an amalgam restoration in the same mouth, but not in contact, are apparently in the neighborhood of 0.5 to 1 microampere or a corresponding electromotive force of approximately 500 millivolts.[7, 8] These currents are somewhat greater when dissimilar metals are present but they also occur between restorations of similar metals, which are never *exactly* comparable in surface composition or structure. A current of less intensity is present even in a single isolated metallic restoration. In the single restoration the cell is created between the two electrolytes, saliva and the "bone fluid."[7] The term "bone fluid" has been used to denote the dentin, soft tissue and blood which provide the means for completing the external circuit.

Although the magnitude of these currents usually diminishes somewhat as the restoration ages, it remains indefinitely at the approximate value cited. The clinical significance of these currents, other than their influence on corrosion, will be discussed later.

A second type of electrolytic corrosion is that due to the heterogeneous composition of the metal surface. A good example of this type is the eutectic alloy. It was previously stated that the corrosion resistance of a eutectic alloy is generally less than that of a solid solution. The reason should now be evident. When the eutectic alloy is immersed in an electrolyte, the metallic grains with the lower electrode potential are attacked and corrosion results. Likewise in a solid solution, any cored structure is less resistant to corrosion than the homogenized structure because of differences in electrode potential caused by segregation and variation in composition between the individual dendrites.

Solder joints may also corrode due to the inhomogeneous composition of the alloy-solder combination. In this case, corrosion is more apt to occur because of the combined effects of dissimilar metals and the difference in composition of the alloy and the solder.

Impurities in any alloy enhance corrosion. They usually collect in the grain boundary, which in itself is more easily attacked by virtue of being in an inherent stressed condition. The impurities, such as mercury contamination of gold, have different potentials from the grains themselves.

A third condition that produces electrolytic corrosion is the presence of an inhomogeneous surface structure. This type is primarily associated with a stress condition in the alloy or metal. For example, even in a pure metal not previously subjected to external forces, a certain amount of stress is always present. The grain boundaries of the pure metal are chemically attacked in preference to the grain itself because of the lattice distortion in the boundary which produces a stressed condition.

Of course, any cold working of an alloy by bending, burnishing or malleting will localize stress in some parts of the structure. A couple composed of the stressed metal, saliva, and the unstressed metal is thus formed. The stressed area is then more readily dissolved by the electrolyte. This is one of the reasons why unnecessary burnishing of the margins of gold foil restorations is contraindicated.

On most dental applicances, the deleterious effect of stress and corrosion are most apt to occur because of fatigue of the metal when associated with a corrosive environment. Repeated removal and insertion of a partial denture, for example, may build up a severe stress pattern in certain types of alloys, especially in those whose grain boundaries are sensitive to corrosion. Combined with an oral condition that would promote corrosion, the stressed appliance develops stress corrosion. Slight surface irregularities at that point, such as a notch or pit, can accelerate the process so that ordinary fatigue starts below the normal limit[9] and failure results.

The fourth type of electrolytic corrosion is called concentration cell corrosion. This situation exists whenever there are variations in the electrolytes, or in the composition of the given electrolyte, within the system. For example, there are often accumulations of food débris in the interproximal areas of the mouth, particularly if mouth hygiene is poor. This débris then produces one type of electrolyte in that area as compared to the normal saliva which provides another electrolyte at the occlusal surface. Therefore, electrolytic corrosion occurs.

A similar type of attack may be produced from differences in oxygen tension between parts of the same restoration. A cell will be produced with the greatest activity occurring around the areas containing the least oxygen. Irregularities, such as pits, contribute to this phenomenon. The areas at the bottom of the surface concavities do not have oxygen since they are covered with food débris and mucin. This area then dissolves as it corrodes, increasing the depth of the existing pits and perpetuating the deterioration. This is one of the primary reasons why a polished amalgam corrodes less than one left unpolished.[4]

Seldom are any of these four types of electrolytic corrosion found alone. Generally two or more act simultaneously and thus compound the problem. This situation can be illustrated by dissimilar metal corrosion between an inlay and an amalgam restoration. Owing to the surface changes that can occur during this type of electrolytic corrosion, differences in oxygen tension arise. At the same time if the tarnish layer is incomplete or porous, as is usually the case with dental alloys, an inhomogeneous surface results which produces new corrosion cells. Likewise, if the tarnished layer is not resistant to mouth fluids, a direct chemical attack may occur. Depending on the location of the phenomena, a concentration cell corrosion may then be initiated.

Such a situation exists when conditions remain constant. Unfortunately the oral environment is not stable due to $p$H fluctuations, oral hygiene habits, characteristics of the saliva and continual stress exerted on the restoration. All of these variables, then, accelerate the multiple corrosion processes.

**Mechanics of Corrosion.**    The actual effect of corrosion on the surface structure is essentially a slow degradation which may occur in a number of ways. It may result in an actual solubility of the alloy itself but solubility of even low carat alloys in mouth fluids is usually negligible. However, localized electrochemical dissolution can produce a metallic taste from certain dissolved ions.[10]

The attack is more apt to be interdendritic, progressing preferentially through areas around the dendrites, or intergranular, advancing along the grain boundaries.[1] Corrosion may also take place in any transgranular cracks caused by shear stress.

**Passivity.**    Certain metals develop a protective coating by oxidation, or some other chemical reaction, which protects them from further corrosion; such a metal is said to be *passive*. Practically it is a form of tarnish in which the adhering coating protects the metal underneath from further tarnish and corrosion.

Chromium is the best example of passivity. This important metal does not readily corrode because it has already corroded so rapidly and so uniformly that the film of corrosion product formed does not mar its reflectivity. It is probable that this film consists of either a continuous layer of adsorbed oxygen or closely packed chromic oxide with each molecule being oriented so that the oxygen is on the outside.[5] Iron, steel and certain other metals which are subject to corrosion may be electroplated with chromium so that they are rendered noncorrosive. The so-called "stainless steels" are alloys of steel with chromium in amounts sufficient to passivate the alloy.

Aluminum is another outstanding example of a passive metal. Aluminum has been used as a denture base material, yet it occurs below hydrogen in the electromotive series. When freshly polished, aluminum exhibits a silvery surface for a very short time only. Because of its affinity for oxygen, it tarnishes rapidly in air, to form a film which is strongly adherent. If the formation of the film is prevented by amalgamating the surface of the metal with mercury, oxidation in air occurs so rapidly as to raise the temperature of the metal, with a feathery growth of oxide occurring in the course of a few minutes.

Passive layers have been attempted on low carat gold alloys. Generally they were ineffective because they were too thin, incomplete or readily attacked by oral fluids.[10-12]

**The Dental Restoration.** It is apparent from the discussion above that the oral environment and dental structures present complex conditions that can promote corrosion and discoloration. The variables of diet, bacterial activity, drugs, smoking and oral hygiene habits unquestionably account for a great portion of the differences in corrosion often noted in different patients where the same dental alloy, handled in the same manner, was employed.

Corrosion resistance is, of course, an important consideration in the composition of the alloy itself. Unfortunately, there is no laboratory test which will duplicate oral conditions exactly and thus predict the susceptibility of the material to corrosion. Various accelerated tests involving hydrogen peroxide, egg yolk and ammonium sulfide have been advocated.[13] The most common test has been the use of a warm sulfurized oil bath. Using these various test methods, it has been shown that the precious metal content, particularly gold, influences the resistance to corrosion. Alloys with a precious metal content below 65 to 75 per cent usually tarnish.[10] For this reason, it is estimated that at least half the atoms in a dental alloy should be gold, with platinum and palladium, to insure against corrosion.[14] Certain base metal alloys, such as the chromium-cobalt alloys to be discussed in Chapter 34, are also especially resistant because of the passivity of the chromium.

In addition to proper compounding of the alloy itself, the surface condition of the restoration must be considered. Before the patient is finally dismissed, the surface of the restoration should be smooth and lustrous. This type of surface is not only desirable esthetically but will also minimize subsequent corrosion. A polished, smooth surface will provide easier cleansing and will minimize accumulation of débris. Likewise the presence of a polished surface, such as with the amalgam restoration, produces a more uniform surface which reduces the possibility of inhomogeneous surface electrolytic corrosion.

As seen earlier, notches, pits and porosity are to be avoided since they provide sources of stress and the risk of stress corrosion.

**Clinical Significance of Galvanic Currents.** The fact that small galvanic currents are continually present in the oral cavity has been proved and their influence on corrosion was discussed earlier. As long as metallic dental restorative materials are employed, there seems to be little possibility that these galvanic currents can be eliminated. The cement base itself, while it is a good thermal insulator, has little effect in minimizing the current that is carried into the tooth and through the pulp.[15] Although many of these base materials are good electrical insulators when dry, they lose this property when they become wet through marginal seepage or from moisture in the dentin. Until materials or technics are developed which will provide perfect adaptation to the cavity walls, the possibility of blocking such currents is highly unlikely. For all practical purposes, the metallic restoration cannot be isolated electrically from the tooth.

Although postoperative pain due to galvanic shock is not a common occurrence in the dental office, it can be a real source of discomfort to an occasional patient. Such postoperative pain usually occurs immediately after insertion of a new restoration and generally it gradually subsides and disappears in a few days. It has often been suggested that the reason why the pain does not last indefinitely is because of the formation of a layer of tarnish on the restoration or that the cement base, such as zinc phosphate cement, becomes a better insulator as setting progresses. However, since it has been clearly shown that these currents continue in old as well as new restorations, and since the cement base itself is not an effective insulator to electrical energy, it is more likely that the physiological condition of the tooth is the primary factor responsible for the pain resulting from this current flow. Once the tooth has responded from the injury of preparing the cavity and returned to a more normal physiologic condition, the same magnitude of current flow then produces no response.

Practically, the best method for reducing or eliminating galvanic shock seems to be the use of an external varnish painted on the surface of the restoration.[15, 16] As long as the varnish remains, the restoration is insulated from saliva and no cell is established. By the time the varnish has worn away, the tooth has usually healed sufficiently so that no pain is evidenced. In the case of the amalgam restoration, polishing of any corroded surface has also been recommended as a possible expedient.[16]

It has been suggested that these currents, or the metallic ions which are liberated from the restoration because of the galvanic current, could account for many types of dyscrasias, such as lesions, ulcers, leukoplakia, cancer and kidney disorders.[17-20] Other research, particularly a statistical analysis of 1,000 patients,[21] has failed to correlate any relationship between dissimilar metals and tissue irritation.

The effects of these currents in pathologic changes in oral, or other, tissues have possibly been exaggerated.[22, 23] The problem will remain controversial as long as there are dissimilar metals used in the mouth, but the efforts which would be necessary to resolve this issue seem not to be worthy of the time and energy required. It is the opinion of the majority of research workers in pathology and dental materials that these currents do exist, but that probably they are deleterious only from the standpoint of possible discomfort to an occasional patient. Until it can be clearly substantiated that there is a correlation between these currents and the many dyscrasias which are attributed to them, it seems logical to assume that such undiagnosed instances are related to more logical, fundamental and established factors.

On the other hand, until the situation is more definitely clarified, it would seem that the conservative procedure would be to avoid situations which might obviously produce an exaggerated condition. For example, the insertion of an amalgam restoration directly in contact with a gold inlay would seem to be contraindicated. Mercury from the amalgam will certainly alloy with the gold alloy and weaken it. A discoloration of both restorations will likely occur. Furthermore, whether it is harmful or not, a metallic taste is always present subsequent to the dental operation, and as previously stated it may persist indefinitely.

## *Literature*

1. American Society for Metals: *Metals Handbook,* Cleveland, Ohio, 1948, p. 15.
2. Stones, H. H.: *Oral and Dental Diseases,* ed. 3, E. & S. Livingstone, Ltd. London, 1954, pp. 504, 513.
3. Hepburn, W. B.: *Report on Structural and Other Changes Arising in Connection with Metals Used in the Mouth.* Trans. Sixth International Dental Congress, The Committee of Organization, London, 1914.
4. Swartz, M. L., Phillips, R. W. and El Tannir, M. D.: *Tarnish of Certain Dental Alloys.* J. D. Res., *37:*837–847 (Oct.), 1958.
5. Burns, R. M. and Bradley, W. W.: *Protection Coatings for Metals,* ed. 2, New York, Reinhold Publishing Corp., 1955, pp. 5–12.
6. Koehler, E.: *Kritische Betrachtungen ueber Messungen Elektrischer Metallpotentiale im Munde.* Deutsche Zahnaerztliche Zeitschrift, Muenchen, Karl Hanser Verlag, (Maerz), 1958, pp. 321, 324–325.
7. Schriever, W. and Diamond, L. E.: *Electromotive Forces and Electric Currents Caused by Metallic Dental Fillings.* J. D. Res., *31:*205–229 (April), 1952.
8. Reed, G. J. and Wilman, W.: *Galvanism in the Oral Cavity.* J.A.D.A., *27:*1471–1475 (Sept.), 1940.
9. Evans, U. R.: *Chemical Behaviors as Influenced by Surface Condition. Properties of Metallic Surfaces.* Institute of Metals, Grosvenor Gardens, London, 1953, p. 264.
10. Souder, W. and Paffenbarger, G. C.: *Physical Properties of Dental Materials.* National Bureau of Standards Circular C433, U. S. Government Printing Office, Washington, D. C., 1942, pp. 24–25.
11. Fischer, H., Hauffe, K. and Wiederholt, W.: *Passivierende Filme und Deckschichten.* Berlin, Springer-Verlag, 1956, p. 300.
12. Schoonover, I. C. and Souder, W.: *Corrosion of Dental Alloys.* J.A.D.A., *28:*1278–1291 (Aug.), 1941.
13. Souder, W.: *Standards for Dental Materials.* J.A.D.A., *22:*1873–1878 (Nov.), 1935.
14. Lane, J. R.: *Survey of Dental Alloys.* J.A.D.A., *39:*421–428 (Oct.), 1949.
15. Phillips, L. J., Phillips, R. W. and Schnell, R. J.: *Measurement of the Electric Conductivity of Dental Cement.* J. D. Res., *34:*839–848 (Dec.), 1955.

16. Nachlin, J. J.: *A Type of Pain Associated with the Restoration of Teeth with Amalgam.* J.A.D.A., *48:*284–293 (March), 1954.
17. Lain, E. S. and Caughron, G. S.: *Electrogalvanic Phenomena of the Oral Cavity Caused by Dissimilar Metallic Restorations.* J.A.D.A., *23:*1641–1652 (Sept.), 1936.
18. Bloodgood, J. C.: *Precancerous Lesions of the Oral Cavity.* J.A.D.A., *16:*1353–1367 (Aug.), 1929.
19. Roome, N. W. and Dahlberg, A. A.: *Electrochemical Ulcer of the Buccal Mucosa: Report of a Case.* J.A.D.A., *23:*1652–1654 (Sept.), 1936.
20. Schell, J. S.: *Galvanic Action of Metals in the Mouth,* J. South. California D. A., *21:*24–26 (Oct.), 1953.
21. Mills, R. B.: *Study of Incidence of Irritation in Mouths Having Teeth Filled with Dissimilar Metals.* Northwestern Univ. Bull., *39:*18–22 (Oct.), 1939.
22. Phillips, R. W.: *An Evaluation of the Problem of Galvanic Currents in the Oral Cavity.* J. Indiana D. A., *37:*8–11 (Jan.), 1958.
23. Loebich, O.: *Unter welchen Umstaenden koennen Metalle im Munde schaedlich sein?* Zahnaerztliche Mitteilungen, No. 6 and 7, vom 15, (April), 1955.

# CHAPTER 22

# Dental Amalgam Alloys.

# Metallography of Amalgam

An amalgam is a special type of alloy in that one of its constituents is mercury. Inasmuch as mercury is liquid, or "molten," at room temperature, its alloying with other metals can be accomplished with the latter in the solid state. This process of alloying is known as *amalgamation*.

Mercury will combine with many metals, but the amalgamation of dental interest is a union with a silver-tin alloy, usually containing a small amount of copper and zinc. This alloy is technically known as the *dental amalgam alloy*.

The amalgam alloy is usually dispensed to the dentist in powder-like filings removed from a cast ingot by a metal cutting tool. In some instances, the filings are pre-weighed and placed in small plastic packets. Another method is to press a certain weight of filings into pellets or "pills." In this latter case, the fine alloy particles are subjected to sufficient pressure to cause them to form a "skin" over the outside and to cohere slightly on the inside, yet the cohesion is not so great that the particles cannot be readily separated when they are amalgamated.

**Dental Amalgam.** The silver-tin-mercury amalgam is used for the restoration of lost tooth structure more than any other dental material. It is estimated that 80 per cent of all restorations are of this amalgam.

The amalgam alloy is mixed with mercury by the dentist, usually in a mortar and pestle. The mixing procedure is technically known as *trituration*. The product of the trituration is a plastic mass similar to that which occurs in the melt of any alloy at temperatures between the liquidus and solidus. The plastic mass is forced into the prepared cavity by a process known as *condensation.* The complete technic will be discussed in detail in a subsequent chapter.

After the condensation, certain metallographic changes take place and new phases appear. These new phases are characterized by solidification temperatures well above any temperature which might occur in the mouth under any conditions. The production of the new phases brings about the *setting* or the *hardening* of the amalgam. The reactions between metals at these low temperatures are unique from a chemical and metallurgical standpoint.

**The Clinical Restoration.** Amalgam is an excellent tooth restorative material. It has been observed[1] that not only is amalgam the most frequently used material in restorative dentistry but also that there is a lower percentage of failure of restorations made with amalgam than with any of the other restorative materials.

One of the reasons for this excellent clinical record may be the tendency of the amalgam restoration to minimize marginal leakage. It has been frequently pointed out in other chapters that one of the greatest hazards of the clinical restoration is the leakage that may occur between the cavity walls and the restoration. No restorative material truly adheres to the tooth structure, consequently penetration of fluids and débris around the margins may be the greatest cause for recurrence of caries and failure.[2, 3, 4]

Amalgam is unique in this respect. Apparently, if the restoration is properly inserted, the leakage becomes less as the restoration ages in the mouth. As seen in Figure 22–1, restorations[4] which have been in service one, two and six months show less penetration of a labeled radioactive isotope than those which are only 48 hours old. The reason for this reduction in leakage may be due to a deposition in this space of corrosion products from the amalgam. At any rate, the reduced leakage may be the significant characteristic which accounts for the optimum clinical results experienced with this material.

However, daily observations in the dental office do reveal many amalgam failures.[5, 6] They are evidenced generally in four ways: (1) by recurrent caries, (2) by fracture, (3) by dimensional change and (4) by excessive tarnish and corrosion.

Since the adoption of an American Dental Association Specification for amalgam, few inferior dental alloys are now marketed, consequently these observed failures may be attributed to factors other than the material itself. Success is dependent upon control of, and attention to, many variables. Each manipulative step from the time the cavity is prepared until the restoration has been polished has a very definite effect upon the physical and chemical properties and the success or failure of the restoration.

The greatest single factor which contributes to recurrence of caries

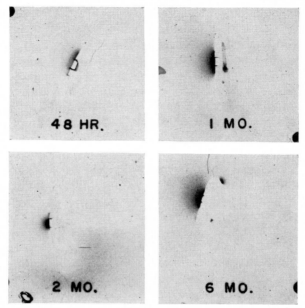

Fig. 22–1. Penetration of Ca⁴⁵ around amalgam restorations which have been in the oral cavity for various periods of time as shown. At the end of 48 hours, complete penetration occurred, but as the restoration aged, the penetration became less.

and/or fracture is, of course, improper cavity preparation. One clinical survey[5] has shown that at least 56 per cent of all amalgam failures may be attributed to violation of the fundamental principles of amalgam cavity preparation,[6, 7] i.e., insufficient provision for bulk, inadequate retentive form and failure to extend the margins to relatively immune areas. Forty per cent of all failures were attributed to faulty manipulation of the amalgam or its contamination at the time of insertion. It is with this 40 per cent that the following discussions will be concerned.

**Physical Properties.** The properties which are most important and which govern the service life of the amalgam restoration are its dimensional stability, strength and flow.

Most metals shrink during solidification. A dental amalgam can either shrink or expand during its solidification, depending upon its composition. The composition of the amalgam alloy is of importance in this connection, and it is determined by the manufacturer. However, the manipulation by the dentist determines the final composition of the amalgam. An inferior amalgam can be produced from the best amalgam alloy if the dentist has not executed the trituration and condensation properly. It is most important that the dentist understand the fundamental principles involved and their effect on the physical properties if the amalgam restoration is to be satisfactory.

The strength of a dental amalgam is generally measured under compression, although under certain conditions its tensile strength may be even more important. Under the best of conditions, the amalgam will flow or "creep" under a comparatively light load, less than its proportional limit. Such a flow may be due to its lack of ability to strain harden. Both the flow and the strength are affected considerably by the composition of the amalgam, and these properties are also under the control of the dentist to a large extent.

**Silver-Tin System.** Since the essential metal components of the alloy are silver and tin, an examination of the constitution diagram for silver and tin is helpful to an understanding of the subsequent reactions. Such a diagram is presented[8] in Figure 22–2.

Although the diagram appears to be somewhat complicated, its interpretation is quite simple.[9] The solidus is represented by the line *ABMCDFEGS*, and the liquidus coincides with the line *AKLES*. It is evident that a eutectic forms at *E*. A cored structure will be present upon rapid cooling, regardless of the composition. This fact is evidenced by the comparatively large solidification range of the alloys, together with the presence of a eutectic in alloys containing more than 27 per cent of tin. If the tin composition of the alloy is greater than that of the eutectic, the structure will consist of a core of tin and a matrix of the eutectic. If the tin composition is less than this, but greater than the composition indicated at *R*, the matrix will also be the eutectic, but an understanding of the structure of the core requires further explanation.

For compositions of tin less than the composition at *R*, the diagram resembles that for the $\alpha$-solid solution of silver and copper (Fig. 20–9), except that more solid-solubility lines are present. Let the alloy compo-

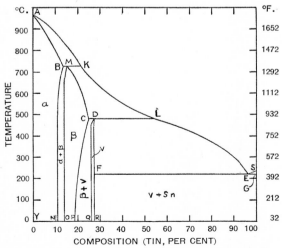

Fig. 22–2. Constitution diagram of the silver-tin alloys.

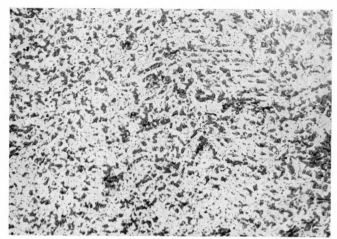

Fig. 22–3. Photomicrograph of the Ag₃Sn phase as cast. ×75. (Courtesy of G. Ryge, Marquette University.)

sitions between *Y* and *N* in Figure 22–2 be considered first. The alloys of this composition solidify along the solidus *AB* to form the *α*-solid solution of silver and tin in which the silver is the solvent. These alloys are solid in the area *ABNY*. The area *ABMK* represents the melt containing a liquid phase of molten metal and solidified *α*-solid solution. At the temperature corresponding to the line *BK* (approximately 725° C.) the *α*-solid solution reacts with the liquid metal to produce a second type of solid solution, with silver as the solvent, known as the *β*-solid solution. The *β*-solid solution crystallizes along the solidus *MC*, and is solid in the area *OMCP*. The transition from the *α*-solution to the *β*-solution is not abrupt, and in the area *NBMO* they exist simultaneously.

The *β*-phase, upon cooling to the temperature indicated by the line *CDL,* reacts with the liquid that is left to form the *γ*-phase, which is solid in the area *QDFR*. Both the *β*- and *γ*-phases are present in the area *PCDQ*.

**Ag₃Sn.** By far the most important constitutent of the silver-tin system, from a dental standpoint, is the *γ*-phase, which has been identified as the intermetallic compound, Ag₃Sn. The composition (by weight) of this phase has been determined[8] as silver, 73.15 per cent, and tin, 26.83 per cent.

A photomicrograph of this constituent is shown in Figure 22–3, obtained from an ingot cooled rapidly. The cored structure is evident. After the alloy has been homogenized at 425° C. (800° F.) for 24 hours, a homogeneous and essentially single-phase structure[10] appears as in Figure 22–4.

If the silver content is increased, so that the *β*-solid solution is present (Fig. 22–2), the amalgam is likely to expand abnormally during hardening. If the silver content is decreased so that the eutectic is present, a contraction of the amalgam results. Actually, the tin content is probably more important than is the silver content so far as the effect on the dimensional stability of the amalgam is concerned. If the tin content is not less than 25 per cent or more than 27 per cent, a very slight expansion of the amalgam can be expected during hardening. A slight expansion of an amalgam restoration during hardening is generally considered to be preferable to a contraction.

As will be noted in the next section, most of the commercial amalgam alloys contain a small amount of copper. The copper presumably replaces the silver in $Ag_3Sn$[11, 12] to form $Cu_3Sn$.

**Composition of Amalgam Alloys.** Modern amalgam alloys which produce dental amalgam restorations with acceptable physical properties are very nearly the same in composition. As previously noted, the amalgam generally contracts when the silver content of the alloy is much below 73 per cent. Usually copper and often zinc are added to the modern alloy in small amount to replace the silver.

The composition range of 51 successful American amalgam alloys has been found to be silver, 67 to 70 per cent, tin, 25.3 to 27.7 per cent, copper 0 to 5.2 per cent, and zinc, 0 to 1.7 per cent.[13] A similar survey in England of 56 amalgam alloys with properties similar to those of the American alloys showed a composition range of silver 67 to 70 per cent, tin, 25 to 29 per cent, copper, 0 to 5.8 per cent, and zinc 0 to 2.0 per cent.[14] It can be seen, therefore, that the limits of the tin content and the silver (plus copper and zinc) content are fairly well confined to the theoretical limits of the $\gamma$-phase as indicated in Figure 22–2.

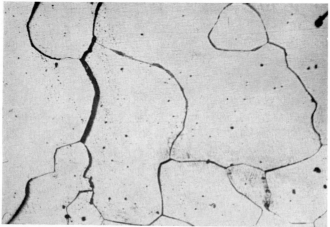

Fig. 22–4.  Same alloy as in Figure 22–3 after homogenizing at 425° C. for 24 hours. ×75. (Courtesy of G. Ryge, Marquette University.)

***Contributions of the Alloy Constituents.***        Silver, the principal constituent, increases the strength of the amalgam and it decreases the flow. Its general effect is to increase the expansion of the amalgam, and, if it is present in excess, the expansion may be excessive. The silver contributes to the resistance of the amalgam to tarnish. In the presence of the tin, it also accelerates the time required for the amalgam to harden.

As previously noted, if the silver content is too low, or if the tin content is too high, a contraction of the amalgam occurs. The tin appears to reduce the expansion or to increase the contraction of the amalgam, and also it reduces the strength and hardness. It increases the length of the hardening time. An advantageous contribution of the tin is to render the amalgamation of the alloy easier because of its affinity for mercury, which is greater than that of either silver or copper.

Copper is added in small amount in replacement of the silver. It tends to increase the expansion of the amalgam in combination with silver. However, if more than approximately 5 per cent of copper is used, an excessive amount of expansion may take place.[15] In addition, the incorporation of copper increases the strength and hardness of the amalgam, and reduces the flow. It also appears to render the amalgam less critical to unavoidable variations in manipulation by the dentist.

The use of zinc in an amalgam alloy is often a subject of controversy. It is seldom present in an alloy to an extent greater than 1 per cent, and in such small quantities it probably exerts only a slight influence on the strength and flow of the amalgam. However, it does contribute to the workability and cleanliness of the amalgam during the trituration and the condensation.

Unfortunately, the zinc, even in small amounts, causes an abnormal expansion of the amalgam in the presence of moisture. Many years ago, it was observed: "Experiments in watching fillings for five years show that one-half of 1 per cent zinc is inadvisable for the reason that the amalgam will continue to change bulk very slowly for that time and perhaps much longer. Though this change is not large, it will finally destroy the usefulness of the filling."[16]

The zinc was first introduced into the alloy to provide a clean ingot after the original fusion of the alloy constituents. The zinc acts as a scavenger in that during fusion it will unite with oxygen and certain other impurities present, and thus the formation of oxides, particularly with tin, is avoided. However, with proper care during the melting procedure, it is possible to make a sound non-zinc alloy. Certainly, zinc is not theoretically essential to the amalgam alloy.

***Manufacture of the Alloy.***        Once an acceptable formula for an alloy has been found, there are a number of factors which must be controlled by the manufacturer.

It is, of course, imperative that metals of complete purity be used.

Furthermore, the metals must be alloyed without oxidation or the incorporation of impurities of any kind.

The same precautions should be observed in the casting of the ingot. The ingot is usually cast in the form of a cylinder, which is comminuted into filings with the proper tools. The filings are then heat treated as described in the next section.

As previously shown, the composition differences in the alloys are small. The difference observed in various commercial amalgam alloys as they are received by the dentist are related almost entirely to the manufacturing process, such as the care during manufacture, the size and shape of the filings, the heat treatments employed, and similar factors. Such a manufacturing process is precise and exacting, and a good product merits the respect of the dentist in its subsequent manipulation.

**Aging of Amalgam Alloys.** Many years ago, it was discovered[17] that freshly cut filings amalgamated much faster, with more mercury required for the amalgamation, than did filings which had been aged at room temperature for several months. It was also found that the same aging effect could be attained by annealing the filings for 30 minutes in boiling water.

Furthermore, it was discovered that the amalgams made with the unaged filings expanded considerably during hardening, whereas the amalgams made with the filings which had been aged on the shelf or annealed either expanded very little, or else they contracted.

It is customary to heat treat or to anneal the filings so that a proper dimensional change and other desirable properties of the amalgam are attained, and, at the same time, to establish a more stable condition that will not change with time. The heat treatment consists of subjecting the filings to a given temperature for a given time, and the process is called *aging*. Aging of the alloy also results in a stronger amalgam with less flow.

Although the effect of aging appears to be connected with the strain hardening of the alloy during the cutting of the filings, it has never been explained. That it is probably related to the strain hardening of the filings is shown by the fact that the affinity of aged filings for mercury can be increased by a strain hardening process.

The effect is also connected with the $Ag_3Sn$ structure of the alloy. For example, the more silver added to the alloy so that the $\beta$-solid solution is present, the less pronounced the aging effect is.

The proper aging of the alloy is an important part of the manufacturing process. An aging procedure should be selected so that the dimensional change of the amalgam will meet the requirements of the American Dental Association Specification No. 1, and yet so that the filings will not age further during storage to produce finally an amalgam which shrinks during hardening. Unless it is definitely known that a certain commercial brand of amalgam alloy has been fully aged, it is best that not more than a three-month supply be kept on hand by the dentist, particularly during the summer months.

**Homogenization.** As can be noted from Figure 22–3, a considerable coring of the alloy ingot is present unless it is homogenized as shown in Figure 22–4. An amalgam made from filings cut from a homogenized ingot differs in certain respects from an amalgam made with filings from an "as cast" ingot of the same composition. The differences with the homogenized filings have been found to be as follows: [18, 19]

1. There is less tendency for the amalgam to expand excessively when it is made with unaged filings. After the filings have been aged, the amalgam exhibits a greater tendency to contract.

2. Less mercury is required for the trituration.

3. Slightly less mercury is retained in the hardened amalgam after the condensation.

4. The amalgam exhibits a greater cohesiveness during condensation.

5. The properties of the hardened amalgam are less affected by variations in the technic.

6. The flow of the amalgam is less, and it exhibits a slightly lower Brinell hardness number.

It will be shown that most of the above factors, with the possible exception of the first, tend to improve the properties of the amalgam restoration.

**Particle Size.** Very likely, the greatest single difference between the various amalgam alloys available to the dentist is in their particle size and shape. The size and shape of the particle is determined by the method of cutting. The alloy ingot is brittle, owing to the $Ag_3Sn$ present, and the filings are apt to be fine, irregular flakes of metal, rather than shavings such as were obtained with the high tin content alloys used 30 to 50 years ago. The size of the particles depends upon the type of cutting tool, the pressure and the rate of feed, as in any metal cutting operation.

The "fine cut" particles shown in Figure 22–5 are definitely smaller than the "coarse cut" particles in Figure 22–6. The particles shown in Figure 22–5 are typical in size but not necessarily in shape. The particles have been treated in a ball mill, and the jagged edges seen on the particles in Figure 22–6 have been rounded off.

In spite of the fact that the particle sizes of the two alloys are so different, dental amalgams of comparable physical properties can be made from either of them. The particle size shown in Figure 22–6 will undoubtedly be comminuted to a smaller size during trituration. Such will likely not be the case with the alloy particles in Figure 22–5, to the same extent at least, since it can be expected that the smoother, smaller particles will be more likely to roll than to be fractured during trituration.

The present trend in amalgam technic appears to favor the use of a small particle size, whether it is the result of the manufacturing or the mixing process.[20-22] Other factors being equal, a smaller particle size tends to produce a more rapid hardening of the amalgam with a greater strength, than do the larger alloy particles.[23] Another objection to the use of a large particle size is that the final mixture of mercury and alloy is apt to lack smoothness, and, as a result, it is possibly more difficult to adapt the amalgam to the cavity walls during the condensation. Furthermore, since the bulk of the finished restoration is composed of particles of the original alloy surrounded by mercury, mercury-tin and mercury-silver phases, the original grain size alters the character of the finished surface.

When the material is partially hardened, the tooth anatomy is

Fig. 22–5.

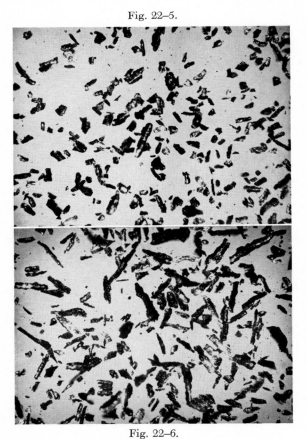

Fig. 22–6.

Fig. 22–5. Alloy particles of a "fine cut" alloy. ×90.
Fig. 22–6. Alloy particles of a "coarse cut" alloy. ×90.

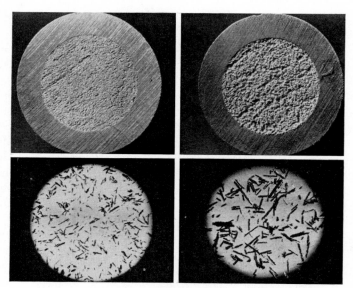

Fig. 22–7. A comparison of the carved surfaces of two dental amalgams made from fine and coarse particle sizes respectively, as shown in the photomicrographs.

carved into the amalgam with a sharp instrument. When an alloy with a large particle size has been used, the filings are apt to be pulled out of the matrix, and the surface of the restoration is roughened. This effect is illustrated in Figure 22–7. The fine particles shown in the photomicrograph (lower left) were amalgamated and condensed into a circular mold. When the surface was carved, a smoother surface resulted than when the surface of an amalgam made from the coarse particles shown at the lower right was similarly treated.[22] It seems logical that the smoother surface produced from the small grain alloy would be less susceptible to tarnish and corrosion in the mouth than would the rougher surface even though both surfaces were subsequently polished.

**Metallography of Amalgam.**     Although a constitution diagram for the silver-tin-mercury system in the region of dental interest is fairly well established,[11] there are a number of important metallographic factors which are a matter of controversy. A complete discussion of the controversial considerations can be found in the literature.[10, 11, 24–26]

The following description is based as much as possible upon fully accepted theories, and it will suffice for the present needs.

The essential component of the silver-tin alloy which enters into the reaction with mercury is the $Ag_3Sn$ ($\gamma$) phase. Any $\beta$-solid solution which may be present only enhances the reactions.

When the alloy is mixed with mercury during trituration, the $Ag_3Sn$ compound dissolves or absorbs mercury, and two crystalline phases result, known as $\gamma_1$ and $\gamma_2$.

The $\gamma_1$ begins to crystallize first.[10] It has been identified[26] as an inter-metallic compound with the formula $Ag_2Hg_3$.

Although the crystals of the $\gamma_2$-phase appear a short time after those of the $\gamma_1$, its rate of growth is more rapid. This phase consists of tin and mercury combined in a hexagonal space lattice.[10] According to some authorities, its composition is $Sn_7Hg$.[24] Actually, the amount of crystallization of both phases will depend upon the amount of mercury present. A reduction of the available mercury present for the reactions causes a greater decrease in the formation of the $\gamma_2$-phase than the $\gamma_1$-phase.

As the crystallization of the $\gamma_1$- and $\gamma_2$-phases proceeds, more of the mercury is dissolved by the $Ag_3Sn$. Presumably, as the $\gamma_1$- and $\gamma_2$-phases form around the alloy particle, they are rubbed off by the trituration process, and further solution of the mercury by the $Ag_3Sn$ phase occurs, and so on. Eventually, there may be insufficient mercury present for the reaction to proceed further, and the crystallization of the $\gamma_1$- and $\gamma_2$-phases terminates. There will remain a certain amount of free mercury, or, more likely, solution of mercury in the $Ag_3Sn$, and it is thought that a third phase may form[11, 24] by a reaction between the solution phase and the remaining $Ag_3Sn$ phase. According to the available evidence,[11] this new phase is a solid solution of mercury in $AgSn_3$, known as $\beta_1$.

The period when the greatest dimensional changes occur in the

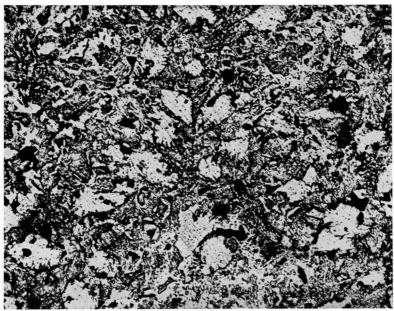

Fig. 22–8. Microstructure of a hardened amalgam. $\times 500$. (Smith, Ferguson and Schoonover, *J.A.D.A.*, Sept., 1953.)

hardening of the amalgam system also coincides with the disappearance of the uncombined mercury.[27] X-ray diffraction studies[28] fail to reveal any uncombined mercury in hardened amalgam below a temperature of 65° C. (149° F.) after this period. The mercury is apparently completely in combination with the other phases present at this stage. These observations, as well as the determination of the phases formed, are also substantiated with measurements of the electrical conductivity during the hardening of the amalgam.[29] The conductivity is markedly influenced by the alloy composition and by the residual mercury content.

Complete equilibrium is probably not attained in practice. Unless an extremely small particle size of alloy is used, some of the alloy particles will be left to form a core. Such a cored structure can be seen in Figure 22–8. The core, or undissolved particles, are surrounded by a matrix which, according to the theory presented, consists of $\gamma_1$, $\gamma_2$, and possibly some $\beta_1$.

## *Literature*

1. Brekhus, P. J. and Armstrong, W. D.: *Civilization—a Disease.* J.A.D.A., *23:*1459–1469 (Aug.), 1936.
2. Hirsch, L. and Weinrab, M. M.: *Marginal Fit of Direct Acrylic Restorations.* J.A.D.A., *56:*13–21 (Jan.), 1958.
3. Nelson, R. J., Wolcott, R. B. and Paffenbarger, G. C.: *Fluid Exchange at the Margins of Dental Restorations.* J.A.D.A., *44:*288–295 (Mar.), 1952.
4. Phillips, R. W., Gilmore, H. W., Swartz, M. L. and Schenker, S. I.: *Adaptation of in Vivo Restorations as Assessed by $Ca^{45}$.* Paper read before Dental Materials Group, 37th Annual meeting of the I.A.D.R., San Francisco, Calif., March, 1959.
5. Healey, H. J. and Phillips, R. W.: *A Clinical Study of Amalgam Failures.* J. D. Res., *28:*439–446 (Oct.), 1949.
6. Wolcott, R. B.: *Failures in Dental Amalgam.* J.A.D.A., *56:*479–491 (April), 1958.
7. Miller, E. C.: *Technique for Building Amalgam Restorations.* J. Pros. Den., *9:*652–667 (July), 1959.
8. Murphy, H. A.: *The Constitution of the Alloys of Silver and Tin.* J. Inst. Metals, *35:*107 (Jan.), 1926.
9. Smith, J. C.: *The Chemistry and Metallurgy of Dental Materials.* Oxford, Blackwell Scientific Publications, 1949, Chapter XIV.
10. Ryge, G., Moffett, J. C. and Barkow, A. G.: *Microstructural Observations and X-ray Diffraction Studies of Silver-tin Amalgams.* J. D. Res., *32:*152–167 (April), 1953.
11. Gayler, M. L. V.: *Dental Amalgams.* J. Inst. Metals, *60:*407–419, 1937.
12. Crowell, W. S.: *The Metallography of Dental Amalgam Alloys.* J. D. Res., *33:*592–595 (Oct.), 1954.
13. Souder, W. and Paffenbarger, G. C.: *Physical Properties of Dental Materials.* National Bureau of Standards Circular C433, Washington, U. S. Government Printing Office, 1942, p. 3.
14. Harvey, W.: *Some Recent Research into Dental Amalgams at the R. A. F. Institute of Aviation Medicine, Farnborough, Hants.* Brit. D. J., *81:*245–255 (Oct. 18), 1946.
15. Gayler, M. L. V.: *The Setting of Dental Amalgams, Part II.* Brit. D. J., *58:*145–160 (Feb. 15), 1935.
16. Black, G. V.: *Operative Dentistry.* Vol. II, ed. 6, Chicago, Medico-Dental Publishing Company, 1924, p. 308.

17. Black, G. V.: *Physical Characters of the Human Teeth.* Dent. Cos., *37:*553–571 (July); 637–661 (Aug.), 1895.

18. Worner, H. K. and Anderson, J. S.: *The Influence of Some Manufacturing Variables on the Properties of Dental Amalgams.* Austral. J. Den., *43:*269–287 (Aug.); 1939.

19. Strader, K. H.: *Amalgam Alloy: Its Heat Treatment, Flow, Mercury Content and Distribution of Dimensional Change.* J.A.D.A., *38:*602–608 (May), 1949.

20. Smith, E. A.: *Particle Size of Dental Amalgam Alloys.* Brit. D. J., *86:*34–41 (Jan.), 1949.

21. Mosteller, J. H.: *An Evaluation of the A.D.A. Specification for Amalgam Alloy in Relation to Particle Size.* Ann. Den., *12:*19–24 (March), 1953.

22. Phillips, R. W.: *Research on Dental Amalgam and Its Application in Practice.* J.A.D.A., *54:*309–318 (March), 1957.

23. Crowell, W. S. and Phillips, R. W.: *Physical Properties of Amalgam as Influenced by Variations in Surface Area of the Alloy Particles.* J. D. Res., *30:*845–853 (Dec.), 1951.

24. Troiano, A. R.: *An X-ray Study of Dental Amalgams.* J. Inst. Metals, *63:*247–259 (Aug.), 1938.

25. Gray, A. W.: *Volume Changes in Amalgams.* J. Inst. Metals, *29:*139–189, 1923.

26. Frankel, C. B. and Fankuchen, I.: *An Investigation of the Chemistry of Dental Amalgam by Roentgen Ray Diffraction.* J.A.D.A., *44:*542–552 (May), 1952.

27. Mitchell, J. A., Schoonover, I. C.; Dickson, G. and Vachec, H. C.: *Some Factors Affecting the Dimensional Stability of the Ag-Sn-(Cu-Zn) Amalgams.* J. D. Res., *34:*273–286 (April), 1955.

28. Mitchell, J. A., Dickson, G. and Schoonover, I. C.: *X-ray Diffraction Studies of Mercury Diffusion and Surface Stability of Dental Amalgam.* J. D. Res., *34:* 744 (Oct.), 1955. Abstract.

29. Schnell, R. J.: *Resistivity of Silver-tin Amalgams.* Master's thesis, Indiana University School of Dentistry, 1958.

# CHAPTER 23

# Dental Amalgam:

# Dimensional Change.

# Strength. Flow

The importance of the manipulation by the dentist to the composition and physical properties of the amalgam was repeatedly emphasized in the preceding chapter. It will be shown in this chapter how and why these factors affect the important physical properties of dimensional change, strength and flow.

## DIMENSIONAL CHANGE

It is generally conceded for testing purposes that an amalgam should expand slightly during hardening.[1] Various limits of expansion have been proposed as acceptable. The present accepted limits appear to be that the dimensional change should not be less than zero nor more than 20 microns per centimeter of length (0.20 per cent) during the first 24-hour period.

**Measurement.** A cylindrical specimen 10 millimeters in length and 5 millimeters in diameter is generally used for the measurement of dimensional change. It is considered that this bulk of amalgam is comparable to that used in a large dental restoration.

In order to measure such small dimensions with sufficient accuracy, a measuring instrument should be used which is capable of accurate measurement to at least 0.5 micron (0.00002 inch). When it is realized that 0.5 micron is approximately comparable to one-eightieth the diameter of a human hair, it is evident that the precision of the measuring instrument must be beyond that of any ordinary micrometer or similar device.

There are several types of measuring instruments which are adequate for the measurement of such dimensional change. Probably the most widely used instrument for this purpose is the dental interferometer and viewing device,[2] shown in Figure 23–1.

The viewing device is essentially a telescope. A discharge tube is used for a source of light, and usually the yellow line of helium, 0.5876 micron, is used. The discharge tube can be seen in Figure 23–1, connected to the high tension wires. The light is collimated and then reflected to the interferometer by a prism situated in the housing at the left end of the viewing device. The returning light beam is focused by the eyepiece at the right end of the viewing device. A light filter is

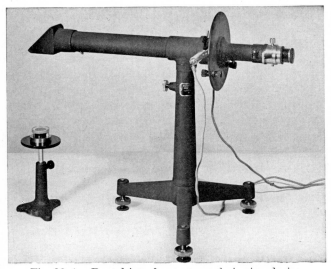

Fig. 23–1. Dental interferometer and viewing device.

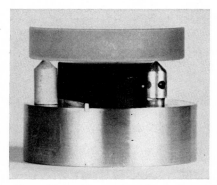

Fig. 23–2. Dental interferometer with amalgam specimen.

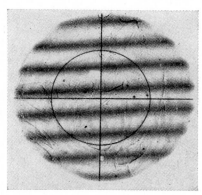

Fig. 23–3. A fringe pattern as seen in the dental interferometer. (Souder and Paffen-barger, *National Bureau of Standards Circular C433.*)

placed in the optical path at some point, in order to provide a mono-chromatic light beam.

The interferometer is shown in detail in Figure 23–2. It consists of two optically flat glass or quartz plates which are placed one above the other, the top plate being supported at three points. One of the sup-ports is the specimen of dental amalgam, which can be seen at the left, under the top plate, in Figure 23–2. The other two supports are posts constructed of invar.

If the plates are placed at a small angle with each other, a parallel, monochromatic light beam is partially reflected from the lower surface of the upper plate and from the top surface of the lower plate. Inter-ference fringes are thus formed at the lower surface of the upper plate, and they appear in the telescope of the viewing device as shown in Figure 23–3.

According to the optics of the system, the greater the angle between the two plates, the more fringes will appear, and vice versa. Since the amalgam forms one of the supports for the upper plate (Fig. 23–2), any change in the dimensions of the amalgam specimen will result in a change in the number of fringes observed in the telescope. The number of fringes present initially can be counted along the vertical line, inside the circle (Fig. 23–3).* As the amalgam specimen changes in dimen-sion, all subsequent countings can be compared with the fiducial read-ing, and the value for the expansion or contraction can be computed mathematically in microns from the constant of the instrument.

The accuracy of the instrument is within ±0.2 micron (0.00001 inch), provided that the dimensional change is not too great. A typical dimensional change curve for an amalgam, observed for a period of twenty-four hours, is shown in Figure 23–4. A short contrac-

* For example, the number of light fringes in Figure 23–3 can be estimated as 4.2 (3 whole fringes plus 0.8 of the top fringe and 0.4 of the bottom fringe).

tion can be noted, followed by an expansion to a maximum. Subsequently, a small contraction may take place for a few hours. When an amalgam has been properly manipulated, no dimensional change of consequence occurs after the first 8 to 12 hours following the condensation.

**Theory of Dimensional Change.** There can be no doubt of the fact that the composition and constitution of the amalgam affect its dimensional change during hardening. It was pointed out in the previous chapter that the most desirable composition for the amalgam alloy is that of the $\gamma$-phase ($Ag_3Sn$). Referring to Figure 22–2, if too much of the $\beta$-phase is present, an excessive expansion will occur, and if free tin is present, a contraction will occur. As previously mentioned, a slight expansion of the amalgam in the tooth is generally considered to be preferable to a contraction.

Such considerations of amalgam alloy composition apply directly to the dimensional change of the amalgam only if the proper components of the silver-tin-mercury system have been produced in proper proportion. In other words, it is entirely possible that a shrinking amalgam can result from an improper trituration and condensation of an amalgam alloy with the proper composition. The phases present in the amalgam restoration are directly related to every detail of its manipulation by the dentist from the proportioning of the alloy and mercury to the condensation.

It is possible to explain the entire curve for dimensional change shown in Figure 23–4 by means of the metallographic changes in the amalgam during hardening, as outlined in the previous chapter. In order for any reaction to take place, the mercury is absorbed by the filings, and a contraction takes place because of the resulting decrease in volume.[3, 4]

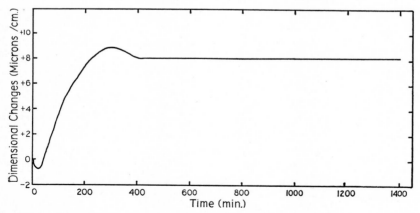

Fig. 23–4. Dimensional change of an amalgam during the first twenty-four hour period after condensation.

The next step is the formation of $\gamma_1$ and $\gamma_2$. When these phases crystallize, they presumably grow in dendritic formation. As the dendrites meet during their crystallization, they exert a certain pressure on each other, and the resultant force is an outward thrust, which results in an expansion (*cf.* the cause of setting expansion of plaster, page 41).

Consequently, any manipulation of the amalgam which increases the amount of solution and decreases the production of $\gamma_1$ and $\gamma_2$ will favor a decreased expansion or a contraction of the amalgam. On the other hand, any manipulation which favors the formation of $\gamma_1$ and $\gamma_2$ will result in increased expansion.

Although the solution of the mercury in $Ag_3Sn$ is considered to take place mainly during the trituration, the disturbance of the mercury-alloy mixture is continued through the condensation, and its termination is indicated by the initial contraction shown in the curve (Fig. 23–4). The contraction is impeded to some extent during this period by the density of the amalgam after condensation. The unreacted alloy particles may actually be touching one another in various areas, and thus a framework may be formed which tends to resist the contraction.[5]

In any event, the crystal growth of $\gamma_1$ and $\gamma_2$ soon nullifies the contraction; an expansion begins and continues for several hours, or until the crystallization is complete. The third phase, $\beta_1$, is then formed. Since the specific gravity of the $\beta_1$ is greater than that of the other phases, a contraction ensues. Since the $\beta_1$ is formed in a comparatively small amount, the final contraction is not great.

All of the variables associated with the manipulation of amalgam determine the final dimensional change in the hardened restoration.[6] However, complete control of these variables by the dentist is impossible. In fact, even in the laboratory, control of these variables to assure uniform and reproducible results is very difficult.

**Effect of the Alloy-Mercury Ratio.** Although the proper alloy-mercury ratio is probably of greater importance in connection with the strength of the amalgam, it also has an effect upon dimensional change. The more mercury that is mixed with the alloy, the greater will be the amount retained in the amalgam,[7, 8] in spite of the fact that one of the objectives of the condensation is to remove a considerable portion of the free mercury.

Since the magnitude of the expansion depends upon the amount of the $\gamma_1$ and $\gamma_2$ phases formed after condensation, it follows that the more free mercury retained in the amalgam, the greater will be the amount of these phases formed. Also the presence of the free mercury weakens the amalgam. Actually, the effect of the free mercury on the strength may be of greater clinical significance than its effect on the dimensional change in certain circumstances. Consequently, the alloy and mercury should be proportioned carefully, by weight, according to the directions of the manufacturer.

***Effect of Trituration.*** Two factors are involved in the trituration of amalgam, both of which exert a pronounced effect upon the dimensional change of an amalgam. The effect of the pestle pressure in breaking up the alloy particles has already been discussed. It will be shown in a subsequent section that the particle size of the alloy exerts a definite influence on the dimensional change.

The other factor involved is the time of trituration. The longer the time of trituration, the less the expansion or the greater the contraction of the amalgam will be. This effect is demonstrated by the dimensional change curves presented in Figure 23–5. As can be noted by a comparison of the legend beneath the figure with the various curves, the longer the trituration time, the less the expansion or the greater the contraction.

The general form of the curves in Figure 23–5 can be predicted from the theory. In the case of curve *1*, the trituration time was so short that a comparatively small amount of solution of mercury in $Ag_3Sn$ occurred. In fact, the initial shrinkage took place before the measurement of the dimensional change began. Such a manipulation suppressed the solution of the mercury in the $Ag_3Sn$ but it favored the crystallization of $\gamma_1$ and $\gamma_2$. The expansion reached a maximum in about 8 hours from the time of trituration, and then a slight contraction ensued as the $\beta_1$ phase appeared.

When the trituration time was increased to 100 seconds, an initial contraction can be observed (curve *2*, Fig. 23–5). The expansion was less, and it reached a maximum in approximately 7 hours. The longer trituration increased the amount and the rate of solution, and the

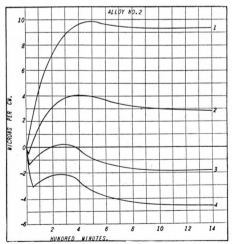

Fig. 23–5. Effect of trituration time on the dimensional change of the amalgam. Curve *1*, 40 seconds. Curve *2*, 100 seconds. Curve *3*, 180 seconds. Curve *4*, 240 seconds. (Ward and Scott, *J.A.D.A.,* Oct., 1932.)

initial contraction is greater than in curve *1*. During the longer trituration, some of the initial reaction product was possibly rubbed off the alloy particles as it formed, and this also caused further solution.

Since the reactions start immediately when mercury comes into contact with the filings, and increase as the trituration continues, it is reasonable to assume that some of the crystals of $\gamma_1$ and $\gamma_2$ may form during the trituration. Any such crystallization during this period cannot be effective in the production of expansion after condensation. Consequently, the observed expansion should be less as the trituration is prolonged, as demonstrated in the curves in Figure 23–5.

Furthermore, the crystals in the condensed amalgam, formed during trituration, may act as nuclei of crystallization for the subsequent crystallization of more $\gamma_1$ and $\gamma_2$. The more nuclei present, the greater the rate of crystallization, and, as a consequence, the earlier the expansion maxima should occur, since the maxima are, in a sense, indicative of the near completion of the crystallization of $\gamma_1$ and $\gamma_2$. The earlier occurrence of the maxima in Figure 23–5 with increased trituration time can be accounted for in this manner.

Whether the final dimension of the amalgam will be the result of an expansion or a contraction depends to some extent upon the magnitude of the initial contraction. If the trituration is too long, the initial contraction may be so great that the subsequent expansion is not sufficient to restore the original dimensions of the amalgam specimen, as in curves *3* and *4*, and an ultimate contraction results.

In any event, it is evident that the trituration should be controlled accurately if the dimensional change of the amalgam is to be controlled. Such control to assure a standardized, uniform mix is one of the cardinal principles of the amalgam technic.

**Effect of Condensation.** If the trituration is held constant, the effect of increased pressure in condensation is to decrease the expansion, as indicated in Figures 23–6 and 23–7. Although none of the curves in the figures exhibit an ultimate contraction with increased condensation pressure, a contraction is possible, although it is not so apt to occur as with overtrituration.

Actually, condensation is a continuation of the trituration so far as the production of $\gamma_1$ and $\gamma_2$ is concerned. The condensation disturbs the mercury-alloy mixture, the initial sheath is rubbed off the alloy particles and more solution can take place. However, as the condensation pressure is increased, the undissolved particles tend to become wedged together, and the initial contraction decreases in magnitude in spite of the fact that the solution continues. This theoretical consideration is borne out by the graphs in Figure 23–6 and 23–7. In Figure 23–6, curve *1*, no condensation pressure was employed and the observed initial contraction was the greatest for the entire series. Under the conditions of the experiment cited, apparently all of the condensing pressures provided sufficient wedging so that there were no appreciable differences in their observed initial contractions. The differences shown were undoubtedly within the experimental error in magnitude.

An increase in condensation pressure removes more mercury from the mass, with the result that less of the $\gamma_1$ and $\gamma_2$ phases is formed. The progressive decrease in expansion with the increase in condensation pressure, as noted in Figure 23–6 and 23–7, can be accounted for in this manner. The maxima for the expansion occur earlier because the

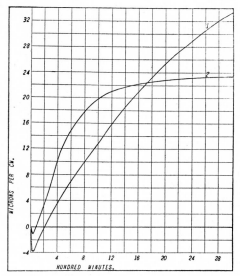

Fig. 23–6. Effect of variation in condensation pressure on dimensional change. Curve *1*, amalgam placed in mold under vibration with no pressure. Curve *2*, amalgam condensed under a pressure of 35 kg. per sq. cm. (500 lb. per sq. in.). (Ward and Scott, *J.A.D.A.*, Oct., 1932.)

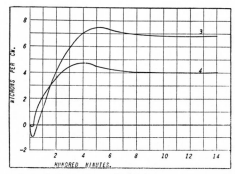

Fig. 23–7. Effect of variation of condensation pressure on dimensional change. Curve *3*, amalgam condensed under pressure of 70 kg. per sq. cm. (1000 lb. per sq. in.). Curve *4*, condensation pressure 140 kg. per sq. cm. (2000 lb. per sq. in.). (Ward and Scott, *J.A.D.A.*, Oct., 1932.)

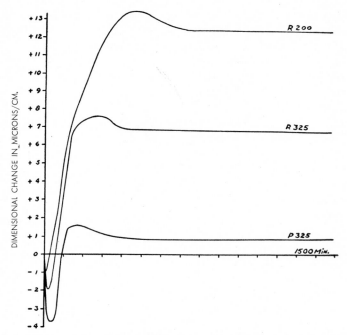

Fig. 23–8. Effect of the alloy particle size on the dimensional change of an amalgam. Curve *R200*, amalgam from alloy particles retained on a 200-mesh sieve; curve *R325*, particles retained on a 325-mesh sieve; curve *P325* particles passed a 325-mesh sieve. (Jarabak, *J.A.D.A.*, April, 1942.)

reactions are accelerated by the more intimate contact between the residual mercury and the other phases as a result of the increased condensation pressure.

Condensation of the amalgam is essential to impart the proper strength and flow, as will be shown in a subsequent section. It is also necessary to prevent excessive expansion as shown in curve *1*, Figure 23–6. At the end of two days (2880 minutes), the expansion was 33 microns per centimeter, and it was increasing at a rapid rate. Although never proved, it is possible that the presence of an excessive amount of free mercury in a poorly condensed filling may cause an expansion sufficient to produce a sensation of pain in the tooth. However, such an effect is more likely to be associated with excessive expansion resulting from moisture contamination. This point will be discussed at length in a subsequent section and in the next chapter.

*Effect of Particle Size.* The effect of varying the particle size of an alloy on the dimensional change of the amalgam is shown in Figure 23–8. It is evident that the smaller the particle size, the less is the expansion for the same technic of manipulation.

Actually, the important consideration is not the size of the particle in terms of its volume, but rather in terms of its surface area.[9] For a given weight of alloy, the greater the surface area of the particles, the greater will be the number of particles, and, generally, the smaller their size. It is evident that an increased surface area resulting in a decrease in particle size will favor more rapid solution of the mercury in the alloy particles during trituration, with the result that a large initial contraction of the amalgam occurs.

The resemblance between the curves in Figure 23–8 and those in Figure 23–5, produced by increased trituration time, is very similar. Both show the same general form, with decreasing expansion maxima which occur at progressively earlier times. In the case of the curves in Figure 23–5, this effect was attributed to overtrituration, and the formation of the crystalline phases in considerable quantity before the condensation was completed. The same reasoning can be employed to explain the curves in Figure 23–8. The amalgams with the smallest particle size were overtriturated in comparison to the trituration of the larger particles. A small particle size amalgam, therefore, should be triturated for a shorter time than an amalgam with a large particle size under the same condition of pressure and similar variables. The general effect of the small alloy particle size is to reduce the hardening time of the amalgam in comparison to that obtained with the larger particle size.[9] It should be noted, however, that the tendency of the small alloy particle to produce a shrinkage of the amalgam can be minimized to some extent by an alteration in its shape, as described in the previous chapter.

If hand trituration with a mortar and pestle is used, the greater the pressure of the pestle on the mortar, the more the particles are broken up, and consequently the less the expansion or the greater the contraction.[6] The manufacturer's directions for a particular alloy in regard to pestle pressure and time of trituration should be followed accurately for the most consistent results.

**Effect of Contamination.** All of the observations thus far presented for the dimensional change of silver amalgams have been for a duration of 24 hours. Although there may be minor expansions and contractions of a few microns for subsequent months and years, the dimensional changes are most minute after 24 hours as shown in Figure 23–9. If, however, the amalgam is contaminated by moisture, a considerable amount of expansion takes place,[10, 11] as shown in Figure 23–10. This expansion usually starts after about 3 to 5 days and may continue for months, reaching values as high as 400 microns per centimeter (0.4 per cent). This type of expansion is known as *delayed expansion* or *secondary expansion*. This type of expansion must not be confused with an excessive expansion caused by too much mercury being retained in the amalgam, as demonstrated by curve *1*, in Figure 23–6.

The delayed expansion is associated with the zinc in the amalgam, as outlined in the previous chapter. However, the zinc content *per se* is

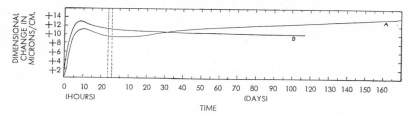

Fig. 23–9. Dimensional change of amalgam *A* which contained zinc (1 per cent) but was not touched with hands or otherwise contaminated during manipulation. Amalgam *B* contained no zinc.

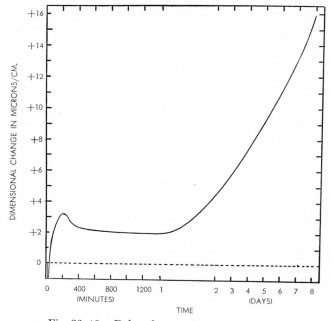

Fig. 23–10. Delayed expansion of an amalgam.

not directly responsible for the delayed expansion. The dimensional changes of two amalgams, one containing zinc and the other with no zinc, are shown in Figure 23–9 for a period of 120 days and longer from the time of trituration. As can be noted, neither amalgam exhibited a noteworthy dimensional change after the first day.

The contamination of the amalgam can occur at almost any time during its manipulation and insertion into the cavity. If the zinc-containing amalgam is touched with the hands during trituration or condensation, skin secretions are likely to be introduced. If the operating area is not kept dry, saliva may be condensed into the restoration along with the amalgam. In short, any contamination of the amalgam with moisture, whatever the source, before it has been inserted into the prepared cavity will cause a delayed expansion if zinc is present.

It is apparent from the foregoing discussion that the effect is due to a corrosion of some sort related to the presence of the zinc. The effect is not present in non-zinc amalgams. It has been clearly demonstrated that the contaminating substance is water, regardless of whether it is pure or contains an inorganic salt.[11]

One of the products of the corrosion was found to be hydrogen. Its evolution was brought about by electrolytic action between the zinc, the electrolyte, and the anodic elements present. For example, some cylindrical specimens (30 millimeters long and 5 millimeters in diameter) of an amalgam containing 1.2 per cent zinc were contaminated with salt solution, and with distilled water. After a storage of twenty days at 37° C., the specimens contaminated with the salt solution were found to contain 6 to 7 milliliters of hydrogen gas measured under normal conditions of room temperature and pressure, and the one to which distilled water had been added contained 4 milliliters of the same gas. The minimum pressures exerted by the gas in the various specimens can be calculated to be between 110 and 155 kilograms per square centimeter (1600 to 2200 pounds per square inch); this magnitude of force is sufficient to cause the amalgam filling to expand by a flow of the amalgam.[11] If the zinc is not present, the expansion will not occur. It should be noted that the contamination must occur *during* the trituration or condensation; once the amalgam is condensed, the surface may come in contact with salt solution, water, saliva, etc., with no ill effect, so far as its dimensional change is concerned.

The amount of delayed expansion is generally associated with the zinc content of the alloy, *i.e.*, the higher the concentration of zinc, the greater is the expansion. It has been reported[12] that delayed expansion can be avoided only when the zinc content is less than 0.01 per cent. It also has been suggested that copper may influence this phenomenon since the higher the copper content, the less is the delayed expansion.[12]

## STRENGTH

It is obvious that sufficient strength to resist fracture is a prime requisite for any restorative material. Fracture, even on a small area, or a fraying of the margins will hasten recurrence of decay and subsequent clinical failure. A lack of truly adequate strength to resist masticatory forces has long been recognized as one of the inherent weaknesses of the amalgam restoration.[13] For this reason, it should be continually stressed that the cavity preparation be designed to provide bulk of amalgam wherever stress is to be applied.[14–16] Furthermore, the amalgam itself should be handled in a manner that will assure maximum strength.

**Measurement of Strength.** The strength of a dental amalgam is usually measured under compressive stress using a cylindrical specimen of dimensions comparable to the volume of a typical amalgam restoration. When measured in this manner, the compressive strength of a satisfactory amalgam probably should be at least 3200 kilograms per square centimeter (45,000 pounds per square inch).

The adequacy of such a test has been questioned[17] so far as clinical interpretation is concerned. The design and shape of a typical amalgam restoration greatly complicates the stress distribution in function in comparison to the distribution during the stressing of a cylinder.

Although the principal stress during mastication might be mainly compressive, the stresses are complex with shear and tensile stress acting as well. For example, on the isthmus of a compound restoration, any compressive stress on the adjacent restored cusp will induce a shear which in turn reacts to produce a tensile stress in the isthmus area.[18, 19] The tensile strength of amalgam is much less than its compressive strength, being approximately 560 kilograms per square centimeter (8,000 pounds per square inch). Since the tensile strength of tooth dentin is estimated to be 2,800 kilograms per square centimeter (40,000 pounds per square inch), the cross section diameter of the isthmus should be kept as great as possible in order to compensate, at least in part, for this weakness. Incidentally, it has been shown that increasing the depth of the isthmus is more effective in this regard than increasing its width.[19]

A third factor to be considered is the dynamic character of the stress induced. The modulus of resilience of dental amalgam is quite low. As a result, the impact energy is likely to become more concentrated in some areas than others, particularly in regions of lesser volume. Marginal areas of amalgam restorations appear to be particularly vulnerable in this regard and frequently fracture or chip.[13] In fact, it has been suggested that this chipping is inherent in amalgam and that it cannot be entirely eliminated.[17]

Probably the true answer to this complex problem of strength evaluation for dental amalgam is related to the term "edge strength" previously described. As stated in Chapter 2, such a strength is difficult to evaluate quantitatively.

Nevertheless, for the comparison of one amalgam specimen to another the test for compressive strength is accepted as standard. The cylindrical specimens can be prepared easily and the test can be duplicated with considerable accuracy.

**Trituration.**    As can be noted from Table 23–1, under-trituration may result in a weaker amalgam and over-trituration may increase the strength slightly in comparison to that of the "normal" mix. However, the trituration time and method are of less importance to the strength of the amalgam than are other factors.

**Mercury Content.**    A very important factor in the control of the strength is the mercury content of the restoration. Although sufficient mercury must be mixed with the alloy to coat the alloy particles and to

*Table 23–1.    Effect of Trituration Time on the Compressive Strength**

| ALLOY NO. | UNDER MIX (KG./CM.²) | (LB./IN.²) | NORMAL MIX (KG./CM.²) | (LB./IN.²) | OVER MIX (KG./CM.²) | (LB./IN.²) |
|---|---|---|---|---|---|---|
| 1 | 2320 | 33100 | 2420 | 34600 | 2500 | 35800 |
| 2 | 2680 | 38400 | 2750 | 39300 | 2860 | 40900 |
| 3 | 2790 | 39900 | 2640 | 37800 | 2680 | 38400 |
| 4 | 2520 | 36000 | 2600 | 37200 | 2620 | 37400 |
| 5 | 2810 | 40100 | 2760 | 39500 | 2770 | 39600 |

* Taylor, Sweeney and Mahler, *J. D. Res.*, June, 1949.

allow a thorough amalgamation, any excess beyond this minimal amount may produce a marked reduction in strength.

There appears to be no important effect of the mercury content on the strength of the amalgam within the limits of approximately 45 to 53 per cent.[20–22] Above approximately 55 per cent mercury content, the strength decreases markedly with increase in mercury content.[8] With 59 per cent mercury, the compressive strength is reduced to 18,000 pounds per square inch (1250 kilograms per square centimeter) from a maximum strength of over 40,000 pounds per square inch (2800 kilograms per square centimeter) with a mercury content of approximately 55 per cent.

The degree of the condensation definitely affects the strength.[21, 23] When dental condensation technics are employed, it is a well-established fact[24, 25] that the higher the condensation pressure, the greater will be the compressive strength. While it is true that the proper packing of the unattacked alloy particles is a factor in the control of the strength,[21] if an insufficient amount of mercury is removed during the condensation, the mercury content becomes the dominant strength factor regardless of the technic employed.

**Rate of Hardening.**    The rate of hardening of the amalgam is of considerable interest to the dentist. A patient may be dismissed from the dental chair within 20 minutes after the trituration of the amalgam, and the question whether or not the amalgam will have gained sufficient strength for its function is a vital one.

The amalgam does not gain strength as rapidly as might be desired. For example, at the end of 20 minutes, its compressive strength may be only 6 per cent of its strength in one week.[25] It is estimated that the amalgam restoration will gain compressive strength at the rate of 6 to 7 kilograms per square centimeter (90 to 100 pounds per square inch) per minute during the first hour.

In any event, the early strength of the amalgam restorations is likely to be low, and the patient should be cautioned not to subject the restoration to a high biting stress for at least 6 to 8 hours after it has been inserted, at which time the amalgam reaches 70 to 90 per cent of its maximum strength. The recommendation of a liquid diet for the next meal is probably a sound safety precaution.

Very likely the magnitude of the early strength is affected by the alloy particle size and shape when the usual condensation technic is employed. For example, fine grain alloys appear to improve early strength.

It is of interest to note that even at the end of a six month period, the amalgams may still be increasing in strength slightly. The change in surface hardness shows a similar relationship with the age of the amalgam.[26] Such observations indicate that the reactions between the mercury and the alloy may continue indefinitely. It is doubtful that equilibrium conditions are ever completely attained.

Rate of hardening or setting is also important in evaluating the "carvability" of the restoration, that is, the time at which the dentist may safely carve the restoration. Indentation tests are not entirely satisfactory for this purpose and it is possible that some type of punch[27] or shear[28] test may prove to be acceptable as a measure of the clinical setting time.

### FLOW

An amalgam exhibits a plastic flow under a static load well below its proportional limit. Usually a cylinder of the amalgam, 4 millimeters in diameter and 8 millimeters in length, is subjected to a given load at a certain time after trituration (usually three hours). The percentage decrease in length during the succeeding 24 hours is called the *flow*. According to the requirements of the American Dental Association Specification No. 1, the flow should not exceed 4 per cent.

If a similar cylinder of gold alloy, for example, is tested in the same way, the metal may flow for a short time (depending on the conditions of the test), after which no more deformation will occur. Furthermore, the applied load necessary in this case approaches or exceeds the proportional limit of the gold alloy. The reason for the lack of flow in this instance is, of course, that the gold alloy becomes strain hardened at the stage when the plastic flow ceases. In industry, such a deformation is known as "creep."

Since the amalgam continues to deform under the static load in comparison to the specimen of gold alloy, it can be assumed that the amalgam does not strain harden as readily as does the gold alloy. Presumably, the amalgam partially strain hardens, however, since its deformation rate under the static load is much lower than that of a metal such as tin which does not strain harden at room or mouth temperature.[29]

As might be expected from the theory of relaxation, the higher the temperature, the greater is the rate of flow. For example, under the testing conditions employed, it has been noted that the flow of an amalgam at body temperature is approximately twice that at room temperature over a period of twenty-four hours.

**Constant Flow.** The flow curve is shown in Figure 23–11 for a typical amalgam tested at 23° C. (74° F.) under the conditions previously noted, with a static load of 250 kilograms per square centimeter (3560 pounds per square inch). As can be noted from the curve, the flow rate becomes constant only after the first 10 to 13 hours after the trituration. It is thought that the initial flow is due to a continuation of the hardening process and that the strain hardening is not the sole factor in the rate of deformation.

On this basis, it has been proposed[29] that the straightline portion of the graph be projected to zero time as shown by the dotted line (Figure 23–11), and that the true flow be measured as the difference between the intercept of the dotted line on the vertical coordinate and the *total flow* value obtained at the end of twenty-four hours. This flow value is termed *constant flow* in contrast to the *total flow*, which value includes the initial non-linear portion as well. On this basis, the total flow of the amalgam specimen employed for the graph in Figure 23–11 would be approximately 2.2 per cent, whereas the constant flow would be in the neighborhood of 1.3 per cent.

Actually, no direct evidence has been encountered to substantiate the fact that the flow of an amalgam is of clinical importance.[17, 30, 31] The low values for constant flow, regardless of the total flow, observed with various amalgams tested[29] appear to corroborate such a finding. The principal merit of the flow test is probably that it provides a satisfactory and convenient way to evaluate the general strength characteristics of this material.

The trituration time has little effect on the flow, other factors being equal,[6, 29] but the effect of an increase in the condensation pressure is to decrease the flow. Even though condensation pressures have been used experimentally far beyond the dental range, the flow is never completely eliminated.[29] Although the removal of the mercury decreases the flow considerably, it is evident that one of the phases in the

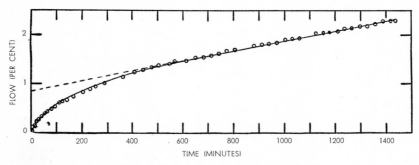

Fig. 23–11. Typical flow curve for an amalgam.

amalgam does not strain harden at normal temperatures, and the amalgam continues to flow or "creep" under a constant load. It is interesting to note that a partial strain hardening occurs, as evidenced by the shape of the flow curve (Fig. 23–11). If no strain hardening were present, the relation between the constant flow and the time would not be that of a straight line.

The laboratory test for flow is a static one, but it has generally been felt that restorations which have a high flow value are more likely to result in failures such as flattened contact points, overhanging margins or even a slight protrusion of the proximal surface in a two- or three-surface restoration.

There is, however, considerable doubt that flow is a true clinical problem with amalgam. Observations on amalgam restorations having flow values as high as 10 per cent have failed to reveal any evidence of flow even when placed in conditions emphasizing traumatic occlusion.[17, 31] Thus the clinical significance of this particular property remains unknown. It would seem that, until proven otherwise, the main merit of the flow test is that it provides a satisfactory and convenient way to evaluate the general strength properties of the amalgam restoration.

## *Literature*

1. Souder, W. and Paffenbarger, G. C.: *Physical Properties of Dental Materials.* National Bureau of Standards Circular C433, Washington, U. S. Government Printing Office, 1942, p. 14.
2. Souder, W. and Paffenbarger, G. C.: *Ibid.,* pp. 6–12.
3. Gayler, M. L. V.: *Dental Amalgams.* J. Inst. Metals, *60:*407–424, 1937.
4. Mitchell, J. A., Schoonover, I. C., Dickson, G. and Vacher, H. C.: *Some Factors Affecting the Dimensional Stability of the Ag-Sn-(Cu-Zn) Amalgams.* J. D. Res., *34:*273–286 (April), 1955.
5. Gray, A. W.: *Volume Changes in Amalgam.* J. Inst. Metals, *29:*139–189, 1923.
6. Ware, A. L. and Docking, A. R.: *Effect of Manipulative Variables on Dental Amalgams.* Parts I, II and III. Austral. J. Den., *58:*283–287 (Oct.), 1954; *58:*355–360 (Dec.), 1954; *59:*167–170 (June), 1955.
7. Phillips, R. W. and Boyd, D. A.: *Importance of the Mercury-alloy Ratio to the Amalgam Filling.* J.A.D.A., *34:*451–458 (April 1), 1947.
8. Swartz, M. L. and Phillips, R. W.: *Residual Mercury Content of Amalgam Restorations and Its Influence on Compressive Strength.* J. D. Res., *35:*458–466 (June), 1956.
9. Crowell, W. S. and Phillips, R. W.: *Physical Properties of Amalgam as Influenced by Variation in Surface Area of the Alloy Particles.* J. D. Res., *30:*845–853 (Dec.), 1951.
10. Phillips, R. W., Swartz, M. L. and Boozayaangool, R.: *Effect of Moisture Contamination on Compressive Strength of Amalgam.* J.A.D.A., *49:*436–438 (Oct.), 1954.
11. Schoonover, I. C., Souder, W. and Beall, J. R.: *Excessive Expansion of Dental Amalgam.* J.A.D.A., *29:*1825–1832 (Oct. 1), 1942.
12. Van Gunst, I. C. A. and Hertog, H. J. P. M.: *On the Relationship between Delayed Expansion of Amalgam and the Composition of Amalgam Alloys.* Brit. D. J., *103:*428–430 (Dec.), 1957.
13. Souder, W. and Paffenbarger, G. C.: *loc. cit.,* p. 32.
14. Wolcott, R. B.: *Failures in Dental Amalgams.* J.A.D.A., *56:*479–491 (April), 1958.

15. Simon, W. J., Ed.: *Clinical Operative Dentistry.* Philadelphia, W. B. Saunders Co., 1956, pp. 14–67.
16. Markley, M. R.: *Restorations of Silver Amalgam.* J.A.D.A., *43:*133–146 (Aug.), 1951.
17. Nadal, R.: *A Clinical Investigation of the Strength Requirement of Amalgam and the Influence of Residual Mercury upon This Type of Restoration.* M. S. D. Thesis, Indiana University School of Dentistry, 1959.
18. Mahler, D. B.: *An Analysis of Stresses in a Dental Amalgam Restoration.* J. D. Res., *37:*516–525 (June), 1958.
19. Mahler, D. B. and Terkla, L. G.: *Analysis of Stress in Dental Structures.* D. Clin. North America, (Nov.), 1958, pp. 789–798.
20. Ryge, G., Dickson, G., Smith, D. L. and Schoonover, I. C.: *Dental Amalgam: The Effect of Mechanical Condensation on Some Physical Properties.* J.A.D.A., *45:*269–277 (Sept.), 1952.
21. Crawford, W. H. and Larson, J. H.: *Dental Restorative Materials: Amalgams, Acrylics.* J. D. Res., *33:*414–424 (June), 1954.
22. Swartz, M. L. and Phillips, R. W.: *Study of Amalgam Condensation Procedures with Emphasis on the Residual Mercury Content of the Increments; I. Strength, Flow and Dimensional Change.* J. D. Res., *33:*12–19 (Feb.), 1954.
23. Skinner, E. W. and Mizera, G. T.: *An Evaluation of the Eames Amalgam Condensation Technic.* Paper read before Dental Materials Group, I.A.D.R., San Francisco, Calif., March, 1959.
24. Ward, M. L. and Scott, E. O.: *Effects of Variations in Manipulation on Dimensional Changes, Crushing Strength and Flow of Amalgams.* J.A.D.A., *19:*1683–1705 (Oct.), 1932.
25. Taylor, N. O., Sweeney, W. T., Mahler, D. B. and Dinger, E. J.: *The Effects of Variable Factors on Crushing Strengths of Dental Amalgams.* J. D. Res., *28:*228–241 (June), 1949.
26. Phillips, R. W.: *Compressive Strength of Amalgam as Related to Time.* J. D. Res., *28:*348–355 (Aug.), 1949.
27. Taylor, D. F. and Margetis, P. M.: *Method for the Measurement of the Setting Time of Dental Amalgams.* I.A.D.R., *34:*81–82, 1956. Abstract.
28. Kumpula, J. W.: *Work in Progress at the National Bureau of Standards.* Washington, D. C.
29. Skinner, E. W.: *Research on the Flow of Dental Amalgam.* J.A.D.A., *25:*1651–1660 (Oct.), 1938.
30. Sweeney, J. T.: *Amalgam Manipulation: Manual vs. Mechanical Aids; Part II.* J.A.D.A., *27:*1940–1949 (Dec.), 1940.
31. Phillips, R. W., Boyd, D. A., Healey, H. and Crawford, W. H.: *Clinical Observations on Amalgams with Known Physical Properties. Final Report.* J.A.D.A., *32:*324–330 (March), 1945.

# CHAPTER 24

# Dental Amalgam:

# Technical Considerations

A good, modern dental amalgam alloy can be manipulated so that an amalgam restoration will be obtained which will be adequate in every respect. If the restoration is defective, in the great majority of the cases the fault is with the dentist and not with the material. As has been mentioned earlier, either the cavity preparation was wrong, or some other factor of design was misjudged, or the amalgam was not manipulated properly. The last factor will be discussed at length in reference to the influence of the technic on the physical properties and thus the clinical success of the amalgam.

## SELECTION AND PROPORTIONING OF ALLOY AND MERCURY

**Selection.** There is only one requisite for dental mercury and that is its purity. Common contaminating elements, such as arsenic, can lead to pulpal damage. Furthermore, a lack of purity may adversely affect the physical properties of the amalgam. Unfortunately, terms such as "pure" or "triple distilled" have no chemical significance. The designation "U.S.P." (United States Pharmacopeia) placed on the mercury container definitely insures a satisfactory purity. This designation indicates that the mercury has no surface contamination and that it contains less than 0.02 per cent nonvolatile residue. This requirement is encompassed in the American Dental Association Specification No. 6 for dental mercury. Consequently, the selection of a mercury which is guaranteed to meet this specification assures the necessary purity.

Likewise, the first criterion in the selection of the alloy is to make sure that it passes the detailed requirements of the American Dental Association Specification No. 1 for amalgam alloy, or a similar specification. As noted, a particular brand of alloy may often be purchased either as a powder or in pellet form. Although one may detect some minor differences in handling characteristics, either form is satisfactory.

The choice of particle size and consistency or smoothness of the mix is likely to be a matter of personal preference. The coarser the particle size, the less plastic the freshly mixed amalgam is apt to be. As noted in the last chapter, the present trend is toward the use of the finer cut alloy or an alloy which breaks up into fine particles of the proper size during trituration. The fine cut alloys provide a smooth amalgam mixture, and the final surface of the restoration can be given a smooth surface and a high polish without great effort.

It is interesting to note that the appearance of the alloy in the bottle is not a certain indication of the fineness of the particle size.[1] The presence of large flakes of alloy mixed with small particles may be difficult to detect visually, yet their presence may affect the amalgam considerably in comparison to the properties contributed by a uniformly fine alloy.

**Proportioning.** The amount of alloy and mercury to be used is usually defined as the *alloy-mercury ratio, i.e.,* the parts by weight of alloy to be combined with the proper amount of mercury. For example, an alloy-mercury ratio of 5/8 indicates that 5 parts of alloy are to be used with 8 parts of mercury by weight.

The manufacturer's directions should be consulted in regard to the correct ratio to be used with any particular alloy. The ratio may vary for different alloy compositions, particle size, heat treatment and even condensation technic. The alloy-mercury ratio generally employed is 5/8, but with the use of finer grained alloys, the ratios of 5/7 or even 5/6 may be prescribed.

A wide variety of alloy and mercury dispensers, or proportioners, is available to the dental profession. They are of two general types. The most common type is the dispenser which is based on volumetric proportioning; the other type is based on measurement by weight.

A study of twenty-five commercially available dispensers was concerned with the accuracy of dispensation of both alloy and mercury.[2] A considerable difference in the degree of accuracy was found and usually those that dispensed by weight were less accurate than were the volumetric dispensers. Probably the average dispenser is sufficiently accurate, provided it is used properly. Most dispensers are not set accurately when received from the manufacturer and should be adjusted by the dentist. With some of the volumetric devices, the alloy tends to cling to the walls and corners, and usually the device should be jarred on the bench or table to insure that all of the alloy is dispensed.

Another disadvantage of the volumetric type of dispenser is that it cannot be used universally with all types of alloy. When the alloy is measured by volume, the weight of the alloy will depend upon its particle size. Consequently, only the alloy should be used for which the dispenser was designed.

As previously noted, probably the best method for the measurement of the alloy-mercury ratio is to employ pre-weighed alloy pellets or packets if available, and to dispense the mercury from a volumetric dispenser regulated to measure the proper amount of mercury per pellet or packet. Since mercury is a liquid, it can be measured by volume without loss of accuracy.

In any event, the proper amount of mercury and alloy must be gauged before the start of trituration. The addition of mercury, once the trituration has started, results in an amalgam which is lacking in strength and resistance to corrosion.

## TRITURATION

Traditionally, the alloy and mercury have been mixed or triturated with a mortar and pestle, but some form of mechanical amalgamation is now more widely used. The object of the trituration is to cause the mercury and the alloy to amalgamate. The alloy particles are coated with a slight film of oxide which it is difficult for the mercury to penetrate. This tarnish must be rubbed off in some manner so that the clean surface of the alloy particle may come into contact with the mercury. Such a procedure is accomplished when the alloy particles and mercury pass under the pestle as it moves over the surface of the mortar.

**Mortar and Pestle Trituration.** The use of the mortar and pestle is likely to introduce variables into the trituration which make it difficult for the dentist to obtain consistent results. The pressure of the pestle on the mortar may break up the particles of alloy as the amalgamation proceeds. The surface roughness of the mortar and pestle may change with use. Also, the human factor enters into the successful completion of the trituration to such an extent that its daily variation may result in certain differences in the consistency of the mix and in the physical properties of the amalgam.

However, the control of the variables can be effected to a large extent by the selection of a proper design of mortar and pestle, by the maintenance of the proper surface on the mortar and pestle, and by the use of a systematic, routine type of trituration.

Mortars and pestles can be purchased in many varieties of shapes. A mortar of any shape which will cause the mercury and alloy to remain under the pestle, and not to travel up its sides during trituration is satisfactory. For example, a mortar with an interior that is parabolic in shape will tend to cause the mercury-alloy mixture to slide constantly toward its bottom.

Another successful mortar has a raised portion in the center, so that the pestle travels over a path formed between the raised portion and the walls of the mortar. Such a design definitely confines the alloy and mercury to the path of the pestle.

Whatever the shape of the mortar, the working surface of the pestle should conform to it. The mortar and pestle seldom fit each other in this manner when they are purchased. Consequently, a new mortar and pestle should always be ground to fit. A paste of 200-mesh carborundum and water may be ground in the mortar and pestle, until the dried surface of the mortar is uniformly abraded in appearance. As the surface wears smooth with use, it should be re-abraded occasionally in the same manner.

It makes little difference whether the mortar is constructed of steel or of glass, provided that the proper care is taken of it.

In any event, all of the alloy particles should be included in the trituration. If any of the particles are inadvertently left unamalgamated, or partially amalgamated in comparison to the rest of the mixture, an inhomogeneous amalgam will result which will exhibit poor resistance to tarnish and corrosion. A proper mixture can be obtained only if all of the alloy and mercury are triturated uniformly.

*Pestle Pressure.* The second factor in the control of the trituration is the pestle pressure. Most manufacturers direct that the pressure of the pestle on the mortar shall be 2 pounds (1 kilogram), but occasionally 4 pounds (2 kilograms) or more is required. It is not easy to estimate these pressures, although if one grasps the pestle by a "pen grip" as shown in Figure 24–1, the pressure is roughly two pounds, provided that the operator holds the pestle firmly but with light pressure, and only guides it over the mercury and alloy. A "fist grip," as shown in Figure 24–2, exerts approximately four pounds pressure when it is held lightly and not consciously forced against the mortar.

There are devices available with a spring arrangement to regulate the exact pressure on the pestle. Although they assist in standardizing this variable, pestle pressure is not so critical provided proper judgment is exercised and only sufficient pressure to assure amalgamation is employed.

*Consistency of the Mix.* It should be evident by this time, that the method of combining the mercury and the alloy is one of the prime manipulative considerations. It is at this stage that the composition of the final amalgam is largely determined, and this composition determines the physical properties. To summarize: too little trituration results in low strength and overexpansion. Overtrituration will likely result in a contraction during hardening and, if too extensive, a reduction in strength as well.

The attainment of a proper mix can be controlled by timing the trituration according to the number of revolutions of the pestle. For

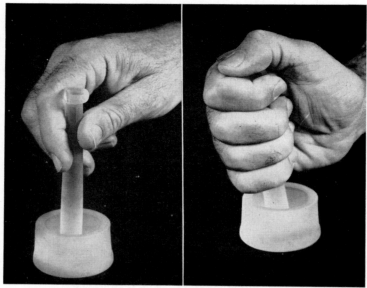

Fig. 24–1.                    Fig. 24–2.

Fig. 24–1. "Pen grip" of the pestle during trituration.
Fig. 24–2. "Fist grip" of the pestle during trituration.

example, a manufacturer may direct that the alloy be triturated for one minute under a pestle pressure of 2 pounds, with the pestle revolving at the rate of 180 times a minute. An amalgam can be overtriturated with a too rapid rate of trituration, as well as when the time is unduly prolonged.

Such a method of timing is satisfactory, provided that the same weights of alloy and mercury are used each time. Usually, a dentist gauges the amount (not the proportion) of the alloy and mercury that he uses according to the size of the prepared cavity. Consequently, in the case of an amalgam that is sensitive to variables in manipulation, a small amount of mercury and alloy could easily be overtriturated with the timing employed for the standard mixture.

If the mortar and pestle have been conditioned as described, the proper trituration can be gauged with sufficient accuracy by the consistency of the mix. However, a certain facility of judgment can be obtained by observation and experience. For example, the somewhat grainy mix shown in Figure 24–3 was undertriturated. Not only will the amalgam restoration made from this mix be weak, but the rough surface left after the carving of this granular amalgam will decrease the tarnish resistance. Furthermore, clinical studies have demonstrated that a marked increase in fractured margins results when such a mix is used.[3–5]

On the other hand, if the trituration is carried to the extent where the amalgam has the general appearance shown in Figure 24–4, the strength of the hardened amalgam will be maximum and the smoother carved surfaces will retain their luster longer after polishing. The consistency shown in Figure 24–4 is readily recognized at the instant the amalgam smooths out with a shiny surface and clings to the mortar. At this stage, when the mortar is jarred repeatedly, the mix coheres into a ball with no trace of amalgam sticking to the mortar. If the mass clings to the mortar to the extent that it cannot be removed readily, the mix has been overtriturated.

Formerly, the amalgamated mixture was mulled in the palm of the hand before it was finally used. Such a practice should not be followed because of the danger of contamination from the skin secretions. With proper trituration, additional mixing should not be necessary. However,

Fig. 24–3.

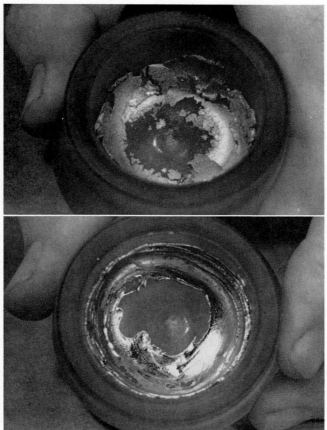

Fig. 24–4.

Fig. 24–3.  Undertriturated amalgam mix.
Fig. 24–4.  Properly triturated amalgam mix.

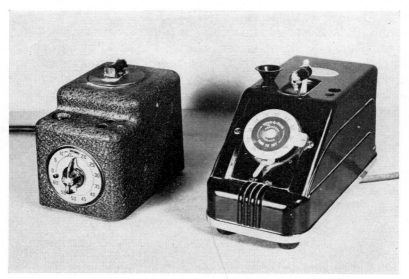

Fig. 24–5.   Two types of mechanical amalgamators.

if desirable, a short mulling period can be employed without contamination of the mix. For example, the mix can be placed in a surgical finger stall or a piece of rubber dam and manipulated with the fingers through the rubber.

**Finger Stall Trituration.**    One of the disadvantages of the use of a mortar and pestle is that all of the particles of alloy are not always in contact with the mercury under the pestle at the same time. Consequently, there is a tendency toward an inhomogeneous amalgamation, regardless of the precautions that are observed. In order to avoid such a situation, it has been suggested[6] that the amalgamation be accomplished in a rubber finger stall.[7]

An alloy-mercury ratio of 4/7 is recommended. The alloy and mercury are placed in a thick rubber thumb or finger stall with friction corrugations, such as might be used for turning the pages of a ledger or book. A surgical finger stall is unsatisfactory for this technic. The alloy and mercury are placed in the stall and kneaded with the fingers through the rubber for one minute. In this manner, it is thought that the amalgamation proceeds more uniformly than with the mortar and pestle, since the filings and mercury are more closely in contact. Furthermore, the original particle size of the alloy is maintained, with the consequent elimination of this variable. This method of trituration is used more extensively in Great Britain than it is in America.

**Mechanical Trituration.**    There are several mechanical amalgamators available, two of which are seen in Figure 24–5. The principle of operation of both types is the same. A capsule can be seen between the arms on top of each machine which serves as a "mortar." A small cylindrical metal or plastic piston of a smaller diameter than the capsule is placed inside the capsule and serves as a "pestle."

The proper quantities of alloy and mercury are placed in the capsule with the piston. The timer, which can be seen in the front of the mortar case, is regulated for the proper timing. The filled capsule is then shaken violently for the automatically controlled time period, and the amalgamation is completed. There are other types of amalgamators and some which operate on somewhat different principles. They vary, not only in efficiency or desirability but also in rate of amalgamation.[8]

Frequently, following trituration, the pestle is removed and trituration without it is continued for a second or two. This procedure is helpful in cleaning the capsule since the amalgam comes out in one piece. If amalgam is permitted to harden in the capsule it will contaminate future mixes.[9]

There are two outstanding advantages of mechanical amalgamation over that by hand. The amalgamation is more uniform from one mix to another.[10] In other words, the personal equation is eliminated. Secondly, the trituration time is reduced from one minute to a few seconds. This advantage is very important in the condensation of complex restorations where several mixes are required.

The chief disadvantage is the tendency to overtriturate in many cases and to cause the amalgam to shrink during hardening. There is probably some advantage to the longer contact of the alloy particles with the mercury during the hand trituration in providing a good consistency of the mix,[8] and for this reason it appears to be necessary in some instances to overtriturate during mechanical trituration in order to obtain a thorough amalgamation. For example, in one investigation,[10] out of twelve commercial amalgam alloys, all of which were satisfactory in dimensional change after trituration with the mortar and pestle, only two expanded on hardening after they had been triturated mechanically to give a consistency comparable to that obtained by hand trituration.

There is little or nothing to be gained in the strength and the flow properties of the amalgam with the use of the mechanical amalgamator over the hand trituration method.[8]

## CONDENSATION

Once the mix is made, amalgam should not be permitted to stand too long before its condensation into the prepared cavity.[3] Amalgam that is over 3 or $3\frac{1}{2}$ minutes old should be discarded and a new mix made.[11] Thus several mixes may be required for a large restoration.

This effect is shown graphically in Figure 24–6 for two amalgam alloys.[11] As can be noted, the longer the time between trituration and condensation, the greater is the loss in strength. The decrease in strength is partially due to the fact that the $\gamma_1$ and $\gamma_2$ phases form

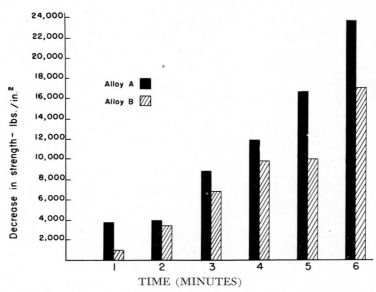

Fig. 24–6. The effect of the elapsed time between trituration and condensation on the decrease in strength of the hardened amalgam. The greater the elapsed time, the less is the strength.

while the amalgam is standing, and the crystals are fractured during the condensation. Also more mercury is retained in the amalgam and the strength is thereby reduced as well.

It follows, therefore, that the condensation should be as rapid as is possible and, in any event, a fresh mix of amalgam should be available if the condensation occupies more than 3 to 4 minutes. In such a case, the use of a mechanical amalgamator becomes imperative.

The purpose of the condensation is to force the remaining alloy particles as closely together as possible and into all parts of the prepared cavity, and, at the same time, to remove as much mercury from the mass as is consistent with good practice. Under the proper conditions of trituration and condensation, there is little danger of removing too much mercury. In other words, the amalgam should be condensed into the prepared cavity so that the greatest possible denseness is attained with sufficient mercury present to insure a complete continuity of the matrix phases between the remaining particles of alloy. The strength is increased by this procedure, and the flow is decreased. The expansion is decreased as the mercury is removed, but if the other factors involved have been properly controlled, such a reduction will not be important from a clinical standpoint.

The field of operation must be kept absolutely dry during the condensation. The incorporation of the slightest moisture at this stage will result in a delayed expansion, and a subsequent failure of the restoration.

Because of the nature of the operation, the condensation must always be accomplished within four walls and a floor; one or more of the walls may be a thin sheet of stainless steel, called a *matrix*. This instrumentation and the discussion of certain extremely important factors of cavity preparation are outlined in textbooks on operative dentistry,[12] or other excellent publications on the use of the matrix.[13, 14] It is never possible to reproduce perfectly the normal contour of the proximal surface but deviations are slight if the matrix band is carefully wedged and contoured.[15, 16]

The condensation can be effected with either mechanical or hand instruments.

**Hand Pressure Condensation.** There are a number of successful condensation technics. The technics differ chiefly in the amount of mercury to be expressed from the mix before condensation and the number and size of the increments of the mix to be condensed.[17] Actually, with the proper judgment, there is little difference in the physical properties of the hardened amalgam prepared with any accepted condensation technic.[18] The basic principles are to remove sufficient mercury from the mix to provide a mass that offers resistance to the condensing instrument, but so much should not be removed that mercury cannot be worked to the surface during condensation. In such case, the sections of the surface do not bond together and a laminated effect occurs which greatly weakens the amalgam. Furthermore, a rough surface will be present on the restoration.[19, 20]

This oldest and most common technic to be described below is often referred to as the "increasing dryness technic." The term "dry" refers to a lack of mercury as opposed to a "wet" mix in which there is so much mercury that the mix appears plashy.

After the amalgam has been triturated, some of the free mercury can be removed at once under pressure in a smooth cloth, known as a "squeeze cloth." The amount of mercury which should be removed at this stage is largely a matter of judgment to be gained by experience. The removal of mercury tends to accelerate the hardening of the amalgam, and it is essential that the mixture be soft and plastic at the time it is condensed into the prepared cavity. Each particle of alloy should be coated with a sheath of $\gamma_1$ and $\gamma_2$, and, as previously stated, sufficient free mercury should be present so that each increment can be condensed thoroughly into the mass already in place.

The freshly mixed amalgam is cut into several pieces, and the excess mercury is removed from the first piece by wringing it in the "squeeze cloth." Sufficient mercury is left in the piece so that slightly more can be expressed under the condensing instrument.

The condensing instrument is similar to the gold foil condenser, except that the amalgam condenser generally is contra-angled toward its working end, and the working point is usually larger than that used for the gold foil condenser.

The piece of amalgam, prepared as described, is then condensed into the prepared cavity by forcing the condenser point into it under hand pressure. The condensation is usually started at the center, and then the condenser point is stepped little by little toward the cavity walls. Any excess mercury or plashy amalgam brought to the surface is removed at once. After the first piece of amalgam has been thoroughly condensed, the mercury is removed from the second piece as before, and the process is repeated. The prepared cavity is thus filled to excess.

After the prepared cavity has been overfilled, more mercury can be blotted out of the top layers by the condensation of some amalgam from which the free mercury has been removed as completely as possible, with pliers, for example. *Such "dry" amalgam should not be left permanently in the restoration,* however, *because of its lack of cohesion caused by a lack of mercury.*

As earlier noted, one of the objectives of the condensation is to remove the excess mercury as the amalgam is condensed. It is evident that the greater the pressure on the amalgam, the greater will be the amount of the mercury removed. Consequently, the method by which the pressure is applied merits special consideration.

**Condensation Pressure.**   The area of the condenser point determines the condensation pressure exerted by the operator. The smallest amalgam condenser point, as designed by Black, is equivalent in area to a circle 1 millimeter in diameter. Dentists differ in their preference for the shape of the condenser point and its size. A condenser point that is unduly small merely punches holes in the amalgam. On the other hand, condensers which are too large do not permit adaptation of the amalgam into the retentive areas and the average operator cannot produce sufficient hand pressure to provide adequate condensation pressure with a condenser point greater than two millimeters.

Probably the average condenser point should be equivalent in area to a circle 1 to 2 millimeters in diameter. The plastic amalgam will offer sufficient resistance to such a point so that the condensation will be effective, and also the proper pressure can be applied manually.

There is a difference between the thrust or force exerted by the operator, and its effectiveness in condensation in terms of its pressure. For example, a thrust of 4.5 kilograms (10 pounds) on a circular condenser point 2 millimeters in diameter would result in a condensation pressure of 140 kilograms per square centimeter (2000 pounds per square inch). In other words, the pressure will vary inversely with the square of the diameter of the condenser point. An example of a large condenser point is a surface equivalent to a circle 3.5 millimeters in diameter. A force of 4.5 kilograms on such a point would produce a pressure of only 47 kilograms per square centimeter (670 pounds per square inch). The greater effectiveness of the small condenser point is evident, provided that it does not penetrate the mass as previously described.

The shape of the condenser point should conform to the area under condensation. For example, a round condenser point would be ineffective adjacent to a corner or angle of a prepared cavity; a triangular or square point would be indicated in such an area. Points of various shapes are, therefore, provided for the most effective condensation.

Although forces as high as 7 kilograms (15 pounds) have been advocated for the thrust of the amalgam condenser, it is doubtful that the average operator can continually condense the amalgam into place, step by step, with a thrust greater than 2 to 4.5 kilograms (5 to 10 pounds). In any event, it is likely that "if the operator's arm does not ache after condensing a large filling, the filling is not well condensed."[13]

**Mechanical Condensation.** There are a number of devices on the market with which the condensation can be effected more or less automatically. For example, the pneumatic gold foil condenser previously described (page 311) has been adapted for use in the condensation of amalgam.[21] In some of the available mechanical condensers, the repeated blows are the result of a rapid vibration, sometimes perpendicular to the direction of condensation, and, in other instruments, parallel to the direction of condensation.

The general principles involved are identical with those outlined for hand condensation. The mercury is removed from each piece of amalgam, which is then condensed with the mechanical condenser. The point is held against the amalgam and moved over its surface without a successive stepping. The advantage of not constantly removing the point and re-setting it is obvious. Also, the manual pressure required is much less than that for the hand condensation, and the operation is less fatiguing to the dentist.

The restoration is gradually condensed piece by piece. Free mercury and "soft" amalgam are removed before the condensation of each succeeding piece, as previously described. Generally, "drier" increments could be employed with mechanical condensation than with hand condensation. Consequently, it is usually not necessary to add the very "dry" amalgam to the overfilled cavity, since the mechanical procedure is quite effective in the removal of mercury at each stage.

The early strength of the amalgam may be increased by mechanical condensation.[22] The final strength of the amalgams from fine cut alloys may be somewhat superior when the mechanical method is used,[10, 22] but in general no important differences in strength are to be expected with the two methods.[8]

The general tendency is for the use of the mechanical condenser to reduce the expansion or to increase the contraction of the amalgam. This effect varies with different amalgam alloys and the different types of mechanical instruments employed. However, any of the instruments can probably be used in such a manner that the amalgam will exhibit the proper dimensional change and other properties.[23]

Similar clinical results can be attained with either hand or mechanical condensation and the selection may depend upon the preference of the dentist. Often mechanical condensation has the advantage of a better standardization of the procedure and it results in less fatigue for the dentist. However, in the case of the impact type of mechanical condenser, care should be observed that the enamel margins of the prepared cavity are not fractured by the blow.[24] In the plastic state, amalgam is incapable of protecting the fragile and brittle enamel walls. Consequently, the amalgam should be kept away from them so that they can be readily seen during the condensation.

A disadvantage of the mechanical condensation is the tendency toward the production of a lamination of the amalgam, as each piece is added to the material already condensed.[8] If too much mercury is removed from each piece, so that no free mercury is present on the surface when an additional piece is added, such a condition may result. Such a lamination indicates a possibility of weakness at the junction of the layers.

If special precautions are observed to correct such faults as have been enumerated, an excellent restoration should result with mechanical amalgamation and condensation.

**Adaptation.**    By adaptation is meant the degree of proximity of the amalgam to the cavity wall. The ideal condition is complete proximity with no space whatever between the hardened amalgam and the cavity wall. Actually, such a condition is impossible of attainment but it can be approached according to the intelligence and skill of the operator. As has been discussed a number of times, all dental restorations are subject to marginal leakage which may or may not be of clinical importance. Certainly, the amalgam restoration is no worse than other types of restoration in this respect. In fact, it is better than some (see page 353). Contrary to what might be expected, an expansion of the amalgam does not necessarily insure a tightly fitting restoration.

It has been shown that superior adaptation is achieved by condensing with small rather than large increments.[25]

Regardless of the particle size of the alloy, and similar factors, the adaptation of the amalgam is largely dependent upon the skill of the operator. The plastic amalgam should be condensed toward the walls and floor of the prepared cavity in such a manner as to insure maximum adaptation. Special care should be taken not to disturb the amalgam already condensed when more is added. The proper technic is attained only as a result of patient and careful practice until skill is acquired.

## *FINISHING*

After the amalgam has been condensed into the prepared cavity, the restoration is carved to reproduce the proper tooth anatomy.

If the proper technic has been followed, the amalgam should be ready for carving soon after the completion of the condensation. The carving should not be started, however, until the amalgam is sufficiently hard to offer resistance to the carving instrument. A scraping or "ringing" sound should be present when it is carved.[13] If the carving is started too soon, the amalgam may be so plastic that it may be pulled away from the margins even with the sharpest carving instrument. Once the condensation is completed, the utmost care should be observed not to disturb the adaptation. A sharp-bladed instrument should be used for carving.

Regardless of how smooth the amalgam surface may appear before hardening, it will exhibit a roughness after twenty-four hours. The smoothest surface after hardening without polishing is probably produced with the amalgams made from a fine grain alloy.

The final polishing of the restoration should be delayed for at least twenty-four hours or preferably one week, in order to allow the amalgam to harden thoroughly. Any attempt to polish the amalgam immediately after it has been carved will result in the burnishing of mercury and soft amalgam over its surface. Subsequently, the surface becomes dull and even rough as the setting reactions proceed.

It is most important to avoid heat during polishing. Any temperature above 65° C. (140° F.) will release mercury and result in weakened areas subject to corrosion or fracture.[26] The use of dry polishing powders and disks can easily raise the surface temperature above this point. A wet abrasive powder in paste form is the agent of choice. The final polish can be obtained with a paste of whiting and water applied with a soft brush.

As will be noted in the next section, the importance of polishing cannot be overemphasized. The restoration is *not* finished until it is polished.

## *CORROSION AND TARNISH*

It is generally recognized that dental amalgam restorations often tarnish and occasionally corrode in the mouth and, as a consequence, their use is generally confined to the posterior teeth. The tarnish layer may render the restoration passive, and no further attack may occur. The tarnish layer in such a case is usually a sulfide.

X-ray diffraction analyses[27] of tarnished amalgams indicate the tarnished layer may be either (Hg, Ag) $S_x$ or $Ag_2S$. At any rate it is predominantly a sulfide. On this basis it might be anticipated that patients on a high sulfur diet or whose mouth hygiene would result in

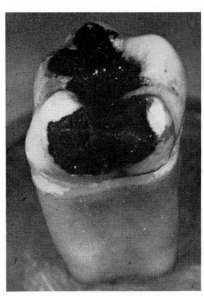

Fig. 24–7. Tarnished amalgam restoration. Discolored layer is probably a sulfur compound.

sulfur accumulation in plaque material would exhibit marked tarnish, as seen in Figure 24–7. This factor might explain the common clinical differences in tarnish of amalgam restorations in individuals even when they are inserted with apparently comparable technics.

According to the theory of electrolytic corrosion presented in Chapter 21, the dental amalgam itself lacks the structural homogeneity to insure corrosion and tarnish resistance. The different phases present in the hardened amalgam exhibit different electrode potentials, and they produce an excellent example of a corrosion cell, with the saliva as the electrolyte. The product of corrosion of this nature is principally tin deposition, with traces of silver and copper.[28]

The homogeneity of the amalgam can be increased by the proper trituration and condensation.[29] For example, if the amalgam is under-triturated, or if some of the alloy particles are not triturated as much as the others, a corrosion of the restoration may be manifested clinically by the presence of pits and a general discoloration.[5] If the mortar and pestle are properly surfaced, as previously described, and if special care is observed to keep the mercury and alloy under the pestle during the trituration, a more homogeneous mixture will result. Also, during condensation if a conservative stepping technic is observed with the condenser point, a greater homogeneity will be obtained.

If an amalgam restoration is highly polished after it has thoroughly hardened, its resistance to corrosion is greatly increased. The presence of the polished surface evidently produces a homogeneous layer which is resistant to chemical attack. The polished surface may tarnish slightly, but it does not usually corrode.[5, 9] Probably polishing of the restoration is as significant a manipulative variable as any other in control of discoloration in the mouth.

In order to provide a tarnish resistance to the amalgam restoration, the polish layer must be uniformly distributed over the entire restoration. In other words, if one small area of the restoration is left unpolished, an electric couple is produced between the unpolished and the polished areas.[28] The result is that the polished area becomes tarnished and even corroded. Eventually, the polarity of the couple is reversed, and the unpolished area begins to corrode. The final result may be a badly pitted and unsightly restoration. The products of the corrosion may be carried into the dentinal tubules, and the entire tooth may appear to be discolored. Such tooth discoloration is evident on the buccal aspect of the amalgam restoration shown in Figure 24–8.

Sometimes the products of corrosion appear to be concentrated at the margin of an amalgam restoration, as manifested by the discoloration of the tooth structure. Such a condition may be caused by a difference in the concentration or nature of the electrolytes. If food débris or acids are concentrated in an open margin of a restoration, the electrolyte formed in the crevice will be chemically and physically different from the saliva. Under such conditions, concentration-cell corrosion takes place, brought about by the difference in electrolytes.[28]

Whenever a gold and amalgam restoration are placed in contact,

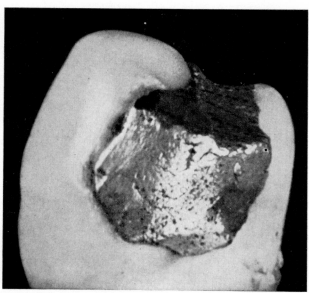

Fig. 24–8. An amalgam restoration which has failed, presumably because of excessive expansion and corrosion. (Courtesy of J. R. Jarabak.)

corrosion of the amalgam restoration can be expected[28] regardless of the condition of its surface. Mercury is usually found in the gold restoration, and the latter may be weakened as a result. Such a practice should be avoided whenever possible.

Galvanic action primarily, then, accounts for tooth discoloration. Although the cement base helps prevent penetration of these ions into the dentin, a cavity varnish may be even more satisfactory.[30]

Mercury, *per se,* does not influence tarnish.[27] In other words, increased mercury does not necessarily produce greater corrosion. However, restorations with high mercury content result in surface deterioration which then accelerates discoloration. So technics designed to minimize the final mercury content of the filling lead to superior tarnish resistance by virtue of the smoother surface and marginal areas.

In general, it can be seen that discoloration is associated with oral environment, galvanic conditions and surface roughness. Anything that can be done to minimize surface irregularities will in turn reduce corrosion. Moisture contamination, high residual mercury, undertrituration and insufficient polishing should all be avoided.

## CLINICAL SIGNIFICANCE OF EXPANSION

A survey[31] of the causes for failures of amalgam restorations has shown that out of 1521 defective restorations, 16.6 per cent failed because of excessive expansion. As outlined in the previous chapter, there are two causes for the excessive expansion of amalgam. One is insufficient trituration and condensation, and the other is the delayed expansion brought about by the contamination of the amalgam during mixing and condensation with moisture. The latter cause is much more frequently responsible for such failures than the former.

According to the accepted theory,[32] the delayed expansion is caused by the internal pressure exerted by the hydrogen which is one of the products of corrosion between the zinc in the amalgam and the incorporated moisture. According to the results obtained with the dental interferometer, the large expansion begins 4 to 5 days after the condensation (see Fig. 23–10). Presumably, the expansion is delayed until the pressure of the hydrogen becomes sufficient to cause the amalgam to flow or expand.

It is customary to undercut the prepared cavity to provide retention. It is conceivable that the undercut portion of the restoration will tend to inhibit the expansion toward the open surface of the restoration. Consequently, a back pressure is built up by the restraining of the expansion. If the floor of the prepared cavity is adjacent to the pulp chamber, as in a gingival third cavity, the back pressure may be transmitted to the pulp. As a result, an excruciating pain may be reported by the patient, approximately ten days after the amalgam has been inserted.[33]

**Clinical Example.**   If the restoration is not removed at this stage, it continues to expand. The final result may be similar to the restoration shown in the extracted tooth in Figure 24–8. Although many factors may have combined to produce the failure shown in Figure 24–8, a possible diagnosis can be related to the faulty manipulation of the amalgam.

For example, perhaps not all of the alloy was amalgamated to the same degree, and localized electric couples caused corrosion as manifested by the pits. Moisture may have been incorporated into the amalgam mix, either from the hands of the operator, or because the field of operation was not kept dry during the condensation. In such a case, excessive expansion of the restoration would ensue, and it would be extruded slightly from the prepared cavity as a result. Since the brittle amalgam margins were then unsupported, they fractured, and the marginal defects resulted. Leakage of the restoration then produced a marginal discoloration with further corrosion and pitting caused by the concentration cells formed.

Another cause for the pitting may have been the escape of the hydrogen gas which collected near the surface. Some of the hydrogen may force its way through the surface of the amalgam and cause blisters, as can be seen[32] in Figure 24–9.

Pitting, regardless of the cause, definitely reduces the strength of the amalgam restoration. If it proceeds far enough, the amalgam may become so pitted as to crumble under stress.[28]

The effect of moisture contamination on an amalgam containing zinc is demonstrated by the graphs[34] in Figure 24–10. As can be noted

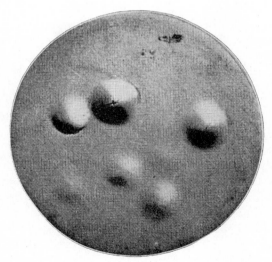

Fig. 24–9.  Blisters formed on the surface of an amalgam disk, caused by escaping hydrogen. (Schoonover, Souder and Beall, *J.A.D.A.*, Oct., 1942.)

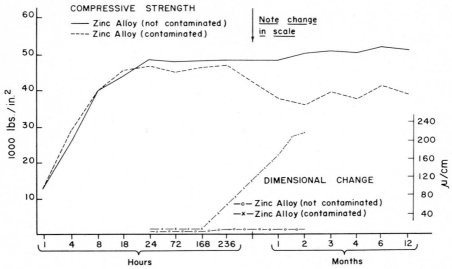

Fig. 24–10.   Effect of moisture contamination on the strength and dimensional change of amalgam.

from the upper curves, contaminated amalgam exhibits approximately the same strength as the uncontaminated amalgam for the first 3 to 4 days, but subsequently it becomes weaker as the hydrogen collects internally. In this instance, the strength decreased about 25 per cent.

As can be noted from the graphs for the dimensional change (Fig. 24–10), the delayed expansion of the contaminated amalgam began at approximately the same time as did the decrease in strength, whereas the dimensional change of the uncontaminated specimens remained constant as predicted in the previous chapter.

**Use of Non-zinc Alloys.**   As might be expected, the deleterious effects of moisture have spurred interest in the non-zinc alloys. Their use is certainly justified in those areas where it is virtually impossible to keep the operating area dry, such as the posterior teeth in the mouth of a child patient.

Formerly, the non-zinc amalgams were extremely dirty to handle. The zinc in the amalgam alloy acts as a scavenger for oxides during the melting and the pouring of the ingot, and, in its absence, considerable oxidation may take place during trituration and condensation with a resulting blackening of the instruments. Modern manufacturing processes appear to have reduced this disadvantage considerably.

Any blackening of the hands or instruments during the manipulation of a non-zinc amalgam apparently has no clinical significance either as to its effect on the tooth structure or its susceptibility to increased tarnish in the mouth.[27]

So far as is known, there are no great differences in the physical

*Table 24–1.* *Comparison of the Compressive Strength and Flow of Zinc-containing and Non-zinc Amalgam Alloys from the Same Manufacturer*

| MATERIAL | COMPRESSIVE STRENGTH | | | | TOTAL FLOW (PER CENT) |
| | ONE HOUR | | 24 HOURS | | |
| | (KG./CM.²) | (LB./IN.²) | (KG./CM.²) | (LB./IN.²) | |
| --- | --- | --- | --- | --- | --- |
| Alloy A | | | | | |
| Zinc | 1,190 | 17,000 | 2,730 | 39,000 | 1.5 |
| Non-zinc | 1,120 | 16,000 | 2,730 | 39,000 | 2.2 |
| Alloy B | | | | | |
| Zinc | 1,220 | 17,500 | 3,000 | 43,000 | 2.0 |
| Non-zinc | 700 | 10,000 | 3,000 | 43,000 | 3.1 |
| Alloy C | | | | | |
| Zinc | 630 | 9,000 | 2,870 | 41,000 | 2.8 |
| Non-zinc | 630 | 9,000 | 2,590 | 37,000 | 3.8 |

properties between the two types of alloys. The compressive strengths of amalgams from zinc and non-zinc alloys manufactured by the same dental companies are presented in Table 24–1. As can be noted for two of the three alloys, there is no significant difference in strength between the zinc-containing amalgams and the non-zinc materials as paired, either at the end of one hour or in 24 hours.

It has been stated[32] that the use of a non-zinc alloy may lead the dentist to a false sense of security and thus eventually to a generally inferior technic. Certainly, a non-zinc alloy should not be preferred solely because it does not exhibit a delayed expansion when contaminated. There is no reason why any amalgam should be contaminated with epidermis and perspiration from the hands, and saliva, blood and similar débris from the mouth, while it is being inserted into the prepared cavity. Professional standards alone should demand a dry, sanitary field of operation regardless of whether or not the amalgam contains zinc.

In any event, if the proper precautions are observed, comparable results can likely be expected from either type of alloy.

## CLINICAL SIGNIFICANCE OF CONTRACTION

It has been pointed out that undertrituration results in reduced strength and possibly too great an expansion during the hardening of the amalgam. It is also true that a slight contraction may occur with some amalgams when they are properly triturated. However, modern alloys are so designed that if the previously presented precautions for trituration with mortar and pestle are followed, or if the timing of the mechanical amalgamator is so regulated as to give a comparable mix in a *minimum time,* no contraction need be expected.

It is obvious that, theoretically at least, a slight expansion is to be

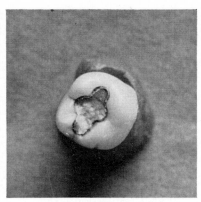

Fig. 24–11. "Ditching" around an amalgam restoration should not be attributed to contraction. (Wolcott, *J.A.D.A.*, October, 1958.)

Fig. 24–12. A common cause for marginal failure. If a feather edge of the amalgam is left overlapping the margin, it fractures during mastication. (Courtesy of G. M. Hollenback.)

preferred to a contraction. However, if there is a choice between increased strength and a *slight* contraction during hardening as tested in the laboratory, the former is to be preferred on the basis of arguments previously advanced. Such a conclusion has been verified by a number of clinical studies.[4, 5, 35–38]

A theoretical calculation can be made of the possible tolerance allowable in dimensional change on the basis of the unavoidable thermal contraction and expansion of the amalgam during the intake of hot or cold foods. For example, on the basis of the thermal coefficient of expansion of amalgam (Table 2–1, p. 28) and the differential thermal dimensional change factor (Table 13–2, page 214), an amalgam restoration five millimeters in linear dimensions might expand or contract as much as three microns at a margin during extremes of temperature change to produce a percolation as discussed in Chapter 13. Consequently, a tolerance of ±6 microns per centimeter might be allowable in the dimensional change of an amalgam restoration within the limits prescribed. As further discussed in Chapter 13, any percolation of an amalgam restoration persists no longer than a few months. Actually, an amalgam from a good modern alloy is not likely to shrink six microns per centimeter in the mouth even under a reasonable amount of abuse during manipulation.

Such theoretical considerations have been correlated with clinical findings.[5] Observations on clinical restorations, placed with thoroughly triturated amalgam which showed a contraction of two to four microns per centimeter measured with the interferometer at room temperature, failed to reveal a single example of marginal contraction after two years. These restorations were actually superior in terms of surface condition and marginal adaptation. Still another study[38] over a three year period resulted in the same conclusion, even though the amalgam (from an alloy specially made for the purpose) contracted as much as 30 microns per centimeter according to an interferometer test.

It is very difficult to estimate whether an amalgam restoration in the mouth has contracted or expanded within the required limits of such dimensional change. When it is recognized that the average human hair is 40 microns in diameter, it is virtually impossible to detect margins which may be open six microns or less, either with the eye or with a dental instrument. In a clinical study previously cited,[31] only 2.5 per cent of the failures of amalgam restorations could be attributed to contraction and all of these were debatable.

The so-called "ditched" filling, an example of which may be seen in Figure 24–11, is often attributed to a contraction of the amalgam. This type of failure is more probably due (1) to leaving a thin feather edge of amalgam after carving (Fig. 24–12); (2) to the presence of unsupported enamel at margins; (3) to inadequate condensation, thus leaving this area mercury rich; or (4) to an actual expansion leaving the margins exposed. Whenever a margin is unsupported for any reason, a fracture results because of the brittleness of the amalgam.

It should be emphasized, however, that these observations should not be construed as a recommendation for a contracting amalgam or a haphazard technic. They merely emphasize that *small* contractions during hardening as measured by laboratory methods may not be clinically significant. They further indicate that there may be a factor of safety if the amalgam is unintentionally or unavoidably abused during its manipulation and insertion, so far as its dimensional change is concerned.

## CLINICAL SIGNIFICANCE OF MERCURY

The amalgam restoration is possible only because of the unique characteristics of mercury. It is this metal which makes possible the plastic mass which can be inserted and finished in the teeth, and which will then harden to a structure that resists the rigors of the oral environment. However, it also is the element which so markedly influences the basic properties necessary to clinical success.

**Toxicity.** From the earliest use of this material, it has been asked whether or not the mercury could produce many local or systemic effects in the human. It is still occasionally conjectured that mercury toxicity from dental restorations is the cause for certain undiagnosed illnesses. It has been further suggested that a real hazard may exist for the dentist or dental assistant where mercury vapor is inhaled during mixing, thus producing an accumulative toxic effect.

It is true that mercury penetrates from the restoration into tooth structure. An analysis of dentin[39] underlying amalgam restorations reveals the presence of mercury, which in part may account for a subsequent discoloration of the tooth. Use of radioactive mercury in silver amalgam has also revealed that some mercury might even reach the pulp.[40] However, the possibility of toxic reactions from these traces of mercury penetrating the tooth, of sensitization from mercury salts dissolved from the surface of the restoration, or from inhalation of mercury vapor[41] is highly improbable. The problem has been well studied in every respect and rather than to review the subject in detail at this time, the student is referred to an excellent monograph.[42]

**Mercury Content.**    Mercury is very important to the clinical success of the individual restoration. The element can be accurately measured either by volatilization in a nitrogen atmosphere[43, 44] or by fluorescent x-ray spectroscopy.[45] Analysis of clinical restorations shows a remarkably wide variation in mercury content[44, 46, 47] which may range as high as 70 per cent in a single restoration. Typical results[44] on ten restorations selected at random from extracted teeth can be seen in Table 24–2. These data include mercury determinations not only in the body or bulk of the restoration, but also in the marginal areas. Mercury in the body portion ranged from 49.5 per cent in one restoration to as high as 60.8 per cent in another.

It is of particular interest that the mercury concentration is characteristically higher in the marginal areas. This observation is true regardless of the method of condensation or the "dryness" of the increments used to build the restoration.[18] An analysis of 100 dental restorations showed an average mercury increase of 2.6 per cent in the marginal areas when hand condensation was used, as compared to an average increase of 2.7 per cent for restorations condensed with three

*Table 24–2.    Mercury Analyses of Ten Amalgam Restorations*

| RESTORA-TION NO. | % Hg AT MARGINS | % Hg IN BULK |
|:---:|:---:|:---:|
| 1 | 54.7 | 52.4 |
| 2 | 58.6 | 58.6 |
| 3 | 58.8 | 56.5 |
| 4 | 56.5 | 55.0 |
| 5 | 53.0 | 56.8 |
| 6 | 49.5 | 49.7 |
| 7 | 55.8 | 53.6 |
| 8 | 58.7 | 60.4 |
| 9 | 60.8 | 60.3 |
| 10 | 55.4 | 54.1 |

automatic condensing devices. There does not seem to be much choice in this respect.

This higher mercury content at the margins is important since it is in these areas, which are critical in terms of fracture, that corrosion and, finally, recurrence of caries may occur.

Most of the amalgam restorations studied in Table 24–2 were judged clinically unsatisfactory by visual examination. Such a judgment is to be expected on the basis of the discussion in the previous chapter in which it was shown that a marked decrease in compressive strength occurred with a mercury content of approximately 55 per cent or over.

In order to test further the influence of mercury content on the clinical performance of amalgam restorations, 200 restorations were inserted in prepared cavities using three technics which were controlled and designed to produce restorations with three mercury contents of approximately 49, 56 and 62 per cent respectively.[48] The restorations were then observed at three-month intervals for one and one-half years.

The influence of the mercury content on the restorations is illustrated typically in Figure 24–13. The restoration in the first molar contained a mercury content of approximately 62 per cent, while the amalgam in the bicuspid contained approximately 49 per cent. The deterioration in the restoration with the higher mercury content at the end of one year is obvious. The margins have broken down and a fracture (*c*) extends across the occlusal surface. Furthermore, a surface roughness

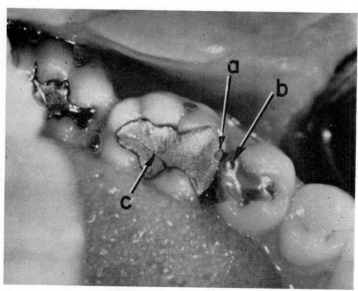

Fig. 24–13. Amalgam restorations after one year in the mouth. The condition of the restoration in the first molar with high mercury content is in contrast to that in the second bicuspid with a lower mercury content. Facets *a* and *b* show the effect of traumatic occlusion. A fracture is seen at *c*.

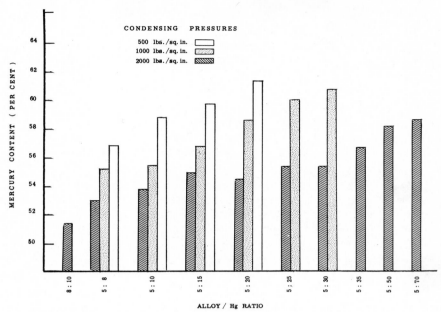

Fig. 24-14. Mercury content of amalgam as influenced by the alloy-mercury ratio with three different condensation pressures.

is evident. This condition is typical of restorations which have a high mercury content. The increased surface roughness, tarnish and particularly the marginal breakdown appeared during the first three months and accelerated as the restoration aged.

**Control of Mercury Content.** In summary of previous discussions, the factors which influence the mercury content of the restoration are (1) the alloy-mercury ratio of the mix, (2) the amount of trituration, and (3) the pressure and time of condensation.

The effect of the original alloy-mercury ratio on the physical properties of the amalgam is of importance. Regardless of the technic employed, the more mercury employed, the greater is the mercury content of the restoration. For example, the lower the alloy-mercury ratio, the greater will be the expansion of the amalgam.

Its effect together with that of the condensation pressure is demonstrated[44] in Figure 24-14. The mercury content is plotted in reference to the alloy-mercury ratio for three different condensation pressures. As can be noted, generally, for a given condensation ratio, the more mercury used in the original mix, the greater is the amount left in the amalgam. Likewise, as previously stated, the greater the condensation pressure for a given ratio, the more mercury will be eliminated during condensation.

Consequently, it can be concluded that the proportioning of the mercury and alloy is important to the success of the restoration.

## COPPER AMALGAMS

Copper amalgam, as the name implies, is an amalgam of copper and mercury. The copper is amalgamated and the mass is allowed to harden. The amalgam is then supplied to the dentist in the form of pellets. The pellets are heated in a test tube or in an iron spoon until the mercury appears in droplets. The mass is then triturated in the usual manner. The composition of nine copper amalgams is shown in Table 24–3.

The copper amalgam usually shrinks during hardening, regardless of the manipulation employed. The contraction is increased, however, the higher the temperature to which the pellets are initially heated.[49] The method or time of trituration appears to have no effect. The copper amalgam hardens slowly over a period of eight to twelve hours. The

*Table 24–3.*     *Composition of Dental Copper Amalgams**

| AMALGAM | MERCURY (%) | COPPER (%) | OTHER METALS |
|---------|-------------|------------|--------------|
| A | 66.3 | 32.5 | Zn, 0.7% |
| B | 61.7 | 37.1 | Zn † |
| C | 67.8 | 32.2 | Trace O$_2$ |
| D | 72.1 | 26.6 | Zn † |
| E | 70.5 | 28.2 | Zn † |
| F | 62.1 | 37.6 | . . . . . . |
| G | 64.1 | 35.7 | . . . . . . |
| H | 67.7 | 30.7 | Sn, about 1.5% |
| I | 69.3 | 28.5 | Sn, about 2% |

\* Contributed by H. K. Worner, formerly Professor of Metallurgy, University of Melbourne.
† Amount not determined.

hardening time as well as the contraction time is increased by raising the temperature during the heating.[50] Consequently, for minimal contraction and hardening time, the pellets should be heated slowly and only until mercury appears on their surface. Once it hardens, its crushing strength is satisfactory and it exhibits no flow whatever when it is tested in the usual manner.

Copper amalgams have been used as restorations in deciduous teeth, but they corrode considerably in the mouth fluids. They have also been used in the construction of dies from impressions of teeth. In recent years, however, their use for this purpose, as well as for restorations in deciduous teeth, has been largely replaced by the silver-tin amalgams.

### Literature

1. Crowell, W. S. and Phillips, R. W.: *Physical Properties of Amalgam as Influenced by Variation in Surface Area of the Alloy Particles.* J. D. Res., 30:845–853 (Dec.), 1951.
2. Ryge, G., Fairhurst, C. W. and Oberbrickling, R. E.: *Proportioning of Dental Amalgam.* J.A.D.A., 57:496–506 (Oct.), 1958.

3. Miller, E. C.: *Clinical Factors in the Use of Amalgam.* J.A.D.A., *34:*820–828 (June 15), 1947.
4. Phillips, R. W., Boyd, D. A., Healey, H. J. and Crawford, W. H.: *Clinical Observations on Amalgam with Known Physical Properties.* J. D. Res., *22:*167–172 (June), 1943.
5. Phillips, R. W., Boyd, D. A., Healey, H. J. and Crawford, W. H.: *Clinical Observations on Amalgam with Known Physical Properties, Final Report.* J.A.D.A., *32:*325–330 (March 1), 1945.
6. Gayler, M. L. V.: *The Setting of Dental Amalgams.* Brit. D. J., *54:*269–288 (March 15), 1933; *56:*605–623 (June 15), 1934; *58:*145–160 (Feb. 15), 1935; *59:*245–251 (Sept. 2), 1935; *60:*605–613 (June 15), 1936; *61:*11–18 (July 1), 1936.
7. Smith, J. C.: *The Chemistry and Metallurgy of Dental Materials.* Oxford, Blackwell Scientific Publications, 1949, pp. 99–100.
8. Taylor, N. O., Sweeney, W. T., Mahler, D. B. and Dinger, E. J.: *The Effects of Variable Factors on Crushing Strengths of Dental Amalgams.* J. D. Res., *28:* 228–241 (June), 1949.
9. Sweeney, J. T.: *Manipulation of Amalgam to Prevent Excessive Distortion and Corrosion.* J.A.D.A., *31:*375–380 (March 1), 1944.
10. Phillips, R. W.: *Physical Properties of Amalgam as Influenced by the Mechanical Amalgamator and Pneumatic Condenser.* J.A.D.A., *31:*1308–1323 (Oct.), 1944.
11. Phillips, R. W.: *Research on Dental Amalgam and Its Application in Practice.* J.A.D.A., *54:*309–318 (March), 1957.
12. Blackwell, R. E.: *G. V. Black's Operative Dentistry, Vol. II,* ed. 9, South Milwaukee, Medico-Dental Publishing Co., 1955, pp. 280–289.
13. Markely, M. R.: *Restorations of Silver Amalgam.* J.A.D.A., *43:*133–146 (Aug.), 1951.
14. Romnes, A. F.: *Amalgam Restorations: A Critical Survey of Present-day Practice.* Internat. D. J., *4:*1–22 (Sept.), 1953.
15. Phillips, R. W., Castaldi, C. R., Rinard, J. R. and Clark R. J.: *Proximal Contour of Class II Amalgam Restorations Made with Various Matrix Band Technics.* J.A.D.A., *53:*391–402 (Oct.), 1956.
16. Castaldi, C., Phillips, R. W. and Clark, R. J.: *Further Studies on the Contour of Class II Restorations with Various Matrix Technics.* J. D. Res., *36:*462–471 (June), 1957.
17. Swartz, M. L. and Phillips, R. W.: *A Study of Amalgam Condensation Procedures with Emphasis on the Residual Mercury Content of the Increments; I. Strength, Flow and Dimensional Change.* J. D. Res., *33:*12–19 (Feb.), 1954.
18. Wilson, R. T., Phillips, R. W. and Norman, R. D.: *Influence of Certain Condensation Procedures Upon the Mercury Content of Amalgam Restorations.* J. D. Res., *36:*458–461 (June), 1957.
19. Miller, E. C.: *Technique for Building Amalgam Restorations.* J. Pros. Den., *9:* 652–667 (July), 1959.
20. Sweeney, J. T.: *Improved Technic for Packing and Condensing Uniform Amalgam Restorations by Hand.* J.A.D.A., *28:*1463–1471 (Sept.), 1941.
21. Sweeney, J. T.: *Uncontrolled Variables in Amalgam with Significant Improvements in the Making of Restorations.* J.A.D.A., *27:*190–197 (Feb.), 1940.
22. Ryge, G., Dickson, G., Smith, D. L. and Schoonover, I. C.: *Dental Amalgam: The Effect of Mechanical Condensation on Some Physical Properties.* J.A.D.A., *45:*269–277 (Sept.), 1952.
23. Skinner, E. W., Marois, P. and Thibault, C.: *A Comparative Study of Mechanical Condensation of Amalgam by Vibration and Hand Condensation.* Actualités Odondo-Stom., *5:*429–438, 1951.
24. Wolcott, R. B.: *Failures in Dental Amalgam.* J.A.D.A., *56:*479–491 (April), 1958.
25. McHugh, W. D.: *Experiments on the Hardness and Adaptation of Dental Amalgam as Affected by Various Condensation Techniques.* Brit. D. J., *99:*44–48 (July), 1955.
26. Mitchell, J. A., Dickson, G. and Schoonover, I. C.: *X-ray Diffraction Studies of Mercury Diffusion and Surface Stability of Dental Amalgam.* J. D. Res., *34:* 273–286 (April), 1955.
27. Swartz, M. L., Phillips, R. W. and El Tannir, M. D.: *Tarnish of Certain Dental Alloys.* J. D. Res., *37:*837–847 (Oct.), 1958.

28. Schoonover, I. C. and Souder, W.: *Corrosion of Dental Alloys.* J.A.D.A., *28:*1278–1291 (Aug.), 1941.
29. Mosteller, J. H.: *The Principles of Condensation of Amalgam.* J. Georgia D. A., *24:*10–14 (July), 1950.
30. Markley, M. R.: *Amalgam Restorations for Class V Cavities.* J.A.D.A., *50:*301–309 (March), 1955.
31. Healey, H. J. and Phillips, R. W.: *A Clinical Study of Amalgam Failures.* J. D. Res., *28:*439–446 (Oct.), 1949.
32. Schoonover, I. C., Souder, W. and Beall, J. R.: *Excessive Expansion of Dental Amalgam.* J.A.D.A., *29:*1825–1832 (Oct.), 1942.
33. Romnes, A. F. and Skinner, E. W.: *A Report of a Study Concerning Post-operative Pain Following Restoration with Amalgam.* Northwest. Univ. Bul., *38:*19–22 (Feb.), 1938.
34. Phillips, R. W., Swartz, M. L. and Boozayaangool, R.: *Effect of Moisture Contamination on Compressive Strength of Amalgam.* J.A.D.A., *49:*436–438 (Oct.), 1954.
35. Roper, L. H.: *Restorations of Amalgam in the Army; An Evaluation and Analysis.* J.A.D.A., *34:*443–450 (April), 1947.
36. Sweeney, J. T.: *Amalgam Manipulation: Manual vs. Mechanical Aid; Part II. Comparison of Clinical Applications.* J.A.D.A., *27:*1940–1949 (Dec.), 1940.
37. Mosteller, J. H.: *Some Important Considerations in the Mixing of Silver Amalgam.* New York J. Den., *24:*310–314 (Aug.), 1954.
38. McDonald, R. E. and Phillips, R. W.: *Clinical Observations on a Contracting Amalgam Alloy.* J. D. Res., *29:*482–485 (Aug.), 1950.
39. Massler, M. and Barber, T. K.: *Action of Amalgam on Dentin.* J.A.D.A., *47:*415–422 (Oct.), 1953.
40. Frykholm, K. O. and Obeblad, E.: *Studies on the Penetration of Mercury Through Dental Hard Tissues Using Hg²⁰³ in Silver Amalgam Fillings.* Acta Odont. Scandinavica, *13:*157–165 (Nov.), 1955.
41. Souder, W. and Sweeney, W. T.: *Is Mercury Poisonous in Dental Amalgam Restorations?* Den. Cos., *73:*1145–1152 (Dec.), 1931.
42. Frykholm, K. O.: *On Mercury from Dental Amalgam. Its Toxic and Allergic Effects and Some Comments on Occupational Hygiene.* Acta Odont. Scandinavica, *15:*7–108, 1957, suppl. 22.
43. Crawford, W. H. and Larson, J. H.: *Residual Mercury Determination Process.* J. D. Res., *32:*713 (Oct.), 1953. Abstract.
44. Swartz, M. L. and Phillips, R. W.: *Residual Mercury Content of Amalgam Restorations and Its Influence on Compressive Strength.* J. D. Res., *35:*458–466 (June), 1957.
45. Ryge, G.: *Mercury Analysis by Fluorescent Spectroscopy.* J. D. Res., *37:*359–367 (April), 1958.
46. Crawford, W. H. and Larson, J. H.: *Dental Restorative Materials: Amalgams, Acrylics.* J. D. Res., *33:*414–424 (June), 1954.
47. Phillips, R. W. and Swartz, M. L.: *Mercury Analysis of One Hundred Amalgam Restorations.* J. D. Res., *28:*569–572 (Dec.), 1949.
48. Nadal, R.: *A Clinical Investigation on the Strength Requirements of Amalgam and the Influence of Residual Mercury Upon This Type of Restoration.* M. S. D. Thesis, Indiana University School of Dentistry, 1959.
49. Wormington, H.: *The Dimensional Changes of a Copper Amalgam Under Various Conditions of Manipulation.* Northwest. Univ. Bul., *40:*10–15 (July), 1940.
50. Anonymous: *Dental Materials: Copper Amalgam.* Austral. J. Den., *58:*321–322 (Oct.), 1954.

# CHAPTER 25

# Dental Casting Gold Alloys

Casting is one of the most widely used methods for the fabrication of metallic restorations outside of the mouth. A pattern of the lost tooth structure or the dental appliance to be reproduced in metal is constructed in wax. The wax is surrounded by an investment which is essentially a mixture of $\alpha$- or $\beta$-hemihydrate of gypsum and silica which is mixed with water in the usual manner. After the investment has hardened, the wax is removed and the molten metal is forced into the space or mold left by the wax. The resulting structure is a remarkably accurate duplication of the pattern, if the proper technic is employed. A complete description of the casting procedure will be presented in the four subsequent chapters.

Since many of the technical considerations of the casting procedure are dependent upon a knowledge of the casting alloy itself, it is necessary to discuss this phase of the subject before the details of the casting procedure are presented. According to the discussion in Chapter 21 of the mouth fluids as a corroding agent, it is not surprising that the metals used most extensively for dental castings are the precious metal alloys. In the present chapter, the composition and significant properties of the gold alloys will be discussed.

**Carat and Fineness.**    The gold content of a dental alloy is often rated according to the carat or fineness of the alloy. The carat of an alloy is the parts of pure gold in the alloy in 24 parts. For example, a 24-carat gold would be pure gold; 22-carat gold is an alloy, 22 parts of which are of pure gold, and the remaining 2 parts of which are composed of other metals. Similarly, 18-carat gold consists of 18 in 24 parts pure gold; 14-carat, 14 parts pure gold, and so on.

A more practical rating for the dentist is by the *fineness* of the alloy.

The fineness of a gold alloy is the parts per thousand of pure gold. For example, if three-fourths of the alloy is pure gold, it is said to be 750 fine. Pure gold is 1000 fine. The percentage gold composition is numerically one-tenth of the fineness rating. The carat rating can be determined from the fineness rating and *vice versa* by a simple direct proportion:

$$\frac{Carat}{24} = \frac{Fineness}{1000}$$

The carat and fineness ratings are of importance to the dentist chiefly as an estimate of the economic value and tarnish resistance of the alloy. They are in most cases of secondary importance as an indication of the mechanical properties of the alloys.

**Composition.** The dental casting gold alloys can be classified according to their composition as it affects their surface hardness.[1] According to current requirements of the American Dental Association Specification No. 5, the classification shown in Table 25–1 likely reflects the most acceptable properties and compositions of modern casting gold alloys. The probable composition limits of the alloys (gold color) commercially available are presented[2] in Table 25–2.

*Table 25–1.* *Classification of Casting Gold Alloys*

| TYPE | GOLD AND PLATINUM GROUP METALS (MINIMUM %) | B.H.N. (SOFTENED) | |
|------|---------|------|------|
| | | MIN. | MAX. |
| I (Soft) | 83 | 40 | 75 |
| II (Medium) | 78 | 70 | 100 |
| III (Hard) | 78 | 90 | 140 |
| IV (Extra Hard) | 75 | 130 | . . . |

*Table 25–2.* *Composition Limits of Dental Casting Gold Alloys (Gold Color)\**

| TYPE | GOLD (%) | SILVER (%) | COPPER (%) | PALLADIUM (%) | PLATINUM (%) | ZINC (%) |
|------|------|------|------|------|------|------|
| A | 79–92.5 | 3–12 | 2–4.5 | 0–0.5 | 0–0.5 | 0–0.5 |
| B | 75–78 | 12–14.5 | 7–10 | 1–4 | 0–1 | 0.5 |
| C | 62–78 | 8–26 | 8–11 | 2–4 | 0–3 | 1 |
| D | 60–71.5 | 4.5–20 | 11–16 | 0–5 | 0–3.5 | 1–2 |

\* Metals Handbook, 1948 edition, American Society for Metals.

It is of interest that although the classification of the alloys by type in Tables 25–1 and 25–2 is relatively the same, not all of the composition ranges shown in Table 25–2 will meet the composition requirements presented in Table 25–1, particularly for the lower gold contents. For example, any alloy of Type A (Table 25–2) with a gold content of less than 83 per cent would not meet the Specification requirements for composition as indicated for a Type I alloy in Table 25–1. For the most reliable results, the dentist should select only those casting gold alloys which are certified to meet the American Dental Association Specification No. 5 for dental casting gold alloys.

One of the important considerations involved in the formulation of a gold alloy for dental use is that sufficient precious metal is employed to insure that the gold alloy restoration will not discolor in the mouth fluids. Furthermore, the melting temperature of the alloy should be sufficiently low so that the alloy can be melted in accordance with the usual dental practice.

The basic alloy is a ternary type of gold, copper and silver, as indicated by the composition limits of the Type A alloys (Table 25–2). Platinum and palladium are rarely added to a Type A or a Type I alloy. As greater strength and hardness are required, platinum and palladium are added to the other types.

**General Effects of Constituents.**     As can be noted from Table 25–2, many of the dental gold alloys are complex, with six or more metallic constituents. It is impossible to study such systems with constitution diagrams, as was done with the binary alloys (Chapter 20). Most of the information concerning the effects of the various constituents is empirical, having been obtained principally from the compositions of a large number of alloys as related to their physical properties.[3, 4] It is largely on the basis of such studies and general experience that the following observations concerning the effects of the various constituent metals on the alloys are made.

*Gold.*     Gold is, of course, the principal constituent of the gold-colored alloys. Its chief contribution is to increase the tarnish resistance of the alloy. As previously indicated in Chapter 21, the tarnish resistance of an alloy is almost a linear function of the gold content when it is combined with base metals. It is estimated that, in general, the number of gold atoms must at least equal the number of base metal atoms for the proper resistance to tarnish and corrosion in the mouth.[5] On such a basis, the gold content of a dental alloy should be at least 75 per cent by weight. However, platinum and palladium can be substituted for gold to a certain extent, as indicated by the American Dental Association Specification requirements.

Gold also contributes ductility to the alloy. It increases the specific gravity, and it is a factor in the heat treatment of the alloy, principally in combination with copper.

*Copper.*     The most important contribution of copper to the gold alloy is to increase the strength and hardness of the alloy. For example, the Brinell hardness number of pure gold may be as low as 32, but the addition of approximately 4 per cent of copper can impart a Brinell number[6] to it as high as 54. The hardness of the gold-silver-copper alloy may be increased in direct proportion to the copper added up to 20 per cent.[7]

The second important contribution of the copper is its role in age hardening in combination with gold, platinum and palladium. More than 4 per cent of copper must be present in an alloy amenable to age hardening heat treatment. If 8 to as high as 25 per cent copper is present, age hardening occurs readily.[5] However, copper lowers the tarnish and corrosion resistance of the alloy, and its use in dental alloys is therefore limited.

Copper generally reduces the melting point of the alloy, and it tends also to reduce the difference in temperature between the upper and lower limits of the melting range. As outlined in Chapter 20, most alloys solidify over a range in temperature, and the less the temperature range generally, the less is the amount of coring to be expected in the alloy.

Within the composition limits of the copper generally used in dental gold alloys, it increases the ductility of the alloy when metals other than gold are added. It tends to impart its own reddish color to the alloy.

*Silver.*     Although silver may affect the heat treatment of an alloy in combination with copper, it is generally somewhat neutral in its effect. It tends to whiten the alloy, and it may enrich the yellow color by neutralizing the reddish color contributed by the copper. In certain instances, it may contribute to the ductility of the gold alloy, particularly in the presence of palladium.

*Platinum.*     Platinum is an even better hardener and strengthener of gold alloys than is copper, and consequently it is used for this purpose. It increases the tarnish and corrosion resistance of the alloy along with gold.

The use of platinum in casting gold alloys is limited by the fact that the platinum increases the melting point. The temperature at which the alloy begins to solidify (liquidus temperature) in the case of dental casting alloys is in the neighborhood of, or less than, 1000° C. (1832° F.), and consequently the maximum platinum content of a dental alloy averages around 3 to 4 per cent.

The platinum tends to whiten the alloy. It reacts with copper to produce an effective age hardening.

*Palladium.*     Because palladium is cheaper in price than platinum, it is often added to alloys to replace the latter. Such a substitution is often successful, since the palladium contributes to the alloy in somewhat the same manner as platinum.

Although the palladium melts at a lower temperature than platinum, it is more effective in raising the melting temperature of the alloy than is platinum. Consequently, it should be used in casting alloys even more sparingly than platinum, all conditions being equal. However, some palladium is generally present in modern alloys of the harder types

(Table 25–2) regardless of the presence of platinum. Palladium is an effective strengthener, hardener and age hardening element, but it is not so effective as platinum in this regard.

The palladium is more effective than any of the other constituents usually employed in dental gold alloys in its ability to whiten the alloy. As little as 5 to 6 per cent of palladium will definitely whiten the alloy. It will be shown in a subsequent section that palladium is the principal active constituent of the "white golds" used in dentistry.

Since the specific gravity of the palladium is less than that of gold and platinum, it can be credited with reducing the weight of the alloy per unit volume.

*Zinc.* Zinc is added in small amounts as a scavenger constituent. It acts to combine with any oxides present, and, thereby, to increase the "castability" of the alloy. It also reduces the melting point.

**Fusion Temperature.** It is important to know the melting range of a casting gold alloy so that the dentist will know the approximate temperature to which the alloy should be heated when it is cast. The alloy must be completely liquid at the casting temperature so that it can be forced into the mold. Consequently, the alloy should be heated slightly above its melting range or liquidus temperature. The temperature range of fusion should be supplied by the manufacturer of the alloy.

It is too complicated a process to obtain the fusion range of an alloy in routine testing. Instead, the *fusion temperature* is routinely determined for dental gold alloys according to the directions presented in the American Dental Association Specification No. 5. The test consists of subjecting a sample of the alloy to a specified tensile stress at progressively higher temperatures. The temperature at which the alloy fractures under the stress is called the *fusion temperature.* The minimum value for this temperature is 940° C. (1725° F.) for a Type I alloy (Table 25–1), 900° C. (1650° F.) for Types II and III, and 870° C. (1600° F.) for a Type IV alloy. The fusion temperature is slightly lower than the complete solidification or solidus temperature. It is of particular value in estimating the maximum temperature for soldering the alloy without melting or softening it unduly.

**Heat Treatment.** Gold alloys can be age hardened according to the theory described in Chapter 20. However, as pointed out in that chapter, the actual solid transformations which take place in an alloy with as many as six metals are complex. Very likely, the hardening may result from several different solid-solid transformations. Because of the complicated nature of the transformations, the final criterion as to the success of an age hardening treatment is its actual trial under testing conditions.

There is sometimes a difference in terminology between the dental and the metallurgical literature. The annealing or solution heat treat-

ment is often called the *softening heat treatment* in the dental literature, and all age hardening treatments are referred to as *hardening
heat treatments*. The student should be familiar with such synonymous
terms.

**Softening Heat Treatment.** A successful solution or softening heat
treatment is that prescribed in the American Dental Association Specification No. 5. The alloy is placed in an electric furnace for 10 minutes
at a temperature of 700° C. (1290° F.), and then it is quenched in
water. During this period, all solid transformations are presumably
changed to a disordered solid solution, and the rapid quenching prevents their re-formation during cooling. The tensile strength, proportional limit, and hardness are reduced by such a treatment, but the
ductility is increased.

The use of a softening heat treatment is indicated for structures
which are to be ground, shaped or otherwise cold-worked, either in or
out of the mouth. An increased ductility improves the "workability,"
for reasons stated in Chapter 18.

**Hardening Heat Treatment.** The age hardening or hardening heat
treatment of dental alloys can be accomplished in any one of three
ways. The alloy can be cooled slowly from red heat (700° C.). Such a
treatment allows time for the proper transformations to take place.

Such a slow cooling treatment can be started at a lower temperature
than red heat. For example, the method prescribed in the American
Dental Association Specification No. 5 is to cool the alloy from 450° C.
(840° F.) to 250° C. (480° F.) over a period of 30 minutes in a furnace,
and then to quench it in water. This method of age hardening is sometimes known as the "oven-cooling" treatment. Such a treatment is
somewhat drastic for many dental gold alloys because they may be
rendered too brittle; it is included in the Specification for testing purposes only. When the "oven-cooling" treatment is used practically,
a shorter cooling time is used, such as 15 minutes, for example.

The third and more practical method used for heat treatment is the
usual age hardening treatment of "soaking" or aging the alloy at a
definite temperature for a definite time before it is quenched. The temperature for aging depends upon the composition of the alloy, but it is
usually between 350° C. (660° F.) and 450° C. (840° F.). The time
required for such age hardening is usually 15 minutes. The proper
method for the hardening heat treatment should be specified by the
manufacturer of the alloy.

In any event, before the alloy is given an age hardening treatment,
it should first be subjected to a softening heat treatment in order to
relieve all strain hardening, if present, and to start the hardening treatment with the alloy as a disordered solid solution. Otherwise, there
would not be a proper control of the hardening process. The increase
in strength, proportional limit, and hardness, and the reduction in

ductility, are controlled by the amount of solid-solid transformations allowed. The transformations, in turn, are controlled by the temperature and time of the treatment.

Since the proportional limit is increased during age hardening, a considerable increase in the modulus of resilence can be expected. The hardening heat treatment is indicated for metallic partial dentures, saddles, and similar structures. In the case of small structures such as inlays, a hardening treatment is not usually employed. An alloy of sufficient resilience in the annealed condition is generally used in such a case.

**Furnaces for Heat Treatment.**   Any annealing treatment is best accomplished in an electric furnace, in order to insure a controlled and uniform temperature. However, a small structure, such as an inlay, can be annealed successfully in a Bunsen burner.

Electric furnaces, equipped with thermoregulators, are available for age hardening treatments of both the aging and the "oven-cooling" type. If the age hardening is to be accomplished at a constant temperature, a salt bath[8] can be used, composed of equal parts of potassium nitrate and sodium nitrate. The mixture melts at 200° C. (400° F.) and may be heated to temperatures ordinarily employed for the age hardening of dental alloys. When the dental structure is placed in such a bath, care should be taken that no moisture or wax is clinging to it. Water and wax are likely to cause explosions and spray molten liquid from the bath as they volatilize at the high temperature.

**Physical Properties of Cast Gold Dental Alloys.**   The range of properties for the alloy compositions given in Table 25–2 are presented in Table 25–3. As can be noted, the range of properties which might be desired is fairly well covered when both the softened and age hardened conditions are considered. The values given in the table are average values, and any gaps can be easily filled by a slight change in composition or heat treatment. The dentist probably has a broader selection of alloys according to their physical properties than does the structural engineer, for example.

A definite relationship exists between the Brinell hardness number of the alloys and their tensile strength. It has been shown[9] that if the Brinell hardness number of an alloy is multiplied by 500, an excellent estimate of its ultimate tensile strength can be obtained in pounds per square inch.* An approximate estimate of the proportional limit of the alloy in pounds per square inch can be obtained by multiplying the Brinell hardness number by 400.

As can be noted from Table 25–3, increases in tensile strength, proportional limit and hardness are generally accompanied by a decrease in ductility. With the proper composition, however, a comparatively

---

* The factor is 35 for the tensile strength and 30 for the proportional limit, if the metric units of kilograms per square centimeter are employed.

*Table 25-3.  Mechanical Properties of Cast Dental Gold Alloys\**

| TYPE† | TREATMENT | B.H.N. | ULTIMATE TENSILE STRENGTH | | PROPORTIONAL LIMIT | | ELONGATION (%) |
|---|---|---|---|---|---|---|---|
| | | | (100 KG./CM²) | (1000 LB./IN.²) | (100 KG./CM²) | (1000 LB./IN.²) | |
| A | Softened | 45–70 | 21–32 | 30–45 | 6–10 | 8–15 | 20–35 |
| B | Softened | 80–90 | 32–38 | 45–55 | 14–18 | 20–25 | 20–35 |
| C | Softened | 95–115 | 34–40 | 48–57 | 16–21 | 23–30 | 20–25 |
| | Age hardened | 115–165 | 42–57 | 60–82 | 20–41 | 29–58 | 6–20 |
| D | Softened | 130–160 | 42–52 | 60–75 | 24–33 | 35–47 | 4–25 |
| | Age hardened | 210–235 | 70–84 | 100–120 | 42–64 | 60–92 | 1–6 |

\* Metals Handbook, 1948 edition.
† Composition given in Table 25-2.

high value for the percentage elongation can be obtained with relatively high strength properties.

**Classification of Dental Casting Gold Alloys.** The alloys listed in Tables 25–2 and 25–3 can be classified according to their use as well as according to their hardness and other properties.

It is generally considered that any alloy with a Brinell hardness number less than 40 is too soft and weak to be used in the mouth. Such alloys will distort permanently under stress until they have become sufficiently strain hardened to resist further stress. The initial distortion is definitely undesirable in an inlay or similar restoration for obvious reasons, and consequently it is to be avoided by the use of stronger and harder alloys.

*Type I.* These alloys should range in hardness (B.H.N.) between 40 and 75, and they should exhibit a percentage elongation of at least 18 per cent. As previously noted, they are essentially alloys of gold, silver and copper, and they seldom or never contain platinum or palladium.

They are quite ductile, and can be burnished readily, but they possess a relatively low proportional limit as indicated by the similar classification shown in Table 25–3 (Type A). They cannot be age hardened. They are quite high melting, and should be heated to temperatures slightly in excess of 950 to 1050° C. (1740 to 1920° F.) for complete fusion.[2]

The Type I alloys are inlay gold alloys to be used in restorations not subject to great stress, such as the restoration of simple proximal incisor and cuspid cavities, and gingival third cavities (Black classification, classes 3 and 5, respectively). The harder members of this type can be used as inlays for prepared cavities in the proximal surfaces of bicuspids and molars, and those occurring in the proximal surfaces of the incisors and cuspids which require the removal and restoration of the incisal angle (Black, classes 2 and 4, respectively).

*Type II.* The alloys belonging to this group have Brinell numbers ranging from 70 to 100, according to the American Dental Association Specification No. 5. Actually, many of the commercial alloys in the similar classification appear to be grouped between Brinell hardness numbers 80 to 90 in the annealed condition (Table 25–3, Type B). This type may contain some palladium and platinum, and the copper content is higher than that of the previous type. These alloys are often classified as "light" and "dark," according to the amount of copper they contain. Their fusion temperature is somewhat lower than that of the Type I alloys. These alloys are completely molten at temperatures in excess of 930 to 970° C. (1700 to 1780° F.).

In spite of the fact that the tensile properties of these alloys are higher than those of the Type I alloys, they possess almost the same values for percentage elongation as the previous group. Many alloys of this type can be age hardened, if it is desirable.

The Type II alloys can be used for any type of inlay, and they are very popular with the dental profession for operative procedures.

*Type III.*    According to the American Dental Association Specification No. 5, the Brinell hardness numbers of this type of alloy should range between 90 and 140 in the softened condition. This group of alloys usually contain the greatest amounts of palladium and/or platinum permissible to allow a fusion temperature within the range of the usual dental gas-air torch. Consequently, these alloys are stronger and harder than the other two types. Because of the platinum and palladium present, they tend to be a lighter yellow in color than the other types of alloy. The percentage elongation of these alloys is lower than that of the previous types (Table 25–3). They are all amenable to age hardening, with a marked decrease in ductility resulting.

Their use is usually confined to crowns, bridge abutments and inlays which are subject to great stress during mastication.

*Type IV.*    A special classification is necessary for those alloys which are suitable for casting large appliances such as saddles, one-piece partial dentures, clasps and lingual bars. Strength and resilience are definitely needed in such alloys, but the fusion temperature cannot be too high, since a considerable weight of the alloy must be fused at one time. Consequently, this type of alloy possesses a fusion temperature generally lower than that of the other types, in the neighborhood of 870 to 985° C. (1600 to 1800° F.).[2]

The fusion temperature is lowered by the introduction of more copper at the expense of the gold content (Table 25–2). Since the alloy is employed for the casting of removable appliances which can be cleansed or polished outside the mouth, a small amount of the protection against tarnish can be sacrificed. The palladium-platinum content can be increased slightly, so that the strongest and hardest alloys of the entire series are included in this type.

The Brinell hardness number of this type of alloy should be 130, or above, after a softening heat treatment. All of the alloys are amenable to age hardening. In fact, their response to age hardening is generally greater than that of any of the other types. Unfortunately, the percentage elongation of this group of alloys is apt to be comparatively low, particularly after age hardening. This lack of ductility should be taken into account during any bending or other adjustment of the appliance after it has been cast.

**"White Gold" Alloys.**    All of the alloys so far described have been "gold-colored," in that the characteristic color of gold generally predominates. As previously noted, the alloy can be rendered "white" or silver-colored by the addition of platinum, palladium, or silver. Nickel can also be employed, but it is generally used sparingly, if at all, in dental casting alloys because of its tendency to embrittle the alloy and to lower its tarnish resistance.

Palladium is the most effective whitener and the dental alloys of this type might well be named "palladium alloys" rather than gold alloys, since the gold content is apt to be at a minimum. For example, one commerical white gold alloy contains gold, 15 per cent; palladium, 24 per cent; silver, 45 per cent; copper, 15 per cent; and zinc, 1 per cent. Typically, however, the better inlay alloys of this type contain gold, 65 to 70 per cent; silver, 7 to 12 per cent; copper, 6 to 10 per cent; palladium 10 to 12 per cent; platinum, 0 to 4 per cent; and zinc, 1 to 2 per cent.[2]

All of these alloys are hard, with Brinell numbers of over 100 in the softened condition. They exhibit generally a low ductility in comparison to the gold-colored alloys, and their tarnish resistance is definitely lower. As might be expected from the high palladium content, the upper limit of their fusion range is high, in the neighborhood of 1025° C. (1880° F.). As a consequence, they are difficult to melt in quantity with the gas-air torch, and unless special care is observed, an oxidation of the palladium may occur. The result of such oxidation is a further reduction in the percentage elongation, an increase in hardness and a reduction in tarnish resistance.

The alloys are amenable to age hardening, but such a treatment may decrease the percentage elongation to as low as 2 per cent.

**Casting Shrinkage.**     As noted in a previous chapter, most metals and alloys shrink when they change from the liquid to the solid state. Gold and its alloys are no exception to this rule.

Such a consideration is of importance in the dental casting procedure. For example, if a mold for an inlay is an accurate reproduction of the missing tooth structure, the gold inlay after casting will be too small by the amount of its casting shrinkage.

The shrinkage occurs in three stages:[10,11] (1) the thermal contraction of the liquid metal between the temperature to which it was heated and the first solidification temperature (liquidus); (2) the contraction of the metal inherent in the change from the liquid to the solid state; and (3) the thermal contraction of the solid metal which occurs to room temperature.

The first-mentioned contraction is probably of no consequence, since as the liquid metal contracts in the mold, more molten metal can flow into the mold to compensate for such a shrinkage. The casting technic, to be described in a subsequent chapter, allows for such a flow of molten metal.

The thermal contraction of a number of dental alloys and gold has been measured, and the results are presented[11] in Table 25-4.

In an attempt to determine the effect of the second stage, various casting alloys were cast by a dental technic into a cylindrical mold, 3.2

millimeters (⅛ inch) in diameter and 76.2 millimeters (3 inches) in length.[11] Since the length of the mold had been carefully predetermined, the percentage shortening of the cast cylinder in comparison to the original length would represent the linear casting shrinkage. Many castings of different dimensions, shapes and compositions were made, and the final value for the casting shrinkage was given[12] as 1.25±0.1 per cent.

It is apparent that the value obtained for the casting shrinkage is less than the linear thermal shrinkage values given in Table 25–4, even though the casting shrinkage as obtained included both the solidification shrinkage and the thermal shrinkage as outlined above.

This seemingly anomalous condition can be accounted for by two logical assumptions.[11] (1) When the mold becomes filled with molten metal, the metal starts to solidify at the walls of the mold, since the temperature of the mold is less than that of the molten metal. (2) During the initial cooling, the first layer of metal to solidify against the walls of the mold is weak, and it will tend to adhere to the mold until it has gained sufficient strength as it cools to pull away. Once it is sufficiently strong to contract independently of the mold, it will shrink thermally until it reaches room temperature.

The important consideration is that the thermal shrinkage of the first weak, solidified layer is initially prevented by its mechanical adhesion to the walls of the mold; during this period, it is actually stretched because of its interlocking with the investment material. Thus, the entire liquid-solid contraction can be eliminated, and part of the thermal contraction can be prevented, with the result that the observed casting shrinkage is less than might be expected on the basis of the three possible stages of the shrinkage as previously stated.

As the first outer layer solidifies, subsequent layers toward the center will solidify against it, until the entire mass is solid.

A further step in the above reasoning indicates that the greater the surface of the casting in relation to its volume, the less will be the casting shrinkage. For example, in a thin casting such as a disk, the increased area of the mold surface may be more effective in stretching

*Table 25–4.* *Percentage Linear Thermal Contraction of Gold Alloys and Gold from Their Melting Points (Solidi)**

| METAL | THERMAL CONTRACTION FROM MELTING POINT TO 25°C. (77°F.) (%) |
| --- | --- |
| Gold (100%) | 1.76 |
| Gold (90%), silver (10%) | 2.03 |
| Gold (90%), copper (10%) | 1.62 |
| Gold (90%), nickel (10%) | 1.91 |

* Coleman, Nat'l. Bur. Standards Research Paper No. 32.

*Table 25–5.*     *Linear Casting Shrinkage of Inlay Casting Gold Alloys*

| METAL | CASTING SHRINKAGE (%) |
|---|---|
| Gold (100%) | 1.67 |
| 22-Carat alloy* | 1.50 |
| Type I | 1.56 |
| Type II | 1.37 |
| Type III | 1.42 |

* Approximate composition: gold, 91.6%; silver, 4.2%; copper, 4.2%.

the freshly solidified metal than a smaller surface surrounding a greater volume, as in the case of a sphere. Consequently, the disk might exhibit less casting shrinkage than the sphere. Similarly, a casting with an irregular shape that would cause the solidifying gold to interlock with the walls of the mold might show less shrinkage than a smooth, cylindrical casting.

A later determination[13] of the casting shrinkage of smooth, cylindrical castings, 6.35 millimeters (¼ inch) in diameter and 25.4 millimeters (1 inch) in length, resulted in the values given in Table 25–5. The last three alloys listed were typical casting gold alloys with compositions in the range given in Table 25–2. The values for the casting shrinkage differ for the different alloys, presumably because of differences in their composition. It has been shown, for example, that platinum, palladium and copper are all effective in reducing the casting shrinkage of an alloy. It is of interest that the value for the casting shrinkage of pure gold (Table 25–5) closely approaches that of its maximum linear thermal contraction (Table 25–4).

None of the values for the linear casting shrinkage in Table 25–5 are as low as the value of 1.25 per cent previously quoted. There may be two reasons for this difference: (1) The modern alloys may exhibit a greater casting shrinkage than those employed for the first determination (*circa* 1928). (2) The cylinder used in the later investigation differed in dimension (6.35 × 25.4 millimeters) from the cylinder formerly used (3.2 × 76.2 millimeters). Since the surface area of the latter cylinder was less in proportion to its volume than that of the first cylinder used, according to the theory previously stated, a greater casting shrinkage should occur in the bulkier cylinder than in the longer and narrower cylinder.

**Porosity in Castings.**     Porosities in gold alloy castings can be classified as follows:[14]

1. Porosities caused by cooling and solidification.
    a. Localized shrinkage porosity.
    b. Microporosity.
    c. Subsurface porosity.

2. Porosities caused by gas.
    a. Pinhole porosity.
    b. Gas inclusions.

The porosity due to localized shrinkage is caused by a lack of molten metal during solidification. As noted in the previous section, during the initial stages of solidification, the solidified metal adheres to the walls of the mold. If the supply of molten metal is cut off at this stage, or before the mold is completely filled, the lack of metal causes voids, particularly near the ingate where the molten metal enters the mold.

This type of porosity can be seen near the ingate in Figure 25–1*a* and in Figure 25–2*C*. As can be noted in Figure 25–2*C*, the porosity occurs in the core area of the dendritic formation. The higher melting constituents solidify but because of insufficient metal, voids form where the lower melting compositions usually surround the dendrites.

If the mold temperature is low, or if the temperature of the molten alloy is near its liquidus temperature, the solidification may occur so rapidly that a shrinkage develops throughout the entire casting to cause the microporosity shown in Figure 25–1*b* and portions of Figure 25–2*A* in the form of small irregular voids.[14]

Subsurface porosity (Figs. 25–1*d* and 25–2*B*) occurs near the border of the casting. This type of porosity is particularly evident in Figure 25–3. The cause is thought to be related to the rate of solidification of the casting.[14] For example, if the molten metal is fed into the mold

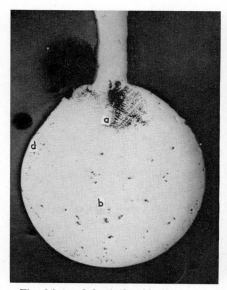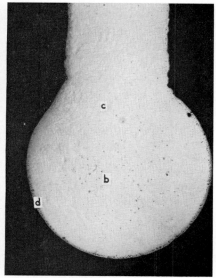

Fig. 25–1. Spherical gold alloy castings. *a.* Localized shrinkage porosity; *b.* microporosity; *c.* pinhole porosity and *d.* subsurface porosity. (Ryge, Kozak and Fairhurst, *J.A.D.A.*, June, 1957.)

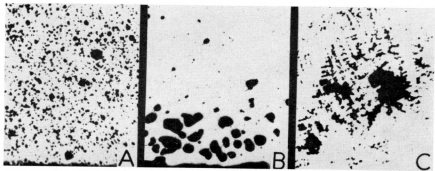

Fig. 25–2. *A.* Microporosity, pinhole porosity and gas inclusions. (Microporosity voids are irregular in shape whereas the other two types tend to be spherical; the largest spherical voids are gas inclusions.) *B.* Subsurface porosity. *C.* Localized shrinkage porosity. (Courtesy of G. Ryge, Marquette University.)

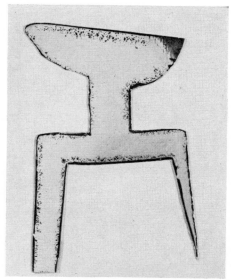

Fig. 25–3. Subsurface porosity around the entire periphery of a casting. (Ryge, Kozak and Fairhurst, *J.A.D.A.,* June, 1957.)

rapidly at a high temperature, the center mass may remain molten longer than the "skin" which solidifies immediately on contact with the mold walls. As already mentioned, this initially solidified layer or "skin" possesses some strength and is mechanically locked to the mold walls. As the center portion then contracts during solidification it may form voids between the "skin" and the interior.

As will be shown in a subsequent chapter, these types of porosity can be minimized by controlling the rate at which the molten metal enters the mold.

The pinhole and gas inclusion porosities are both related to the entrapment of gas during solidification. They are both characterized by a spherical contour but they are decidedly different in size. The gas inclusion porosities are usually much larger than the other type as indicated in Figure 25–2A.

Many metals dissolve or occlude gases while they are molten. For example, both copper and silver will dissolve oxygen in large amounts in the liquid state. Molten platinum and palladium have a strong affinity for hydrogen as well as oxygen. Upon solidification, the absorbed gases are expelled and the pinhole porosity results. The larger voids (Fig. 25–2A) may also result from the same cause, but it seems more logical to assume that such voids may be caused by gas mechanically trapped by the molten metal in the mold or else carried in during the casting procedure.

All castings probably contain a certain amount of porosity as exemplified by the photomicrograph shown in Figure 25–4B. However, the porosity should be kept to a minimum since it deleteriously affects the physical properties of the casting.[3, 15, 16]

**Corrosion.**    As noted in Chapter 21, a gold alloy can tarnish or corrode in the mouth under certain conditions. For example, as previously noted, the precious metal content (gold, platinum and palladium) must be sufficient to prevent corrosion which may be related to the composition of the alloy. This factor should be unimportant if the gold alloy is certified to meet the composition requirement of the American Dental Association Specification No. 5 for dental inlay casting gold alloys.

Electrolytic tarnish and corrosion can occur if the gold alloy restoration is in contact with a restoration of a dissimilar metal such as an amalgam. The theory of such corrosion is understood, but there are many variables which may complicate the basic phenomenon.[17] As a result of the electrolytic corrosion, mercury and other elements may be dissolved by the gold alloy from the amalgam. Both the resulting inhomogeneity of the gold alloy and its solution potential in relation to that of the amalgam result in corrosion products of varying colors depending on the chemical compounds formed.

It is possible that a gold alloy restoration may tarnish in the mouth even though no other restorations are present. In such a case, surface inhomogeneity of the alloy due to coring is one of the main causes to be suspected.

Coring can occur for many reasons, but as previously described, a slow cooling of the alloy between its liquidus and solidus and to room temperature in the solid state, aids greatly in the homogenization of the coring. Such a procedure would be inconvenient and impractical with the dental casting technics employed at the present time. Furthermore, as explained in Chapter 17, an undesirably large grain structure of the casting would result.

**Other methods for the reduction of coring are by altering the alloy**

A

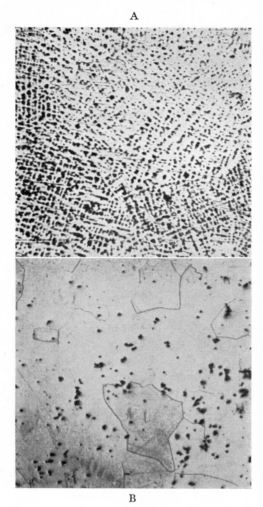

B

Fig. 25–4. *A*. Grain structure of a Type III gold alloy as cast. *B*. Same alloy after homogenizing at 725° C. (1337° F.) for 70 minutes. Pinhole porosity can be noted in *B*. (Courtesy of B. Hedegård, University of Umeå.)

compositions so that a small fusion range in temperature will occur during solidification. In this respect, the gold-copper alloys are excellent. Little or no coring will occur regardless of the cooling rate, within practical limits at least. As can be noted from the gold-copper constitution diagram (page 335), a small fusion range is present with these alloys regardless of the composition.

The addition of other metals, particularly platinum and palladium, may alter the situation under certain conditions and may produce an objectionable amount of coring. A superior dental gold alloy, therefore, should exhibit a minimum amount of coring during solidification under the conditions employed by the dentist in casting, in addition to its other desirable properties.

As described in Chapter 20, it is possible to homogenize a cast dental restoration by heating it to a temperature near its solidus for a specified time. Such a procedure may be indicated in the case of metallic dental prostheses, according to a clinical study in this regard.[18]

A Type III gold alloy was employed for the construction of dental bridges in the mouths of 53 patients. The gold alloy selected had a fusion range of 945 to 880° C. (1732 to 1612° F.). Its microstructure as cast is shown in Figure 25–4A and, after a homogenization at 725° C. (1337° F.) for 70 minutes, the recrystallized grain structure is shown in Figure 25–4B. Twenty-six of the patients received bridges which were inserted as cast, and the bridges for the other 27 patients were homogenized before insertion. The cases were observed for three years and a marked difference was noted in the tarnish or discoloration of the bridges in two groups. In the case of the group with the inhomogeneous restorations, all crowns, bridges and soldered joints were discolored. In the other group, 12 cases exhibited no discoloration whatever. There was a slight discoloration observed with the bridges in the mouths of the remaining 15 patients, usually on a surface in contact with an amalgam restoration or at a soldered joint. It is unlikely that the solder would homogenize as readily, if at all, as did the casting gold alloy.

It was also noted that subjective symptoms such as an increase in salivation, prickling sensation in the tongue and general oral discomfort were more frequent in the cases of patients with the inhomogeneous bridges than with the other group. Lesions of the mucous membrane were observed in three patients with inhomogeneous bridges. The lesions disappeared in two to four months after the inhomogeneous bridges were replaced with temporary acrylic resin bridges.[18]

The preceding research has been described at some length, since it is the only systematic clinical investigation on record of a situation which should be more widespread according to the theoretical considerations involved. The clinical evaluation of this study by other observers is yet to be done.

Although the occurrence of pathologic tissue changes may be rare, the discoloration of the gold alloy on the surface of the bridge or inlay is unpleasant to look at, and it cannot be removed by the patient with ordinary methods of mouth hygiene. Although polishing during periodic prophylaxes might maintain the rich gold color of the exposed surfaces of the bridge, it cannot remove the gradually intensified gray color of a plastic facing occasioned by a tarnish of the gold alloy behind the facing,[18] for example.

**Remelting of Casting Alloys.** There is always a surplus of gold alloy which is detached from the casting before the restoration or appliance is placed in the mouth. If this surplus can be re-cast, a considerable economic saving can be effected.

It has been shown[19] that an alloy can be remelted two or three times before any important change in its composition occurs. The only element that is likely to be volatilized during heating is the zinc. As previously noted, the chief function of the zinc is to act as a scavenger for the oxides. As the zinc content decreases, the tendency for the alloy to oxidize during melting becomes greater. Usually this lack of zinc can be remedied sufficiently by the addition of new alloy to the remelted metal as it is necessary.

Any surplus gold alloy should be saved and segregated according to its type. It is an obvious fact that the use of nondescript "scrap gold" for casting purposes is definitely not indicated.

## Literature

1. Souder, W. and Paffenbarger, G. C.: *Physical Properties of Dental Materials.* National Bureau of Standards Circular C433. Washington, U. S. Government Printing Office, 1942, pp. 188–191.
2. Wise, E. M.: Cast Gold Dental Alloys, in *Metals Handbook,* 1948 edition. Cleveland, American Society for Metals, 1948, p. 1121.
3. Coleman, R. L.: *Physical Properties of Dental Material.* National Bureau of Standards Research Paper No. 32. Washington, U. S. Government Printing Office, 1928, p. 893.
4. Souder, W. and Paffenbarger, G. C., *loc. cit.,* pp. 37,57.
5. Lane, J. R.: *A Survey of Dental Alloys.* J.A.D.A., *39:*421–437 (Oct.), 1949.
6. Coleman, R. L., *loc. cit.,* p. 907.
7. Vines, R. F. and Wise, E. M.: *Age Hardening Precious Metal Alloys.* A.S.M. Symposium, 1939, pp. 190–230.
8. Paffenbarger, G. C., and Sweeney, W. T.: *Dental Research at the National Bureau of Standards in Relation to Orthodontia.* Int. J. Ortho., *20:*1166–1172 (Dec.), 1934.
9. Souder, W. and Paffenbarger, G. C., *loc. cit.,* pp. 64–65.
10. *Ibid.,* pp. 69–73.
11. Coleman, R. L., *loc. cit.,* 908–911.
12. Souder, W.: *Fifteen Years of Dental Research at the National Bureau of Standards.* J.A.D.A., *21:*58–66 (Jan.), 1934.
13. Hollenback, G. M., and Skinner, E. W.: *Shrinkage During Castings of Gold and Gold Alloys.* J.A.D.A., *33:*1391–1399 (Nov. 1), 1946.
14. Ryge, G., Kozak, S. F. and Fairhurst, C. W.: *Porosities in Dental Gold Castings.* J.A.D.A., *54:*746–754 (June), 1957.
15. Peyton, F. A.: *Flexure Fatigue Studies of Cast Dental Alloys.* J.A.D.A., *21:*394 (March), 1934.
16. Crawford, W. H.: *Selection and Use of Investments, Sprues, Casting Equipment and Gold Alloys in Making Small Castings.* J.A.D.A., *27:*1459–1470 (Sept.), 1940.
17. Swartz, M. L., Phillips, R. W. and El Tannir, M. D.: *Tarnish of Certain Dental Alloys.* J. D. Res., *37:*837–847 (Oct.), 1958.
18. Hedegård, B.: *Homogenization.* Dept. Pros., Royal Sch. Dent., Stockholm (1958).
19. Coleman, R. L., *loc. cit.,* p. 897.

# CHAPTER 26

# Inlay Casting Wax

The first procedure in the casting of an inlay is the preparation of a wax pattern. The cavity is prepared in the tooth and the pattern is carved, either directly in the tooth or on a die which is a reproduction of the tooth and the prepared cavity. If the pattern is made in the tooth itself, it is said to be prepared by the *direct technic*. If it is prepared on a die, the procedure is called the *indirect technic*. There are other modifications of the technics, but these two classifications are sufficient for the present purpose.

However the pattern is prepared, it should be an accurate reproduction in form of the missing tooth structure. The wax pattern forms the outline of the mold into which the gold alloy is cast, and consequently the casting can be no more accurate than the wax pattern, regardless of the care observed in subsequent procedures. Therefore, the pattern should be well adapted to the prepared cavity, properly carved and the distortion factors minimized.

Wax patterns are used in the casting of many complex restorations other than inlays and crowns, but the present discussion will be limited to the construction of restorations employed in operative dentistry.

**Composition.** A number of formulas for inlay wax have been published,[1-5] some of which are quite complex. The essential ingredients of a successful inlay wax are paraffin wax, gum dammar and carnauba wax, with some coloring material. All of these substances are of natural origin derived from mineral or vegetable sources.

Paraffin wax is generally the main ingredient, usually in a concentration of 40 to 60 per cent. Paraffin is derived from the high-boiling fractions of petroleum. It is composed mainly of a complex mixture of hydrocarbons of the methane series, together with a minor amount of amorphous or microcrystalline phases. The wax can be obtained in a wide melting or softening range depending upon the molecular weight of the constituents. The melting range can be determined by means of a time-temperature cooling curve as shown in Figure 26–1 for an inlay wax containing paraffin. The time-temperature relationship during cooling indicates the successive solidification of progressively lower molecular weight fractions. Such a condition is desirable from a dental standpoint, since it imparts a moldability to the wax below its temperature of liquefaction.

Unfortunately, the paraffin wax is likely to flake when it is trimmed, and it does not present a smooth, glossy surface, which is a desirable requisite for an inlay wax. Consequently, the other waxes and natural resins to be mentioned are added as modifying agents.

Gum dammar, or dammar resin, is a natural resin derived from a certain variety of pine tree. It is added to the paraffin to improve the smoothness in molding, and to render it more resistant to cracking and flaking. It also adds to the toughness of the wax, and it enhances the smoothness and luster of the surface.

Carnauba wax occurs as a fine powder on the leaves of certain tropical palms. This wax is quite hard, and it is relatively high melting. It is combined with the paraffin to decrease the flow of the latter at mouth temperature. It possesses an agreeable odor, and it also contributes to the provision of a glossy surface on the wax, even more than the dammar resin.

Candelilla wax can also be added to replace the carnauba wax, in part or entirely. The candelilla wax contributes much the same general qualities as the carnauba wax, but its melting point is lower, and it is not so hard as carnauba wax.

In modern inlay waxes, the carnauba wax is often replaced in part with certain synthetic waxes which are compatible with paraffin wax. At least two waxes of this type can be used. One is a complex nitrogen derivative of the higher fatty acids, and the other is composed of esters of acids derived from montan wax, a petroleum derivative, and other sources. As in the case of impression compound, the use of a synthetic wax is preferable to that of a natural wax because of the greater uniformity of the former. Because of the high melting point of the synthetic waxes, more paraffin can be incorporated and the general working qualities of the product are improved.

**Desirable Properties.**    There are a number of desirable properties of inlay waxes, some of which are difficult to obtain. For example, it is necessary to soften the wax under heat and then to insert it in the prepared cavity. During this period it should not become flaky or exhibit laminations when it is bent and formed. It should remain plastic when it is heated, and it should be of a smooth texture at all times.

When the direct technic is used, the wax should be sufficiently plastic at a temperature slightly above that of the tooth so that it can be forced into the prepared cavity to reproduce every minute detail. If the softening temperature is too high, the patient will suffer discomfort or a permanent injury to the pulp of the tooth. On the other hand, the wax should be rigid when it is cooled to the temperature of the mouth, so that the finished pattern can be withdrawn from the prepared cavity without distortion or flow.

When the indirect technic is used, a wax of a lower solidification temperature is employed. Since the wax is adapted to a die at room temperature, the lower temperature provides for less distortion by temperature change,[6] easier manipulation and carving. The temperature at which the wax hardens should not be so low that the wax will draw under the carving instrument or flow upon removal from the die preparatory to the investing procedure. According to the current American Dental Association Specification No. 4 for inlay casting wax, the wax employed for the direct technic should not flow more than 1 per cent when tested according to the Specification. Probably the wax for the indirect technic should exhibit the same flow property at 30° C. (86° F.). Such a requirement would assume that the wax for the direct technic would be used at room temperatures greater than 30° C. Other than the different temperature requirement, the requisites of the wax for indirect work are essentially the same as for the wax used in the direct technic.

After the wax has hardened in the tooth or on the die, it is carved to reproduce the missing tooth anatomy. The wax should be capable of being carved to the thinnest margin without distorting, flaking or chipping under the sharp blade of the carving instrument.

The color of the wax should be in sharp contrast to that of the mouth tissues or the die material in order to aid visibility during carving.

In the direct technic, the pattern should not change in dimension greatly when it is removed from the mouth to room temperature. In other words, the wax should have a low thermal coefficient of expansion and contraction.

A common method for the elimination of the wax from the mold is to ignite it. Consequently, the wax should vaporize completely under such a condition, without leaving a residue which might clog the mold and prevent the egress of air and other gases as the molten gold enters. The American Dental Association Specification No. 4 requires that the melted wax, when vaporized at 500° C. (932° F.), shall leave no solid residue in excess of 0.10 per cent of the original weight of the specimen.

*Flow.*     As noted in the previous section, one of the desirable properties of the inlay wax is that it exhibit a marked plasticity or flow at a temperature slightly above that of the mouth. The tempera-

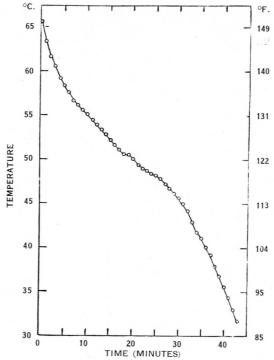

Fig. 26–1.   Time-temperature cooling curve for an inlay wax.

tures at which the wax is plastic are indicated by the time-temperature cooling curve shown in Figure 26–1. The interpretation of this curve is the same as that for its counterpart—a typical time-temperature cooling curve for a solid solution alloy. The wax begins to harden when the curve first departs from a straight line at approximately 56° C. (133° F.), and it is solid below approximately 40° C. (104° F.), when it again cools at a constant rate. When the wax is heated between those two temperatures, the microcrystalline portions and some of the low molecular weight fractions melt, and any amorphous constituents soften.

The American Dental Association Specification No. 4 provides certain requirements for the flow properties of inlay waxes. Cylindrical specimens are prepared, 6 millimeters (0.236 inch) in altitude and 10 millimeters (0.394 inch) in diameter. The specimens are subjected to a load of 2 kilograms (4.4 pounds) for ten minutes at various temperatures, and the flow is measured as the percentage shortening in length. The generally accepted requirement for the flow of direct (Type I) waxes is that it should not be less than 70 per cent at 45° C. (113.0° F.). At approximately this temperature the wax is inserted into the prepared cavity and if it does not have sufficient plasticity, it will not flow into all of the detail in the preparation.

For example, wax No. 5 in Figure 26–2 exhibits a flow of 73 per cent at a temperature of 45° C. However, at a temperature only 8° C. (14° F.) lower, the flow is very small. According to the Specification the flow must not be more than 1.0 per cent at 37° C. (99° F.), which is approximately the temperature of the pattern on the tooth, although the open mouth temperature has been estimated[7] as being 35° C. (95° F.). As previously noted, the wax should be rigid at mouth temperature. It has been shown by experiment[8] that it is impossible to cool the pattern appreciably below mouth temperature while it is in the tooth. The temperature of the wax always returns to that of the tooth before it can be removed from the prepared cavity.

The wax No. *1* in Figure 26–2 might be satisfactory for use in the indirect technic, but it would be too soft at mouth temperature (37° C.) to be withdrawn from the tooth without flow and a consequent change in form. Wax No. *13* in Figure 26–2 softens at too high a temperature for use as an inlay pattern in any accepted type of wax pattern technic.

**Thermal Properties.** As previously noted, the inlay waxes are softened with heat, forced into the prepared cavity, and cooled. The thermal conductivity of the waxes is low, and time is required both to heat them uniformly throughout and to cool them to body or room temperature.

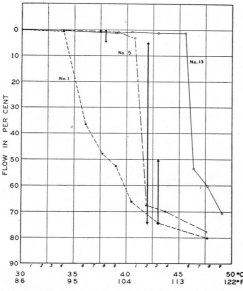

Fig. 26–2. Flow of a soft (*No. 1*), a medium (*No. 5*) and a hard (*No. 13*) inlay wax, tested according to the method described in A.D.A. Specification No. 4. (Souder and Paffenbarger, *National Bureau of Standards Circular C433.*)

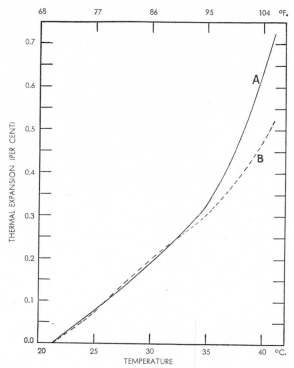

Fig. 26–3. Thermal expansion of an inlay wax. Curve *A* represents the thermal expansion when the wax was held under pressure while it was cooling from the liquid state. When the same wax was allowed to cool without pressure and again heated, curve *B* resulted.

The linear thermal coefficient of expansion of inlay wax is quite high in comparison to most substances. As can be noted from Figure 26–3, the wax may change linearly as much as 0.7 per cent with an increase in temperature of 20° C. (36° F.). Thus, its average linear coefficient of expansion over such a temperature range is 0.00035 per degree Centigrade. A comparison with the linear coefficients of thermal expansion of dental materials given in Table 2–1 indicates that the inlay wax expands and contracts thermally per degree change in temperature more than any other dental material. Inasmuch as the pattern may be formed in the mouth at a temperature of 37° C. (99° F.) and subsequently cooled to the temperature of the room (20° C.), the errors involved in the thermal dimensional changes of the wax may be of considerable importance.

The amount of the thermal change may be affected by the previous treatment of the wax. Curve *A* in Figure 26–3 represents the thermal expansion of an inlay wax which had been previously cooled under pressure. As can be observed, the expansion rate increases abruptly above a temperature of approximately 37° C. (99° F.). The temperature at which the change in rate occurs is known as the transition temperature, or transition point. It is analogous to the transition point described for the synthetic resins (p. 176), and its general effect is very similar. Some constituents of the wax probably change crystalline form at this temperature, and the wax is more plastic at higher temperatures. Not all waxes exhibit transition temperatures; the transition point shown in Figure 26–3 appears to be characteristic of a paraffin wax.[9]

It is of interest to note that when the wax is allowed to cool without being placed under pressure, upon re-heating the transition temperature is not so pronounced, nor is the change in the linear coefficient of expansion so great, as shown in curve *B*, Figure 26–3.

**Wax Distortion.** Probably distortion is the most serious problem faced during the forming and removal of the pattern from the mouth or die. Such distortion arises from thermal changes and from the release of the internal stress always present in the pattern. These stresses are induced from (1) natural tendency of the wax to contract upon cooling, (2) change in shape of the wax during molding and (3) manipulative variables such as carving, pooling and removal. The amount of residual stress and resulting distortion will thus be governed by the method of forming the pattern, its handling and the length of time and temperature at which it is stored. All of these factors will be discussed in the following sections.

The change in dimension or distortion of a wax pattern during relaxation, as with any thermoplastic material, may be considerable as the stress unavoidably induced in the wax during manipulation is released. The condition is similar but more critical than that discussed in connection with impression compounds (p. 65). In the case of the impression compound, as it is used for the impression of an edentulous mouth, the soft tissues might compensate for slight errors in the denture base, caused by the relaxation of the compound. In the case of an inlay wax, however, any warpage of the pattern whatever will be reflected in the misfit of the rigid metallic inlay on the unyielding, hard tissue of the tooth.

An example of a poorly fitting crown is shown in the casting on the right in Figure 26–4. Both castings were made at the same time to fit two shoulder crown dies. As can be noted, the casting on the left in Figure 26–4 fits the shoulder crown die, but the casting on the right is too small. The difference is caused entirely by a difference in the manipulation of the wax in the formation of the patterns.

In the case of the casting on the left (Fig. 26–4), the wax pattern was formed under pressure. A thin cylinder of copper, known as a *matrix band,* was adapted about the die so that the crown preparation was completely surrounded. The wax was melted, and the matrix band was filled with liquefied wax so that the crown preparation was com-

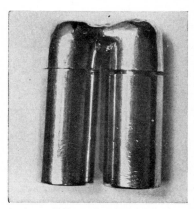

Fig. 26–4.  Castings made from differently manipulated wax patterns. (Courtesy of P. B. Taylor.)

pletely covered. The wax was immediately placed under pressure and immersed in cold water until it solidified. The pattern for the casting on the right was prepared in the same manner, except that the wax was allowed to cool to room temperature without chilling and without being held under pressure.

In the first case, the pressure on the wax introduced compressive stresses into the wax during cooling. Since the wax was confined, the stresses would tend to be hydrostatic in nature, at least above the transition point or before sufficient solidification took place to resist the pressure. After the wax was cooled and the matrix band was removed, the relaxation of the compressive stresses would tend to expand the pattern slightly. Consequently, the casting should fit the crown die, or perhaps it might be a trifle large, depending upon the casting technic.

On the other hand, once the pattern cooled to its transition point without pressure, it would tend to be stretched around the die as it cooled further. Consequently, any relaxation of this pattern would tend to relieve the tensile stresses induced. The pattern would, therefore, contract and the casting would be too small, as shown in the casting on the right, Figure 26–4.

The differences in the thermal expansion curves in Figure 26–3 can now be explained. Both of the wax specimens expanded thermally at the same rate until the transition point was reached. Above the transition temperature, the stresses were released. Since the wax employed in obtaining the data for curve *A* was previously cooled under pressure, when the compressive stresses were relieved, a greater expansion would be expected than if no stresses were present. In the case of the specimen cooled without pressure, its adhesion to the walls of the mold would introduce tensile stresses, with the result that its thermal expansion would be less when such stresses were relaxed. Had the specimen been stretched while it solidified originally, it might exhibit a decrease in length with increase in temperature, since it is possible that the tensile stresses and strains, when relieved, might be sufficient to overcome the natural thermal expansion.[10]

If the conditions are reversed, and if the wax is compressed when it is soft and then cooled, it is possible that the thermal contraction may be nullified by the relaxation. And if the wax is stretched while it is soft, the contraction during cooling may be greater than the normal thermal contraction. Such consideration should always be taken into account when the dentist is obtaining a wax pattern.

According to the theory of relaxation, the higher the temperature, the less is the time required for relaxation. Consequently, it is to be expected that a wax pattern will distort more at mouth temperature than at a normal room temperature in a given time.

The time required for relaxation increases as the temperature decreases. For example, wax patterns were prepared by melting the wax and cooling it under pressure as previously described. Steel dies were used, similar to the one shown on the right in Figure 9–3. The patterns were removed from the dies and stored at room temperature for various periods of time before they were invested. The resulting castings are shown[11] in Figure 26–5. As can be observed, the longer the patterns were stored, the less satisfactory was the fit of the casting. Furthermore, the higher the room temperature during storage, the poorer was the fit of the casting. The maximum time that such wax patterns can be stored at a normal room temperature without noticeable distortion of the casting is approximately 45 minutes.[11]

Naturally, the configuration of the prepared cavity will influence the degree of distortion. While a slight amount of dimensional change does not greatly interfere with the visible fit of a casting made from a simple two-surfaced pattern, a corresponding distortion of the long, nearly parallel walls of an m.o.d.* pattern would result in a gross inaccuracy of the casting. It should be a paramount rule that, regardless of its type, the pattern should be invested as soon as possible after

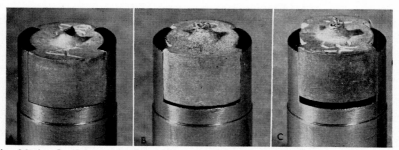

Fig. 26–5. Castings made from patterns prepared with melted wax, cooled under pressure. *A.* Pattern invested immediately. *B.* Pattern stored for 2 hours before investing. *C.* Pattern stored for 12 hours before investing.

* Mesio-occluso-distal.

removal from the die. Even with indirect technics where the pattern has been stored overnight on the die, all margins should be carefully checked just before removal. Although the die itself will prevent distortion in certain directions, distortion may occur in the unconfined directions such as the proximal walls.

On occasion, it may not be feasible or possible to invest the direct wax pattern immediately. In those cases, it is best to store the pattern at a low temperature such as in a refrigerator. As previously noted, the flow is lower and yield point higher at decreased temperatures so distortion will be less.[11] Too often, the pattern is placed next to a burner or oven and the distortion is increased tremendously. The storage environment itself, whether it be water or air, is immaterial. Release of stress and the accompanying distortion is a function of time and temperature. Certainly, the preferred procedure is to invest the pattern shortly after it is finished regardless of the technic employed. Once the investment mold has formed, there can be no further distortion of the pattern *per se.*

**Effect of the Method of Heating.** The stresses introduced into the wax are also dependent upon the method of heating it. Commonly, the wax in stick form is softened over a Bunsen burner. Such a method of softening seldom produces a uniform temperature and plasticity throughout the wax, and, as a result, a considerable amount of stress may be present which cannot be controlled and the molded pattern tends to return to the original stick form. An experimental method for a qualitative estimation of the possible distortion caused by such stresses has been devised.[12] A wax pattern is obtained by any selected technic, and an enlarged optical image is projected onto a piece of paper, where its outline can be traced. Any changes in the shape of the pattern as relaxation occurs can be observed by a comparison with the original outline. There are several other methods for studying the possible distortions of the wax pattern,[13, 14] but probably the method to be described is the simplest.

The tracings obtained during the relaxation of a mesio-occluso-distal pattern from a wax softened over a Bunsen burner and chilled under pressure, as previously described, is shown[15] in Figure 26-6. The time for relaxation was decreased by raising the temperature of the pattern. As can be noted, the left step portion distorted outward and the right step portion distorted inward. With such a manipulation of the wax, the direction of the relaxation was found to be unpredictable.

When the same experiment was repeated, using the technic first described of melting the wax and allowing it to solidify under pressure, the results shown in Figure 26-7 were obtained. The relaxation is definitely less in this case, and that the stresses are better controlled is evidenced by the fact that the two step portions both distorted outwards slightly each time the experiment was performed.

Naturally, the residual stress is less in the poured type pattern since there is no tendency for the wax to return to its original form as in a plastic or molded pattern. As it congeals, the molecules align themselves to the shape of the prepared cavity and will attempt to maintain that configuration. Thus the poured pattern will distort less on storage[11, 14] and small additions of wax in building a pattern on a die will produce less distortion than use of large additions.[14] Furthermore, the softer waxes, preferred for indirect pattern technics, distort less. It is apparent then that the pattern formed on the indirect die is superior in terms of reduced residual stress and exhibits less distortion if stored.

The technic of using melted wax for the pattern cannot be employed

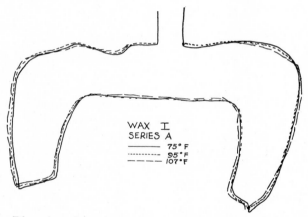

Fig. 26–6.    Distortion of a wax pattern obtained with wax softened over a flame. The relaxation was obtained by increasing the temperature of the pattern as indicated. (Lasater, *J.A.D.A.*, April, 1940.)

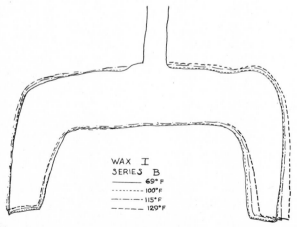

Fig. 26–7.    Distortion of a wax pattern prepared by cooling the wax under pressure after melting. (Lasater, *J.A.D.A.*, April, 1940.)

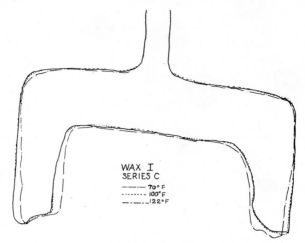

WAX I
SERIES C
——— 70° F
········ 100° F
—·—·—122° F

Fig. 26–8.  Distortion of a wax pattern prepared from wax which was uniformly soft-ened at a temperature of 52° C. (125° F.). (Lasater, *J.A.D.A.*, April, 1940.)

with the direct technic because of the high temperatures involved in melting the wax. Further studies along the same line as described[15] indicated that there are optimum temperatures at which the wax can be manipulated in the plastic condition, provided that it is heated uniformly throughout. Such a method of heating entails the use of a heater of some kind at a constant temperature for as long as 20 minutes. The relaxation of a pattern obtained by such a method is indicated in Figure 26–8. The relaxation is small, and it can be noted that when the pattern distorts, the step portions move inward. Unfortunately, the optimum manipulation temperature for certain inlay waxes appears to be somewhat critical. The optimum temperature is generally in the upper part of the softening range (Fig. 26–1). For example, the optimum temperature for the manipulation of the wax employed in obtaining the data for Figures 26–6, 26–7 and 26–8 was 52° C. (125° F.). Many inlay waxes can be manipulated approximately at this temperature with success, provided that the properties of the wax meet the requirements of the American Dental Association Specification No. 4.

**Distortion by Flow.**    Distortion of the pattern may occur for another reason quite aside from that of relaxation. The pattern may become distorted by a flow of the wax upon its removal from the tooth or die.

If the pattern is stored at room temperature, particularly in the summer, a flow of the wax may occur under its own weight and the higher the temperature, the greater is the flow. Such a flow can be easily demonstrated with a stick of inlay wax. The stick of wax should first be tested for straightness by rolling it along a smooth surface. If the wax is now supported at its two ends for several days, or even over-night during hot weather, it will sag under its own weight, as deter-mined by again rolling it along a smooth surface.

**Theory of Wax Distortion.** Wax pattern distortion is a typical example of relaxation, and the theory of relaxation (p. 26) applies precisely in this case. However, the reasons for the differences in amount of stress release with different methods of manipulation require further elaboration.

The effect of the pressure on the wax during cooling has already been explained by the production of compressive stresses which are later re-lieved. It should be emphasized, however, that the pressure throughout the liquefied wax should be uniform during its solidification. Otherwise, a subsequent distortion of the pattern may be expected. A minimum amount of distortion should result under a uniform stress, since the crystals of wax can form in the position in which the pattern will finally solidify, and a condition should result analogous to that de-scribed for a cast metal.

On the other hand, when the wax is manipulated in the plastic con-dition, certain of the crystals may become distorted or, in a sense, strain hardened. Such stresses may be released by a subsequent relaxa-tion. However, it is conceivable that the stressed condition may be minimized to some extent if the plastic wax is at a constant tempera-ture throughout. For example, under the manipulation described for the conditions pictured in Figure 26–8, probably only the lower molec-ular weight, microcrystalline and amorphous constituents have been melted or softened. It is, therefore, conceivable that these lower melting constituents may act as plasticizers or lubricants for the unmelted phases to roll over one another into new positions during molding, without being strained or deformed.

However, if the temperature is not uniform, and if some of the larger crystals in certain areas are melted along with the lower melting phases, a condition of stress can be imagined to occur during cooling, owing to the cramping or inhibiting of the growth of the larger crystals which were melted.

**Manipulation of Inlay Wax.** However the wax is softened, it should be carried out with "dry heat." The use of a water bath for the softening of inlay wax is not indicated. The lower melting con-stituents are leached out by the water, and possibly a plasticization occurs as in the case of impression compound. In any event, some inlay waxes become crumbly and unmanageable after they have been softened in warm water for any length of time. With the direct technic, the use of a constant temperature device for softening the wax offers the advantage that the wax is always ready for use, in addition to the fact that the uniformity of texture results in less subsequent distortion.

If the wax is to be softened over a flame, care should be taken not to volatilize any of the constituents. The safest method is to hold a stick of wax above the flame, and to rotate it rapidly until it becomes plastic. At no time should it be allowed to melt, as indicated by a shiny surface with molten wax flowing over it. The wax is then kneaded and shaped approximately to the form of the prepared cavity. The plastic mass is then inserted into the prepared cavity at as high a temperature as possible, and held under pressure while it solidifies. Pressure may be applied either with the finger or by the patient biting on the wax. It is not necessary to chill the pattern with water, but if water is used, low temperatures should be avoided. The best procedure is to allow the pattern to cool gradually by itself to mouth temperature.

Whatever the method employed, it should be accomplished with the aim that as little carving and repairing is to be done subsequently as possible. Any addition of wax to the pattern after the initial cooling introduces stresses caused by the unequal cooling of the added wax against the wax already solidified. In other words, part of the wax has solidified under pressure, and the added wax solidifies without pressure. Furthermore, the heat of the added wax may cause the temperature of the already solidified wax to increase to the extent that a relaxation of the latter takes place. Such procedures as melting or "pooling" the wax in various areas, presumably to relieve stressed conditions, are definitely not indicated.[11]

Considerable care should be observed in the removal of the pattern from the prepared cavity so as not to distort it. It can be attached to a heated sprue pin, cooled with water, and withdrawn, or it can be removed with the point of a sharp explorer provided it can be removed in a direction parallel to the axial walls of the prepared cavity. Under no circumstances should it be hooked with the explorer point and rotated out of the prepared cavity. A complicated pattern, such as for an m.o.d. cavity, can best be removed by luting a staple to the pattern so that each prong is fastened above a corresponding step portion. The pattern can then be removed with dental tape looped through the staple.[16] In this manner, the pattern can be withdrawn in a direction parallel to the axial walls with a minimum of distortion.

However it is removed, the pattern should never be touched with the hands, as such a procedure introduces an additional and unnecessary temperature change. Unnecessary temperature changes should be avoided in order to minimize the relaxation. Such precautions are necessary whether the direct or the indirect technic is employed.

For fabricating the indirect pattern, the die is first lubricated to prevent the wax from sticking. The liquid wax may be poured onto the preparation in small increments or, in the case of the full cast crown, the die may be dipped into liquid wax.

Since the type and amount of relaxation are dependent upon factors not always under the control of the operator, the best procedure is to invest the pattern as soon as possible after it has been removed from the mouth as already discussed. In a well organized dental office, it should not be a problem to invest the pattern within 15 to 20 minutes after it has been removed from the prepared cavity.

## *Literature*

1. Coleman, R. L.: *Physical Properties of Dental Materials.* National Bureau of Standards Research Paper No. 32. Washington, U. S. Government Printing Office, 1928, p. 912.
2. Smith, J. C.: *The Chemistry and Metallurgy of Dental Materials.* Oxford, Blackwell Scientific Publications, 1949, p. 226.
3. Grossman, L. I.: *Dental Formulas.* Philadelphia, Lea & Febiger, 1952, pp. 62–65.
4. Bennett, H.: *Commercial Waxes.* Brooklyn, Chemical Publishing Co., 1944, p. 268.
5. Overberger, J. E., Taylor, D. F., Brauer, G. M. and Davenport, R. M.: *Investigation of Selected Waxes for Possible Use in Dentistry.* National Bureau of Standards Report No. 5757, December 31, 1957.
6. Smyd, E. S.: *Wax, Refractory Investments and Related Subjects in Dental Technology.* J. Pros. Den., *5:*514–526 (July), 1955.
7. Coy, H. D. and Hall, S. G.: *Hygroscopic Investment Expansion for Small Castings.* D. Clin. North America, November, 1958, pp. 625–636.
8. Taylor, N. O. and Paffenbarger, G. C.: *A Survey of Current Inlay Casting Technics.* J.A.D.A., *17:*2058–2081 (November), 1930.
9. Bennett, H., *loc. cit.,* p. 50.
10. Taylor, P. B.: *Inlay Casting Procedure—Its Evolution and the Effect of Manipulatory Variables.* Proc. Dent. Centenary Celebration, 1940, pp. 214–224.
11. Phillips, R. W. and Biggs, D. H.: *Distortion of Wax Patterns as Influenced by Storage Time, Storage Temperature and Temperature of Wax Manipulation.* J.A.D.A., *41:*28–37 (July), 1950.
12. Maves, T. W.: *Recent Experiments Demonstrating Wax Distortion on All Wax Patterns When Heat Is Applied.* J.A.D.A., *19:*606–613 (April), 1932.
13. Hollenback, G. M.: *A Study of the Behavior of Pattern Wax.* J. South California D. A., *27:*298–308 (Sept.); 419–434 (Dec.), 1959.
14. Mahler, D. B. and Miller, G. E.: *The Dimensional Behavior of Wax Patterns Made to Gypsum Dies.* J. D. Res., *38:*756–757 (July-Aug.), 1959. Abstract.
15. Lasater, R. L.: *Control of Wax Distortion by Manipulation.* J.A.D.A., *27:*518–524 (April), 1940.
16. Markley, M. R.: *The Wax Pattern.* D. Clin. North America, November, 1958, pp. 615–623.

# CHAPTER 27

# Gypsum Investments for

# Inlay Casting Procedures

After the wax pattern has been obtained, a *sprue former* or *sprue pin* is attached to it and it is surrounded with an investment, as previously described. The investment consists essentially of a mixture of α- or β-hemihydrate of gypsum and a form of silica. It is mixed with water in the same manner as plaster or dental stone, placed around the pattern, and allowed to set. After it hardens, the sprue former is removed, the wax is also removed, and the molten metal is forced into the mold left by the wax, through the *sprue* or *ingate* formed by the sprue former. These procedures will be described in detail in the next two chapters.

**Composition.**   As already noted, the essential ingredients of the dental inlay investment are a hemihydrate of gypsum and a form of silica. Although a few commercial investments employ plaster, most of them contain α-hemihydrate, since greater strength is obtained in this manner. The gypsum product serves as a binder in the investment, to hold the other ingredients together and to provide rigidity. The strength of the investment is dependent upon the amount of binder present. The investment may contain 25 to 45 per cent of the gypsum product.

The remainder of the investment consists of silica, certain modifying agents, coloring matter, and reducing agents, such as carbon or powdered copper. The reducing agents are used in some investments in an attempt to provide a reducing atmosphere in the mold at the time the gold alloy is cast.

Unlike the dental stones, a setting expansion is usually desirable in an investment, and accelerators or retarders are employed to regulate the setting expansion and the setting time. However, such added constituents, including the reducing and stabilizing agents, generally are present in amount not greater than 2 per cent, the remaining constituents being α- or β-hemihydrate and silica.

**Silica.** Silica, $SiO_2$, is added for two reasons: (1) to provide a refractory during the heating of the investment, and (2) to regulate the thermal expansion. Usually, the wax pattern is eliminated from the mold by heat. During the heating, the investment is expected to expand thermally in order to compensate partially or totally for the casting shrinkage of the gold alloy. As can be noted from Figure 27–1, gypsum, regardless of whether it is set plaster or stone, shrinks considerably when it is heated. The shrinkage occurs between the temperatures at which the water of crystallization is given off. As can be noted from the figure, the castings are too small when they are made in a mold formed by gypsum alone.

If the proper form of silica is employed in the investment, such a

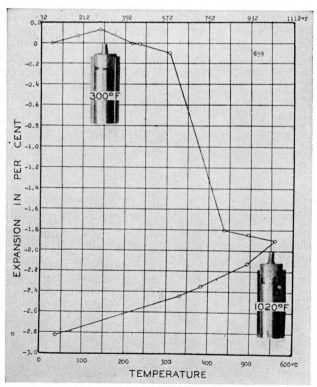

Fig. 27–1. Thermal expansion of gypsum made from plaster of paris. (Souder and Paffenbarger, *National Bureau of Standards Circular C433*.)

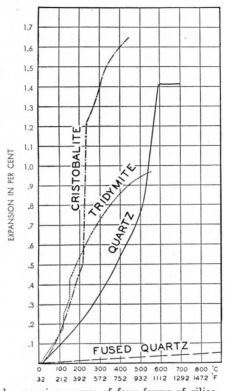

Fig. 27–2.   Thermal expansion curves of four forms of silica. (Volland and Paffenbarger, *J.A.D.A.*, Feb., 1932.)

contraction can be eliminated and changed to an expansion during heating. Silica exists in at least four allotropic forms: quartz, tridymite, cristobalite and fused quartz. The first three are of particular dental interest.

When either quartz, tridymite or cristobalite is heated, a change in crystalline form occurs at a transition temperature characteristic of the particular form of silica. For example, when quartz is heated, it inverts from a "low" form, known as $\alpha$-quartz, to a "high" form, called $\beta$-quartz at a temperature of 575° C. (1070° F.). In a similar manner, cristobalite undergoes an analogous transition between 200° C. (390° F.) and 270° C. (520° F.) from "low" or $\alpha$-cristobalite to "high" or $\beta$-cristobalite. Two inversions of tridymite occur at 117° C. (243° F.) and 163° C. (325° F.), respectively. The $\beta$-allotropic forms are stable only above the transition temperatures noted, and an inversion to the lower or $\alpha$-form occurs upon cooling in each case.

The change in crystalline form is occasioned by a shift in the direction of the valence bonds of the oxygen. In the $\alpha$-form, the valence bonds are roughly at a tetrahedral angle, whereas in the $\beta$-form, the valence bonds may be directly opposite to each other.[1] It is evident that such a change can result in an increase in volume. The linear expansion of the four forms of silica previously mentioned are shown in Figure 27–2. The change in the magnitude of the linear coefficient of expansion at the inversion temperature in each case is quite evident.

Fused quartz is amorphous and glasslike in character, and it exhibits no inversion at any temperature below its fusion point. It possesses the lowest known linear coefficient of expansion. It is of little use in connection with dental investments.

Either quartz or cristobalite, or both, may be used in a dental investment. Tridymite is useful in combination with cristobalite for the control of the thermal expansion. Since the inversion temperatures of the two substances are so nearly alike, the tridymite can be added to the cristobalite for the purpose of reducing its linear expansion.

**Setting Time.** The setting time of an investment can be measured in the same manner as for plaster (p. 36). Furthermore it can be controlled in the same manner as well.

According to the American Dental Association Specification No. 2 for dental inlay casting investment, the setting time should not be less than 5 minutes, nor more than 30 minutes. Usually the modern inlay investments set initially in 7 to 12 minutes. Sufficient time should be allowed for mixing and investing the pattern before the investment sets.

**Normal Setting Expansion.** A mixture of silica and either type of gypsum hemihydrate results in an increased setting expansion beyond that of the gypsum product when it is used alone.[2b] Very likely, the silica particles interfere with the intermeshing and interlocking of the crystals as they form. Thus the mixture is held in a semisolid state for a longer time, and the outward thrust of the crystals during growth is more effective in the production of an expansion.

As a rule, the resulting setting expansion is too high. The setting expansion of a modern investment of this type is usually regulated between 0.1 and 0.45 per cent by means of retarders and accelerators, as described for the plasters and stones (p. 40). The investments are, therefore, usually "balanced" in that their setting time is not affected by a normal mixing time when a given W/P ratio is employed.

The purpose of the setting expansion is to aid in the enlarging of the mold in order to compensate partially for the casting shrinkage of the gold. There is some doubt that all of the setting expansion is effective in expanding the wax pattern. It has been shown[3] that the part of the setting expansion that is effective may be due to the thermal expansion of the pattern brought about by the heat of reaction which occurs at the same time the setting expansion of the investment is taking place. It is reasoned that under such circumstances, the setting expansion is not confined by the wax pattern, and a uniform expansion of the mold may occur. It follows from such a theory that the setting expansion will be effective only to the extent that the exothermic heat is transmitted to the pattern. Since the amount of such heat present depends upon the gypsum content of the investment, the setting expansion of an investment with a comparatively high gypsum content will be more effective in enlarging the mold than will a product with a lower gypsum content.

**Hygroscopic Setting Expansion.**     The hygroscopic setting expansion was previously described in connection with the setting of dental plaster and stone (p. 45). It was pointed out that the hygroscopic setting expansion differs from the normal setting expansion described in the previous section in that it occurs when the gypsum product is allowed to set under or in contact with water and that it is greater in magnitude than the normal setting expansion.

The hygroscopic setting expansion was first discovered in connection with an investigation of the dimensional changes of a dental investment during setting.[4] As illustrated in Figure 27–3, the hygroscopic setting expansion may be six or more times the normal setting expansion of a dental investment. As a matter of fact, when it is measured on a mercury bath (see p. 121), it may be as high as 4 to 5 per cent linear.[2a] As will be shown in the next chapter, the hygroscopic setting expansion is one of the methods for expanding the casting mold to compensate for the casting shrinkage of the gold alloy.

Different commercial investments exhibit different amounts of hygroscopic expansion.[2c] Although all investments appear to be subject to hygroscopic expansion, the expansion in some cases is not sufficient for practical use.[5] In general, a number of factors are probably of importance in the control of the hygroscopic expansion.

*Effect of Composition.*     The magnitude of the hygroscopic setting expansion of a dental investment is generally proportional to the silica content of the investment, other factors being equal.[2c, 5] The finer the particle size of the silica, the greater will be the hygroscopic expansion. [2c, 6] In general, the $\alpha$-hemihydrate is apt to produce a greater hygroscopic expansion in the presence of silica than is the $\beta$-hemihydrate, particularly when the expansion is unrestricted.[2c] As previously stated in Chapter 3, the hygroscopic expansion of the stone or plaster alone is very slight.[7]

In a dental investment, there must be sufficient hemihydrate binder with the silica to provide sufficient strength after a hygroscopic expansion. Otherwise, a shrinkage will occur during the subsequent drying of the set investment. Approximately 15 per cent of binder at least is necessary to prevent a drying shrinkage.[5]

*Effect of the W/P Ratio.*     The higher the W/P ratio of the original hemihydrate-water mixture, the less will be the hygroscopic setting expansion.[2c, 8] This effect is more marked in some commercially available investments than in others.[9]

*Effect of Spatulation.* With most investments, the shorter the mixing time, the less is the hygroscopic expansion.[10, 11] It should be noted that this factor is important in connection with the control of the normal setting expansion as well.

*Shelf-Life of the Investment.* The older the investment, the less will be its hygroscopic expansion.[10] Consequently, the dentist should limit the amount of investment he purchases at one time.

*Effect of the Temperature of the Immersion Water.* With some investments, the higher the temperature of the added water to 40° C. (104° F.), the greater will be the hygroscopic setting expansion.[5] The change in expansion is likely to be less from this cause than from other factors. With some investments, such a change is not evident.[9]

*Effect of Time of Immersion.* The greatest amount of hygroscopic setting expansion is observed if the immersion takes place before

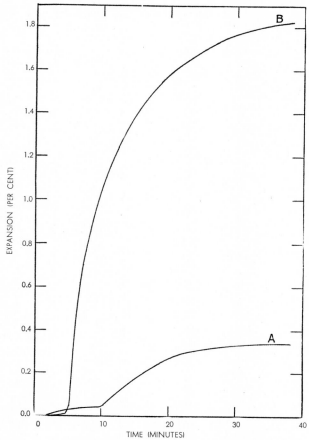

Fig. 27–3. Curve *A*, normal setting expansion. Curve *B*, hygroscopic setting expansion, water added 5 minutes after the beginning of mixing. W/P ratio–0.30.

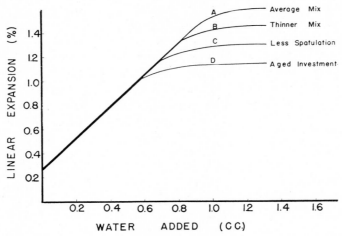

Fig. 27–4. Graphic representation of the relation of the linear hygroscopic setting expansion and the amount of water added as influenced by certain manipulative factors. (Asgar, Mahler and Peyton, *J. Pros. Den.*, Sept., 1955.)

the initial set.[5] The longer the immersion of the investment in the water bath is delayed beyond the time of the initial set of the investment, the less will be the hygroscopic expansion.[2c, 4, 9]

*Effect of Confinement.* Both the normal and hygroscopic setting expansions are confined by opposing forces such as the walls of a wax pattern or a container, as previously described. However, the confining effect on the hygroscopic expansion is much more pronounced than the confining effect on the normal setting expansion.[5] The effective hygroscopic setting expansion is, therefore, likely to be less in proportion to the expected expansion than is the normal setting expansion.

*Effect of the Amount of Added Water.* In the previous discussions, it has been assumed that the investment was immersed in a water bath, and that it could sorb as much water as necessary to effect the expansion. It has been shown that the magnitude of the hygroscopic setting expansion can be controlled by the amount of water added.[6, 7, 10, 11]

It has been proved that the magnitude of the hygroscopic expansion is in direct ratio to the amount of water added during the setting period until a maximum expansion occurs. No further expansion is evident regardless of any additional amount of water added.[10]

The effect of some of the factors previously discussed (W/P ratio, mixing and shelf-life) on the maximum hygroscopic setting expansion is illustrated[10] in Figure 27–4 in reference to the amount of water added. As can be noted, the effect of these factors on the maximum expansion are as predicted.

The important consideration to be noted in Figure 27–4 is that, within the limits of the investigation, below the maximum expansion the magnitude of the hygroscopic setting expansion is *dependent only on the amount of water added,* and is independent of the W/P ratio, the amount of mixing and the age or shelf-life of the investment.[10] This finding serves as the basis for a mold expansion technic to be described in the next chapter.

**Theory of Hygroscopic Expansion.** A number of theories to account for the hygroscopic setting expansion of gypsum products have been advanced.[4, 5, 7, 12-14] The theory to be presented herewith probably represents the present thought on the subject.

The presence of the quartz is a matter of introducing a filler of some nature to act as a "wick" or path for the added water to penetrate the investment during setting. Acrylic resin pearls[7] galena crystals[6] and similar inert fillers have been added to the hemihydrate as a substitute for the quartz, and a hygroscopic expansion occurred of the same nature as when the quartz was present. If the filler was a water repellent, the hygroscopic expansion was reduced.[7]

It has been further demonstrated that water need not be added to the setting investment to provide hygroscopic setting expansion. For example, oils, glycerine and alcohol can be added in place of water and the normal setting expansion is increased according to the liquid properties of the additive.[12]

It has also been shown that the dihydrate formed from the hemihydrate is no greater in amount during hygroscopic setting expansion than during the normal setting expansion.[12]

All of these facts considered collectively indicate that the hygroscopic setting expansion can be accounted for on the basis of a physical reaction or combination, rather than by a chemical reaction or any crystalline change differing from that which occurs during the normal setting expansion. As a matter of fact, the hygroscopic setting expansion can be considered as a normal setting expansion in which the growth of the dihydrate crystals is not inhibited.

As previously described, the silica particles in the investment enhance the magnitude of the expansion in both cases. It has been proposed[14] that the phenomenon can be explained on the basis of surface tension action. The theory is illustrated diagrammatically in Figure 27–5. In step I, shown at the top of the Figure, the initial mix is represented by the three round particles, or nuclei, of crystallization. They are surrounded by water. In step II, the reaction to the dihydrate has started and the crystals of the dihydrate are starting to radiate from the nuclei with the normal setting expansion (left diagrams, Fig. 27–5), the water around the crystallizing particles is reduced by the formation of the dihydrate and the particles are drawn closer together by the surface tension action of the water (cf. action of surface tension in the condensation of porcelain, p. 274). In the case of the hygroscopic ex-

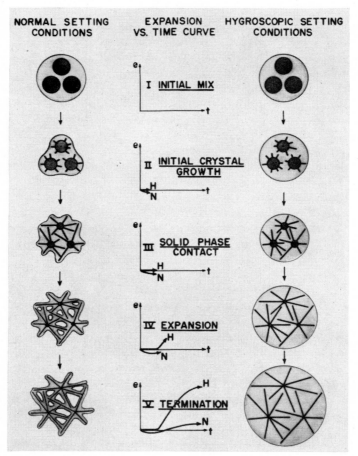

Fig. 27–5. Diagrammatic representation of the setting expansion of plaster. Left: the surface tension of the excess water crowds the crystals together and inhibits growth. Right: water added during setting relieves action of surface tension by forming a continuous film. Crystallization is not inhibited. (Mahler and Ady, *J. D. Res.*, May-June, 1960.)

pansion (right, Fig. 27–5), the added water replenishes that used in the reaction, and the particles remain the same distance apart as before.

In step III, the solid phases make contact, and no further contraction by surface tension can occur. In step IV, the setting expansion begins as the crystals intermesh and collide, thus providing an outward thrust according to the theory for the setting expansion (p. 41). In the case of the normal setting expansion (left, Fig. 27–5), as the water is used up in the reaction, less water surrounds the growing crystals and they tend to be packed more closely together. On the other hand, in the case of the hygroscopic expansion (right, Fig. 27–5), the added water continues to compensate for the water lost in the reaction and more space is provided for outward crystal growth. Finally, in step V, the maximum crystal growth occurs, and the more uninhibited and longer crystals formed during the hygroscopic expansion produce a greater amount of expansion than do the inhibited crystals in the case of the normal setting expansion.

As a further proof of this theory, the setting expansion can be increased as the surface tension of the gauging water is reduced.[14] A surface tension regulator was added to the gauging water in various concentrations so as to reduce its surface tension before mixing with the investment. As can be noted from the results in Table 27–1, the lower the surface tension, the greater is the hygroscopic expansion of the investment. In other words, the magnitude of the normal setting expansion can be increased in an amount comparable to that of the hygroscopic expansion by reducing the surface tension of the gauging water and without the addition of water during setting.

The influence of all of the factors previously described can be related to the theory presented. The greater the amount of the silica or the inert filler, the more easily the added water can diffuse through the setting material and the greater will be the expansion for the same reason as previously described for the normal setting expansion of investment. The W/P ratio affects the hygroscopic expansion for the same reason that it affects the normal setting expansion in the same manner. The higher the temperature of the immersion water, the less its surface tension and, as a result, the hygroscopic expansion tends to be slightly greater at 37° C. (98.6° F.) than at room temperature. The later the water is added to the investment, the less is the hygroscopic setting expansion because part of the crystallization has already started in a "normal" fashion. Some of the crystals have intermeshed and will inhibit further crystal growth after the water is added. On the same basis, the less water added, the lower will be the expansion, *i.e.*, there will be less counteraction of the surface tension action.

Finally, it should be noted that the term "hygroscopic" in its strict sense is a misnomer. Although the added water may be drawn into

*Table 27–1.*    *Effect of Surface Tension of Gauging Water on the Setting Expansion of an Investment\**

| SURFACE TENSION (DYNES/CM.) | SETTING EXPANSION (PER CENT) |
|---|---|
| 72 | 0.49 |
| 56 | 0.50 |
| 44 | 0.56 |
| 36 | 0.61 |
| 31 | 0.84 |
| 28 | 1.07 |
| 26 | 1.17 |

\* Mahler and Ady, *J. D. Res.*, May–June, 1960.

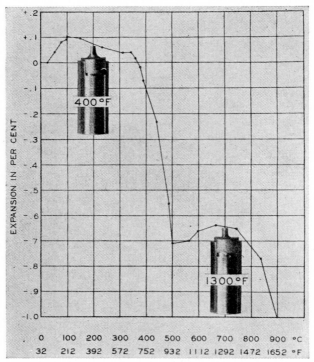

Fig. 27–6.   Thermal expansion of an investment which contained plaster of paris, 55 per cent, and quartz, 45 per cent. (Volland and Paffenbarger, *J.A.D.A.*, Feb., 1932.)

the setting material by capillary action and changes in true volume,[12] the effect is not a matter related to hygroscopy. Furthermore, on the basis of the theory, the hygroscopic setting expansion is as "normal" a phenomenon as that which occurs during what is designated as "normal setting expansion." However, the terms have gained general acceptance by usage even though they may be inaccurate on the basis of theoretical considerations.

**Thermal Expansion.**   As noted in a previous section, the thermal expansion of the investment is directly related (1) to the amount of silica present and (2) to the type of silica employed.

The effect on the thermal expansion of an investment caused by the inversion of the quartz during heating is illustrated in Figure 27–6. Forty-five per cent of quartz was added to 55 per cent of plaster of paris to form the investment. A comparison of Figure 27–1 with Figure 27–6 indicates that the contraction of the plaster is not as great when the quartz is present. Furthermore, approximately at the transition temperature of the quartz, a slight increase in dimension occurs until the casting temperature (700° C.) is reached. As might be expected, castings made with this investment do not fit because of the contraction of the mold during heating.

A considerable amount of quartz is necessary to eliminate the contraction of the gypsum during heating. Even when the quartz content of the investment is increased to 60 per cent, with the balance being hemihydrate binder, the initial contraction of the latter is not eliminated, as shown in Figure 27–7. Although a thermal expansion of the investment occurs above the inversion temperature, it is not sufficient to compensate for the casting shrinkage.

The contraction of the gypsum is entirely eliminated when the quartz content is increased to 75 per cent (Fig. 27–8). If a sufficient amount of setting expansion had been present, the casting made at 700° C. (1292° F.) would probably have fit the die reasonably well.

The effect of cristobalite as compared to that of the quartz is strikingly demonstrated in Figure 27–9. Owing to the much greater expansion which occurs during the inversion of the cristobalite, the contraction of the gypsum during heating is easily eliminated. Furthermore, the expansion occurs at a lower temperature (*cf.* Fig. 27–8)

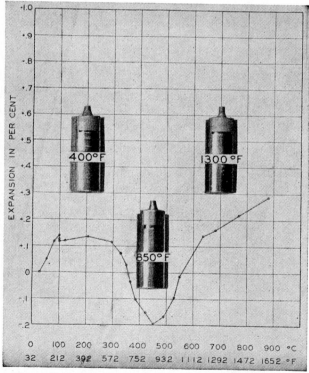

Fig. 27–7. Thermal expansion of an investment which contained plaster of paris, 40 per cent, and quartz, 60 per cent. (Volland and Paffenbarger, *J.A.D.A.*, Feb., 1932.)

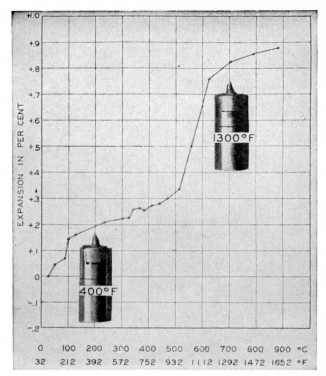

Fig. 27–8. Thermal expansion of an investment which contained plaster of paris, 25 per cent, and quartz, 75 per cent. (Volland and Paffenbarger, *J.A.D.A.*, Feb., 1932.)

because of the lower inversion temperature of the cristobalite in comparison to that of quartz. As can be noted (Fig. 27–9), a reasonably good fit of the castings occurred when the gold alloy was cast into the mold at temperatures between 500° C. (930° F.) and 900° C. (1650° F.).

The desirable magnitude of the thermal expansion of a dental investment depends upon its use. If the hygroscopic setting expansion is relied upon to compensate for the gold alloy shrinkage, a linear thermal expansion of approximately 0.5 to 0.6 per cent is adequate. However, if the thermal expansion is employed for this purpose together with the normal setting expansion, the investment should expand linearly 1.0 per cent or more.

Another desirable feature of an inlay investment is that its maximum thermal expansion be attained at a temperature not greater than 700° C. (1292° F.). This temperature is normally the mold temperature in the casting of gold alloy when an investment thermal expansion technic is employed. As will be shown later, the gold alloy is apt to be contaminated at a mold temperature higher than 700° C.

*Effect of the W/P Ratio.*    Since the magnitude of the thermal expansion is related to the amount of silica present, it is to be expected that the more water used in mixing the investment, the less will be the thermal expansion. This effect is demonstrated by the curves shown in Figure 27–10. It is imperative, therefore, that the water and powder be measured accurately, if the proper compensation is to be realized.

*Effect of Chemical Modifiers.*    A disadvantage of an investment which contains sufficient quartz to prevent any contraction during heating is that the weakening effect of the quartz in such quantities is apt to be too great. It has been found[15] that the addition of the chlorides of sodium, potassium or lithium in small amounts to the investment will eliminate the contraction caused by the gypsum and will increase the expansion without the presence of an excessive amount of quartz.

The effect of sodium chloride in this connection is shown in Figure 27–11. The original investment, containing 45 per cent plaster of paris and 55 per cent quartz, exhibited only a small thermal expansion between room temperature and 700° C. (1292° F.), as can be noted from the lowest broken line curve. The addition of 0.4 per cent sodium

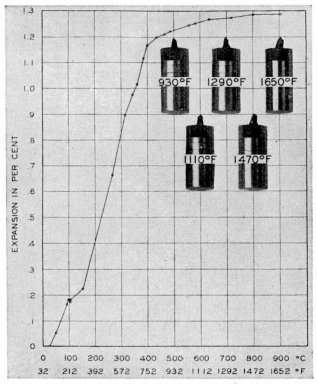

Fig. 27–9.  Thermal expansion of an investment containing cristobalite instead of quartz. (Volland and Paffenbarger, *J.A.D.A.*, Feb., 1932.)

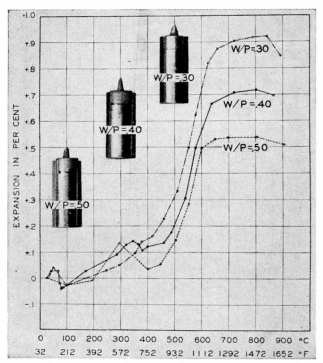

Fig. 27–10. Effect of the W/P ratio on the thermal expansion of an investment containing plaster of paris, 20 per cent, and quartz, 80 per cent. (Volland and Paffenbarger, *J.A.D.A.*, Feb., 1932.)

chloride to replace the same amount of silica eliminated the contraction and increased the thermal expansion. As can be noted from the Figure, additions of sodium chloride in excess of 0.8 per cent had little effect on the total thermal expansion. However, the total thermal expansion can be made to approach that of the cristobalite investment (*cf.* Fig. 27–9) by the addition of this chemical modifier.

Boric acid has somewhat the same effect. It also acts to harden the set investment. However, it apparently disintegrates during the heating of the investment and a roughened surface on the casting may result.

**Thermal Contraction.**    When an investment is allowed to cool from 700° C. (1292° F.), its contraction curve follows the expansion curve during the inversion of the β-quartz or cristobalite to its stable form at room temperature. A thermal contraction curve for a quartz–α-hemihydrate investment containing sodium chloride is shown in Figure 27–12. After the inversion, the investment contracts to less than its original dimension as shown.

If the investment is reheated, it will expand thermally to its original dimensions. However, in practice the investment should not be heated a second time because of the internal cracks which develop during the first cooling and a second heating.

**Strength.** The strength of an investment is usually measured under compressive stress. The compressive strength is increased according to the amount and the type of the gypsum binder present. For example, the use of α-hemihydrate instead of plaster definitely increases the compressive strength of the investment. The use of chemical modifiers as described in the previous section also aids in increasing the strength, since more of the binder can be used without a marked reduction in the thermal expansion.

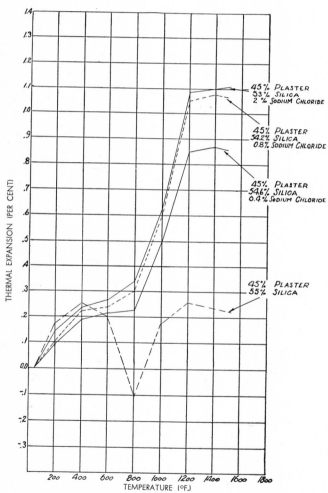

Fig. 27–11. Effect of sodium chloride on the thermal expansion of an investment. (Courtesy of the Ransom and Randolph Co.)

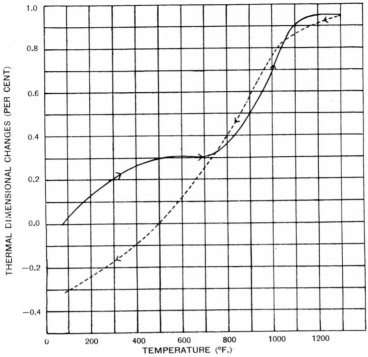

Fig. 27–12. Thermal contraction (dotted line) of an investment.

According to the American Dental Association Specification No. 2, the compressive strength should not be less than 24.5 kilograms per square centimeter (350 pounds per square inch). Any investment which meets this requirement should possess adequate strength for the casting of an inlay. However, when larger complicated castings are made, a greater strength is necessary.

The strength of the investment is affected by the W/P ratio in the same manner as any other gypsum product; the more water employed in mixing, the lower is the compressive strength. Heating of the investment to 700° C. (1292° F.) does not greatly lower its strength below that at room temperature.[16] However, after it has cooled to room temperature, its strength decreases considerably, presumably because of fine cracks which form during cooling.

**Fineness.**    The fineness of the investment may affect its setting time and other properties. It was previously noted that a fine silica results in a higher hygroscopic expansion than when a coarse silica is present. A fine particle size is preferable to a coarse one. The finer the investment, the smaller will be the surface irregularities on the casting.

The requirements for fineness of the American Dental Association Specification No. 2 are that the investment powder shall pass a No. 30

standard sieve, 95 per cent shall pass a No. 100 standard sieve, and 85 per cent must go through a No. 200 sieve.

**Porosity.** During the casting, the molten metal is forced into the mold under pressure. As the metal enters the mold, the air must be forced out ahead of the metal in order to prevent a back pressure. The common method for venting the mold is through the pores of the investment.

In general, the more gypsum crystals present in the set investment, the less is its porosity. It follows, therefore, that the less the hemihydrate content and the greater the amount of gauging water used to mix the investment, the more porous it will be.

The particle size of the investment is also a factor. The more uniform the particle size, the greater is its porosity. This factor is of greater importance than is the actual particle size. A mixture of coarse and fine particles will exhibit less porosity than will an investment composed of a uniform particle size.[17]

**Technical Considerations.** The same precautions for storage of an investment should be observed as for plaster or dental stone. Under conditions of high relative humidity, the setting time may change for the reasons given in connection with the storage of plaster and stone (p. 57). Under such conditions, the setting expansion and the hygroscopic expansion may change in value, so that the entire casting procedure may be adversely affected. The investment should, therefore, be stored in air-tight and moisture-proof containers. During use, the containers should be opened for as short a time as possible.

The selection of an investment by the dentist is largely a matter of choice, provided that the investment meets the requirements of the American Dental Association Specification No. 2. Some investments are formulated for casting inlays employing thermal expansion as the main factor for casting shrinkage compensation and others are intended for use with hygroscopic setting expansion. A third type is intended for use with large dental castings. Consequently, the choice by the dentist is limited in part according to the purpose for which the investment is to be used.

As previously noted, the investment should be weighed and the water should be measured with a graduate, or weighed also, in the proportioning of the investment mix. Only in this manner can the dentist expect to control the setting expansion or the thermal expansion in relation to the compensation needed for the casting shrinkage, and other important properties. The accuracy of the weighing should be at least to 0.1 gram.

Some dental manufacturers supply their investment in pre-weighed packages so that the dentist need only measure the gauging water.

The mixing and subsequent manipulations of the investment will be described in the next chapter.

## Literature

1. Kracek, F. C.: "Phase Transformations in One-Component Silicate Systems," in *Phase Transformations in Solids*. New York, John Wiley & Sons, Inc., 1951, p. 258.
2. *a*, Docking, A. R.: *The Hygroscopic Setting Expansion of Dental Casting Investments, Part I*. Austral. J. Dent., *52:*6–11 (Jan.), 1948; *b, Part II*, with Chong, M. P., and Donnison, J. A.: *Ibid.*, *52:*160–166 (May), 1948; *c, Part III, Ibid.*, *52:*320–329 (Sept.), 1948; *d, Part IV*, with Chong, M. P.: *Ibid.*, *53:*261–271 (*Sept.*), 1949.
3. Skinner, E. W.: *The Role of Investment Setting Expansion in Gold Compensation Casting Techniques*. Den. Cos., *75:*1009–1018 (Oct.), 1933.
4. Scheu, C. H.: *A New Precision Casting Technic*. *J.A.D.A.*, *19:*630–633 (April), 1932.
5. Skinner, E. W. and Degni, F.: *Hygroscopic Expansion of Dental Investments*. J.A.D.A., *54:*603–608 (May), 1957.
6. Donnison, J. A., Chong, M. P. and Docking, A. R.: *The Effect of the Surface Area on the Hygroscopic Setting Expansion and Strength of Casting Investments*. J. D. Res., *36:*967–973 (Dec.), 1957.
7. Lyon, H. W., Dickson, G. and Schoonover, I. C.: *The Mechanism of Hygroscopic Expansion in Dental Casting Investments*. J. D. Res., *34:*44–50 (Feb.), 1955.
8. Hollenback, G. M.: *Simple Technic for Accurate Castings: New and Original Method of Vacuum Investing*. J.A.D.A., *36:*391–397 (April-May), 1948.
9. Langren, N. and Peyton, F. A.: *Hygroscopic Expansion of Some Casting Investments*. J. D. Res., *29:*469–481 (Aug.), 1950.
10. Asgar, K., Mahler, D. B. and Peyton, F. A.: *Hygroscopic Technique for Inlay Casting Using Controlled Water Additions*. J. Pros. Den., *5:*711–724 (Sept.), 1955.
11. Asgarzadeh, K., Mahler, D. B. and Peyton, F. A.: *The Behavior and Measurement of Hygroscopic Dental Casting Investment*. J. D. Res., *33:*519–530 (Aug.), 1954.
12. Ryge, G. and Fairhurst, C. W.: *Hygroscopic Expansion*. J. D. Res., *35:*499–508 (Aug.), 1956.
13. Fusayama, T.: *Proposition of a Theory on the Mechanism of the Hygroscopic Expansion of Gypsum Products*. Bull. Tokyo Med. and Den. Univ., *4:*225–229, (July), 1957.
14. Mahler, D. B. and Ady, A. B.: *An Explanation for the Hygroscopic Setting Expansion of Dental Gypsum Products*. J. D. Res., *39:*578–589 (May-June), 1960.
15. Moore, T. E.: *Method of Making Dental Castings and Compositions Employed in Said Method*. U.S. Patent No. 1,924,874 (Aug. 29), 1933.
16. Souder, W. and Paffenbarger, G. C.: *Physical Properties of Dental Materials*. National Bureau of Standards Circular C433. Washington, U.S. Government Printing Office, 1942, p. 88.
17. Taylor, N. O., Paffenbarger, G. C. and Sweeney, W. T.: *Dental Inlay Casting Investments: Physical Properties and a Specification*. J.A.D.A., *17:*2266–2286 (Dec.), 1930.

# CHAPTER 28

# Gold Inlay Casting Procedures:

# Theoretical Considerations.

# Investment Expansion Technics.

# Investing Procedures

Although gold castings can be made of any size from a denture base to the smallest inlay, only the procedure employed for the construction of an inlay will be discussed. However, the fundamental principles are the same, regardless of the size of the casting, and the technics differ only in minor details.

**Theoretical Considerations.** The sole objective of the casting procedure is to provide a metallic duplication of missing tooth structure, with as great an accuracy as possible. The tolerance limits of the dental inlay are not known, although it has been stated that an error of ±0.2 per cent cannot be detected clinically.[1] However, in all probability the accuracy should be greater than can be detected by the eye or by the ordinary methods of clinical testing with instruments. At the margins a thin line of cement is always present, even though it may not be readily visible. The solubility and deterioration of cement in the oral cavity has been stressed in Chapter 14. Thus, the less accurate the casting and the greater the amount of cement exposed, the more likely is the restoration to fail. Certainly, absolute accuracy of fit cannot be realized continuously under mouth conditions because of the differential thermal dimensional changes between the tooth and the gold inlay. It stands to reason, however, that the more accurate the fit of the inlay in the prepared cavity, the less will be the likelihood of leakage.

Assuming that the wax pattern is satisfactory, the procedure then becomes a matter of the enlarging of the mold uniformly and sufficiently to compensate for the casting shrinkage of the gold alloy.

Theoretically, if the shrinkages of the wax and the gold alloy are known, the mold can be expanded an amount equal in magnitude to such a shrinkage, and the problem is solved. Unfortunately there are variables in the behavior of the materials involved, especially the wax, that cannot be rigidly controlled. The over-all dimensional accuracy possible with current technics has never been clearly defined. Although minimum deviations of approximately 0.1 per cent,[2] or even 0.05 per cent,[3] have been reported, there may be variations as high as 1.0 per cent.[2] Thus, neither the allowable tolerance of accuracy in the fit of the casting nor that obtainable during the casting procedure is known. In the last analysis, the casting procedure is partly empirical and a matter of routine procedure, which should be rigidly adhered to.

There are, however, many steps in the procedure concerning which a considerable number of facts are known; their application will be discussed in subsequent sections. There are also certain ramifications of the technics here described which will produce equally satisfactory results. However, any technic involves strict adherence to certain fundamentals that are common to all. It is these fundamentals which will be stressed.

**Compensation Technics.**     The compensation for the shrinkages inherent in the technic may be obtained by any one, or combinations of, the following three methods:

1. Thermal expansion of the wax pattern.
2. Setting expansion or hygroscopic expansion of the investment.
3. Thermal expansion of the investment.

The thermal expansion of the wax pattern can be obtained by maintaining the temperature of the water-investment mixture at 40 to 42° C. (104 to 108° F.) after the pattern has been invested, before the investment sets. As might be predicted from the discussion of wax distortion (pp. 437–443), such a treatment produces a relaxation of the wax and a consequent distortion. For this reason, this technic is no longer employed.

The two types of casting technic employed at present are known as the *investment thermal expansion technic* and the *investment hygroscopic expansion technic*. As can be deduced from their names, the principal mold compensation in the first mentioned technic is by the thermal expansion of the investment from room temperature to a high temperature (700° C. or 1292° F.) at which the casting is made. In the second technic, the main mold compensation is realized by means of the hygroscopic expansion of the investment. In the latter case, the mold is heated only to 430° to 480° C. (800° to 900° F.). On the basis of their respective mold temperatures at the time of casting, the two methods are often designated as *high heat* and *low heat* casting technic, respectively.

Aside from the differences mentioned, the operations involved are quite similar and the two technics will be described simultaneously. If no differentiation is made, it can be assumed that the procedures described are common to both technics.

**Preparation of a Die.** In the indirect technic, the pattern is prepared on a die which is a replica of the tooth and the prepared cavity. The preparation of a die from an impression is a matter to be considered carefully, if the desired accuracy is to be obtained.

Before the advent of the elastic impression materials, the die was formed in the impression, usually with copper amalgam. Amalgam dies are still used to an extent, although silver amalgam has largely replaced the use of copper amalgam for this purpose. The accuracy of such a die is dependent upon the usual factors which affect the dimensional stability of the amalgam.

Dental stone is usually employed as a die material, with impressions made with the elastic impression materials. The use of a stone die was discussed in connection with the subject of hydrocolloid and rubber impression materials. Undoubtedly an accurate die can be obtained in this manner, particularly when the Class II dental stones are employed. However, the likelihood of removing some of the stone surface during the carving of the wax pattern is apt to be a source of error unless extreme care is used. There is one advantage of the stone die over a metal die and that is that the thermal conductivity of the latter may introduce additional stresses in the wax pattern during cooling.[4]

**Electroplated Dies.** The electroplating of the impression in compound or wax is an excellent means for providing a hard surface on a die. There are several modifications of this technic, and the literature[5-9] should be consulted for a complete account.

The first step in the procedure is to treat the surface of the impression material so that it will conduct electricity. This process is referred to as *metalizing*. A thin layer of metal is deposited on the compound or wax. This metal layer determines to a large extent the surface character of the finished die. Various metalizing agents are available, including bronzing powder suspended in oil of almonds, suspensions of silver powder and powdered graphite. Any of these agents can be burnished on the surface of the impression with a camel's-hair brush. Particularly dense and accurate deposits are possible by the chemical reduction of an aqueous solution of silver nitrate.[9]

The electroplating bath itself is primarily an acid solution of copper

*Table 28–1.* *Composition of an Electroplating Bath for Wax or Compound Impressions*

| | |
|---|---|
| Copper sulfate, anhydrous | 225–250 gm. |
| Sulfuric acid, concentrated | 75 ml. |
| Phenol | 10 ml. |
| Ethyl alcohol | 25–50 ml. |
| Distilled water | 1,000 ml. |

sulfate, containing certain other added ingredients. For example, phenol and ethyl alcohol tend to increase the hardness and ductility of the electrodeposited copper.[10] The greater the concentration of the copper sulfate, the faster will copper be deposited, whereas the acid content increases the *throwing power*, a term which refers to the ionic penetration of the electric field in a concave structure such as an impression for a full crown. Dental impressions of teeth generally have walls with a relatively long depth to the occlusal area. A considerable amount of throwing power is, therefore, desirable.

A compromise is usually effected between the rate of the electrodeposition and the throwing power by regulating the composition of the electroplating bath. The composition presented in Table 28–1 is recommended.[9] The bath should be allowed to stand for several days after mixing before it is used.

An electrical contact is made between the copper matrix band or the metal tray and the metalized surface of the impression, which is made the cathode in the electroplating bath. A piece of copper is used for the anode. All parts not to be electroplated are insulated with wax or a similar nonconductor. A direct current of 0.1 ampere per square centimeter of surface is applied for approximately 10 hours.

Hydrocolloid impressions are difficult to electroplate and the process is not feasible for dental use. Although silicone rubber impressions can be electroplated, it is not recommended because of the distortion which may occur during the time required for the plating process.[11] The electroformed die made from the polysulfide rubber impression is clinically acceptable when a silver cyanide bath is used, although it is not as accurate as a stone die properly constructed. As shown in Chapter 9, although the dimensional stability of a polysulfide rubber impression is much superior to that of an impression with silicone rubber, a slight change in dimension occurs during the time of plating.

The polysulfide rubber impression is cleaned thoroughly and dried. It is then metalized with a fine silver powder. Although other metalizing agents can be used, the silver powder results in a superior surface on the electroplate.

A silver cyanide bath is preferred to the use of an acid copper bath. The reliability and throwing power of the silver bath appear to be better. Also, it is possible that the dimensional stability of the poly-

*Table 28–2.* *Composition of a Silver Cyanide Bath for Electro-plating Polysulfide Rubber Impressions*

| | |
|---|---|
| Silver cyanide | 36 gm. |
| Potassium cyanide | 60 gm. |
| Potassium carbonate | 40 gm. |
| Distilled water | 1,000 ml. |

sulfide rubber is better in the alkaline silver cyanide bath than in the acid copper sulfate medium.[12]

A formula for a satisfactory silver cyanide[11] bath is given in Table 28–2. Special care should be observed so that acid or other chemicals do not inadvertently contact this solution. Acids in particular may produce fumes of the extremely toxic hydrocyanic acid. As a precautionary measure, the bath should be kept in a well ventilated environment.

An anode of pure silver, at least twice the size of the area to be plated, is employed and the electroplating is carried out as before for approximately 10 hours using 5 to 10 milliamperes per square centimeter of cathode surface.

Whatever the plating method, the electroplated die is filled with dental stone. After the stone sets, the impression material is removed.

**Indirect vs. Direct Technic.** It is assumed in the preceding section that the indirect technic is to be used. The indirect technic is indicated particularly in connection with crown and bridge construction, whereas the direct technic is primarily designed for work in operative dentistry. Since the introduction of the elastic impression materials, many dentists are employing the indirect technic for all restorative work.

The chief advantage of the indirect technic so far as accuracy is concerned, is that all of the areas of the wax pattern are in the direct field of vision of the operator. Many areas in the mouth, particularly in the posterior region, are difficult of access, and the accurate carving of the pattern is not easy because of this lack of direct vision as well as access.

The disadvantage of the indirect method is the cumulation of errors from three different materials and manipulations: the impression material and technic, the construction and material of the die, and the preparation of the wax pattern. Only the errors introduced by the inlay wax and its manipulation are inherent in the direct technic.

**The Sprue Former.** The purpose of the sprue former or sprue pin is to provide an ingate or sprue in the investment through which the molten alloy can reach the mold after the wax has been eliminated. It is usually constructed of metal, although a wax or a plastic may be employed.

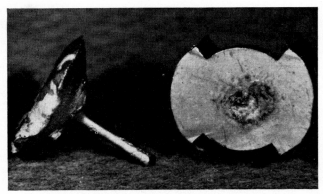

Fig. 28–1. Localized shrinkage caused by the use of an improper sprue diameter.

### Table 28–3.    Diameter of Sprue Former for Various Uses*

| DIAM. OF SPRUE FORMER (B. AND S. GAUGE) | APPROXIMATE DIAMETER (MM.) | COMMENTS |
|---|---|---|
| 16 | 1.3 | Thin inlays only; may need reservoir on sprue |
| 14 | 1.7 | Largest size for air pressure castings |
| 12 | 2.1 | Best for most inlays |
| 10 | 2.6 | Use on heavy crowns only |

* Sausen, R. E. and Serr, H. H., *D. Clin. North America*, Nov., 1958.

The size of the sprue former depends to a considerable extent on the type and size of the pattern, the type of the casting machine to be used, and the dimensions of the flask or ring in which the casting is to be made.

The diameter of the average sprue pin may vary between Brown and Sharpe gauge No. 10 and No. 16 (0.259 and 0.129 centimeter). If the pattern is small, the sprue pin itself must be small since use of a large sprue former attached to a thin, delicate pattern would cause a distortion. Likewise, if the gold is to be melted directly above the sprue or ingate, as in the air pressure casting machine to be described in the next chapter, the use of extremely large sprues is to be avoided in order to prevent the molten gold from flowing into the ingate under its own weight, before the pressure is applied. If the gold is to be melted in a separate crucible as in a centrifugal casting machine, then any diameter compatible with the size of the pattern may be used. Generally, however, for the average size pattern, sprue formers smaller in diameter than 15 gauge are contraindicated. If the sprue is too small, the molten metal will freeze completely in this area first and localized shrinkage porosity as shown in Figure 28–1 will result. Suggestions as to the proper diameters for sprue formers are given in Table 28–3.

A *reservoir* can be used as an added precautionary measure. The reservoir is a piece of wax attached to the sprue former approximately 1 millimeter from the pattern. An example may be seen at *c* in Figure 29–3 in the diagrammatic representation of the various components involved in the investing procedure. It is also seen attached to the casting in Figure 29–4. The purpose of the reservoir is, of course, to prevent localized shrinkage porosity. When the molten gold alloy pours into the mold, the fused metal in the reservoir should be the last to solidify so that any voids in the mold caused by shrinkage will be immediately filled from the reservoir. Thus, the importance of providing a greater bulk of gold in the reservoir than in the thickest cross section of the casting becomes evident, as does the necessity for placing the reservoir as close to the pattern as possible so that the alloy in the connecting ingate will not solidify first. Consequently, the reservoir should be within one millimeter of the pattern and it should be larger than the adjacent portion of the pattern.

The use of a reservoir is a necessity only with sprue formers of very small diameter. If an ample size sprue pin is used a reservoir may be unnecessary.

The sprue pin is usually heated and attached to the pattern by a localized melting of the wax. Care must be exercised to avoid overheating the pattern and thus distorting an adjacent margin. A hollow sprue pin is especially good from this standpoint, since its heat capacity is lower than that of a solid sprue. It is also helpful to attach a drop of wax to the pattern and attach the sprue pin to this added wax. Once attached, wax should be used to build up the sprue pin at this point so that it flares out slightly in the direction of the pattern. The sprue former should never taper toward this area so that the movement of the entering metal is restricted. Flaring of the sprue former may act in much the same way as a reservoir, and it facilitates the flow of molten metal into the cavity.[13]

The position of the sprue former attachment is often a matter of individual judgment in relation to the shape and form of the wax pattern. Some prefer the occlusal surface while others may wish to preserve the anatomy of the pattern, thus they may sprue on the proximal wall. As a general rule, it is desirable to sprue at the point of greatest bulk in the pattern. In that case, there is less chance of distortion upon attaching the sprue, and the molten metal will be more apt to remain liquid in this area until the entire mold is filled.

The direction of the sprue former is also important. It should never point directly toward a thin or delicate part of the mold since the molten metal, as it rushes in, may abrade or fracture the investment in this area and a misfitting casting may result.

If the sprue pin is attached at a right angle to a broad flat surface of the mold, the entering gold may develop a *turbulence* in that it must turn at right angles to the direction of flow. Such turbulence

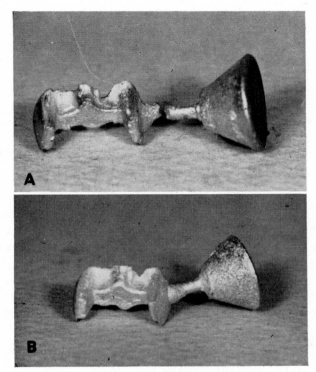

Fig. 28–2. *A.* Detached sprue indicates severe porosity at point of attachment because of turbulence occasioned by improper sprue angle. *B.* Sound casting results with
sprue at 45 degrees to proximal wall.

delays the filling of the mold and a localized shrinkage porosity may
develop. This effect is illustrated in Figure 28–2*A.* Fortunately, the
flaring of the sprue as shown prevented the localized shrinkage from
occurring in a critical area. When the same pattern was sprued at an
angle of 45 degrees to the proximal wall, a satisfactory casting was
obtained as presented in Figure 28–2*B.*

The length of the sprue former depends upon the length of the
casting ring. If the sprue is too short, the mold may be so far removed
from the end of the casting ring that it is difficult for the gases to be
vented so that the metal will fill the mold completely. If the gases
are not completely eliminated, a type of porosity referred to as *back
pressure porosity* develops.[13, 14, 15] This effect will be discussed in
greater detail in the following chapter. A good rule to follow is to
adjust the sprue length so that the portion of the wax pattern farthest
from the sprue pin is within 6 to 8 millimeters (¼ inch) of the open
end of the ring. Such a proper location is shown in Figure 28–3 where
an invested wax pattern with a wax sprue former has been sectioned.

The material of which the sprue former is made is important. A carbon steel or iron sprue pin is apt to rust in contact with the wet investment. When it is withdrawn, iron rust will likely cling to the walls of the ingate, later to contaminate the gold alloy.

The sprue former should be heated as little as possible before it is attached to the pattern. However, care should be taken that it is firmly attached to the pattern so that it will not pull loose during the investing procedure. A hollow sprue pin is especially recommended because of its greater retention to the pattern.

The sprue pin is best attached to the pattern while the latter is in position on the die or in the tooth, provided that it can be attached so that the pattern can be removed directly in line with the principal axis of the tooth or the prepared cavity. In such a case, any visible distortion of the pattern can be detected and repaired. If the direction of the sprue pin after attachment is such that the pattern cannot be removed from the prepared cavity without a tipping or a twisting, the pattern should be removed with a sharp explorer point or a U-shaped staple as previously described, and the sprue former should be attached to the pattern after it has been laid on the bench or table.

The sprue former with the pattern is then attached to the *sprue base* or *crucible former*. A typical crucible former can be seen, with the pattern attached, in the hand of the operator in Figure 28–4.

Provision must be made for the setting expansion. If the pattern is invested in a solid ring or casting flask, it has been shown[16] that the mold is made smaller rather than larger by the reverse pressure caused by the confinement of the setting expansion. This disadvantage can be overcome by the use of a three-part split ring or by the use of very

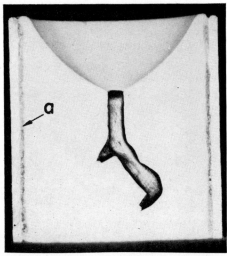

Fig. 28–3. Cross section of an invested wax pattern with the extreme end of the pattern near the end of the ring opposite the ingate for the gold. *a.* Asbestos liner.

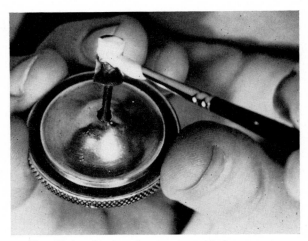

Fig. 28–4. Coating the pattern with investment.

flexible rubber rings,[17] either of which can be increased in volume by the force of the setting expansion. Possibly the most effective and widely used means of preventing the confinement of the setting expansion is to line the casting ring with a sheet of asbestos to form a cushion or liner for the setting expansion. Such an asbestos liner can be seen at *a* in Figure 28–3.

In general, the asbestos liner should extend to within 3 to 4 millimeters ($\frac{1}{8}$ inch) of the ends of the ring.* It is imperative that the liner not extend to the end of the ring if the molten alloy is to be forced into the mold under air pressure. Otherwise the air will leak out through the asbestos and the alloy will not be forced into the mold. It has been shown, however, that if the asbestos liner is carried to the ends of the ring, more longitudinal setting expansion occurs than if the liner is slightly shorter than the ends of the ring.[18] The expansion lateral to the ring is unaffected.

It has been recommended that the thickness of the asbestos layer should not be less than approximately 1 millimeter.[19] Certainly, thicker asbestos or use of two layers will provide even greater expansion.[20] Not only does the liner afford greater normal setting expansion in the investment, but also the water absorbed by the asbestos causes a hygroscopic expansion as it is drawn into the investment during setting.

**Investing.** The investment and water should be proportioned accurately for the reasons outlined in the previous chapter. The same precautions should be observed in mixing the water and investment as were outlined for the mixing of plaster or stone. The investment powder should be sifted into the water so that the least possible amount of air

* It is assumed throughout this discussion that the dimensions of the ring are approximately 35 millimeters ($1\frac{3}{8}$ inches) in length. With shorter rings, the distance from the ends should be reduced proportionately.

will be introduced at this stage. The mixture can then be vibrated to remove any large air bubbles. If the mixing is to be done by hand, the mixture should not be whipped during the process.

The use of a mechanical mixer, either hand or motor driven, is recommended. A typical hand-operated mixer is shown in Figure 28–5. The revolution of the paddle is so rapid that any air bubbles are broken up to the extent that their effect on the surface roughness of the casting is minimized. The investment is then vibrated a second time after it has been mixed.

The casting ring is now filled and the pattern carefully painted with a soft brush, as shown in Figure 28–4. The investment should be flowed from the brush onto the pattern evenly from one area only. If it is painted or flowed on from two parts of the pattern, bubbles may be trapped at the spot where the two portions of investment meet. A further aid in minimizing any trapped air is to blow off the excess investment gently, so as to leave a thin film of investment over the pattern, and then to repaint it.

Since the surface of the wax is a water repellent, it is difficult to coat the pattern evenly without the entrapment of air or water. Before the painting begins, it is often customary to cover the pattern with a wetting agent in order to overcome the adverse effect of the surface tension of the water and the water repellency of the wax. Many wetting agents are retarders for the setting of the investment, and the surface of the casting may be roughened by their use. Even the best wetting agent should be used sparingly for this reason.[21] The wetting agent is spread over the pattern, and the investment is applied immediately as described.

There are two methods for investing the painted pattern. One is to place the pattern in the inlay ring and flow investment around it until the ring is filled. The second method, as seen in Figure 28–6, tends to minimize entrapment of air voids within the mass of investment and the collection of air bubbles on the wax pattern. The crucible former

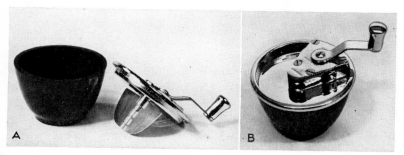

Fig. 28–5. A mechanical mixer. *A.* The paddle for mixing and the cover are shown separated from the rubber mixing bowl. *B.* The cover on the bowl, to show the handle with which the paddle is rotated.

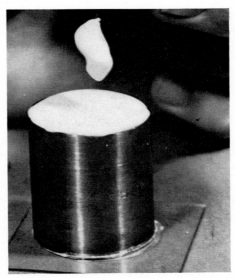

Fig. 28–6. The pattern covered with investment is forced gently into the investment-filled ring.

with the attached pattern is gently forced, with slight agitation, into the filled ring until the former and ring are in contact. If the proper W/P ratio of the investment has been employed, there is adequate time to carry out the procedure without the investment setting to the point where the pattern might be distorted or broken off as it is forced into the filled ring. The ring and crucible former are then inverted so that the crucible former rests on the bench, with the open end of the ring free for the setting expansion to take place.

If the hygroscopic technic is to be employed, the casting ring is immediately immersed in a water bath at a temperature of 37° C. (98.6° F.). For the investment thermal expansion technic, the investment is allowed to harden in the ring seated on the bench. In either case, the wax elimination described in the next chapter is not started for at least one hour after investing the pattern.

**Double Investment Technic.** This method of investing is used only for the investment thermal expansion technic. The preceding method of investing is sometimes known as the *single investment technic,* since the same W/P ratio was used throughout. With some investments, the W/P ratio to effect the proper mold compensation may be so low that the thick mixture would be difficult to paint on the pattern.

In such a case, the thinner mix is applied to the pattern and its W/P ratio is reduced by dusting the applied investment with dry investment powder. The process may be repeated several times until a core, or "cherry," is built around the pattern. The coated pattern is then invested as usual in the thinner mix of investment. Since two different consistencies of investment are present, the technic is called the *double investment technic.*

Although the porosity of the core will be greater than that of the surrounding investment[22] and thus a better venting of the mold is provided, this technic is not used greatly at the present time. Modern dental investments provide sufficient mold compensation at a convenient W/P ratio so that the single investment technic is usually satisfactory.

**Control of the Shrinkage Compensation.** The setting, hygroscopic and thermal expansions of investments can be controlled to a certain extent by a variation of the W/P ratio. The less the W/P ratio, the greater is the shrinkage compensation and conversely. For example, one experiment demonstrated that a difference in the fit of a casting could be detected when the gauging water was changed only 0.5 cubic centimeter.[23]

However, there is a limit to which the W/P ratio can be reduced. If the mix is too thick, it cannot be applied to the wax pattern without a likelihood of distorting the pattern and of producing air voids during the investing. There is also a practical limitation on how much the water-powder ratio can be increased in order to reduce the expansion. If the water-investment mixture is too thin, a rough surface on the casting will result.

The problem of too much expansion of the mold in the case of the thermal expansion technic using cristobalite investment may be important. As can be noted from Figure 27–9, a thermal expansion of 1.3 per cent may take place with such an investment. If an effective setting expansion of 0.3 to 0.4 per cent is added to such a thermal expansion, a total linear expansion as high as 1.7 per cent may be obtained. Such an expansion is definitely higher than the average casting shrinkage of the gold alloy (see Table 25–5), and, as a result, the casting may be too large.

The thermal expansion of the cristobalite investment can be reduced either by increasing the W/P ratio or by combining it in specified ratios with a specially prepared lower expanding investment containing quartz.[24] The greater the amount of the quartz investment blended with the cristobalite investment, the less is the resulting thermal expansion. The shrinkage compensation thus can be controlled without changing either the W/P ratio or the setting expansion.

A simple scale can be procured with which to weigh the water, quartz investment and cristobalite investment in the proper proportions to obtain any desired shrinkage compensation within practical limits. Once the ingredients are measured, the remainder of the technic is as described for the single investment technic.

In addition to the control of the hygroscopic expansion by means of the W/P ratio, the hygroscopic expansion can be regulated either by reducing the time of immersion of the setting investment or by controlling the amount of water to be added during the setting. The longer the delay in time before the investment is immersed in the water bath, the less is the hygroscopic expansion. This procedure was the first method employed for the control of the shrinkage compensation in the hygroscopic technic.[25]

In most of the modern investment hygroscopic expansion technics, the shrinkage compensation is controlled by the regulation of the W/P ratio, although in one technic it is controlled by the addition of water during the setting of the investment[26] as described in the preceding chapter. This method is usually referred to as the *controlled water added technic.*

**Controlled Water Added Technic.** As shown in Figure 27–4, the linear hygroscopic expansion increases according to the amount of water added until a maximum expansion is attained. The investments for use with the water added hygroscopic casting technic are so composed that their maximum expansion during immersion in water is in excess of the desired mold compensation. The desired amount of hygroscopic expansion is then obtained by adding only the amount of water to the investment which will provide the desired expansion.

As stated in the previous chapter, the W/P ratio of the investment mix is not important in this technic so far as the compensation factor is concerned, but it is important in regard to strength and the surface smoothness of the casting. Consequently, the proportioning of the powder and water is important but not so critical as with other technics.

A soft, flexible rubber ring is employed instead of the usual asbestos-lined metal ring. The pattern is invested as usual. A specified amount of water is then added on the top of the investment in the rubber ring and the investment is allowed to set, usually at room temperature.[26] The crucible former, the sprue former and the rubber ring are removed, ready for the elimination of the wax.

Thus many ways exist for varying the shrinkage compensation, and different types of restorations may require varying degrees of investment expansion. Although one level of compensation may be found to provide proper dimensional fit for most preparations, there will be certain types of patterns that require somewhat less or somewhat greater expansion in the investment. For example, restorations such as the full cast crown or the large m.o.d. inlay usually involve walls that are long and parallel. If the casting is slightly undersize, frictional retention will prevent it from seating. In those cases, greater compensation may be required than in a preparation involving short or converging walls. Furthermore, the configuration of the pattern may also influence the effective setting or hygroscopic expansion. The proximal walls of a thin delicate pattern offer less resistance and are more readily expanded during the setting of the investment than if the walls are bulky or continuous as in the full cast crown.

**Vacuum Investing.**   One of the defects of a casting is likely to be the presence of nodules on its surface, caused by the collection of air bubbles during the investing. If the precautions outlined in a previous section are observed, there is no reason why an excellent surface on the casting cannot be obtained routinely, particularly after a certain amount of skill and experience has been acquired.

However, if the personal equation in this regard is to be eliminated, the logical solution is to subject the water-investment mixture to a vacuum during the investing procedure, in order to remove the air bubbles.

A vacuum equivalent to a negative mercury pressure of 680 to 740 millimeters (27 to 29 inches) at sea level is necessary to remove the air effectively. In the simplest equipment, the investment is mixed in the usual manner and poured into a casting ring containing a pattern sprued as usual. An extension is usually placed on the open end of the ring by means of wax or a short length of rubber tubing, to allow for the increase in volume of the investment while it is in the vacuum.[27]

The filled ring is then placed under a bell jar or a similar type of vacuum chamber. It is important that a small vacuum chamber be used, since the time of evacuation should be held to a minimum so that the investment will not begin to set. As the vacuum is applied, the boiling point of the mixture decreases. When the air pressure is sufficiently reduced, the water in the investment starts to boil violently; any air bubbles have been enlarged by the reduction in pressure and the escaping water vapor carries the air with it. The vacuum is held for about 10 seconds, and then the air is let in rapidly so that the water vapor bubbles are condensed, and the investment is forced into intimate contact with the wax pattern by the atmospheric pressure. Vibration of the ring during the procedure aids in obtaining a dense investment.[28]

A water aspirator (filter pump) can be used to obtain the vacuum if the water pressure is sufficient,[21, 27] or a motor driven vacuum pump can be used.[29] There are a number of types of dental vacuum investing equipments available, one of which is shown in Figure 28–7.

The sprue base and former are fitted to the casting ring so that the junctions are air-tight. The properly proportioned mixture of investment and water is mixed mechanically. During the mixing, the casting ring is removed and the orifice connecting the ring with the rubber bowl is closed with a rubber stopper. The mechanical mixing is effected by engaging the shaft on the mixing bowl with that of the rotating motor which can be seen just below the hand of the operator (Fig. 28–7).

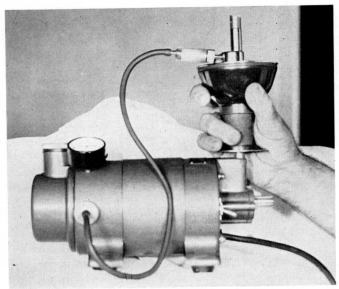

Fig. 28–7. A vacuum investing unit.

The equipment is then assembled as shown in Figure 28–7 and the investment is vibrated from the mixing bowl into the casting ring while the vacuum is maintained by the vacuum pump through the rubber tube leading to the mixer. The vibration is supplied by the motor to the platform on which the sprue base is seated.

The porosity of the investment is definitely reduced by vacuum investing,[28] presumably because of the increased density obtained. As a result, the texture of the surface of the casting is somewhat smoother with better reproduction of fine detail. The compressive strength of the investment is increased slightly by the vacuum investing.

Not all of the air is removed under the vacuum treatment. The amount removed will depend somewhat upon the consistency of the mix. The more viscous the mix, the more air bubbles will remain in the investment.[21] However, a thick mix is usually necessary because of the desired shrinkage compensation, and because of the poor surface texture which is obtained with a thin mix.

Apparently air bubbles can be entrapped on flat or concave surfaces facing away from the direction of the air evacuation. In order to minimize this effect, the pattern should be tilted whenever possible so that the water vapor bubbles, during the boiling, can stream across all of the surfaces of the pattern as they rise to the top, and thus remove any clinging air bubbles. However, the method of spruing should be carefully evaluated, since improper spruing may result in a distortion of the wax pattern when the air enters after the evacuation.[28]

As previously stated, equally good results can be obtained with hand investing as with vacuum investing. However, the latter method is probably more dependable in the prevention of surface nodules. In a comparison of the two methods, a study indicated that 95 per cent of the vacuum-invested castings made were free from nodules, whereas only 17 per cent of the castings made from hand-invested patterns by the same operators were entirely free from nodules.[30] Freedom from surface imperfections is highly important, as even a tiny nodule on an inlay casting may damage a frail enamel margin when the casting is tried in the prepared cavity. The finished casting should always be checked under magnification for such defects.

**Influence of Relative Humidity.** Regardless of the method used for investing the pattern, a minimum period of time should be employed for the process. Not only is the investment likely to thicken if too much time elapses, but also the cooling effect brought about by the evaporation of the water from the investment mix will cause a thermal contraction of the pattern. During the investing at atmospheric pressure, the relative humidity of the room will be a factor in connection with the cooling effect. The relative humidity of the average dental office in most climates is apt to be low during most of the seasons, and the cooling caused by the increased rate of evaporation under such a condition could cause the pattern to shrink 0.1 to 0.3 per cent during a prolonged investing period. Once the pattern is invested, no further temperature change of significance need be expected.

During a vacuum investing, considerable evaporation of the water may occur because of the induced vapor pressure, with a consequent reduction in temperature of the pattern. However, if the vacuum is applied for a short period of time, *e.g.*, 10 seconds, approximately 0.3 cubic centimeters of water will evaporate from an average size inlay ring, with a temperature decrease of the pattern of 1° C. (2° F.).[28] Such changes are not practically significant, but if the time in the vacuum is prolonged, the temperature of the pattern may be reduced as much as 4° C. (7° F.), which would cause the wax pattern to shrink approximately 0.15 per cent, an amount which is significant[28] (see p. 436).

## Literature

1. Herbert, W. E. and Thompson, A. R. F.: *Research on Gold Casting.* Proc. Roy. Soc. Med. (Sec. Odont.), *30:*13–30 (Jan.), 1937.
2. Suffert, L. W. and Mahler, D. B.: *Reproducibility of Gold Castings Made by Present-day Dental Casting Technics.* J.A.D.A., *50:*1–6 (Jan.), 1955.
3. Fusayama, T.: *Factors and Technique of Precision Casting; Parts I and II.* J. Pros. Den., *9:*468–497, (May), 1959.
4. Smyd, E. S.: *Physics and Techniques of Metal Inlay Laboratory Procedures.* J. Pros. Den., *3:*434–438 (May), 1953.
5. Frankel, C. B.: *A Scientific Approach to the Solution of Practical Problems Encountered in Electroforming Copper Dies.* J.A.D.A., *32:*1130–1138 (Sept. 1), 1945.

6. Ellis, R.: *Electrodeposition and Its Application in Dentistry*. Issued by the Canadian Dental Research Foundation, Toronto, Canada, 1943.

7. Rosenstiel, E.: *Improvements in Electroforming Dental Dies*. Brit. D. J., *88:*269–275 (May 19), 1950.

8. Novak, A.: *Copper Electroformed Dies*. New York J. Den., *22:*286–291 (Aug.), 1952.

9. Phillips, R. W. and Dettman, F. P.: *A Study of Some Variables Associated with Copperplating of Dental Impressions*. J. Pros. Den., *6:*101–113 (Jan.), 1956.

10. Blum, W. and Hogaboom, G. B.: *Principles of Electroplating and Electroforming*, ed. 3, New York, McGraw-Hill Book Co., Inc., 1949.

11. Phillips, R. W. and Schnell, R. J.: *Electroformed Dies from Thiokol and Silicone Impressions*. J. Pros. Den., *8:*992–1002 (Nov.), 1958.

12. Skinner, E. W. and Cooper, E. N.: *Desirable Properties and Use of Rubber Impression Materials*. J.A.D.A., *51:*523–536 (Nov.), 1955.

13. Asgar, K. and Peyton, F. A.: *Pits on the Inner Surfaces of Cast Gold Crowns*. J. Pros. Den., *9:*448–456 (June), 1959.

14. Phillips, R. W.: *Studies on the Density of Castings as Related to Their Position in the Ring*. J.A.D.A., *35:*329–342 (Sept. 1), 1947.

15. Strickland, W. D. and Sturdevant, C. M.: *Porosity in Full Cast Crowns*. J.A.D.A., *58:*69–78 (April), 1959.

16. Suffert, L. W.: *Influence of the Asbestos Liner on the Setting Expansion of Investment*. Rev. Assoc. Paulista de Cir. Dent., *4:*19–25 (March-April), 1951.

17. Peyton, F. A., Mahler, B. D. and Asgar, K.: *Controlled Water-addition Technic for Hygroscopic Expansion of Dental Casting Investment*. J.A.D.A., *52:*155–161 (Feb.), 1956.

18. Palmer, D. W., Romnes, A. F. and Skinner, E. W.: *The Effect of the Asbestos Liner on the Dimensions of the Investment Mold*. Paper presented to the Den. Mat. Group, I.A.D.R. Annual Meeting, 1960.

19. Fusayama, T., Sakurai, S. and Suzuki, E.: *Expansion of Investment in Casting Rings*. Bull. Tokyo Med. and Dent. Univ.., *4:*327–341, 1957.

20. Gustafsson, C. G. and Hedegård, B.: *Investing and Casting Technique*. Acta Odont. Scandinavica, *12:*233–250 (Feb.), 1955.

21. Ireland, J.: *Vacuum Investing and Its Relation to Cast Surfaces*. Brit. D. J., *86:*111–118 (March 4), 1949.

22. Sturdevant, R. E.: *A Simple Control for Practical Castings*. J.A.D.A., *24:*231–238 (Feb.), 1937.

23. Martin, K. H.: *An Investigation of the Effect of the Water/Powder Ratio on the Accuracy of the Fit of Gold Alloy Castings*. Austral. D. J., *1:*202–203 (Aug.), 1956.

24. Phillips, D. W.: *A Scientifically Correct Inlay Technique*. Dent. Digest, *39:*72–81 (Feb.), 1933; *Controlled Casting*. J.A.D.A., *22:*439–451 (March), 1935; *Present-day Precision Inlay Investing and Casting Technic*. J.A.D.A., *24:*1470–1479 (Sept.), 1937.

25. Scheu, C. H.: *A New Precision Casting Technic*. J.A.D.A., *19:*630–633 (April), 1932.

26. Asgar, K., Mahler, D. B. and Peyton, F. A.: *Hygroscopic Technique for Inlay Casting Using Controlled Water Additions*. J. Pros. Den., *5:*711–724 (Sept.), 1955.

27. Estes, G. D.: *The Casting Process*. J.A.D.A., *32:*1377–1382 (Nov., Dec.), 1945.

28. Phillips, R. W.: *Relative Merits of Vacuum Investing of Small Castings as Compared to Conventional Methods*. J. D. Res., *26:*343–352 (Oct.), 1947.

29. Hollenback, G. M.: *Simple Technic for Accurate Castings: New and Original Method of Vacuum Investing*. J.A.D.A., *36:*391–397 (April-May), 1948.

30. Lyon, H. W., Dickson, G. and Schoonover, I. C.: *Effectiveness of Vacuum Investing in the Elimination of Surface Defects in Gold Castings*. J.A.D.A., *46:*197–198 (Feb.), 1953.

# CHAPTER 29

# Gold Inlay Casting Procedures:

# Wax Elimination and Casting.

# Defective Castings

After the investment has hardened for at least one hour, the wax elimination and heating of the investment to the casting temperature can be started. The crucible former is removed carefully so that the sprue former remains in the investment. Any loosely attached investment around the edge of the ring is removed with a pointed instrument as shown in Figure 29–1. The sprue former is then carefully removed so that the surface around the ingate is not chipped. The ring should then be inverted and any small particles of investment in the area of the ingate removed with a camel's-hair brush. As an added precaution, the inverted ring should be rapped sharply on the top of the laboratory bench to remove any particles which may have fallen into the ingate.

**Wax Elimination and Heating.**    There are at least two methods by which the wax can be removed from the mold. One method is to remove it by flushing the mold with boiling water.[1] The invested pattern and ring are placed in boiling water for three to four minutes. The liquefied wax is then drawn out by suction. Since some of the water is also drawn out, the mold is thoroughly washed free of wax. A disadvantage of the method is that some of the very fine detail of the mold may be lost by a solution or a disintegration of the gypsum binder.[2]

In most of the technics under discussion, the wax pattern is eliminated by heat. In the case of the investment thermal expansion technic,

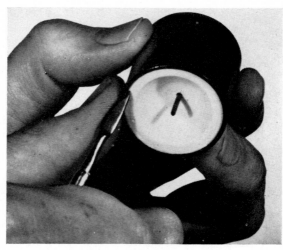

Fig. 29–1. Any loose pieces of investment around the edge of the ring should be carefully removed.

the casting ring containing the invested pattern is heated slowly to the temperature at which the maximum thermal expansion of the investment is obtained, usually 700° C. (1292° F.).

As the temperature is increased, the wax melts, boils and finally ignites. Some of the melted wax is absorbed by the investment and the residual carbon from the ignition becomes trapped in the investment. If the investment thermal expansion technic is employed, the mold is heated to 700° C. (1292° F.), and a great deal of the carbon is removed in the form of carbon monoxide or dioxide. Provided that the mold is not overheated, a slight amount of carbon remaining is advantageous in that it may aid in the production of a reducing atmosphere when the molten gold alloy enters the mold.

In the case of the investment hygroscopic technic, the ring is heated to no higher than 480° C. (900° F.) since an appreciable thermal expansion of the investment is not desired. Even though the mold is usually held at this temperature for 60 to 90 minutes, there remains the possibility that the carbon will be retained in sufficient quantity to prevent an adequate venting of the mold. In this case, the use of the boiling water method for the elimination of the wax may offer a certain advantage over the dry heat method.

The rate of the heating of the investment is a factor in the production of a smooth surface on the casting. If the heating is too rapid at the start, the steam resulting from the elimination of the water of crystallization may cause the walls of the mold to flake off as it emerges from the investment. In extreme cases, the steam pressure may build up in the interior of the investment and cause an explosion.

A further result of too rapid heating may be the production of cracks in the investment. In such a case, the outside layer of the investment becomes heated before the center portions. Consequently, the outside layer starts to expand thermally, with the result that radial cracks are transmitted to the mold and the casting may exhibit fins or spines similar to those shown in Figure 29–2. Such a condition is especially likely to be present after a too rapid heating when a cristobalite investment is employed for expanding the mold thermally. The comparatively low inversion temperature of the cristobalite, and the rapid rate of expansion during the inversion (see Fig. 27–9) makes it especially important to heat the investment slowly.[3] A safe heating period for any inlay investment is not less than 60 minutes and preferably longer. The complete amount of the thermal expansion may not be realized with continuous rapid heating. For example, it has been shown that when a certain quartz investment was heated to 700° C. (1292° F.) in three hours, its linear thermal expansion was 1.15 per cent, but when the same investment was heated to the same temperature in thirty minutes, its expansion was only 0.89 per cent.[4]

Although a gas elimination furnace can be used if special care is observed in the regulation of the heat, an electric furnace is more easily controlled. In an electric furnace, the top, bottom and sides of the muffle are generally heated. In such a case, it is best to invert the ring so that the crucible end will be in contact with the heated surface on the bottom of the muffle. It is advantageous to have the crucible end *slightly* hotter than the opposite end of the mold so that there will be

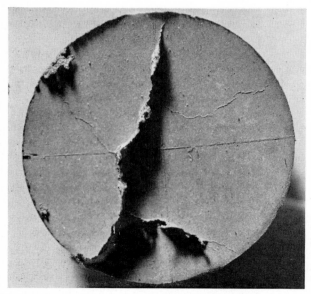

Fig. 29–2. Fins on the surface of a casting formed as a result of cracks in the investment.

less chance of the molten alloy solidifying prematurely in the ingate. Whenever the source of heat is at the side of the ring, it should rest crucible end up, so that the heat can rise to the top of the ring during heating, as in a gas furnace.

The heating is continued until a temperature of 700° C. (1292° F.) is reached, as indicated by a pyrometer. At this temperature, the sprue exhibits a cherry-red color when it is viewed in a shadow. A cherry-red color in direct light is an indication of a temperature much higher than 700° C. If the investment is heated to too high a temperature, a rough casting will result, as well as a possible contamination of the gold alloy with sulfur, due to the chemical disintegration of the investment.

Contamination of the gold alloy and a resulting brittleness in the casting, because of a breakdown of dental investments, probably is more common than heretofore realized. Several investigators[5, 6] have noted that sulfur gases are given off by gypsum investments when heated above 700° C. (1292° F.). The mechanism of this investment decomposition and alloy contamination is related to a chemical reaction between the residual carbon and the calcium sulfate binder.[7]

Calcium sulfate *per se* will not decompose unless heated to about 1200° C. (2100° F.). However, the reduction of calcium sulfate by carbon takes place rapidly above 700° C. in accordance with the following reactions:

$$CaSO_4 + 4C \rightarrow CaS + 4CO$$
$$3CaSO_4 + CaS \rightarrow 4CaO + 4SO_2$$

Thus this reaction will take place whenever gypsum investments are heated above 700° C. in the presence of carbon. The sulfur dioxide as a product of this reaction contaminates gold castings and makes them extremely brittle. This fact places emphasis, then, upon complete wax elimination, and avoiding burn-out temperatures above 700° C., particularly if the investment contains graphite.

Consequently, the wax elimination furnace should be equipped with an accurate pyrometer and thermocouple. Furthermore, once the casting temperature has been obtained, the casting should be made immediately. A maintenance of the high casting temperature for any considerable period may result in a sulfur contamination of the casting as indicated and also a rough surface on the casting owing to the disintegration of the investment.

Obviously, with a mold temperature of 430° to 480° C. (800° to 900° F.), as is employed with the low heat technic, the danger of contamination of the gold alloy because of the disintegration of the investment is non-existent despite any excessive amount of carbon present. Furthermore, with quartz investments there is no limit to the rate of heating the investment with this technic since the quartz inversion occurs above this temperature.

A diagrammatic representation of a longitudinal section of the mold as it should appear after elimination of the wax is shown in Figure 29–3. The entire mold, including the reservoir and ingate, is filled with molten alloy, with sufficient metal left over in the crucible to form the *button*, which can be seen attached to two of the castings in Figure 29–4. Before the inlay is placed in the mouth, the sprue portion is cut through close to the casting, and the excess metal is saved for recasting.

**Time Allowable for Casting.** As noted in a previous chapter (Fig. 27–12), the investment contracts thermally as it cools. When the investment thermal expansion or high heat technic is used, it can be expected, therefore, that once the heated ring is removed from the furnace to be placed in the casting machine, the investment will lose

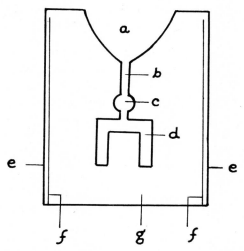

Fig. 29–3. A diagrammatic representation of an inlay casting mold. *a.* Crucible; *b.* ingate or sprue; *c.* reservoir; *d.* inlay mold; *e.* casting ring; *f.* asbestos liner; *g.* investment.

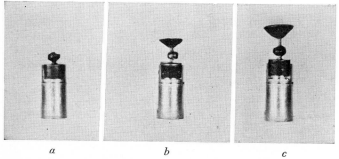

*a*　　　　　　*b*　　　　　　*c*

Fig. 29–4. *a.* Casting completed in one minute after the ring was removed from the furnace; *b.* casting completed in two minutes; *c.* casting completed in three minutes.

heat, and the mold will contract. Owing to the presence of the asbestos liner, and to the low thermal conductivity of the investment, a short period of time can elapse before the temperature of the mold is appreciably affected. Under average conditions of casting, approximately one minute can elapse without a noticeable loss in dimension as evidenced by the fit of the casting.[8] For example, the castings shown in Figure 29–4 were cast one, two and three minutes, respectively, after the mold was removed from the furnace. As can be observed, only the casting made at the end of one minute fits the steel die.

The completion of the casting within one minute is not difficult if the proper routine is employed. If the gold alloy is to be melted in the crucible formed in the investment, the alloy is premelted on a charcoal block before the ring is removed from the furnace. The ring is then placed in position in the casting machine. The melted gold alloy has meanwhile solidified sufficiently so that it can be transferred to the crucible with tongs. It is again quickly melted, and the casting is completed.

If the gold alloy is to be melted in a crucible separated from the investment, the process is simplified, since the metal can be preheated in the crucible, and, with the aid of an assistant, it can be maintained in the molten state while the heated ring is transferred to the machine.

In the case of the low heat casting technic, the temperature gradient between the investment mold and the room is not so great as that employed with the high heat technic. Also, the investment thermal expansion is not so important to the shrinkage compensation. Consequently, more time can be allowed for the casting without appreciable loss of dimension. Nevertheless, the procedure should not be too leisurely. A cold mold is not indicated for dental casting under any circumstances where the conventional investing and spruing procedures have been followed. Although the mold temperature is comparatively low, its maintenance insures a sound casting with less danger of premature solidification. Furthermore, the thermal expansion, though small, may be necessary for shrinkage compensation.

**Casting Machines.** There are two general types of casting machines in use at the present time. In one type, illustrated in Figure 29–5, the gold is forced into the mold under air pressure as described in the legend beneath the figure. Usually at least 0.7 kilograms per square centimeter (10 pounds per square inch) gauge pressure is required to complete the casting.[9]

One type of centrifugal casting machine is shown in Figure 29–6. In this case, the gold alloy is fused in a crucible separated from the ring. In the type of machine shown, the arm is revolved by a spring. The gold is fused, and the spring is released. The first movement is to whip the "broken arm" into line with the main arm, and the two arms remain in line during the revolution. The gold is thrown into the mold under centrifugal force. The force or pressure on the molten alloy in this case will depend upon the angular speed of the revolving arm, its radius and the weight of the gold. The mathematical relationship between these quantities is.

$$F = 0.004 \, \pi^2 \, n^2 \, mr$$

Where F = centrifugal force in grams at any instant
$\pi$ = 3.1416
n = speed in revolutions per second
m = weight of the gold alloy in grams
r = radius of the arm of the machine in centimeters.

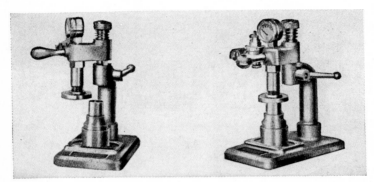

Fig. 29–5.   An air-pressure casting machine. The picture on the left shows the ring in position. The gold alloy is melted directly in the crucible formed in the investment. After melting, the arm is swung over the ring as shown at the right; the plunger immediately covers the top of the ring and the molten alloy is forced into the mold under air pressure. (Courtesy of the Kerr Dental Mfg. Co.)

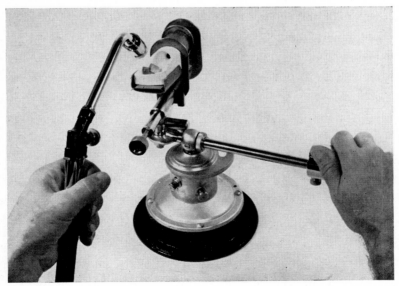

Fig. 29–6.   Casting with a centrifugal casting machine.

It is evident from the formula that the most important quantity in the determination of the force is the speed of revolution. This quantity is determined by the tension in the spring. The spring is placed under tension by revolving the arm backward a specified number of turns. Usually, 3 to 4 such manual revolutions of the arm are sufficient for the casting of an inlay.

The third type of casting machine makes use of the vacuum principle in that the gold is drawn into the mold under reduced air pressure instead of increased air pressure. One of these units is a combination of vacuum and centrifugal force. Otherwise, either a vacuum alone or a combination of increased air pressure (above that of the atmosphere) and a vacuum are used. It should be noted that when the vacuum is used, it is actually the normal pressure of the atmosphere which forces the molten alloy into the mold. Consequently, all such types can truly be classified as air-pressure casting devices.

So far as is known, there is little practical difference in the physical properties or accuracy of the inlay castings obtained with either type of machine, and the choice between the various types is a matter of personal preference. In fact, any method is satisfactory by which the molten alloy can be forced into the mold under sufficient pressure so that the pressure can be maintained for at least four seconds after the gold has been cast.[9]

**Fusing the Gold Alloy.**   The alloy is best melted by placing it on the side of the crucible. In such a position, the operator can better observe the progress of the melting, and there is a greater opportunity for any gases in the flame to be reflected from the surface of the metal rather than to be absorbed.

The fuel employed in most cases is a mixture of natural or artificial gas and air, although oxygen-air and acetylene can also be used. The temperature of the gas-air flame is greatly influenced by the nature of the gas and the proportions of gas and air in the mixture. Considerable care should be taken to obtain a nonluminous brush flame, with the different combustion zones clearly differentiated. Two types of flame which can be obtained with the gas-air blowpipe are shown in Figure 29–7. The air supply for the lower flame is excessive, and incomplete combustion and a lower temperature result. This type of flame is likely to be favored by the beginner because the roaring sound which accompanies this flame adjustment "sounds hot."

The upper brush flame (Fig. 29–7) indicates the proper adjustment for maximum efficiency and temperature. The parts of the flame can be identified by the conical areas. The first long cone emanating directly from the nozzle is the zone in which the air and gas are mixed before combustion. No heat is present in this zone. The next cone, green in color and immediately surrounding the inner cone, is known as the *combustion zone*. Here, the gas and air are in partial combustion. This zone is definitely oxidizing and it should be kept away from the metal during fusion at all times.

The next zone, dimly blue in color, is the *reducing zone*. It is the hottest part of the entire flame and is just beyond the tip of the green combustion zone. It is this area which should be kept constantly on the metal during fusion. The outer cone (*oxidizing zone*) is the area where combustion occurs with the oxygen in the air. Under no circumstances should this portion of the flame be employed to fuse the alloy. Not only is its temperature lower than that of the reducing zone, but also its use will cause oxidation of the metal.

With a little practice, the proper zone in contact with the metal can be readily detected by the condition of the metal surface. When the reducing zone is in contact, the surface of the alloy will be bright and mirror-like as indicated in Figure 29–8*A*. Furthermore, the surrounding environment will radiate the maximum intensity of temperature color possible, quite in contrast to the duller halo shown in Figure 29–8*B* with the dull, non-reflecting surface on the molten metal which occurs when the flame is applied improperly.

Although care should be taken not to overheat the alloy, there is generally more danger from underheating when the gas-air flame is used. The alloy first appears to be spongy, and then small globules of fused metal will appear. A gradual spheroiding of the bulk of the alloy then occurs as indicated in Figure 29–8*A*. At the proper casting temperature, the molten alloy is a light orange color and tends to spin or follow the flame when the latter is moved slightly. Ideally at this point, the metal should be approximately 38° to 65° C. (100° to 150° F.) above its liquidus temperature.[10] The casting should be made immediately when the proper temperature is reached.

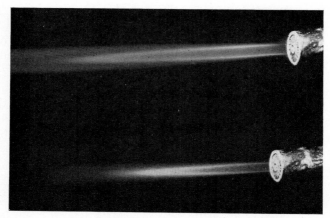

Fig. 29–7. Two types of nonluminous flame showing combustion areas. The upper flame should be employed for fusing the gold alloy. The lower flame results from too much air.

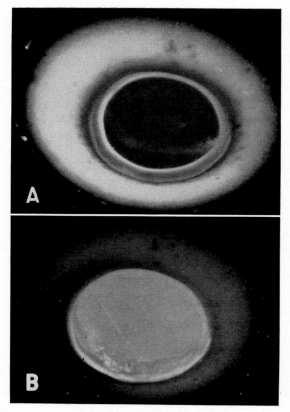

Fig. 29–8. *A.* Mirror-like surface indicates proper fusion. *B.* Cloudy surface indicates surface oxidation by blowpipe flame.

It is always desirable to use a flux to aid in minimizing porosity. Properly employed, the flux increases the fluidity of the metal and the film of flux formed on the surface of the molten alloy helps to prevent oxidization. Reducing fluxes containing powdered charcoal are often used, but small bits of carbon may be carried into the mold and cause a deficiency at a critical margin. Although such reducing fluxes are excellent for cleaning up old metal, a better flux for the casting procedure itself may be made from equal parts of fused borax powder ground with boric acid powder. The boric acid retains the borax on the surface of the metal better. The flux is added when the alloy is completely melted and should be used with either old or new metal.

As pointed out in Chapter 25, old sprues and buttons from the same alloy may be recast provided they are not contaminated or have not been unduly abused. The metal is placed on a charcoal block, melted and adequately fluxed, in this case with a reducing flux containing powdered charcoal (Fig. 29–9). A common mistake is to remove the blowpipe at this time which permits the molten metal to absorb gas from the atmosphere, with a resulting oxidation of the metal. Proper procedure (Fig. 29–10) is to turn the air off and allow the luminous gas flame to protect the surface until the solidification is complete.

**Cleaning the Casting.** After the casting has been completed, the ring is removed and quenched in water as soon as the button emits a dull red glow. There are two advantages to be gained in quenching: (1) The gold alloy is left in an annealed condition for burnishing, polishing and similar procedures. (2) When the water contacts the hot investment, a violent reaction ensues. The investment becomes soft and granular, and the casting is more easily cleaned.

Many times the surface of the casting will appear dark with oxides and tarnish. Such a surface film can be removed by a process known as *pickling*, which consists of heating the discolored casting in an acid. Probably the best pickling solution is made from one part concentrated hydrochloric acid and one part water. The hydrochloric acid will aid in the removal of any clinging investment as well as of the oxide coating. The disadvantage to the use of hydrochloric acid is that the fumes from the acid are likely to be corroding in their action on office and laboratory metal furnishings. The use of a similar solution of sulfuric acid is more advantageous in this respect. Its action can be increased by the addition of a small amount of potassium dichromate.

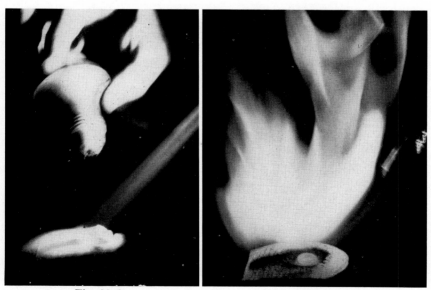

Fig. 29–9. Fig. 29–10.

Fig. 29–9. Melting "scrap gold" on a charcoal block. Plenty of reducing flux is used.

Fig. 29–10. After the "scrap gold" has been fused, it should be cooled in a luminous gas flame to prevent oxidation and gas occlusion.

The best method for pickling is to place the casting in a test tube or dish, and pour the acid over it. It may be necessary to heat the acid, but boiling should be avoided because of the considerable amount of acid fumes evolved. After pickling, the acid is poured off and the casting is removed. The pickling solution should be renewed frequently, as it is likely to become contaminated with use.

In no case should the casting be held with steel tongs so that both the casting and the tongs come into contact with the pickling solution. If this is done, the casting may become contaminated. The pickling solution usually contains small amounts of copper dissolved from previous castings. When the steel tongs contact this electrolyte, a small galvanic cell is created and copper will be deposited on the casting at the point where the tongs grip it. This copper deposition extends into the metal and will be a future source for discoloration in the area.

It is a common practice to heat the casting and then drop it into the pickling solution. The danger of such a method is that a delicate margin may be fused in the flame or the casting may be distorted by the sudden thermal shock when plunged into the acid.

After the pickling, the casting should be washed thoroughly in running water, and then may be immersed for a short time in a solution of sodium bicarbonate to insure that the acid is thoroughly removed or neutralized before the inlay is placed in the tooth.

## CAUSES FOR DEFECTIVE CASTINGS

An unsuccessful casting may result in considerable trouble and loss of time. In almost all cases, defects in castings can be avoided by a strict observance of procedures governed by certain fundamental rules and principles. Seldom is a defect in a casting attributable to other factors than the carelessness or ignorance of the operator. With present technics, casting failures should be the exception, not the rule.

Defects in castings can be classified under four headings: (1) distortion, (2) surface roughness, (3) porosity and (4) incomplete or missing detail. Some of these factors have been discussed in connection with some of the phases of the casting technics. The subject will now be summarized and analyzed in some detail.

**Distortion.** Any marked distortion of the casting is most likely related to a distortion of the wax pattern as described in Chapter 26. This type of distortion can be minimized or prevented by the proper manipulation of the wax and the handling of the pattern.

Unquestionably some distortion of the wax pattern occurs as the investment hardens around it.[2, 11, 12] The setting and hygroscopic expansion of the investment produce an uneven movement of the walls of the pattern. The change in shape can be measured in various ways, such as imbedding small metal workers in the pattern and using x-rays to study the movement,[11] or by placing sharp lines on the metal die and measuring their reproduction by carefully sectioning the hardened investment.[2]

The type of distortion is a tendency to move the proximal walls outward unevenly in the three-surface restoration. The gingival margins are forced apart by the mold expansion while the solid occlusal bar of wax resists expansion during the early stages of setting. The configuration of the pattern, type of wax and thickness all influence the distortion which occurs. For example, it increases as the thickness of the pattern decreases.[11] As would be expected, the smaller the setting expansion of the investment, the less will be the distortion.

Unfortunately, there is probably not a great deal that can be done to control this phenomenon. Generally, it is not a serious problem except that it accounts for some of the unexplained inaccuracies that may occur in small castings. It is possible that the greater the amount of residual stress present in the pattern, the greater might be the distortion upon setting of the investment. Thus minimal residual stress, as discussed in Chapter 26, may be of importance in this regard.

Evidence has been presented that a further distortion of the mold may occur during the thermal expansion of the investment in the high heat technic.[13] Consequently, although the distortion during the hygroscopic expansion may be greater than that which occurs during normal setting expansion, the over-all distortion may be of somewhat the same magnitude in both the low heat and the high heat technics. In any event, this type of distortion is small and its effect can be generally disregarded as a cause when it is necessary to re-make a casting because of a gross distortion.

**Surface Roughness.** The most probable causes for surface roughness, and their remedies, are as follows:

*Air Bubbles.* Small nodules on a casting are caused by air bubbles which became attached to the pattern during or subsequent to the investing procedure. The air bubbles can be removed from the water-investment mixture most surely by the use of a vacuum investing technic. If the manual method is used, various precautions can be observed to eliminate air from the investment mix before the investing. As previously outlined, the use of a mechanical mixer, and vibration both before and after mixing, should be practiced routinely. However, the vibration should not be sufficiently drastic to cause the investment particles to settle and to produce a thin mixture or water film at the surface of the mixed investment.

The use of a wetting agent may be helpful in the prevention of the collection of air bubbles on the surface of the pattern, but it is by no means a certain remedy.

Vibration during the painting of the pattern is an aid in obtaining good contact between the pattern and the investment. But after the pattern has been inserted in the ring, any vibration causes the bubbles present to circulate in the viscous investment mix, and some of them are almost sure to cling to the pattern.

*Water Films.* Wax is repellent to water, and if the investment becomes separated from the wax pattern in some manner, a water film may form irregularly over the surface. Occasionally, this type of roughness appears as minute ridges or veinings on the surface.

If the pattern is moved slightly after investing, jarred, or vibrated, or if the painting procedure does not result in an intimate contact of the investment with the pattern, such a condition may result. The use of a wetting agent is of aid in the prevention of such a type of roughness.

*Too Rapid Heating.* This factor has been discussed in a previous section. It results in "fins" or spines on the casting similar to those pictured in Figure 29–2. Or a characteristic surface roughness may be evident owing to a flaking of the investment when the water or steam poured into the mold. Furthermore, such a surge of steam or water may carry some of the salts used as modifiers into the mold, which are left as deposits on the walls after the water evaporates. As previously mentioned, the mold should be heated gradually. At least 60 minutes should elapse during the heating of the investment-filled ring from room temperature to 700° C. (1292° F.). The greater the bulk of the investment, the more slowly it should be heated.

*W/P Ratio.* The higher the W/P ratio, the rougher is the casting.[14] Presumably, the use of too much water is not conducive to a dense surface against which the gold is cast. However, if too little water is used, the investment may be unmanageably thick, so that it cannot be applied to the pattern properly. Or, in the case of a vacuum investing, the air may not be sufficiently removed. In either case, a surface roughness of the pattern may result.

As so often emphasized, the amount of water and investment should be measured accurately. Although in the case of the controlled water added technic this factor is not critical so far as mold compensation is concerned, it is important for the surface smoothness of the casting.

*Prolonged Heating.* When the high heat casting technic is used, a prolonged heating of the mold at the casting temperature will likely cause a disintegration of the investment and the walls of the mold will be roughened as a result. Furthermore, the products of decomposition are sulfur compounds which may contaminate the gold alloy to the extent that the surface texture is affected. Such contamination possibly is the reason why the surface of the casting sometimes will not respond to pickling. When the investment thermal expansion technic is employed, the mold should be heated to the casting temperature, not greater than 700° C. (1292° F.), and the casting should be made immediately.

*Temperature of the Gold Alloy.* If the gold alloy is heated to too high a temperature before casting, the surface of the investment will likely be attacked, and a surface roughness of the type described in the previous section may result. As previously noted, in all probability the alloy will not be overheated with a gas-air blowpipe which uses the gas supplied in most localities. If other fuel is used, special care should be observed that the color emitted by the molten gold alloy is not lighter than a light orange.

*Casting Pressure.*    Either too low or too high a pressure[14] during casting will produce a rough surface on the casting. A gauge pressure of 0.7 to 1 kilogram per square centimeter (10 to 15 pounds per square inch) in an air pressure casting machine or 3 to 4 turns of the spring in an average type of centrifugal casting machine is sufficient for the purposes of inlay casting.

*Composition of the Investment.*    The ratio of the binder to the quartz influences the surface texture of the casting[14] Also a coarse silica will cause a surface roughness. If the investment meets the American Dental Association Specification No. 2 for inlay investment, the composition will probably not be a factor in the surface roughness.

*Foreign Bodies.*    When foreign substances get into the mold, a surface roughness may be produced. For example, a rough crucible former, with investment clinging to it, may roughen the investment upon its removal so that bits of investment are carried into the mold with the molten alloy[3] Carelessness in the removal of the sprue former may be a similar cause.

Usually contamination results not only in surface roughness but also in incomplete areas or surface voids. An example may be seen in Figure 29–11. Any such casting which shows sharp, well-defined deficiencies indicates the presence of some foreign particles present in the mold, such as pieces of investment or bits of carbon from the

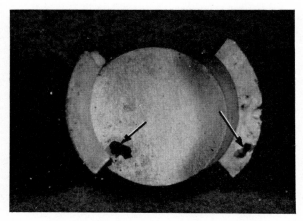

Fig. 29–11.    Irregular surface voids as shown by arrows indicate the inclusion of foreign bodies present in the mold.

flux. Bright appearing concavities may be the result of flux being carried into the mold with the metal.

Surface discoloration and roughness can result from sulfur contamination, either from investment breakdown at elevated temperatures or from a high sulfur content of the blowpipe flame. Black castings result which are brittle and do not clean readily during pickling.

*Impact of Molten Alloy.* It was pointed out that the direction of the sprue former should be such that the molten gold alloy would not strike a weak portion of the mold surface. Occasionally, the molten gold may fracture or abrade the mold surface as it strikes it regardless of its bulk. Unfortunately, sometimes the abraded area is smooth so that it cannot be detected on the surface of the casting. Such a depression in the mold is reflected as a raised area on the casting, often too slight to be noticed, yet sufficiently large to prevent the seating of the casting. This type of surface roughness or irregularity can be avoided by proper spruing so as to prevent the direct impact of the molten metal at an angle of 90 degrees with the investment surface. A glancing impact is likely to be less damaging and at the same time an undesirable turbulence is avoided.

*General Causes.* There are certain surface discolorations and roughnesses which may not be evident at the time the casting is completed, but which may appear during service. For example, various gold alloys, such as solders, bits of wire or various types of casting alloys should never be melted together and re-used. The resulting mixture not only would not possess the proper physical properties, but also might form eutectic or similar alloys with low corrosion resistance. Later discoloration and corrosion generally result during service.

Contamination with copper during improper pickling as previously discussed may be a factor in future surface change.

A source of discoloration often overlooked is the surface contamination of a gold alloy restoration with mercury. Mercury penetrates rapidly into the alloy and causes a marked loss in ductility and a greater susceptibility to corrosion. Completed castings should never be placed in contact with amalgam dies or on a bracket table where amalgam scrap may be lying. As previously stated in Chapter 21, it is not a good practice to place gold alloy restorations in contact with amalgam restorations for this and other reasons.

**Porosity.** Porosity may occur both internally and externally. The latter is a factor in surface roughness, but also it is generally a manifestation of internal porosity. Not only does the internal porosity weaken the casting,[3,15] but also, if it appears on the surface, it may be a cause for discoloration and, if severe, it could produce leakage and recurrent caries. Although the porosity in a casting cannot be prevented entirely, it can be definitely minimized by a proper technic. There are numerous causes for porosity, and some of them will be discussed in detail.

As previously stated (p. 424), internal porosity can be classified mainly as being caused (1) by method of solidification of the metal and (2) by occlusion of gas while molten.[10]

*Control of Solidification.* As previously discussed, three types of porosity result from improper control of the solidification of the molten metal. One type, localized shrinkage (Fig. 25–1*a* and 25–2*C*), is caused by a lack of flow of molten metal into the mold during solidification. The use of an adequate size sprue will minimize such porosity, or a reservoir may be employed close to the casting (p. 471). Even with either of these precautions, if the investment adjacent to the ingate is not heated sufficiently, the alloy may solidify prematurely. Such a condition of uneven heating is more likely to occur if the elimination is accomplished with gas heat, particularly with a Bunsen burner.

As previously noted, microporosity is occasioned by underheating the metal prior to casting. The temperature of the metal should be 38° to 50° C. (100° to 150° F.) above its liquidus temperature when the casting is made.

The effects of the various factors involved in the minimization of this general type of porosity are summarized in Table 29–1.

The subsurface porosity, produced by the bulk of the molten gold alloy pulling away from the "skin" portion first to solidify, can be largely prevented by not overheating either the melt or the investment mold. Thus, a more uniform solidification of the molten metal tends to occur.

*Occluded Gases.* Oxygen is dissolved by some of the metals in the alloy while they are in the molten state. During solidification, the gas is expelled to form blebs and pores in the metal. As was pointed out earlier, this type of porosity may be attributed to abuse of the metal. Castings severely contaminated with gases usually come out of the investment black (Fig. 29–12) and do not clean up easily on pickling. The porosity which extends to the surface is usually in the form of

*Table 29–1.* *Effects of Technical Factors on the Porosity Resulting from Metal Solidification\**

| TYPE OF POROSITY | INCREASED SPRUE THICKNESS | INCREASED SPRUE LENGTH | INCREASED MELT TEMPERATURE | INCREASED MOLD TEMPERATURE |
|---|---|---|---|---|
| Localized shrinkage porosity | Decreased | Increased | Decreased | Decreased |
| Subsurface porosity | Increased | Decreased | Increased | Increased |
| Micro-porosity | No effect | No effect | Decreased | Decreased |

\* Ryge, Kozak, and Fairhurst, *J.A.D.A.,* (June), 1957.

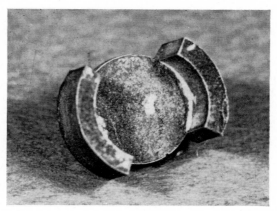

Fig. 29–12. A black-coated casting caused either by sulfur contamination or oxidation during melting.

small pin point holes (Figs. 25–1c and 25–2A). When they are polished out, others appear.

Larger spherical porosities (Fig. 25–2A) may be caused by gas occluded from a poorly adjusted blowpipe flame, or if the reducing zone of the flame is not used.

These types of porosity can be minimized by pre-melting the gold alloy on a charcoal block if the alloy has been used before, and by a correct adjustment and positioning of the blowpipe flame during melting.

*Back Pressure.* A type of porosity may be found on the casting owing to the back pressure of the air at the time the molten metal enters the mold. Back pressure porosity[9, 16, 17] may well be the most common type of porosity seen in dental castings, although it is often blamed on other causes. The modern dense investments, the increase in mold density effected by vacuum investing and the tendency for the mold to clog with residual carbon with the use of the low heat technic, all increase the difficulty in venting the gases from the mold during casting. Such porosity is especially common on the cavity side of the full cast crown or the m.o.d. inlay (Fig. 29–13) where the plug of investment in this location magnifies the problem. It may exhibit itself in ways other than these porous concavities. Rounded margins, holes extending through the casting and holes or incomplete areas in the button itself are other possible manifestations of this phenomenon.

Venting the mold by inserting a wax rod in the investment close to the pattern is inadequate.[16] This type of porosity can be avoided by using a sprue long enough that the outer end of the casting is within six millimeters (¼ inch) of the open end of the ring, the use of sufficient casting pressure and flaring the sprue at the point of attachment to the pattern.

***Incomplete Casting.*** Occasionally, only a partially complete casting, or perhaps no casting at all, will be found after the ring has been quenched and its contents examined. The obvious cause for such a condition is that the molten alloy has been prevented, in some manner, from completely filling the mold. There are at least two factors which might inhibit the ingress of the liquefied metal:[10, 18] (1) insufficient venting of the mold, and (2) a high viscosity of the fused metal.

The first consideration, *i.e.,* insufficient venting, is directly related to the back pressure exerted by the air in the mold. If the air cannot be vented with sufficient rapidity, the molten alloy will not fill the mold before it solidifies.

In such a case, the magnitude of the casting pressure should be suspected. If insufficient casting pressure is employed, the back pressure cannot be overcome. Furthermore, the pressure should be applied for at least 4 seconds. The mold is filled and the metal is solidified in approximately 1 second or less,[18] yet it is very soft during the early stages, and the pressure should be maintained for a few seconds beyond this point. An example of an incomplete casting because of insufficient casting pressure is seen in Figure 29–14. These failures are usually exemplified in rounded, incomplete margins.

A second common fault for an incomplete casting is an incomplete elimination of the mold. If too many products of combustion remain in the mold, the pores in the investment may become filled so that the air cannot be vented. If actual particles of wax remain, or moisture, when the molten alloy contacts either of these foreign substances an explosion may occur which can produce sufficient back pressure to prevent the mold from being filled. An example of a casting failure due to incomplete wax elimination can be seen in Figure 29–15. Although similar to the incomplete casting in Figure 29–14, it will be noted that the rounded margins are quite shiny rather than dull. This shiny condition

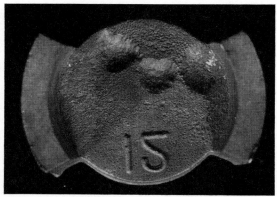

Fig. 29–13.   Concavities on cavity side of casting due to back pressure porosity.

Fig. 29–14.

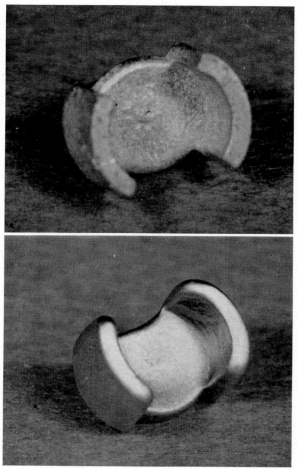

Fig. 29–15.

Fig. 29–14.  Rounded, incomplete margins due to insufficient casting pressure.
Fig. 29–15.  Incomplete casting caused by incomplete wax elimination, character-ized by roundness of margins and shiny appearance.

of the metal is due to the strong reducing atmosphere created by the carbon monoxide left by the residual wax.

The possible influence of the W/P ratio of the investment has already been discussed. The lower the W/P ratio, the less will be the porosity of the investment. A greater pressure during casting is indicated in such a case.

It is probable that different gold alloy compositions exhibit varying viscosities in the molten state. However, both the surface tension and the viscosity of a molten alloy are decreased with an increase in temperature; so far as is known, an incomplete gold alloy casting resulting from too great viscosity of the casting metal can be attributed to insufficient heating. The temperature of the alloy should be raised higher than its liquidus temperature so that its viscosity and surface tension will be lowered, and so that it will not solidify prematurely as it enters the mold. Such premature solidification may account for the greater susceptibility of the white gold alloys to porosity,[16] since their liquidi are higher in temperature and thus they are more difficult to melt with gas-air fuel.

The surface tension is also important, inasmuch as a high surface tension may cause rounded margins and corners on a casting which might otherwise be satisfactory. Such defects can be remedied by heating the gold alloy to a higher temperature before casting.

## *Literature*

1. Hollenback, G. M.: *Simple Technic for Accurate Castings: New and Original Method of Vacuum Investing.* J.A.D.A., *36:*391–397 (April-May), 1948.
2. Mumford, G. and Phillips, R. W.: *Dimensional Change in Wax Patterns During Setting of Gypsum Investments.* J. D. Res., *37:*351–358 (April), 1958.
3. Crawford, W. H.: *Selection and Use of Investments, Sprues, Casting Equipment and Gold Alloys in Making Small Castings.* J.A.D.A., *27:*1459–1470 (Sept.), 1940.
4. Osborne, J. and Skinner, E. W.: *Physical Properties of Gypsum Model Investments.* J.A.D.A., *59:*708–715 (Oct.), 1959.
5. Souder, W. and Paffenbarger, G. C.: *Physical Properties of Dental Materials.* National Bureau of Standards Circular C433, U. S. Government Printing Office, Washington, D. C., 1942, p. 91.
6. Brumfield, R. C.: *Dental Gold Structures.* New York, J. F. Jelenko Co., 1953, p. 103.
7. O'Brien, W. J. and Nielsen, J. P.: *Decomposition of Gypsum Investments in the Presence of Carbon.* J. D. Res., *38:*541–547 (May-June), 1959.
8. Skinner, E. W.: *Contraction of the Investment Mold During Casting.* Northwestern Univ. Bull. Dent. Res., *38:*12–16 (Nov.), 1937.
9. Phillips, R. W.: *Studies on the Density of Castings as Related to Their Position in the Ring.* J.A.D.A., *35:*329–342 (Sept.), 1947.
10. Ryge, G., Kozak, S. F. and Fairhurst, C. W.: *Porosities in Dental Gold Castings.* J.A.D.A., *54:*746–754 (June), 1957.
11. Van Aken, J.: *Distortion of Wax Patterns as Influenced by Setting and Hygroscopic Expansion of the Investment.* In press.
12. Jørgensen, K. D.: *Investigations on Dental Precision Casting Technic.* Göteborgs Tandläkare-Sällskaps Artikelserie, *36:*1–45 (Jan.), 1953.
13. Mumford, G. M. and Phillips, R. W.: *Measurements of Thermal Expansion of Cristobalite Type Investments in the Inlay Ring—Preliminary Report.* J. Pros. Den., *8:*860–864 (Sept.-Oct.), 1958.
14. Pomes, C. E., Slack, G. L. and Wise, M. W.: *Surface Roughness of Dental Castings.* J.A.D.A., *41:*545–556 (Nov.), 1950.
15. Peyton, F. A.: *Flexure Fatigue Studies of Cast Dental Gold Alloys.* J.A.D.A., *21:* 394–415 (March), 1934.
16. Strickland, W. D. and Sturdevant, C. M.: *Porosity in the Full Cast Crown.* J.A.D.A., *58:*69–78 (April), 1959.
17. Asgar, K. and Peyton, F. A.: *Pits on Inner Surface of Cast Gold Crowns.* J. Pros. Den., *9:*448–456 (May), 1959.
18. Herbert, W. E. and Thompson, A. R. F.: *Research on Gold Casting.* Proc. Roy. Soc. Med. (Section Odont.), *30:*13–30 (Jan.), 1937.

# CHAPTER 30

# Dental Gold Alloy Wires

The general use of wrought metal in the mouth has declined steadily since the advent of precision casting procedures. At one time, metallic dentures bases, saddles, and similar structures were constructed of gold alloy plate metal. The plate was swaged onto a cast made with low fusing alloy.

In modern dentistry, wire is the principal form in which wrought metal is used extensively. Gold alloy wires are occasionally employed for the construction of clasps. They also are used for the construction of orthodontic appliances.

**Composition.** The composition limits in eight groupings or types, which represent the compositions of modern dental gold alloy wires,[1] are given in Table 30–1. Since the wires should possess a relatively high fusion temperature, platinum and palladium can be used in much greater amount than in casting gold alloys (*cf*. Table 25–2). In fact, the alloys included in type No. 1, Table 30–1, contain gold in a minor amount in comparison to their platinum and palladium content. Alloys of type No. 8 in the same table contain no gold; the principal elements in this case are palladium (42 to 44 per cent) and silver (38 to 41 per cent). The alloys in this classification are the counterparts of the "palladium alloys" for casting discussed on page 421. The wires of this composition range are more successful in use than are the similar alloys for casting purposes.

According to the American Dental Association Specification No. 7 for dental wrought gold wire alloys, the gold, platinum and palladium content should total at least 75 per cent. All of the alloys listed in Table 30–1 can be formulated within such a composition range, with the exception of type No. 8 and possibly type No. 6.

**General Effects of the Constituents.**   As in the case of the casting alloys, extensive composition and physical property data for the gold alloy wires have been published[2] so that certain empirical relationships can be obtained between the chemical composition of the alloy and its chemical and physical properties.

As might be expected, the contributions of the individual metals are essentially the same as outlined for the casting gold alloys (p. 414). The presence of the platinum and/or palladium in considerable amount insures that the wire will not fuse during soldering operations. Furthermore, the platinum and the palladium, to a lesser extent, insure a fine grain structure and a high recrystallization temperature.

With the exception of alloy types Nos. 4 to 6 inclusive in Table 30–1, all of the wires are "white" or platinum colored.

The chief function of the copper is to contribute to the ability of the alloy to age harden. It is probably present in considerable amount in alloys No. 5 and 6 in order to aid in strengthening the wire in the absence of a considerable amount of platinum and palladium. It is noteworthy that the silver content of these alloy types is high as well, presumably to mask the reddish cast produced by the copper.

Nickel is sometimes included in wrought precious metal alloys in a small amount. It is a strengthener of the alloy, although it tends to reduce the ductility.[3] Also, the inclusion of a considerable amount of nickel tends to reduce the tarnish resistance of the alloy[4] and to change its response to age hardening.[5] In the amounts given in Table 30–1, any deleterious effects of the nickel are not likely to be present.

At first thought it might seem that the use of zinc as a scavenger agent is unnecessary in wrought alloys, since they are not melted by the dentist. However, the alloys are originally cast into ingots before the wires are drawn, and the use of zinc aids in the obtaining of oxide-free castings during the process of manufacture.

**Fusion Temperature.**   The fusion temperature of the wires is de-

*Table 30–1.   Composition Limits of Dental Gold-Alloy Wire\*†*

| TYPE NO. | GOLD (%) | PLATINUM (%) | PALLADIUM (%) | SILVER (%) | COPPER (%) | NICKEL (%) | ZINC (%) |
|---|---|---|---|---|---|---|---|
| 1 | 25–30 | 40–50 | 25–30 | ... | ... | ... | ... |
| 2 | 54–60 | 14–18 | 1–8 | 7–11 | 11–14 | 0–1 | 0–2 |
| 3 | 45–50 | 8–12 | 20–25 | 5–8 | 7–12 | ... | 0–1 |
| 4 | 62–64 | 7–13 | 0–6 | 9–16 | 7–14 | 0–2 | 0–1 |
| 5 | 64–70 | 2–7 | 0–5 | 9–15 | 12–18 | 0–2 | 0–1 |
| 6 | 56–63 | 0–5 | 0–5 | 14–25 | 11–18 | 0–3 | 0–1 |
| 7 | 10–28 | 0–25 | 20–37 | 6–30 | 14–21 | 0–2 | 0–2 |
| 8 | ... | 0–1 | 42–44 | 38–41 | 16–17 | 0–1 | ... |

\* Fractional percentages of iridium, indium and rhodium have not been included.
† Metals Handbook, 1948 edition.

*Table 30–2.*     *Fusion Temperatures (Wire Method) of Dental Gold Alloy Wires**

| TYPE NO.† | FUSION TEMPERATURE (°C.) | (°F.) |
|:---:|:---:|:---:|
| 1 | 1500–1530 | 2730–2790 |
| 2 | 1000–1100 | 1840–2010 |
| 3 | 1060–1120 | 1950–2050 |
| 4 | 945–1020 | 1730–1860 |
| 5 | 900–930 | 1650–1710 |
| 6 | 880–900 | 1610–1650 |
| 7 | 940–1080 | 1725–1975 |
| 8 | 1050–1080 | 1910–1970 |

\* Metals Handbook, 1948 edition.
† Composition limits given in Table 30-1.

termined as described in Chapter 25 (p. 416). Probably the fusion temperature should not be less than 954° C. (1750° F.). This lower limit of the fusion temperature is established in order to insure that the wires will not melt during normal soldering procedures.

The general limits of the fusion temperatures of the wires of the compositions given in Table 30–1 are presented in Table 30–2. It is interesting to note that none of the wires of types Nos. 5 and 6 meet the minimum requirement for fusion temperature. A comparison of Tables 30–1 and 30–2 indicates the general trend of the increase in fusion temperature as influenced by the platinum and palladium content. For example, type No. 1 contains the greatest platinum and palladium content, and these alloys exhibit the highest fusion temperatures. The alloys of types Nos. 5 and 6 contain the least palladium and platinum, and they exhibit the lowest fusion temperatures. The influence of the high palladium content of the wires of type No. 8 on the fusion temperature is evident.

**Mechanical Properties.**     A wire of a given composition is generally superior in mechanical properties to a casting of the same composition. The casting contains unavoidable porosity which produces a weakening effect. When the cast ingot is drawn into a wire, the small pores and blebs may be collapsed, and welding may occur so that such defects disappear in the wire. If the casting defects of this type are so large that they do not disappear when the wire is drawn, the wire will be definitely weakened.

Some of the mechanical properties of the alloys with the composition given in Table 30–1 are indicated[1] in Table 30–3. The tensile strength of a gold alloy wire probably should be not less than 10,500 kilograms per square centimeter (150,000 pounds per square inch), and its yield point should not be less than 8750 kilograms per square centimeter (125,000 pounds per square inch) after the wire has been age hardened by an "oven-cooling" treatment. After a softening heat treatment the elongation of the wire should be at least 15 per cent, and after an "oven-cooling" treatment, the value for the elongation should not be less than 4 per cent.

The values for the proportional limit and tensile strength obtained after an age-hardening treatment are not included in Table 30–3, since they can be estimated from the values for the Brinell hardness numbers by the usual method of calculation (p. 418). Probably formulations can be made from the alloy compositions indicated in Table 30–1 so that the requirements for both yield point and tensile strength can be met. The same observation holds for the values for the elongation in the "softened" (solution or softening heat treatment) condition, with the possible exception of the alloys included in type No. 3 (Table 30–3). However, after an "oven-cooling" heat treatment, alloy types Nos. 5 and 6 are probably too brittle.

The proportion between the Brinell hardness number and the proportional limit or the tensile strength of gold alloy wires is the same as described for the casting gold alloys (p. 418). Also, there appears to be a relationship between the proportional limit and strength of these alloys when they are tested under tension. As a rule, the value for the proportional limit will be approximately two-thirds that of the tensile strength value.[6]

The values of the mechanical properties presented in Table 30–3 can generally be predicted from the compositions presented in Table 30–1. The mechanical properties of the type No. 8 alloys which contain no gold are of interest. These alloys possess mechanical properties quite similar to the gold-containing alloys. In fact, they exhibit the greatest ductility after an oven-cooling treatment of any of the alloys (Table 30–3).

**Heat Treatment.** The methods for heat treatment of the gold alloy wires are the same as described for the casting gold alloys (p. 416). The considerations for solution heat treatment and age hardening are also the same.

All of the alloys with the compositions presented in Table 30–1 can be age hardened with the exception of type No. 1. The alloys of type No. 1 contain no copper, and, although age hardening is theoretically possible, they do not always respond to the usual age hardening treatments. However, the large amount of platinum and palladium contribute sufficient strength properties to the alloy so that it is equivalent in this respect to the other alloy types after age hardening (Table 30–3). Since the ductility of this type of alloy is sufficiently high, it can be strain hardened and annealed without fear of fracture or recrystallization, even though its proportional limit and strength are considerable.

As can be noted from Table 30–3, the "oven-cooling" age-hardening treatment results in a considerable decrease in the values for elongation

*Table 30–3.   Mechanical Properties of Gold Alloy Wires\**

| TYPE† NO. | PROPORTIONAL LIMIT‡ (100 KG./CM.²) | (1000 LB./IN.²) | TENSILE STRENGTH‡ (100 KG./CM.²) | (1000 LB./IN.²) | BRINELL HARDNESS NO. SOFTENED‡ | HARDENED§ | ELONGATION SOFTENED‡ (%) | HARDENED§ (%) |
|---|---|---|---|---|---|---|---|---|
| 1 | 56–105 | 80–150 | 87–126 | 125–180 | 200–245 | .... | 14–15 | .... |
| 2 | 50– 71 | 72–102 | 77– 91 | 110–130 | 150–190 | 240–285 | 12–22 | 5–10 |
| 3 | 77– 84 | 110–120 | 98–105 | 140–150 | 210–230 | 250–270 | 8–10 | 7– 9 |
| 4 | 38– 56 | 55– 80 | 63– 80 | 90–115 | 166–195 | 240–295 | 14–26 | 2– 8 |
| 5 | 37– 51 | 53– 73 | 57– 84 | 82–120 | 135–200 | 230–290 | 14–20 | 1– 3 |
| 6 | 36– 41 | 52– 58 | 59– 70 | 84–100 | 138–170 | 220–280 | 20–28 | 1– 2 |
| 7 | 42– 80 | 60–115 | 67–103 | 96–148 | 150–225 | 180–270 | 9–20 | 1– 8 |
| 8 | 44– 61 | 63– 87 | 70– 77 | 100–110 | 150–200 | 235–270 | 16–24 | 8–15 |

\* Metals Handbook, 1948 edition.
† Composition limits given in Table 30–1.
‡ After a softening heat treatment.
§ Age hardened by "oven-cooling."

from the "softened" condition. Such a treatment is somewhat drastic, and it is not recommended for practical cases. It is an excellent testing criterion, however, since the alloy can withstand almost any amount of abuse by heat treatment if it can be heat treated by "oven-cooling" without reducing the elongation to less than 4 per cent.

The directions of the manufacturer should be followed in heat treating procedures, particularly for age hardening. The optimum age hardening temperature depends upon the composition of the alloy, and it may be a narrow or a broad range.

The dependence of the age hardening temperature range upon the composition of a gold alloy is illustrated in Figure 30–1. Two gold alloy wires (K and R) were given a solution heat treatment at 700° C. (1292° F.) for ten minutes and were then quenched. Their respective Vickers hardness numbers after this treatment are indicated by the horizontal lines. The wires were then age hardened for 60 minutes at each of the temperatures indicated and their hardness was again measured.[5]

The composition by weight of alloy K was gold 60.3 per cent, silver 15.2 per cent, copper 9.0 per cent and platinum 15.5 per cent, whereas that of alloy R was gold 63.3 per cent, silver 12.4 per cent, copper 14.9 per cent, platinum 4.3 per cent, palladium 4.5 per cent and zinc 0.6 per cent. The maximum hardness for alloy R can be obtained by age hardening it at any temperature between 250° C. (480° F.) and 400° C. (750° F.), whereas in the case of alloy K the temperature range for maximum hardness is between 350° C. (660° F.) and 400° C. (750° F.). It follows, therefore, that alloy R can be age hardened at any temperature between 250° C. and 450° C., whereas the effective age hardening

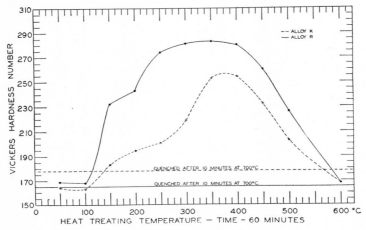

Fig. 30–1. Change in hardness of two gold alloy wires after being age hardened for 60 minutes at the temperatures indicated, preceded by a solution heat treatment. (Paffenbarger, Sweeney and Isaacs, *J.A.D.A.*, Dec., 1932.)

temperature range for alloy $K$ is only 50° C., between 350° C. and 400° C. Also, the response of alloy $R$ to the "oven-cooling" treatment is much greater than that of alloy $K$, since the temperature range of the "oven-cooling" treatment (450° to 250° C.) is entirely within the age hardening temperature range for alloy $R$, but not for alloy $K$.

**Microstructure.**     The microstructure of a wire was previously discussed in Chapter 18. The elongated grain structure shown in Figure 18–4 is usually characteristic of a wire. It is caused by the deformation of the grains in the direction of working when the alloy is drawn through a die below the recrystallization temperature.

The structure shown in Figure 18–4 is characteristic of an alloy which contains platinum and perhaps palladium in substantial amount.[6] It can be assumed that all wires exhibit a banded or elongated structure of this nature when they are first drawn, but if the recrystallization temperature is sufficiently low, an equiaxed structure may be formed during the solution heat treatment. Such a structure tends to reduce the tensile and bending properties of the wire in the solution heat treated condition in comparison to the wires whose banded structure has been preserved to any extent.[7] After age hardening, the tensile properties of the wires with equiaxed grain structure appear to be comparable with those of the wires with the banded structure, with the exception of the elongation, which is reduced to an extent that such wires are definitely brittle.[7] These effects are clearly demonstrated in the wire types Nos. 5 and 6 in Table 30–3. These types are low in platinum group metals (Table 30–1), and they exhibit comparatively low tensile properties and surface hardness after a solution heat treatment. After age hardening, their surface hardness is comparable with that of the other alloy types, but their ductility is greatly reduced.

Consequently, on the basis of present research findings and general experience as indicated by the type of wires usually employed by orthodontists, for example, it can probably be concluded that the banded or elongated structure provides a better wire functionally in dental appliances. Such a conclusion implies that the wire should contain sufficient platinum and/or palladium to preserve a refined grain structure during all heating operations, and that the wire should not be heated above its recrystallization temperature.

## Literature

1. Taylor, N. O.: *High-Strength Precious Metal Wires.* Metals Handbook, 1948 edition. Cleveland, American Society for Metals, 1948, p. 1120.
2. Souder, W. and Paffenbarger, G. C.: *Physical Properties of Dental Materials.* National Bureau of Standards Circular C433. Washington, U. S. Government Printing Office, 1942, pp. 38, 60.
3. Souder, W.: *Nickel in Dental Alloys.* Metals and Alloys, 6:194 (July), 1935.
4. De Wald, L. N.: *Nickel in Precious Metal Alloys.* Metals and Alloys, 6:331 (Nov.), 1935.

5. Paffenbarger, G. C., Sweeney, W. T. and Isaacs, A.: *Wrought Gold Wire Alloys: Physical Properties and a Specification.* J.A.D.A., *19:*2061–2086 (Dec.), 1932.
6. Bush, S. H., Taylor, D. F., and Peyton, F. A.: *Comparison of the Mechanical Properties, Chemical Compositions, and Microstructures of Dental Gold Wires.* J. Pros. Den., *1:*177–187 (Jan.-March), 1951.
7. *Ibid., cf.* Tables I, II and III, Figs. 1 and 2.

CHAPTER 31

# Gold Alloy Solders.

# Soldering Procedures

Solders are used in dentistry for joining parts of an assembly, as in the assembling of a bridge, and for building up or adding to the bulk of certain structures, such as the establishment of proper contact areas on inlays and crowns with adjacent teeth. Solder used for the latter purpose is sometimes known as a *building solder*. Building solders were formerly used extensively in dentistry for the actual formation of crowns.

Solders are used extensively in orthodontics for the joining of wrought metal parts such as wires and bands. Because of the possible structural changes in wrought metal, such as recrystallization and grain growth, orthodontic soldering procedures may be more critical than when castings are joined. Both types of soldering will be considered.

**What is "Soldering"?**    There are a number of terms which are used in connection with the joining of metals, such as *soldering, brazing* and *welding*. The three operations differ from one another as follows:

*Soldering* is the joining of metals by the fusion of intermediary alloys which are of a lower melting point. The lower fusing metal, or solder, is fused to the parts to be joined. In industrial procedures, if the solder possesses a melting temperature greater than 425° C. (800° F.), the process is known as *brazing*. In dentistry, however, such a distinction is not made, and all such operations are known as soldering, regardless of the temperature of the solder.

*Welding* is a process used to join metals, usually with heat. *Fusion*

**Page 512**

*welding,* which includes *gas* and *arc welding,* requires that the parts to be joined be melted and fused together, without the use of a solder. In *pressure welding,* the joining is accomplished with pressure and, usually, with heat, but the parts are not melted; they recrystallize across the interface between them in some manner. As noted in Chapter 19, gold foil can be welded under pressure at room temperature; most metals and alloys require both heat and pressure for such a method of joining.

**Requisites for a Dental Solder.** Dental solders are classified metallurgically as *hard solders* in contrast to the low melting *soft solders* used by plumbers and tinsmiths. The hard solders are generally high fusing and more resistant to tarnish, and stronger than the soft solders.

The following general properties may be listed[1] as being important in a hard solder to be used for dental purposes:

1. The fusion range of the solder must be lower than that of the parts to be soldered so that the parts will not be melted, and in order that the solder may be "easy flowing" over the work when it is fused. This factor is controlled by the composition of the solder. The fusion temperature of the solder is often at least 100° C. (180° F.) below the fusion temperature of the work, although technicians expert in the art often join parts with solders possessing a fusion temperature of 50° C. (90° F.) or less below that of the work.

2. The composition of the solder should be such that it is "free-flowing," that is, so that it will flow freely, once it is melted. The term covers certain characteristics of the solder which are related to its fluidity and surface tension, as well as its ability to alloy superficially with the work to be soldered. For example, if the solder alloys too readily with the metal to be soldered, it may "soak in" instead of flowing along the surface. A freely flowing solder will spread easily and quickly over clean metal surfaces; it will penetrate small openings, and follow along points of contact by capillary action.

The flowing property and a physical adhesion of the solder to the metal are extremely important. Without true adhesion there is no actual soldering action, but only a mechanical anchorage to surface irregularities. The molten solder physically adheres when it leaves a continuous permanent film on the surface of the alloy instead of merely rolling over it. For such adhesion to occur, there must be a stronger attraction between the atoms of the liquid solder and those of the metal surface than between the atoms of the solder itself. The minimum temperature of adhesion does not, however, always correspond exactly with the liquidus of the particular solder. Adhesion is thus a complex property related to the composition of the solder, its melting range and the thermal conductivity of the metal being soldered.[3]

3. The solder should not cause pitting of the soldered joint. Unfor-

tunately, pitting is one of the most prevalent flaws encountered in soldering procedures, and it is usually the result of improper technic on the part of the operator. However, pits may be more prevalent when solder is used which contains a considerable amount of base metal. On overheating, the base metals volatilize and the vapor creates pits.

Pitting is also related to the distance, or gap, between the parts to be soldered.[2]

4. The strength of the solder should be at least as great as that of the parts to be soldered. The hardness and strength of the gold alloy solders increase as the gold content or fineness of the solder decreases. Solders above 650 fine should not be used when considerable stress is involved.[1]

5. The color of the solder should match that of the parts to be soldered. However, after a soldered joint has been polished, it usually is not noticeable, even though there may be considerable difference in color between the solder and the work, provided that the proper soldering technic has been employed.

6. The solder should be resistant to tarnish and corrosion in the mouth fluids. Undoubtedly, the solders of higher fineness are superior in this respect to the solders with the lower gold content. The choice of a solder, so far as tarnish resistance is concerned, depends upon the type of restoration. If the restoration can be removed from the mouth, a solder with a lower fineness can be used so that strength need not be sacrificed. Likewise, if the appliance is a temporary one and not in the anterior part of the mouth, as with orthodontic appliances, then a solder of lower fineness is indicated. Strength is maintained and the risk of failure because of any loss in properties of the metals being soldered is minimized. However, if the restoration is permanent and is not going to be removed and polished frequently, then a solder of higher fineness is indicated. The exact minimum gold and platinum group metal content which is necessary in the solder to resist corrosion is not known. Although 580 fine has been suggested[4] as the minimum fineness for permanent use in the mouth, probably a solder of at least 680 fineness is safer so far as the prevention of discoloration is concerned.[5, 6]

**Composition** The basic composition of a gold solder is similar to that of a casting alloy, namely, gold, silver and copper. Zinc and tin are added to reduce the fusion temperature of the solders, since the addition of copper is not sufficient for this purpose. For each 1 per cent of such base metals added the liquidus temperature may be reduced approximately 10° C. (18° F.) and the solidus, 24° C. (43° F.) when the gold content is 625 fine or lower. In the case of solders of higher fineness, the reduction of the liquidus is about 5° C. (9° F.) more, but the solidus change is approximately the same as for alloys of lower fineness. Such figures are only estimates, however, since the various combinations of precious metals employed may change such relationships considerably.

In addition to the base metals, phosphorus may be added in a small amount as a deoxidizer to improve the resistance of the solder to oxidation while it is fused.

If a "white" colored solder is required, nickel is added to replace the copper. The copper and silver content can be varied, with the gold and base metal content held constant, to modify the color of the solder from a rich gold-color contributed by the copper to a light gold-color contributed by the silver.

Such a variation in the copper and silver content of the solder should be controlled so that properties other than color may not be adversely affected. For example, the higher the silver content, the less is the melting range, and conversely, when a considerable amount of copper is used at the expense of the silver, the fusion range may be so large that the solder melts partially and penetrates the part to be soldered, instead of flowing.[4] The result is that more than a superficial alloying between the parts and the solder takes place, and the general composition of both the solder and the part may be changed. Such solders are sometimes called "sticky," since they appear to melt but do not flow. Such solders may be good building solders, however.

On the other hand, solders containing silver in predominance to copper, other conditions being equal, will adhere to the metal to be soldered and they will flow freely over the surface. Such solders are preferable in most cases.

The compositions[7] of five dental gold solders are presented in Table 31–1. The first three solders are of a lower fineness than the last two. Only in the case of solder *B* is the copper content greater than the silver content.

The gold composition of the solder is properly designated by its fineness, as it has been designated in the previous discussion. Gold manufacturers, however, may designate their solders as "14-carat," "18-carat," etc. Such a designation does not indicate the gold content of the solder, but rather the carat of the gold alloy on which the solder is intended to be used. For example, an "18-carat solder" does not contain 18 parts in 24 parts of pure gold; rather it is a solder to be used with a gold alloy of 18-carat. In Table 31–1, solders *A*, *B*, and *C* are "18-carat" solders, and the other two solders are "20-carat." In connection with modern dental alloys, which may contain platinum and palladium in addition to the gold, such a designation becomes meaningless, since the melting point and other properties have been completely altered by the additions.

**Fusion Temperature.**     As previously noted, the upper limit of the fusion temperature (liquidus) of the solder should be less than the solidus temperature of the parts to be soldered. In the case of gold

### Table 31–1. Composition of Dental Gold Solders*

| SOLDER NO. | GOLD (%) | SILVER (%) | COPPER (%) | ZINC (%) | TIN (%) |
|---|---|---|---|---|---|
| A | 65.4 | 15.4 | 12.4 | 3.9 | 3.1 |
| B | 66.1 | 12.4 | 16.4 | 3.4 | 2.0 |
| C | 65.0 | 16.3 | 13.1 | 3.9 | 1.7 |
| D | 72.9 | 12.1 | 10.0 | 3.0 | 2.0 |
| E | 80.9 | 8.1 | 6.8 | 2.1 | 2.0 |

\* Coleman, R. L., *National Bureau of Standards Research Paper No. 32.*

### Table 31–2. Melting Ranges of Dental Gold Solders*

| SOLDER NO.† | MELTING RANGE (°C.) | (°F.) |
|---|---|---|
| A | 745–785 | 1375–1445 |
| B | 750–805 | 1385–1480 |
| C | 765–800 | 1410–1470 |
| D | 755–835 | 1390–1535 |
| E | 745–870 | 1375–1595 |

\* Coleman, R. L., *National Bureau of Standards Research Paper No. 32.*
† Compositions given in Table 31–1.

alloy wires, the fusion temperature of the solder should be less than the recrystallization temperature of the wire for reasons explained in the previous chapter.

As a general rule, the greater the gold content of the solder, the higher its fusion temperature is expected to be. Such a condition does not necessarily follow, however, by merely increasing the gold content. For example, although the gold content of solders D and E in Table 31–1 is progressively higher than that of the first three solders tested, their fusion temperatures (Table 31–2) are not appreciably different from those of the lower gold-content solders, A, B, and C.

It is desirable that the fusion temperatures of different solders vary progressively from a low temperature to a high temperature. Occasionally, in the construction of complicated dental appliances it may be necessary to solder a part of the appliance to another part, which has already been soldered. In such a case, a lower fusing solder than the first one used is necessary. A third soldering procedure may be required, and a still lower fusing solder must be used, and so on. It is possible to formulate satisfactory dental solders with graded fusion temperatures if the proper proportions of the constituent metals are employed.[1]

As a general rule, it is wise to select a solder which melts not less than approximately 80° C. (150° F.) below the lower limit of the melting range of the parts to be soldered.

*Table 31–3.* *Tensile Properties of Gold Solders**

| SOLDER NO. † | HEAT TREATMENT | PROPORTIONAL LIMIT (KG./CM.²) | (LB./IN.²) | TENSILE STRENGTH (KG./CM.²) | (LB./IN.²) | ELONGATION (%) |
|---|---|---|---|---|---|---|
| A | Softened | 1,890 | 27,000 | 2,980 | 42,500 | 14 |
|   | Hardened | 3,850 | 55,000 | 4,400 | 63,000 | 1 |
| B | Softened | 2,060 | 29,500 | 3,120 | 44,500 | 12 |
|   | Hardened | 5,420 | 77,500 | 5,850 | 83,500 | <1 |
| C | Softened | 2,100 | 30,000 | 3,080 | 44,000 | 9 |
|   | Hardened | 5,400 | 77,000 | 6,450 | 92,000 | <1 |
| D | Softened | 1,680 | 24,000 | 2,520 | 36,000 | 7 |
|   | Hardened | 4,300 | 61,500 | 4,900 | 70,000 | <1 |
| E‡ | Softened | 1,440 | 20,500 | 2,620 | 37,500 | 18 |

* Coleman, R. L., *National Bureau of Standards Research Paper No. 32.*
† Composition given in Table 31–1.
‡ Not appreciably affected by age hardening.

**Heat Treatment and Mechanical Properties.** The mechanical properties of the solders with the compositions given in Table 31–1 are presented in Table 31–3. The heat treatment designated as "softened" consisted of quenching the alloy in water from a temperature of 700° C. (1292° F.), and, when the alloy was "hardened," it was age hardened by cooling it slowly from 450° C. (840° F.).

The proportional limits and tensile strength of the solders (Table 31–3) are comparable in value to the similar properties of a type *B* or *C* cast gold alloy (Table 25–3), but they are generally less in magnitude than the similar properties of a gold alloy wire (Table 30–3). It is axiomatic, therefore, that a soldered joint should not be introduced into a wire appliance at a point of great stress.

The values for the elongation of the solders are definitely lower than those of any of the other types of gold alloy.

The gold solders are generally amenable to age hardening, although solder *E* in the accompanying tables is an exception. Often, the solders age harden quite radically, and the values for the elongation may be so low after such a heat treatment that the soldered joint is quite brittle.

**Fluxes.** As will be emphasized frequently in later sections, the parts to be joined must be free of oxides or any other impurity, or the solder will not flow or adhere to the surface. In order to keep the surface clean at the soldering temperature, it is covered with a *flux* before the solder is applied.

The soldering fluxes are ceramic materials which will melt and flow over the parts to be soldered at a temperature well below the fusion temperature of the solder. Since they are solvents for the metallic oxides, or reducing agents, they keep the parts clean while the heat is being applied during the soldering procedure. However, the film of flux should be capable of being separated from the solid metal by the molten solder.

There are a number of high melting salts, notably borax, or boric acid, which can be used individually as fluxes. However, since each chemical of this type exhibits certain fluxing characteristics of its own, they are usually combined so that a superior flux can be produced with the good characteristics of each of the ingredients. A formula for a soldering flux which is quite efficient is:[8]

| | | |
|---|---|---|
| Borax glass | 55 | parts |
| Boric acid | 35 | parts |
| Silica | 10 | parts |

The ingredients may be fused together, and then ground to a fine powder.

Borax glass, or sodium pyroborate ($Na_2B_4O_7$), is preferable to ordinary borax, or sodium tetraborate ($Na_2B_4O_7 \cdot 10H_2O$), for fluxing purposes. Borax effloresces when it is heated on the work as its water of crystallization is driven off, and, as a result, a part of the surface may be exposed, and a pit may result.

The boric acid reduces the fusion point of the flux so that it will flow smoothly over the work at a low temperature. The silica contributes a viscosity or toughness to the film after fusion so that it will stay on the work.

The flux can be employed in a powdered form or as a paste. If it is used as a paste, alcohol should be used as the liquid agent rather than water. A paste formed by mixing fused borax in water will result in a hydration of the sodium pyroborate to common borax, and the efflorescence previously described will be troublesome.

One method for the forming of a paste which has been highly successful, is to mix the powdered flux with an inert grease or plastic gel such as petrolatum. The grease protects the flux from the air, and when the organic petrolatum is fused on the wire along with the flux, it carbonizes and is eliminated into the air or flame.

The soldering flux presented above can also be used in fluxing the molten metal during casting (p. 492).

An *antiflux* is any material which may be placed on the work, before the soldering flux is applied, to confine the flow of the molten solder. If the soldering temperature is not too high, such an area can be marked off with a lead pencil. The molten solder will not flow across the graphite line, unless a temperature is reached where the carbon combines with the oxygen and thus is removed from the surface. Another effective means for the production of such a barrier is to paint the work with a suspension of iron rouge or whiting in alcohol.

### INVESTMENT SOLDERING

Usually the units of a bridge, such as the inlay or crown abutments and the pontics, are soldered together rather than to cast the entire bridge in one piece. The intricacy of the procedure can be realized when it is considered that the bridge abutments are expected to fit the tooth with the usual precision of an inlay or crown. Furthermore, the structures between the abutments must fit the vacant space formerly occupied by the missing teeth so precisely that no lateral stress is induced in the supporting teeth.

Cleanliness is the first requisite for a successful solder joint. The parts must not only be free of oxides incurred from casting but also from any polishing agents which contain oil, wax or grease. When such agents have been used, the restorations should be scrubbed with soap and water and then pickled. Crowns or bands which have been previously fitted on fusible metal or amalgam dies should be boiled in nitric acid to remove traces of the contaminating metal.

In brief, the technic is as follows: The bridge is usually assembled on a master cast and fastened together with "sticky wax," a wax composition containing rosin, in order to increase its mechanical adhesion. The assembly is then carefully lifted from the master cast and imbedded in an investment with only the joints exposed. The wax is then eliminated with boiling water. The investment is heated, and the parts are brought to the soldering temperature with a gas-air blowpipe and the soldering is completed.

**Gap Distance.** The correct gauging of the distance between the parts to be soldered is a matter of importance for the prevention of warpage.

Theoretically, the distance between the parts should be related to three factors: (1) the thermal expansion of the investment during heating, (2) the thermal expansion of the parts and (3) the shrinkage of the solder during solidification. During heating, the thermal expansion of the investment will cause the parts to move further apart, but the thermal expansion of the metal parts themselves will tend to close this gap and partially or totally neutralize the expansion effect of the investment. The shrinkage of the solder during solidification is presumably of the same order of magnitude as the casting shrinkage of a casting gold alloy.[9]

Unfortunately, the above relationships have not been subjected to detailed analyses, as has been done with the inlay casting procedure. One investigation has shown that the parts should not be in contact before the investment is heated. With the materials employed, it was demonstrated that the parts should be separated at least 0.1 millimeter (0.005 inch) in order to prevent warpage.[2]

**Soldering Investment.** The composition of the soldering investment is much the same as that of a quartz casting investment. In fact, the stronger casting investments can sometimes be used as a soldering investment. An investment containing quartz is preferable to a cristobalite investment because of the lower thermal expansion of the former.

Furthermore, an investment with a low normal setting expansion is preferred to one with a high setting expansion.[2] The setting expansion tends to change the spacing of the parts and even causes a warpage. Under no circumstances should the investment come in contact with water during setting because this will cause a hygroscopic setting expansion.

A third requisite of a soldering investment is that it withstand the heat of the blowpipe during soldering without cracking.

**Investing.**    The parts of the bridge should be securely fastened together with the wax before the assembled bridge is removed from the master cast and invested. If this factor is controlled, there should be no appreciable error involved during the investing procedure.[2]

No ring or supporting medium need be used for the investing procedure. The investment is mixed to a thick consistency with the proper W/P ratio as indicated by the manufacturer. The investment can be poured on a glass plate and the appliance seated in it. The investment is carefully removed from above and underneath the joints so that there is free access.

After the investment has set, the wax is then flushed with boiling water until the parts are completely free of both wax and adhering investment.

If an antiflux is desired to confine the flow of the solder, it can be applied at this time. Also, there is a certain advantage to the application of a paste flux while the parts are still hot.[2]

**Heating.**    Although the investment can be heated prior to the soldering operation with a blowpipe or Bunsen burner, the safest method is to heat the investment to about 430° C. (800° F.) in an elimination furnace as in the casting technic. There will be less chance of weakening or cracking the investment during soldering. Any fracturing of the investment during heating with the blowpipe is likely to cause a warpage of the bridge. Excessive heating of the investment may cause a sulfur contamination of the gold alloy and solder.

The purpose of the preheating is to eliminate moisture from the investment and, as previously mentioned, to provide a certain amount of thermal expansion.

**Soldering.**    If the flux has not already been applied, it should be spread thoroughly but not excessively over the parts to be joined. It should be confined to the joint area only.

The exposed parts should be heated gradually with the reducing flame until the flux is seen to flow. The temperature is then elevated rapidly to the soldering temperature which can be observed as yellowish red heat, observed in diffused light. As can be noted from Table 31–2, the melting range of the solder is between approximately 750° C.

and 870° C. (1385° F. and 1595° F.). As in the case of the heating of casting gold, only the reducing flame should be used. At this stage, the area of the flame should be adjusted to as small a cone as possible so as to confine the heating to the area to be soldered.

The solder is then applied without removing the flame. If the operation has been properly completed, the solder should flow at once, and the flame is immediately removed.

If the solder does not immediately flow smoothly over the area to be soldered, the soldering operation should be discontinued. Further heating will volatilize the base metals in the solder, thus raising its fusion temperature, and the parts themselves may melt. With the proper solder, the only cause for "balling" of the solder on the work is that the surface of the latter has become contaminated in some manner, either with oxide or it was not properly prepared at the start.

The solder flows between the flux and the metal, thus the metal surface is protected from oxidation throughout the soldering procedure. The direction of flow is affected by gravity, temperature and capillary action in addition to the adhesive forces between the solder and the work.

Solder will flow toward the area with the highest temperature. Consequently, a flame of small area is indicated so that the flow can be directed. The less the distance between the parts to be soldered, within limits, the greater will be the attraction by capillary action.

The gap distance, however, can be too small. In such a case, porosity in the soldered joint is considerably increased.[2] When the surfaces are in direct contact at the time of soldering, the solder may not flow at the point of contact.[10] These considerations are illustrated in Figure 31–1 which shows a solder joint after it was pulled apart. The lack of solder at the points of contact is evident. Also, considerable porosity is evident in the small gap distance immediately surrounding the point of contact.

**Structure of the Soldered Joint.**      As previously noted, the union of the solder with the work is the result of physical adhesion. However,

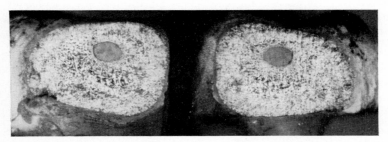

Fig. 31–1   Soldered proximal surfaces of two bridge units which were soldered in contact. The two units were in contact in the area with no solder. (Courtesy of G. Ryge, Marquette University.)

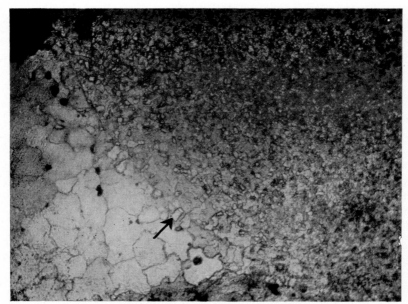

Fig. 31–2. Cross section through a wire on which solder has been flowed (solder structure at the left). The arrow indicates a grain in the wire which may have been a nucleus of crystallization for the solder. Note the banded wire structure in cross section. ×200. (Courtesy of R. L. Coleman, J. M. Ney Co.)

it has been shown that the strength of the joint, particularly when the higher fusing solders are used, is influenced by the composition of the parts.[11] Such an observation indicates that a limited atomic diffusion may possibly occur between the parts and the solder and *vice versa.*

It is also possible that the grains in the soldered part may act as nuclei of crystallization for the solder. The grain indicated by the arrow in Figure 31–2 is evidence for such a theory.

If the solder is overheated, a diffusion of the solder occurs into the work as can be noted[2] in Figure 31–3. The proper soldering temperature for the solder employed for the joints in Figure 31–3 was 760° C. (1400° F.). The metallographic structure of the properly soldered joint is indicated by the upper left photomicrograph in Figure 31–3. The dendritic structure of the solder is evident adjacent to the cast structure, with no *visible* diffusion between the two. When the solder is overheated to a temperature of 815° C. (1500° F.), the diffusion of the solder into the grain boundaries of the bridge unit becomes evident, as well as a tendency for the diffusion of the cast structure into the solder. As the soldering temperature increases, the atomic diffusion continues until at a temperature of 900° C. (1650° F.), the solder and the parent alloy completely fuse. The composition of both the solder and the gold alloy has been changed, with the result that the mechanical properties of the joint are no longer under the control of the operator. Not only is the bridge weakened and embrittled by the overheating, but a warpage also results.[2]

The same effect can occur at lower temperatures, although not as readily, if the heating is sufficiently prolonged. If follows, therefore, that the soldering should be accomplished at the lowest temperature and in the least time possible.

**Heat Treatment.** As can be noted from Table 31–3, gold solders are, in general, markedly susceptible to age hardening heat treatment, particularly in relation to their reduction in ductility. Such an obser-

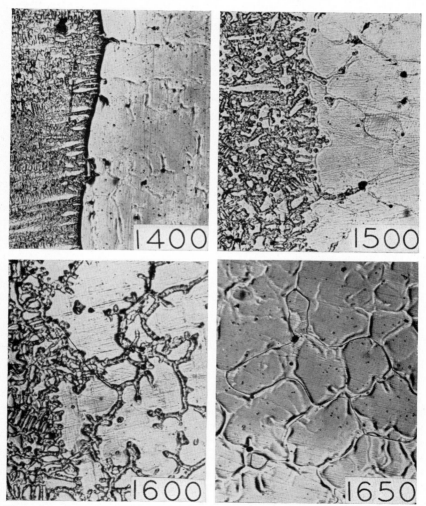

Fig. 31–3. Diffusion of gold solder at various temperatures as indicated in lower right hand corner (° F.) of photomicrographs. (Ryge, *D. Clin. North America*, November, 1958.)

vation indicates that the soldered joint should be quenched from the soldering temperature in order to prevent the precipitation of the keying phases. In practice, however, such a procedure is not indicated because of the warpage which will occur if the invested bridge is plunged into water at the soldering temperature. Furthermore, subsequent heat treatments after removal from the investment are also likely to result in a warpage of the bridge.[2, 12]

As a compromise, the bridge can be allowed to cool in the investment for five minutes and then quenched. With such a treatment, the danger of warpage is minimized and, at the same time, the mechanical properties are improved without a great reduction in percentage elongation.

**Strength of Soldered Joints.** The tensile strength of the soldered joints in a bridge assembly is not greatly affected by the gap distance between the parts, at least within practical limits. If the gap is excessively large, the solder will need to be built up to bridge the gap. Molten solder, like a drop of water, tends to be spheroid because of its surface tension. The higher the temperature of the fused solder, the less is its surface tension. Consequently, on overheating, a film of solder occasionally breaks between two adjacent widely separated parts, and the parts are not joined.

Furthermore, the surface tension action may cause the solder to decrease in cross section area if the parts are too widely separated, much as will a drop of water if it is "stretched" between the ends of two glass rods. The result is a reduction of area with a consequent loss of strength at the joint. However, if the parts are spaced approximately 0.1 millimeter (0.005 inch), as previously advised, these effects should not be troublesome.

So far as the composition of the solder itself is concerned, the general trend is for increased strength with compromise between tarnish resistance and strength. As previously noted, if the dental appliance is removable, a solder of lower fineness can be used than if the appliance is fixed in the mouth. In the former case, any tarnish spots will be noticed by the patient and can be removed by polishing. If the appliance is fixed, the ordinary habits of mouth hygiene are usually insufficient to prevent corrosion.

Inasmuch as a marked increase in proportional limit and strength by an age hardening heat treatment is not feasible for reasons previously stated, an adequate strength in the quenched condition is highly desirable.

**Porosity.** Probably the greatest single factor affecting the strength of a soldered joint is the presence of porosity in the solder after solidification. In summary, improper cleaning, fluxing, spacing of the parts, and application of the soldering flame as previously discussed may cause porosity. Overheating may cause pits and porosity. In addition to the pits and porosity caused by the volatilization of base metals, the borax flux may fuse with the metal and the solder will not flow over the area.

Even the method of applying the molten solder to the work may cause porosity. For example, if the solder is placed in the joint before heating, the porosity of the joint will be greater than if the solder is applied after heating as described.[2]

**Corrosion.** As might be expected because of its composition, the solution potential of the soldered joint is generally less than that of the work. Consequently, the solder will be more susceptible to electrolytic tarnish and corrosion than will the gold alloy bridge unit.

Another factor is the alloy type present in the solder. Most of the gold alloy solders, particularly the lower fusing types, undoubtedly contain eutectic phases. Because of the resulting general lack of surface homogeneity, electrolytic couples are present in the solder itself which promote discoloration and corrosion in the mouth.

As in the case of the silver amalgam restoration, a highly polished surface on the soldered joint will greatly improve its resistance to tarnish and corrosion. Furthermore, because of its susceptibility to tarnish and corrosion, the solder should be confined as much as possible to the joint and should not be allowed to spread over adjacent surfaces. As previously noted, the solder can be confined by the use of antifluxes and the proper direction of the flame on the work.

## FREE-HAND SOLDERING

When wires or bands are soldered for orthodontic appliances, the volume and linear dimensions of the parts are such that a gold alloy wire can be contoured to shape and then soldered to another part by holding the two parts in contact in the flame with the hands or tweezers. The solder is then applied as described for the cast bridge.

Although most of the principles described for investment soldering apply equally well to orthodontic or clasp soldering, the use of wrought metal structures complicates the situation because of the danger of weakening the joint by recrystallization and grain growth of the wires during soldering.

**Application of the Flux.** The same type of flux can be used for orthodontic soldering as for investment soldering. The use of antiflux is seldom necessary, however.

For the sake of simplicity, the soldering of two wires in an end-to-end, or butt, joint will be described. The same principles can be applied to other types of joints as well.

Whenever a wire is to be soldered, ideally it should first be subjected to a solution heat treatment. Furthermore, as repeatedly stated, a wire can be bent and contoured much more readily in this condition. A previously annealed wire structure is much less apt to warp by relaxation during the soldering procedure even though the wires are strain hardened to an extent during shaping.

As with investment soldering, cleanliness is one of the first requisites. The parts of the wires to be soldered should be free of oxides or any other surface impurities.

The application of the flux is confined as much as possible to the area to be soldered. The ends of the wires are then heated until the flux is seen to flow.

**Soldering.**    As previously noted, since the orthodontic appliance can be removed and cleaned periodically, it is customary to use 450 fine solders or even lower fineness in certain instances. Solders with a gold content greater than 650 fine are never used in orthodontic soldering. In this manner, considerable strength of the joint is assured.

Usually the parts are held in contact during free-hand soldering. Because of the much smaller areas involved, there is little danger that the solder will not flow throughout the joint area. Owing to the sharp peripheral edges of the wire ends, the surface tension of the solder may cause a decrease in diameter of the joint if any appreciable gap is present. Contrary to the situation found with the soldered bridge parts, the closer in apposition the parts before soldering, the stronger is the soldered joint.[13]

The flame used in soldering wires should be needle-like in thinness. A special orthodontic blowpipe is used. The blowpipe rests on the bench so that the hands are free. The needle-like flame is essential so that the heat can be confined to the joint. As usual, only the reducing flame is used in heating and soldering.

Very likely, the solder should be added to the heated joint as directed for investment soldering, but usually this procedure is not feasible since both hands of the operator are already occupied in holding the work. A more practical method is to attach the solder to the end of one wire and then to re-fuse the solder with the end of the other wire in contact. Again, because of the small volumes involved, this procedure appears to be sound in orthodontic soldering.

As in all soldering operations, the solder should fuse and flow immediately and the work should be removed from the flame at once before metallic diffusion and grain growth can occur. Since the work held in the hands cannot be moved until the solder completely solidifies, it is customary to blow out the flame without moving the hands.

**Metallographic Structure.**    The metallographic structure of a properly soldered orthodontic joint is shown in Figure 31–4. There is no evidence of diffusion of the solder into the wires, nor has the characteristic band structure of the latter been altered.

However, with overheating, not only does a solution of the solder and the parts occur as in Figure 31–3, but also the grain structure of the wire can be changed. Both effects will result in a weak soldered joint.

The recrystallization and grain growth of a wire because of over-

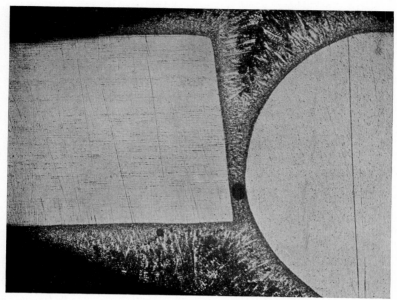

Fig. 31–4. Cross section through an arch wire and a finger spring of an orthodontic appliance which had given good service. The solder has not diffused into the wire, nor has the structure of the latter been changed. The two blebs are probably unavoidable gas inclusions. (Courtesy of R. L. Coleman, J. M. Ney Co.)

Fig. 31–5. Microstructure of a high fusing wire. ×500. (Courtesy of R. L. Coleman, J. M. Ney Co.)

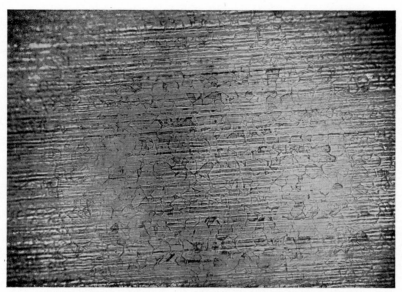

Fig. 31–6.   Microstructure of same wire (Figure 31–5) after being heated at 954° C. (1750° F.) for five minutes. ×500. (Courtesy of R. L. Coleman, J. M. Ney Co.)

Fig. 31–7.   Microstructure of same wire (Figure 31–5) after being heated to 1010° C. (1850° F.) for five minutes. ×500. (Courtesy of R. L. Coleman, J. M. Ney Co.)

heating are shown in Figures 31–5 to 31–7. The microstructure of the original wire is shown in Figure 31–5. The wire contained considerable platinum and/or palladium with a fusion temperature of 1050° C. (1925° F.), high above the melting temperature of a dental gold solder (Table 31–2).

Nevertheless, if this wire is overheated during soldering, a recrystallization and grain growth can occur as shown in Figures 31–6 and 31–7. The photomicrograph of a practical case in which grain growth occurred in the wire is shown in Figure 31–8.

Even though the solder may not be heated to the recrystallization temperature of the wire, a prolonged application of the heating can cause a solution of the wire in the solder as indicated in Figure 31–9. The reduction in area of the wire decreases the mechanical properties of the joint drastically.

If the joint is overheated for too long a time, the structure shown in Figure 31–10 will result. As in the case of the overheated soldered joint in the investment soldering technic (Fig. 31–3), the solder and the gold alloy wire have fused together. The structure is no longer that of a wire, and a cast structure is present. The mechanical properties of the joint are definitely reduced.

**Heat Treatment.** Whenever possible, the soldered joint should be quenched immediately after removal from the flame in order to provide a solution heat treatment. It is often an advantage in an orthodontic appliance to be able to bend the wire close to the joint and, in such an instance, ductility in the solder is advantageous. Furthermore, it is not always feasible to place the soldered joint at a point of minimum stress. The increased ductility of the solder obtained by

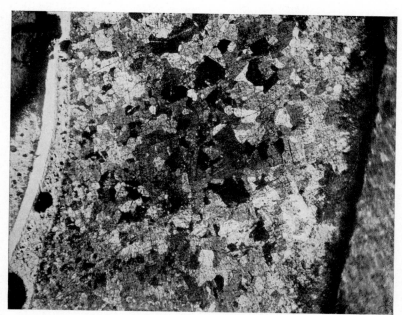

Fig. 31–8. Microstructure of a wire which broke in service. The grain growth indicates that the wire was heated to a relatively high temperature for too long a time during soldering. ×100. (Courtesy of R. L. Coleman, J. M. Ney Co.)

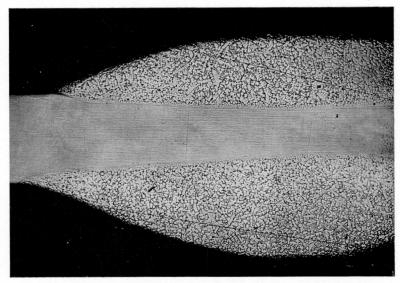

Fig. 31–9.  Solder was flowed onto a wire and kept molten for 45 seconds before the flame was removed. ×30. (Courtesy of R. L. Coleman, J. M. Ney Co.)

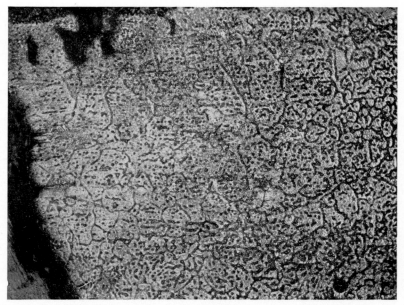

Fig. 31–10.  Microstructure of a wire which broke in service near the soldered joint. The solder has dissolved in the wire and a cast structure replaced the banded structure of the wire. ×500. (Courtesy of R. L. Coleman, J. M. Ney Co.)

quenching is thus an additional insurance against fracture of the joint during service.

It is usually not feasible to heat treat the entire orthodontic appliance for the usual reason of stress relaxation and warpage. However, little advantage would be gained by an age hardening treatment as indicated in Figures 31–11 and 31–12.

Stress-strain curves under bending stress for a gold alloy clasp wire and a soldered joint made between two lengths of the same wire[14] are shown in Figure 31–11. The solder employed was 490 fine. Both the soldered joint and the wire were given a softening heat treatment (held at 700° C. for ten minutes and quenched).

As can be noted from Figure 31–11, the modulus of elasticity and the proportional limit of the soldered joint under a bending load were definitely less than the similar properties for the wire alone. After the soldered joint and the wire were given an age hardening treatment, the bending properties of the wire increased as shown in Figure 31–12. Although the proportional limit of the wire was increased, that of the soldered joint was scarcely changed from the solution heat treated condition (Fig. 31–11) because of the embrittlement of the solder by the age hardening heat treatment. The age hardening treatment employed was an aging at 500° C. (930° F.) for 15 minutes.

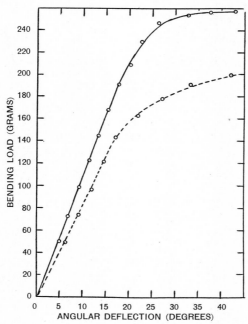

Fig. 31–11. Stress-strain curve under a bending stress. Solid line indicates orthodontic wire. Dotted line indicates soldered joint. Both wire and soldered joint were previously subjected to a softening heat treatment.

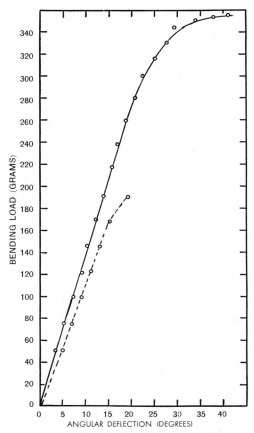

Fig. 31–12. Same type wire and soldered joint as in Figure 31–11 after being subjected to age hardening.

***Tensile Properties of Soldered Joints.*** Although the strength of
the solder is important in estimating the strength of the soldered joint,
it is necessary to test the joint itself if its true strength is to be determined.

The tensile strength of a number of soldered joints[11] are plotted in
Figure 31–13. Three wires (*A*, *B* and *C*), of the same gauge but different compositions, were each soldered end to end with a low-fusing
solder, 490 fine, and a high-fusing solder, 650 fine. The wires were
soldered and air cooled; the tensile strengths for this group of joints
are plotted at the left in the figure. The joints were given a solution
heat treatment, or annealing, by holding them at 700° C. (1292° F.)
for 10 minutes, and then quenching; the tensile strengths for this group
are shown by the center points in Figure 31–13. The third group of
joints were age hardened by "oven-cooling," and their tensile strengths
are plotted at the right in the figure. The broken lines connect the

strength values of the joints soldered with the 650-fine solder, and the solid lines indicate similarly the strengths obtained with the 490-fine soldered joints. The tensile strength of the 490-fine solder itself in the age-hardened ("oven-cooling") condition was 5150 kilograms per square centimeter (73,800 pounds per square inch), and that for the 650-fine solder after a similar heat treatment was 4350 kilograms per square centimeter (62,100 pounds per square inch).

According to the results presented in Figure 31–13, the strengths of the soldered joints were greater in almost every instance than the strengths of the solders themselves. Furthermore, it is evident that the natural cooling of the soldered joints from the soldering temperature resulted in generally erratic values for the strength. Such a scattering of the data indicates that such a practice is not controlled, and, therefore, is unreliable.

After the soldered joints were given a solution heat treatment as described, the strengths of the joints made with the 490-fine solder were approximately the same, regardless of the type of wire employed. In

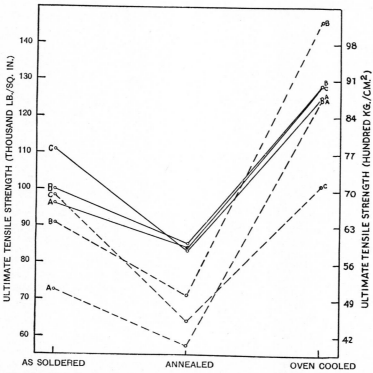

Fig. 31–13. Tensile strengths of soldered joints with three different orthodontic gold alloy wires (*A, B* and *C*) and two types of gold solder. Broken lines indicate joints soldered with 650-fine solder, and solid lines indicate those soldered with 490-fine solder.

the case of the joints soldered with the 650-fine solder, the tensile strengths varied considerably between the various wires.

After the age hardening treatment, the strengths of the joints made with the 490-fine solder were increased uniformly and independently of the composition of the wires employed. On the other hand, a considerable variation in the strengths of the joints occurred after the "oven-cooling," according to the wires employed.

Such results indicate that, in certain instances, there may be a diffusion of atoms during soldering from the metal soldered to the solder, as well as from the solder to the metal. In such a case, the composition of the solder may be altered sufficiently to change its response to heat treatment quite markedly. It is further evident from the greater variations in strength with the different wire compositions when 650-fine solder was used, that the effect of composition was more pronounced with the higher fusing solder than with the lower fusing 490-fine solder.

## Literature

1. Taylor, N. O., and Teamer, C. K.: *Gold Solders for Dental Use.* J. D. Res., *28*:219–227 (June), 1949.
2. Ryge, G.: *Dental Soldering Procedures.* D. Clin. North America, November, 1958, pp. 747–757.
3. Lewis, W. R.: *Notes on Soldering.* Tin Research Institute, Battelle Memorial Institute, Columbus, Ohio, 1948, pp. 17–18.
4. Crowell, W. S.: *Dental Gold Solders.* Metals Handbook, 1948 edition. Cleveland, American Society for Metals, p. 1104.
5. Souder, W., and Paffenbarger, G. C.: *Physical Properties of Dental Materials.* National Bureau of Standards Circular C433. Washington, U. S. Government Printing Office, 1942, p. 42.
6. Spreng, M.: *Metallkunde fuer den Zahnarzt.* Basel, Schweiz. Appollonia-Verlag., 1940.
7. Coleman, R. L.: *Physical Properties of Dental Materials.* National Bureau of Standards Research Paper No. 32, Washington, U. S. Government Printing Office, 1928, p. 894.
8. Weinstein, L. J.: "Dental Metallurgy," in Peeso, F. A.: *Crown and Bridgework,* ed. 2, Philadelphia, Lea & Febiger, 1924, pp. 461–463.
9. Anonymous: *Gold.* Hartford, The J. M. Ney Co., p. 57.
10. Ryge, G.: *Dental Bridge Soldering Procedures.* Paper read before the American Academy of Crown and Bridge Prosthodontics, September 12, 1959.
11. Turbyfill, W. J.: *Heat Treatment of Orthodontic Soldered Joints.* Thesis, Northwestern University Dental School, 1939.
12. Steinman, R. R.: *Warpage Produced by Soldering with Dental Solders and Gold Alloys.* J. Pros. Den., *4*:384–395 (May), 1954.
13. Wesselhoeft, H. D.: *Physical Properties of Soldered Joints in Orthodontic Appliances with Especial Reference to Heat Treatments.* Thesis, Northwestern University Dental School, 1934.
14. Stone, F. W.: *Heat Treatment of Orthodontic Soldered Joints.* Thesis, Northwestern University Dental School, 1939.

# CHAPTER 32

# Steel: Its Constitution

# and Heat Treatment

The dentist is seldom called upon to work or to cast carbon steel in any manner. However, practically all of the cutting tools used in dentistry are of some form of carbon steel. In order to handle such tools intelligently, the dentist should know something of their metallurgy and metallography, particularly in regard to their heat treatment. Many times excellent dental tools are ruined inadvertently because of ignorance in regard to their proper treatment.

The steels to be discussed in the present chapter are essentially alloys of carbon and iron, and for this reason they are known as *carbon steels* to distinguish them from the *stainless steels* to be discussed in the next chapter.

The metallurgy of steel is a subject in itself. Alloys of carbon and iron have received more study by far than any single non-ferrous alloy because of the commercial importance of the ferrous alloys. The subject is treated very superficially in these pages. Only those factors are considered which may be of immediate interest to the dentist.

**Constitution Diagram for Steel.**     The alloys of iron and carbon may be classified as of the mixed type, and their constitution diagram resembles to some extent that of the silver-copper system in Figure 20–9 (p. 332). Carbon is soluble in iron to the extent of 1.7 per cent by weight. The alloys in this range of solubility are known as *steel*. When the carbon content exceeds 1.7 per cent, a eutectic alloy is formed, known as *cast iron*. Cast iron is so brittle that it cannot be wrought to

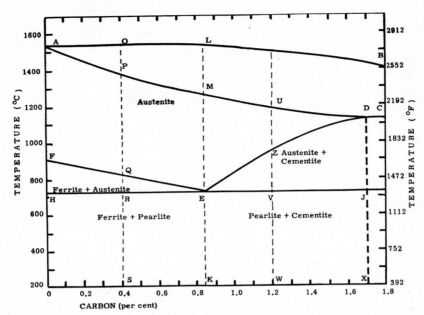

Fig. 32–1.   A simplified constitution diagram for carbon steel.

the same degree as the steel, and, consequently, the difference between the two types of alloy is considerable from a commerical standpoint.

The constitution diagram for carbon steel is presented in Figure 32–1. The eutectic point is not included, since its carbon content is greater than that of steel. The liquidus is the line *AOLB* in the figure, and the solidus is the line *APMUDC*. The remaining lines indicate solubility and transformation limits, and they require further explanation.

The remainder of the diagram can be simplified considerably, if the student will block out the liquidus and solidus lines with a piece of paper for the time being. The resemblance of the remainder of the diagram to that of the constitution diagram of a eutectic alloy system is evident (*cf.* Fig. 20–5, p. 328). It is as though the line *FQEZD* were a liquidus, the line *FHREVJD* were a solidus, and the point *E* a eutectic. Although the entire area described is solid, the analogy between the lines indicated with the liquidus and solidus of a eutectic alloy system is complete.

In order to understand the constituents present, a review of the allotropic forms of iron will be given. At ordinary room temperature, iron exists in the α-form. Alpha-iron possesses a body-centered cubic space lattice, and it is magnetic. Metallographically, it is termed *ferrite*. As the iron is heated, it loses its magnetism. The non-magnetic iron is known as β-iron. Since there is no change in space lattice between the α- and the β-form, β-iron is not differentiated as an allotropic form. At a slightly higher temperature, a true allotropic change takes place to a face-centered cubic space lattice known as $\gamma$-iron. The carbon is more soluble in the $\gamma$-iron than other forms. The $\alpha$- and $\gamma$-forms are important in explaining the heat treatment of steel.

The carbon combines with the iron to form an intermetallic compound, $Fe_3C$, known as iron carbide or *cementite*, which is hard and brittle.

Referring again to Figure 32–1, the solid solution phase of the steel is represented in the area between the pseudo-liquidus lines *FQEZD* and the true liquidus. The $\gamma$-iron acts as a solvent for the cementite in this area to form a solid solution known metallographically as *austenite*.

**Eutectoid Steel.**    The structures involved in the various transformations and precipitations indicated in the constitution diagram can best be illustrated by examples. For example, assume that an alloy of iron 99.16 per cent and carbon 0.84 per cent is allowed to cool slowly from the liquid state along the line *LMEK*. At the temperature indicated by *L* (approximately 1525° C.), the first solid will form as austenite. The solidification will be complete at the temperature corresponding to *M* (approximately 1310° C.). No further change occurs until a temperature corresponding to *E* (approximately 725° C.) is reached, when a metallographic change takes place to an intimate mixture of ferrite and cementite, known as a *eutectoid* rather than a eutectic. The steel of this particular composition is known as a *eutectoid steel*.

The intimate mixture of cementite and ferrite consists metallographically of alternate laminations of ferrite and cementite as shown in Figure 32–2. The cementite is the dark constituent, and the ferrite is light. The cementite is much harder than the ferrite, and, during the polishing in the preparation of the metallographic specimen, the laminations of the cementite are made to stand out slightly above the ferrite phase. After the specimen has been etched, the ridges of cementite cause the light from the microscope to be diffused and diffracted in such a manner

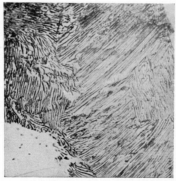

Fig. 32–2.   Microstructure of pearlite obtained with a slow cooling of carbon steel from above the critical temperature. ×100. (Greaves and Wrighton: *Practical Microscopical Metallurgy*, Chapman and Hall, Ltd.)

that the surface appears in the microscope to be pearl-like in texture. For this reason, the eutectoid structure is termed *pearlite*. The temperature at which the change to pearlite occurs is known as the *critical temperature*.

**Hypoeutectoid Steel.**     If a steel containing 0.4 per cent carbon and 99.6 per cent iron is allowed to cool slowly along the line *OPQRS*, the austenite is present as before until a *critical temperature* corresponding to *Q* (approximately 820° C.) is reached. The composition of the first precipitated phase can be found as described in Chapter 20 for the gold-silicon system (p. 328). If a line is drawn through *Q* parallel to the base line to intersect the solidus, the composition of this precipitated phase can be seen to be 0 per cent carbon and 100 per cent iron. In other words, ferrite is precipitated from the austenite which is analogous to the liquid phase of a eutectic system. As the temperature decreases, more ferrite is precipitated until finally the eutectoid composition remains, and pearlite finally precipitates.

A steel in which a mixture of free ferrite is found in a mixture with pearlite is known as a *hypoeutectoid steel*.

**Hypereutectoid Steel.**     If a steel containing carbon, 1.2 per cent, and iron, 98.8 per cent, is allowed to cool slowly along the line *UZVW*, the solid structure is austenite until the critical temperature corresponding to *Z* (approximately 950° C.) is reached, when cementite is precipitated from the austenite. As the temperature decreases, the cementite continues to precipitate until the eutectoid composition is reached, when pearlite is formed. A carbon steel with a metallographic structure consisting of a mixture of pearlite and cementite is known as a *hypereutectoid steel*.

Since the cementite is hard, it can be expected that the hypereutectoid steels are harder than the hypoeutectoid steels. The latter are more ductile, however.

**Heat Treatment.**     A slow cooling leaves the steel in the softest and most ductile condition possible for its composition. It should be noted that such a heat treatment produces the opposite effect in a gold alloy which can be age hardened.

If the steel is cooled instantaneously from above its critical point, the austenitic structure will be preserved. In practice, an instantaneous cooling is impossible, and, regardless of the rapidity of the cooling, some precipitation occurs. The phase precipitated upon rapid cooling is known as *martensite*. It is a very hard substance, possibly keyed with cementite. The Brinell hardness number of martensite may be 400 to 700, depending upon the amount of carbon present. The greater the amount of carbon in the steel, the harder the structure will be.

These two heat treatments are basic for the practical heat treatments for steel. There are three heat treatments of interest to the dentist.

1. *Annealing* consists of cooling the steel slowly from above its critical temperature as described.

2. *Hardening,* or *hardening heat treatment,* consists of quenching the steel in water or oil from above its critical temperature to produce a martensitic structure. The hardness is too great in most cases, and the structure is usually softened slightly before it is used.

3. *Tempering* is the relief of the hardening to an extent which is needed for the particular tool or structure. It is accomplished by raising the temperature of the hardened steel sufficiently to allow a desired amount of precipitation of ferrite, cementite or pearlite to occur, depending upon the type of steel.

In order to discuss these heat treatments in more detail, it will be assumed that it is desired to heat treat a dental carbon-steel enamel chisel. Although the process can be completed as will be described, the result will not be so satisfactory as the original heat treatment given by the manufacturer, since certain refinements will have been omitted.

**Annealing.**     The purpose of the annealing is to relieve all strains and to render the steel as ductile as possible for purposes of machining. Very likely, the chisel is a hypereutectoid steel with a carbon content of approximately 1.1 per cent. In order to anneal it, it should be cooled slowly from above 900° C. (1650° F.).

The chisel should not be heated too high above its critical temperature (900° C.) at any time. If grain growth is allowed to occur in the austenitic condition, its physical properties will be impaired. Although an accurate temperature control is highly desirable, as a makeshift the blade of the chisel can be heated in the reducing zone of a non-luminous gas-air flame to a yellowish-orange color. The color should be viewed in a shadow against a dark background. Once the proper temperature is attained for a few seconds, the chisel is immediately plunged into heated sand or a similar thermal non-conductor, and it is allowed to cool slowly to room temperature.

While the instrument is in this comparatively soft, malleable condition any necessary machining is accomplished. Nicks in the blade are filed out and the chisel is re-contoured to any desired shape.

**Hardening Heat Treatment.**     The blade and shank are again heated above the critical temperature as before, but this time the work is quenched, usually in water, and maintained in the quenching medium until it has thoroughly cooled.

The result of the quenching process depends considerably upon the quenching medium. Water is not so efficient in this respect as certain other mediums. When the orange-hot steel is immersed in the water, steam forms around the metal. Since the steam is a poor thermal conductor, the cooling rate is retarded. A medium with a higher boiling point would, therefore, be generally superior, since a harder steel would result.

*Table 32–1.*   *Temper Colors for Carbon Steel\**

| TEMPERATURE °C. | °F. | COLOR | PROPER TEMPER FOR: |
|---|---|---|---|
| 220–238 | 428–461 | Straw | Lancets, razors, surgical instruments, enamel chisels |
| 243 | 470 | Full yellow | Excavators, small cold chisels |
| 254 | 488 | Brown | Condensers (foil and amalgam), scissors, penknives |
| 265 | 509 | Brown with purple spots | Axes, hacksaws, cold chisels |
| 276 | 529 | Purple | Table knives, large shears |
| 287 | 549 | Bright blue | Swords, watch springs |
| 292 | 558 | Full blue | Fine saws, augers |
| 315 | 600 | Dark blue | Handsaws |

\* Hodgen, *Practical Dental Metallurgy*, 7th ed., C. V. Mosby Co.

**Tempering.**   As previously noted, the cutting edge of the enamel chisel is too hard and brittle after a hardening heat treatment to be of practical use. Any attempt at cutting with such a tool would result in a chipping or a fracturing of the edge. The blade of the chisel is toughened by allowing a controlled amount of the cementite to be precipitated by a tempering process.

The higher the temperature of the hardened steel is raised, the greater is the atomic diffusion, and, consequently, the greater the amount of the precipitation.

As the temperature of the steel is raised, an oxide coating will form on its surface, and the thickness of the coating as indicated by its color is an excellent indication of the degree of tempering for a carbon steel. Such colors are known as *temper colors*.

The tempering temperatures and temper colors used for various instruments and tools are presented in Table 32–1. As can be noted from the table, the first color to appear at the lowest temperature is a straw color. As the temperature rises, the oxide coating thickens, and a yellow color appears. At a higher temperature, the color changes to a brown, then to a purple, which is followed by a series of blues as the temperature progressively increases. As noted, each color indicates a certain amount of ferrite or cementite precipitated.

The proper temperatures can also be gauged by the use of a temperature indicator in a molten salt or low-fusing metal bath and a greater precision of control can be obtained than by observation of the temper colors. The sodium-potassium nitrate bath described on p. 418 can be used, for example.

Contrary to previous heat treatments, the tempering of the chisel should be carried out in a direct light of considerable intensity. The reducing zone of a Bunsen burner can be employed for heating.

In order to obtain more resilience in use, the shank of the tool is tempered to a bright blue color, whereas the blade should be a straw color as noted in Table 32–1. The instrument should be smooth and polished so that the colors can be observed readily.

The blade of the chisel should be grasped with a pair of smooth-nosed pliers so that the heat will be conducted away while the shank is being heated. The shank is held in the flame until a purple color is observed. It is then removed from the flame and the blade is released from the pliers. The residual heat will be conducted into the blade. The instant the blade exhibits a straw color, the instrument is quenched in water or oil and cooled thoroughly. Meanwhile, the shank will have turned to a bright blue color. If the operation has been properly accomplished, the blade can be sharpened to a keen edge, which should hold without dulling for a considerable time.

**Practical Considerations.** By this time, the student should realize the folly of heating a tempered cutting instrument for any purpose whatever. For example, heating a knife blade or any tempered instrument while cutting wax should never be done. The heating changes the temper of the steel so that the knife cannot maintain a cutting edge. The knife blade was originally tempered properly by the manufacturer, and any further heating will result in a softening.

The same observations hold for all types of steel tools used by the dentist. Wax carvers and similar instruments used with heat are made from some alloy which is not readily changed by heating. During sharpening procedures, or any other manipulation which is likely to heat the tool, care should be taken to avoid overheating. If necessary, such operations should be carried out under oil or water, or in an air stream, so that the heat evolved can be conducted away. When tools are handled properly and with respect, the dental operation can proceed with the minimum pain to the patient and time of the dentist.

**Modifying Elements.** Usually a carbon steel will contain one or more modifying elements to alter its properties in one way or another. For purposes of illustration, the modifying elements in a steel composition for dental tools will be discussed, according to the compositions given in Table 32–2.

*Table 32–2.* *Composition of Steels for Dental Instruments**

| MODIFIER | DENTAL INSTRUMENTS (%) | FORCEPS (%) |
|---|---|---|
| Carbon | 1.1–1.2 | 0.4–0.5 |
| Chromium | 0.2–0.3 | 0.4–0.5 |
| Manganese | 0.2–0.3 | 2.0–2.3 |
| Silicon | 0.4 | 0.1–0.2 |
| Molybdenum | | 0.5 |
| Iron | Balance | Balance |

* Cleveland Dental Manufacturing Co.

In the first place, it should be noted that the dental instruments, including cutting instruments, foil and amalgam condensers, etc., are made from a hypereutectoid steel, whereas the forceps, which should be less brittle in order to impart toughness, are of the hypoeutectoid type, or perhaps very close to a eutectoid type on the basis of certain considerations to be outlined.

Both types of steel contain a small amount of chromium. Chromium forms a solid solution in $\alpha$-iron in all proportions. One of the chief effects of the chromium is to increase the tarnish resistance by a process of passivation. This effect is not great in such small quantities, however. The chromium also tends to reduce the critical temperature of the steel, and to lower the carbon content of the eutectoid. It enhances the hardness, strength and elastic limit of the steel.

The manganese is added chiefly as a scavenger for oxides during the original melting process. Most steels contain a small amount of manganese. The manganese forms a solid solution with pure iron, although if carbon is present, it will form a carbide more easily than will iron. It is also a hardener of the steel. It tends to reduce the critical temperature.

The molybdenum is also a hardening agent, and it will form carbides as well. It aids in the prevention of grain growth in the austenite at high temperatures. It tends to reduce the critical temperature of the alloy.

The silicon is added as a scavenger agent and deoxidizer, along with the manganese.

Since all of the elements added, with the possible exception of silicon, tend to reduce the critical temperature and the amount of carbon in the eutectoid, in all probability the steel used for forceps is close to being a eutectoid steel rather than a hypoeutectoid steel. Also, since some of the modifying agents, particularly chromium, tend to inhibit the oxidation of the alloy, it follows that the temperatures at which the temper colors appear may be changed. The operator, therefore, should always know the composition of the steel and regulate the tempering processes accordingly.

## Literature

1. Smith, J. C.: *The Chemistry and Metallurgy of Dental Materials.* Oxford, Blackwell Scientific Publications, 1949, pp. 126–130.

CHAPTER 33

# Wrought Base Metal Alloys.

# Orthodontic Wires.

# Welding.

There are a number of wrought base metal alloys which are used in dentistry, mainly as wires for orthodontic treatment. As in the case of the carbon steels, the metallography of these alloys is extremely complex. Only applications of practical interest will be discussed. Chromium and nickel are present in most of the alloys such as the *80–20 nickel-chromium alloys*. In addition, the *stainless steels* contain carbon and iron.

## STAINLESS STEEL

**Chromium Steels.** As noted in the previous chapter, the addition of chromium to steel definitely lowers the carbon content of the eutectoid. In other words, point $E$ in Figure 32–1 is shifted to the left. If sufficient chromium is added, the structure upon slow cooling will be mainly cementite. In such a case, the austenite will be a solid solution of iron, carbon and chromium. The presence of the chromium renders the transformations from austenite during cooling somewhat sluggish.

The chief contribution of the chromium is to render the steel resistant to oxidation by virtue of the passivity of the chromium, and it is because of this contribution that the term "stainless steel" is applied.

In order for a steel to be "stainless," at least 12 per cent chromium must be present, with a carbon content of approximately 0.5 per cent.

Cutlery steels may contain more chromium than this. Stainless steel dental instruments are available which may contain as much as 17 per cent chromium.

The heat treatment of such steels is complex, and generally it should not be attempted by the dentist. The temperature for a hardening treatment is much higher than that of a carbon steel, and, as previously noted, the transformations on cooling are sluggish owing to the lack of atomic diffusion in the amount usually present in the carbon steels. Although a tempering heat treatment can be employed, it usually is not necessary, since the structure of the proper hardness may be obtained on rapid cooling.

***18–8 Stainless Steel.***    The numbers "18–8" refer to the chromium and nickel content of this type of steel. The chromium is present to the extent of approximately 18 per cent with 8 per cent nickel; the remainder of the composition is carbon (approximately 0.5 per cent or less), iron and possibly some modifying elements in minor amount. The 18–8 stainless steels are very resistant to corrosion. When the maximum passivity exists, these steels are between copper and silver in the electromotive series as regards their solution potential. The stainless steels can be drawn into wires which are used extensively in orthodontic appliances. Unless otherwise specified, in subsequent discussions the term "stainless steel" will refer to the 18–8 variety.

With 18 per cent chromium present, the eutectoid critical point $E$ exists at such a low carbon content that for all practical purposes only a cementitic structure is possible upon slow cooling. The nickel present contributes to corrosion resistance other than oxidation, and this variety of stainless steel is, therefore, highly resistant to corrosion.

If this type of stainless steel is cooled rapidly from a temperature of 1050 to 1100° C. (1920 to 2000° F.), a homogeneous austenitic structure persists at room temperature, owing to the lack of atomic diffusion. The austenite is a solid solution of chromium, nickel, and carbon in iron. This structure is relatively soft (B.H.N. 100 to 200). No hardening or tempering treatments are practical with this type of steel.

***Stabilized Stainless Steel.***    The 18–8 stainless steel may lose its resistance to corrosion if it is heated between 400 and 900° C. (750 and 1650° F.), the exact temperature depending upon its carbon content. Since such temperatures are definitely within the range used by the orthodontist in soldering and welding, this effect merits further discussion.

The reason for such a decrease in corrosion resistance is the precipitation of chromium carbide at the grain boundaries at the high temperatures. When the chromium combines with the carbide in this manner, its passivating qualities are lost, and, as a consequence, the corrosion resistance of the steel is reduced. Since the center of the grain is the portion generally "robbed" of chromium to produce the carbide, an intergranular corrosion occurs, and a partial distintegration of the metal may result with a general weakening of the structure.

There are several methods by which such a condition can be minimized. An obvious method from a theoretical standpoint would be to reduce the carbon content of the steel to an extent that such carbide precipitation cannot occur. However, such a remedy is not commercially possible because of the increased cost of manufacture.

If the stainless steel is severely cold worked, the carbides will precipitate along the slip planes. As a result, the distribution of the areas deficient in chromium will be less localized, or, in other words, the carbides will be more uniformly distributed so that the resistance to corrosion will be greater than when the grain boundaries only are involved. Such a method is presumably relied upon in orthodontic stainless steel wires.

The method employed most successfully is the introduction of some element which will precipitate as a carbide in preference to chromium. For example, titanium is often used for this purpose. If titanium is introduced, in amount approximately six times the carbon content, the precipitation of chromium carbide can be inhibited for a short time at the temperatures ordinarily encountered in soldering procedures. Stainless steels which have been treated in this manner are said to be *stabilized*. Unfortunately, very few, if any, of the stainless steel structures used in orthodontics are so stabilized.

**General Causes for Corrosion.** As previously noted, the function of the chromium is to prevent corrosion by oxidation. The situation as regards the prevention of electrolytic corrosion is somewhat analogous to that of dental amalgam discussed in Chapter 24.

Any surface inhomogeneity is a potential source of tarnish or corrosion. Severe strain hardening may produce localized electric couples in the presence of an electrolyte such as saliva. Any surface roughness or unevenness may allow corrosion cells to form. Not only should the stainless steel orthodontic appliance be polished for the comfort of the patient, but also so that it will keep cleaner and freer from tarnish or corrosion during use.

A common cause for the corrosion of a stainless steel is the incorporation of bits of carbon steel or similar metal in its surface. For example, if the stainless steel wire is manipulated carelessly with carbon steel pliers, it is conceivable that some of the steel from the pliers may become imbedded in the stainless steel. Or if the stainless steel appliance is abraded or cut with a carbon steel bur or similar steel tool, some of the steel from the tool may also become imbedded in the stainless steel. Such a situation results in an electric couple which may cause considerable corrosion.

**Mechanical Properties.** The general range of the mechanical properties of 18–8 stainless steel is presented[1] in Table 33–1. Regard-

*Table 33–1.* *Mechanical Properties of 18–8 Steel\**

| PROPERTY | UNITS | ANNEALED | COLD ROLLED |
|---|---|---|---|
| Yield strength | 100 Kg./Cm.$^2$ | 24–32 | 35–105 |
| | 1000 Lb./In.$^2$ | 34–45 | 50–150 |
| Tensile strength | 100 Kg./Cm.$^2$ | 56–63 | 70–125 |
| | 1000 Lb./In.$^2$ | 80–90 | 100–180 |
| Elongation | Per Cent | 60–55 | 50–10 |
| Brinell hardness number | | 135–185 | 190–330 |

\* Metals Handbook, 1948 edition.

less of their treatment, the stainless steels are definitely not as strong or hard as many of the carbon steels. An interesting feature of the data in Table 33–1 is the large increase in hardness and strength properties upon cold rolling in comparison to the annealed condition. For all practical purposes, the mechanical properties of the cold-rolled steel can be assumed to be identical with those of a "hard drawn" wire for orthodontic purposes.

The property of being readily strain hardened is a characteristic of stainless steel. Unfortunately, after strain hardening, a stainless steel wire can become fully annealed in a few seconds at a temperature of 700 to 800° C. (1292 to 1470° F.). After such an annealing, it has lost much of the stiffness or "springiness" so necessary to a satisfactory orthodontic appliance. Since the annealing temperatures involved are in the soldering and welding temperature ranges normally employed, such an unavoidable softening of the wire during normal heating operations is a decided disadvantage, unless the wire can be subsequently strain hardened.

Such a disadvantage can be minimized by the use of low-fusing solders, and by confining the time for soldering and welding procedures to a minimum. Any softening which occurs under such conditions of heating can be remedied to a considerable extent by the strain hardening incurred in subsequent operations such as contouring and polishing.

**Solders for Stainless Steel.** As previously noted, it is important that the stainless steel wire not be heated to too high a temperature, in order to minimize carbide precipitation, and to prevent an excessive softening of the wire so that its usefulness is lost. The requirement of a low temperature soldering technic generally rules out of consideration any of the gold solders normally employed with gold alloy wires, since their melting points are generally too high. Furthermore, the union between the stainless steel and a gold solder is not so strong as it is when a silver solder is used.[2] In order for a gold solder to be sufficiently low melting for the soldering of stainless steel, a fineness of approximately 250 (10-carat solder) is necessary. With such a low corrosion resistance, it makes little difference in this respect from a practical standpoint whether such a gold solder or a silver solder is used.

*Table 33–2.* Composition and Fusion Ranges of Silver Solders

| SOLDER NO. | SILVER (%) | COPPER (%) | CADMIUM (%) | ZINC (%) | NICKEL (%) | MELTING RANGE (°C.) | (°F.) |
|---|---|---|---|---|---|---|---|
| 1 * | 56 | 22 | — | 17 | — | 622–668 | 1152–1230 |
| 2 | 50 | 15.5 | 16 | 15.5 | 3 | 646–688 | 1195–1270 |
| 3 | 45 | 15 | 24 | 16 | — | 607–618 | 1125–1145 |
| 4 † | 67 | — | — | — | — | 724‡ | 1335‡ |
| 5 | 50 | 15.5 | 18 | 16.5 | — | 630–640 | 1160–1175 |
| 6 * | 56 | 22 | — | 17 | — | 630–650 | 1165–1200 |
| 7 § | 42 | 31 | 7 | 20 | — | — | — |

\* Contains tin, 5 per cent.
† Contains copper and indium, amounts not specified.
‡ Liquidus temperature.
§ Experimental solder by P. B. Taylor.

Although such solders definitely corrode in use since they are cathodic to the stainless steel, in orthodontic appliances such a condition is not too objectionable. The appliance is a temporary structure, not to be worn in the mouth for more than 6 to 12 months, and, since frequent inspections are necessary by the orthodontist, the appliances are regularly cleaned and polished.

The compositions of a number of commercial silver solders as supplied by the manufacturers are given in Table 33–2, along with their melting ranges. The solders are essentially alloys of copper and zinc to which silver is added to reduce the melting temperature and to increase the tarnish resistance. Phosphorus is sometimes added to aid in the elimination of oxidation during soldering.

The melting ranges of the solders are reasonably small. This is an important characteristic of the solder for free-hand soldering as normally practiced by the orthodontist. In free-hand soldering, the solder should harden promptly when the work is removed from the flame. Otherwise, the operator tires and unavoidably moves the work before the solder has completely solidified, and the joint is thus weakened.

**Fluxes.** In addition to the usual reducing and cleaning agents incorporated in a flux, a flux used for soldering stainless steel also contains a fluoride to dissolve the passivating film supplied by the chromium. The solder will not unite with the metal when such a film is present. Potassium fluoride is one of the most active chemicals in this respect.[3]

There are a number of commercial fluxes available for use in either powder or paste form. The following flux appears to operate reasonably well in practice:

| | | |
|---|---|---|
| Potassium fluoride | 50 per cent |
| Boric acid | 34 " " |
| Borax glass | 8 " " |
| Sodium carbonate or silica | 8 " " |

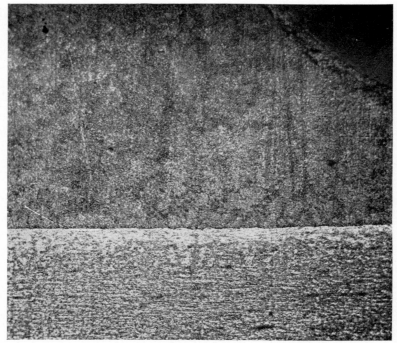

Fig. 33–1. Photomicrograph of a soldered joint between a stainless steel orthodontic wire and a silver solder. ×200.

The ingredients are fused together and then ground to a fine powder. The flux can be used dry or as a paste in alcohol or petrolatum.

The flux is somewhat similar to that recommended for gold soldering, with the exception of the addition of the potassium fluoride. The boric acid is used in a greater ratio to the borax than in the flux for gold soldering because it lowers the fusion temperature. Sodium carbonate can be used to replace the silica, and the fusion point of the flux will be reduced thereby. However, the silica can be used if the annealing temperature of the wire is not too low.

**Technical Considerations.** The free-hand soldering operation with stainless steel is not greatly different from that of gold soldering described in Chapter 31. The minimum time should be employed for the soldering of stainless steel. A needle-like, non-luminous, gas-air flame may be used. The thinner the diameter of the flame, the less the metal surrounding the joint will be annealed. The work should be held about 3 millimeters (1/8 inch) beyond the tip of the blue cone, in the reducing zone of the flame. The soldering should be observed in a shadow, against a black background, so that the temperature can be judged by the color of the work. The color should never exceed a dull red.

The solder should be applied first to the part with the heavier gauge. The flux is applied, and the work is placed in the flame. The instant the flux melts, a small bit of solder should be added, instead of waiting until its fusion temperature is reached. The solder will remain on the work, and time can be saved at the higher temperature. After the solder has flowed, the work should be quenched in water.

The other part is now fluxed, and the two pieces are held in apposition until the solder again flows between the pieces. The work is removed from the flame and held rigidly for approximately one second before it is again quenched.

**Metallography of the Soldered Joint.** A photomicrograph of the junction of a silver solder with a stainless steel wire used for orthodontic purposes is shown[4] in Figure 33–1. Solder No. 1 in Table 33–2 was employed. The photomicrographs seem to show that a superficial alloying occurs between the wire and the solder as described for the gold soldered joints. However, the point is controversial according to other evidence which supports the theory that the union is only mechanical in nature.[5] Evidence has also been presented that the fluoride salt in the flux may remain between the solder and the stainless steel after soldering and may initiate a corrosion of the joint during service.[6]

The tensile strengths of soldered joints made between stainless steel

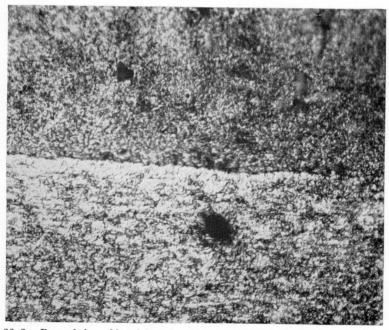

Fig. 33–2. Part of the soldered junction in Figure 33–1 under higher magnification. ×800.

*Table 33–3.*     *Tensile Strength of Stainless Steel Soldered Joints*

| SOLDER NO.* | ULTIMATE TENSILE STRENGTH | |
|---|---|---|
| | $(KG./CM.^2)$ | $(LB./IN.^2)$ |
| 1 | 6820 | 97,500 |
| 2 | 5470 | 78,200 |
| 3 | 5050 | 71,980 |
| 4 | 4950 | 70,060 |
| 7 | 6650 | 95,000 |

\* Composition given in Table 33–2.

wires with some of the silver solders, the compositions of which are presented in Table 33–2, are given in Table 33–3. The tensile strength of a silver solder is less than 4900 kilograms per square centimeter (70,000 pounds per square inch), and all of the values for tensile strength given in Table 33–3 are higher than the tensile strength of the particular solder employed. It can possibly be concluded from such observations that an atomic diffusion occurs from the wire to the solder during soldering, as well as from the solder to the wire. The situation is similar to that described for the gold soldered joints between gold alloy wires (p. 510).

## WELDING

Base metal orthodontic appliances are welded together more often than soldered. The basic fundamentals of welding are more complex than those related to soldering procedures and only a superficial discussion can be given here.

The welding process employed by the orthodontist is known as *resistance welding* or *spot welding*. The two pieces to be welded are held under pressure and an electric current is applied for a given period of time. The electrical resistance of the juncture of the two parts causes a rise in temperature and a localized fusion of the metal parts occurs. This process differs from other forms of welding in that no extraneous materials such as fluxes or brazing alloys are used. Inasmuch as the parts are under pressure during the welding, the process also differs from *fusion welding* in which no pressure is used. In some respects, resistance welding approaches mechanical forging in theory.

The following discussion is largely confined to the welding of stainless steel parts, orthodontic bands in particular, since more information is available in this connection than for other similar procedures. However, most of the discussion can undoubtedly be related to other types of orthodontic alloys and structures as well.

**Welding Unit.** A simplified circuit diagram of a resistance welder is shown in Figure 33–3. The alternating current is received from the service line as indicated at *S*, either 110 volts or 220 volts. A timing switch (*T.S.*) determines the length of time that the current is supplied to the primary (*P*) of the transformer. Since the current produces the desired heat for molding, a step down transformer is used to deliver a high current value with a low voltage. Usually, 250 to 750 amperes are used with a voltage of 2 to 6 volts.

The relation between the current and the heat generated is expressed by the familiar formula:

$$E = 0.24 \ I^2Rt \tag{1}$$

where

    E = electrical energy expressed in calories.

  0.24 = constant of equivalence between electrical and heat energy.

    I = current in amperes.

    R = resistance of the circuit in ohms.

    t = time or duration of the current.

As can be noted from the formula, the heat generated is proportional to the *square* of the current.

The resistance of the joint is, of course, fixed according to the work to be welded. This factor cannot be controlled by means of the welding unit. However, the length of time can be, and is, controlled by the welding unit. Since the length of time the current is applied is directly proportional to the heat generated, its accurate regulation is also of extreme importance. The welding time may vary from 1/25 to 1/50 second.

Another function of the welding unit is to hold the work under the proper contact and pressure. This factor is controlled by the electrodes shown at *E* in Figure 33–3.

In brief, a properly welded joint is effected by heating the parts under pressure to the temperature at which a *localized melting* occurs at the point of juncture so that the parts are fused. Ideally, the melting is confined to the junction area and can be observed metallographically in cross section as a *nugget* of resolidified cast structure, which is elliptical in shape with a characteristically uniform symmetry (Figure 33–4). The grain structure of the wire surrounding the nugget should not be affected. All of the variables, particularly the current, should be controlled accurately to prevent overmelting and burning or undermelting, either of which will produce an unsatisfactory weld.

In practice, a circuit of much greater complexity than that shown in Figure 33–3 is required. One type of an electric welder suitable for

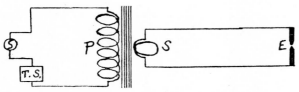

Fig. 33–3. Circuit diagram for a resistance welder.

Fig. 33–4.

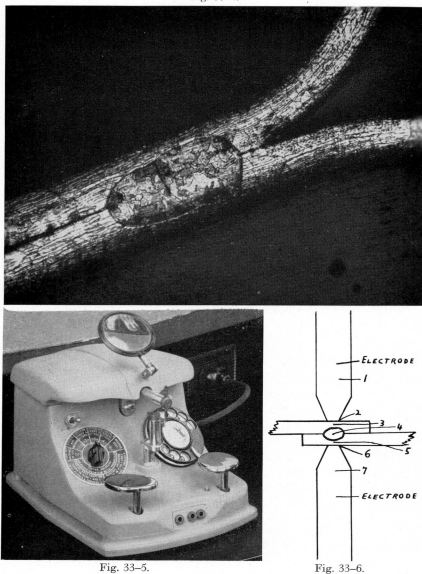

Fig. 33–5.                                        Fig. 33–6.

Fig. 33–4.   Metallographic structure of a welded joint. ×90.

Fig. 33–5.   A resistance welder for use in the fabrication of an orthodontic appliance.

Fig. 33–6.   Position for welding a lap joint. Electrodes, (1) and (7); contact of electrodes with work, (2) and (6); upper sheet (3) in lap contact with lower sheet (5); interface and position of nugget after welding (4).

orthodontic purposes is shown in Figure 33–5. The electrodes can be seen in the center of the figure. They can be adjusted as to position and pressure by various levers, two of which can be seen in the foreground toward the front of the unit. The left dial determines the heat or current employed by changing the number turns of the primary circuit. The current can be supplied in one impulse or a number of successive pulsations which provide welding and cooling impulses. The number of pulsations is controlled by the telephone dial at the right.

**Preparation of the Joint.** As in soldering procedures, the parts to be welded must be clean and free from surface oxides for a properly welded joint to be obtained. Blood, dried saliva or oxides increase the electrical resistance of the circuit and cause the wrong part of the joint to become heated.

In order to simplify the discussion, the welding of two flat surfaces such as an orthodontic band in a lap joint will be described.

The proper position for the parts to be welded between the electrodes is shown[7] in Figure 33–6. The lap between the parts should provide enough area for the application of the copper electrodes (1 and 7), but should be short enough that the ends beyond the weld will not be so long as to be a hindrance in subsequent operations.

The parts should be in complete apposition at their common point of contact, as well as at their points of contact with the electrodes. The pressure of the electrodes should be sufficient to prevent movement during the application of the current.

**Electrical Resistance.** It is evident from Ohm's law that the current will be the same throughout the secondary circuit. In the secondary circuit of the wiring diagram in Figure 33–3, the current will be determined not only by the ratio of the coils in the primary of the transformer to those in the secondary, but also by the resistance of the secondary circuit.

According to formula (1) above, the heat generated in any part of the circuit will depend upon the electrical resistance of that portion of the circuit. Referring again to the secondary circuit shown in Figure 33–3, it follows that if the electrical resistance of the entire circuit can be kept low in comparison to the resistance of the parts to be welded between the electrodes $E$, the heat generated at $E$ may be sufficient to effect a weld with a minimum of heat in the remaining part of the circuit. Any heat generated in parts of the circuit other than $E$ will be wasted energy.

In practice, the resistance of the circuit outside the weld area is reduced by using large diameter copper conductors and electrodes throughout and by keeping the length of the conductors as short as possible.

Since all of the resistances in the circuit are in series, their sum determines the total resistance. On this basis, the resistance of the metallic junction at the interface (4) in Figure 33–6 should be greater than any other part of the circuit to provide a weld.

The resistance of the electrodes (1) and (7) can be neglected. The electrodes are usually constructed of copper wire or rod of as large a diameter as is practical.

The first resistance to be encountered is the junction of the electrodes with the work at (2) and (6). The resistance at these points should be minimized as much as possible. It should be noted that the electrodes taper to the area desired for the weld. Whatever the area of contact, it should be complete over the entire surface contacted to prevent arcing.

The area of contact affects the resistance. The smaller the area of contact, the greater the resistance and *vice versa*. Consequently, the smaller the area of contact, the greater will be the amount of heat generated in the weld. On the other hand, the smaller the area of contact, the weaker the weld will be within certain practical limits.[7] Also, if the area is too small, the metal may be over-fused or burned. Consequently, with a considerable reduction in contact area, the current must be reduced as well, and, therefore, nothing is gained.

The area of contact is determined not only by the area of the electrode point, but also by the pressure of the electrodes. The greater the pressure of the electrodes, the greater will be the area of contact by the electrodes and also between the work at (4) as well, and the less will be the heat generated. On the other hand, insufficient pressure may result in a poor weld since the resistance at (2) and (6) may be increased to the extent that the welds may occur between the work and the electrodes instead of at the desired interface (4).

With the proper control of the other factors, the greatest pressure should occur at the point of welding (4). The copper electrodes are softer than the work pieces and under pressure the electrodes fill in all the minute irregularities on the surface of the steel. Consequently, the area of contact is greater at (2) and (6) than at the interface (4). It is for this reason that the nugget forms only at (4) under the proper conditions.

**Current and Time.** As previously noted, the magnitude of the current is of prime consideration, with the control of its period of application almost equal in importance. Too high a current or too long a time of application will produce too much heat and the work will be burned or over-fused, and a condition of grain growth in the surrounding area will result. With too low a current, either no weld or a defective weld will occur.

**Arcing.** It is a well-known fact that if an electric potential between two areas becomes too great, the current will arc, *i.e.*, an electrical discharge will occur through the air between the two areas. The temperature of the arc is extremely high, and a fusion or burning of the metal at the arc contacts generally occurs, with a grain recrystallization and growth around the fused area. Consequently, arcing should be avoided under all circumstances.

As previously noted, arcing may occur when the electrodes or the parts are not in intimate contact during welding. As might be expected, the shorter the distance between the gaps of the parts involved, the greater is the tendency for an arc to form. Consequently, *complete* contact is essential.

It follows, therefore, that the contour of the electrode tip should conform to that of the work. Various shapes and sizes of electrode tips are generally supplied for this reason.

This problem becomes particularly critical when two circular wires are to be welded. One wire may be of a different gauge than the other and possibly they are to be welded at right angles. Assuming that the electrodes can be fitted to the contour of the wires, the junction area between the crossed wires will be only slightly greater than a point with no dimensions. The surface of each wire will curve gradually from that of the other, providing an almost infinitely small space between the wires near their point of contact. As a result, a certain degree of arcing cannot be avoided during the welding unless a precise control of the variables is employed. This situation is one of the reasons why the welding of curved orthodontic structures is apt to be less successful than the welding of plane surfaces where intimate contact is not a problem.

**Metallographic Structure.** The metallographic structure of a welded joint is presented in Figure 33–4. A lap joint of two stainless steel orthodontic bands was welded.[7] The nugget is characterized by the equiaxed grain structure in contrast to the plate metal structure.

Ideally, when the nugget forms and solidifies, the heat should be dissipated immediately into the surrounding metal and electrodes. Actually, such a condition does not occur, and a recrystallization of the surrounding metal occurs. The beginning of such a recrystallization is evident in the metal surrounding the nugget even in the properly welded union shown in Figure 33–4. If too much current had been used, complete grain growth and an oxide inclusion would be evident.

**Strength.** The strength of the welded joint is more directly related to the metallographic structure around the nugget than to the nugget itself. Welded orthodontic joints seldom fracture through the nugget itself.[7]

As might be expected, the greater the weld area, the greater is the strength, other conditions being equal.[7]

**Corrosion.** Welded stainless steel joints generally corrode in the mouth. As previously noted, orthodontic stainless steel structures are seldom stabilized against carbide precipitation. Since the welding temperatures occur in the region of rapid precipitation of chromium car-

*Table 33–4.* *Mechanical Properties of Nickel-Chromium (80–20) Alloy Wires**

| PROPERTY | UNITS | ANNEALED | HARD | "EXTRA SPRING" |
|---|---|---|---|---|
| Tensile strength | Kg./Cm.$^2$ | 6,650 | 11,540 | 14,000 |
|  | Lb./In.$^2$ | 95,000 | 165,000 | 200,000 |
| Modulus of elasticity | Kg./Cm.$^2$ | 2,170,000 | — | — |
|  | Lb./In.$^2$ | 31,000,000 | — | — |
| Elongation | Per cent | 25–35 | 0–1 | 0 |
| B.H.N. |  | 142–157 | 201–225 |  |

* Metals Handbook, 1948 edition.

bide, precipitation of such carbides and less passivity can be expected under the best of conditions. Obviously, the higher and more prolonged the welding temperatures, the greater will be the carbide precipitation.

Even though there was no carbide precipitation, a tendency to tarnish and corrode would be present because of the differences in grain structure brought about by the welding. However, this factor is negligible compared to carbide precipitation.

### WROUGHT NICKEL-CHROMIUM ALLOYS

Another type of base metal wire which has become very popular with the orthodontists for the construction of arch wires and similar appliances is the nickel-chromium alloy composed of nickel, 80 per cent, and chromium, 20 per cent. These wires are part of a general classification of heating element wires, used for heating elements in toasters, wax elimination furnaces and similar electrical heating devices.

One of the reasons for the popularity of these wires in orthodontics is their high resistance to corrosion and tarnish. Their chromium content results in a passivation which enables the wire to resist oxidation, and the presence of the nickel minimizes any electrolytic corrosion. In an orthodontic appliance which is cleaned and polished periodically, the wires remain bright and free from corrosion.

**Mechanical Properties.** The general range of mechanical properties of the alloys under discussion is given[8] in Table 33–4. The only heat treatment for these wires is an annealing treatment between 870° C. (1600° F.) and 1040° C. (1900° F.). Any increase in hardness and strength is obtained by strain hardening as with the stainless steels.

It is interesting to note (Table 33–5) that, after annealing, the strength of the nickel-base wire is approximately the same as that of 18–8 stainless steel after strain hardening (*cf.* Table 33–1). It is this property of not softening markedly during soldering and similar heat treatments which also has contributed to the popularity of these wires. The recrystallization temperature of the wires is quite high, and since their melting temperature is approximately 1400° C. (2550° F.), any

*Table 33–5.*     *Tensile Strength of Nickel-Chromium (80–20) Alloy*
*Wires as Used by the Orthodontist*

| ALLOY NO. | ULTIMATE TENSILE STRENGTH | | | |
| | AS RECEIVED | | "SOFTENED" * | |
| | (KG./CM.$^2$) | (LB./IN.$^2$) | (KG./CM.$^2$) | (LB./IN.$^2$) |
|---|---|---|---|---|
| 1 | 15,400 | 220,600 | 10,200 | 145,400 |
| 2 | 13,000 | 186,200 | 8,950 | 127,500 |
| 3 | 10,400 | 148,000 | 6,800 | 97,100 |
| 4† | 13,100 | 187,100 | 8,850 | 126,400 |
| 5 | 9,120 | 130,200 | 8,850 | 126,400 |
| 6 | 15,700 | 225,200 | 8,390 | 119,900 |
| 7 | 11,500 | 164,100 | 10,000 | 142,900 |

\* Heated at 700° C. (1292° F.) for 10 minutes and quenched in water.
† Specially marketed for orthodontic use.

danger from any reasonable amount of overheating is minimized considerably.

The tensile strengths of seven commercial wires of the 80–20 composition are presented[9] in Table 33–5, as they were received from the manufacturer, and after they were given a "softening heat treatment" as prescribed for dental gold alloy wires (p. 507). Assuming that the soldering temperature is the same for these wires as for the 18–8 stainless steel wires, heating at 700° C. (1292° F.) for 10 minutes should represent an excessive amount of heating during normal soldering operations.

According to the results presented in Table 33–5, none of the wires was appreciably affected by the heat treatment so far as their "activation" as an orthodontic spring might be concerned. The different wires present different strengths "as received," probably because of differences in manufacture. Alloy No. 4 is of special interest in that it is supplied to the orthodontist "hard drawn" in one-foot lengths. After the "softening heat treatment," its strength was the same as wire No. 5. In fact, two wires were found to be identical,[9] except that wire No. 5 was dispensed on a spool and wire No. 4 was supplied straightened at a much higher cost.

**Soldering.**     Because of the passive surface of the 80–20 nickel-chromium wires, the problems in soldering are essentially the same as those outlined for the soldering of stainless steel wires. However, with the 80–20 nickel-chromium wires, a higher soldering temperature can be used.

Although the soldering procedures described for 18–8 stainless steel wires with silver solder are much easier to perform, gold solders can be used with the nickel-chrome wires. Whatever the type of solder, a borax fluoride flux must be employed. The strengths of soldered joints made with 450-fine and 282-fine solders using five commercial 80–20 nickel-chromium wires are presented[10] in Table 33–6.

*Table 33–6.* *Tensile Strength of Soldered Joints in Nickel-Chromium (80–20) Alloy Wires, Using Gold Solder*

| | ULTIMATE TENSILE STRENGTH | | | |
|---|---|---|---|---|
| WIRE NO. | GOLD SOLDER, 450 FINE | | GOLD SOLDER, 282 FINE | |
| | (KG./CM.²) | (LB./IN.²) | (KG./CM.²) | (LB./IN.²) |
| A | 5350 | 76,600 | 4930 | 70,400 |
| B | 4210 | 60,300 | 4050 | 57,800 |
| C | 5700 | 81,400 | 3680 | 52,500 |
| D | 4300 | 61,500 | 3790 | 54,100 |
| E | 4420 | 63,300 | 3430 | 49,000 |

It is interesting to note that the strength of the joint made with wires *A* and *B* did not vary greatly with the fineness of the solder employed. In all other cases, stronger joints were obtained with the 450-fine solder, possibly because of the greater atomic diffusion at the higher soldering temperature. Wire *C* is identical with wire 5 in Table 33–5. All of the soldered joints were stronger than the solders themselves.

The wires can be welded together in the same manner as the stainless steel wires.

### WROUGHT COBALT-CHROMIUM ALLOYS

Cobalt-chromium alloys drawn into wire form can be used successfully in orthodontic appliances. These alloys were originally developed for use as watch springs,[11] but their properties are also excellent for orthodontic purposes.

The wires are furnished to the orthodontist in a number of different shapes with differing physical properties as well. Their resistance to corrosion and tarnish in the mouth is excellent. Furthermore, they can be subjected to the same welding and soldering procedures as described for the other orthodontic base metal wires.

**Composition.** The alloys contain cobalt, chromium, nickel, beryllium, iron, molybdenum, manganese and carbon.

The cobalt is present in amount from 28 to 45 per cent.[11] It is the chief strengthener in the alloy and aids in the age hardening heat treatment.

As might be expected, the chief contribution of the chromium is to passivate the alloy to provide resistance to tarnish and corrosion. The preferred range is 20 to 26 per cent.[11]

Nickel is present in amounts from 15 to 30 per cent. Nickel and iron are supplementary to each other, although more nickel is usually employed than iron. Preferably the iron content is kept below 15 per cent.[11] These metals improve the quality of the alloy during rolling and drawing.

Although the beryllium content is limited to 0.02 to 0.09 per cent, depending upon the carbon content, it is an important constituent so far as strength properties are concerned, particularly after an age hardening treatment.

Molybdenum is also a strengthener of the alloy when it is present in an amount of 6 to 7 per cent.

Manganese is added in an amount of about 0.5 to 2 per cent and probably acts as a scavenger for oxides during fusion and also improves the properties of the alloy during its fabrication into wires and sheets.

The carbon content should be kept low in order not to reduce the ductility of the alloy. The usable range is about 0.05 to 0.30 per cent.[11] As in the case of steel, it acts to harden and strengthen the alloy.

**Heat Treatment.**     The solution heat treatment of the alloy consists in heating to temperatures of 1100° C. (2000° F.) to 1200° C. (2200° F.) and then quenching rapidly.

The fabricated structure can then be age hardened at temperatures between 260° C. (500° F.) and 650° C. (1200° F.). The usual age hardening treatment is to heat the alloy at 480° C. (900° F.) for five hours.[11]

Neither of these heat treatments is usually employed by the orthodontist; rather the structures are pre-heat treated by the manufacturer, if necessary.

**Physical Properties.**     As previously noted, the tarnish and corrosion resistance of the alloy is excellent.

After a solution heat treatment, the Brinell hardness number is in the neighborhood of 250 with an ultimate tensile strength of approximately 8750 kilograms per square centimeter (125,000 pounds per square inch).[11] The properties are increased considerably by cold working. For example, the average value of the proportional limit may be as high as 10,000 kilograms per square centimeter (145,000 pounds per square inch), with a modulus of elasticity of 1,700,000 kilograms per square centimeter (24,00,000 pounds per square inch) and a tensile strength of approximately 18,000 kilograms per square centimeter (260,000 pounds per square inch).

These properties may be further increased by as much as 50 per cent by subjecting the cold worked structure to a solution heat treatment followed by an age hardening treatment as previously described.[11] However, since the latter heat treatment reduces the ductility, in all probability the wires are supplied to the dentist mainly in a cold worked condition.

## LOW TEMPERATURE HEAT TREATMENT

A certain increase in the elastic properties of an orthodontic wire can be effected by heating it to comparatively low temperatures after it has been cold worked by bending during the fabrication of an appliance.[12-16] The temperatures involved are in the neighborhood of 370° C. (700° F.) to 480° C. (900° F.). The proportional limit, modulus of elasticity and modulus of resilience are increased,[15, 16] but the ductility is reduced.[14]

The amount of the increase appears to depend upon the degree of strain hardening before the heat treatment. For example, no effect was found when an 18–8 stainless steel wire as received was heat treated in comparison to an untreated specimen. Yet when eight V-shaped bends were placed in the wire, a decided increase in the modulus of elasticity was noted after the structure was heat treated at 454° C. (850° F.) for three minutes.[13]

When closing loops were used in an 18–8 stainless steel wire,[12, 14] an improvement of as high as 39 per cent in elastic properties was reported[14] after the bent wire was heat treated at 480° C. (900° F.) for three minutes. On the other hand, when a similar wire with a circular loop was treated in the same manner, the effect was found to be negligible so far as its clinical importance was concerned.[15, 16]

The 80–20 nickel-chromium wires and the cobalt-chromium wires appear to respond to this type of heat treatment much better than do the 18–8 stainless steel wires,[14–16] with a definite increase in all elastic properties. For example, when a cobalt-chromium wire was held at 480° C. (900° F.) for 3 minutes, its resistance to permanent deformation was increased 55 to 66 per cent in comparison to its condition before heat treatment. The ductility, however, was reduced 60 to 77 per cent. No change in ductility occurred when the 18–8 stainless steel closed loop was heat treated.[14]

It was noted by two investigators that the duration of the heat treatment was not a factor up to 15 minutes.[15, 16]

As in the case of the 18–8 stainless steel wires, the increase in the elastic properties of the 80–20 nickel-chromium wires and the cobalt-chromium wires effected by heat treatment varied with the amount of strain hardening. In other words, the increase appeared to be greater with the closed loops than when a circular loop was employed. Such an observation appears to indicate that the phenomenon may be related to a partial stress relief rather than to a precipitation hardening of some nature.

Other evidence to support such a theory of a partial stress relief as being the controlling factor is that the 18–8 stainless steel bent wire structures changed form during the heat treatment, thus indicating a relaxation.[15, 16] Such a change in form is, of course, disadvantageous so far as maintaining the proper relations between the parts of the orthodontic appliance is concerned. However, no change in form was observed with the 80–20 nickel-chromium wire.[15]

In summary, probably the best method for heat treatment is to heat the wire to 480° C. (900° F.) for three minutes and then to cool it in the air. Although temperatures higher than 480° C. for a shorter time do not harm the 80–20 nickel-chromium wires or the cobalt-chromium wires, the higher temperatures will cause a definite decrease in the elastic properties of the 18–8 stainless steel wires.

The heat treatment can be accomplished in an electric furnace or by means of an electric current. The latter method is very convenient, particularly with the 80–20 nickel-chromium wires and the cobalt-chromium wires, both of which are high in electrical resistance. Some of the orthodontic welding units are provided with attachments specifically for this purpose.

## *Literature*

1. Parmitter, O. K.: *Wrought Stainless Steels,* Metals Handbook, 1948 edition. Cleveland, American Society for Metals, 1948, pp. 553–556.
2. Vosmik, C. J. and Taylor, P. B.: *Some Facts and Observations Related to the Soldering of Chrome Alloys.* Int. J. Ortho. and Oral. Surg., *22:*705–715 (July), 1936.
3. Subcommittee on Brazing: *Brazing, Silver Brazing, Copper-Hydrogen Brazing and Related Joining Methods,* Metals Handbook, 1948 edition. Cleveland, American Society for Metals, 1948, pp. 78–81.
4. Henns, R. J.: *A Metallographic Study of the Bond between Stainless Steel and Silver Solder.* Thesis, Northwestern University Dental School, 1951.
5. Ayers, H. D. and Bien, S. M.: *Comparison of Solder Joints in Precious Metal Alloys and Rustless Metal Alloys.* I.A.D.R., *34:*90, 1956. Abstract.
6. Bien, S. M. and Ayers, H. D.: *Autoradiographs of Solder Joints with Fluorine[18].* J. D. Res., *38:*428–435 (May-June), 1959.
7. Vassar, R. J.: *A Metallographic Study of the Welded Bond between Two Pieces of Stainless Steel Band Material.* Thesis, Northwestern University Dental School, 1957.
8. Gatward, W. A.: *80 Ni–20 Cr,* Metals Handbook, 1948 edition. Cleveland, American Society for Metals, 1948, p. 1060.
9. Cleek, L. D.: *Physical Properties of Heating Element Wires with a View to Their Use in Orthodontic Appliances.* Thesis, Northwestern University Dental School, 1941.
10. Duncan, C. R.: *Physical Properties of Soldered Joints in Resistance Wires.* Thesis, Northwestern University Dental School, 1946.
11. Harder, O. E. and Roberts, D. A.: *Alloys Having High Elastic Strengths.* U.S. Patent 2,524,661, Oct. 3, 1950.
12. Backofen, W. A. and Gales, G. F.: *Heat Treating Stainless Steel for Orthodontics.* Am. J. Orthodont., *38:*755–765 (Oct.), 1952.
13. Funk, A. G.: *The Heat Treatment of Stainless Steel.* Angle Orthodont., *21:*129–138 (July), 1951.
14. Denver, P. I.: *Heat Treatment of Orthodontic Steel Wire.* Thesis, Indiana University School of Dentistry, 1958.
15. Kemler, E. A.: *A Study of the Effect of Low Temperature Heat Treatment on the Physical Properties of Orthodontic Wire.* Thesis, Northwestern University Dental School, 1955.
16. Mutchler, R. W.: *The Effect of Heat Treatment on the Mechanical Properties of Orthodontic Cobalt-Chromium Steel Wire as Compared with Chromium-Nickel Steel Wire.* Thesis, Northwestern University Dental School, 1959.

CHAPTER 34

# Cobalt-Chromium Alloys

# for Dental Castings

Cobalt-chromium alloys are used for casting dental appliances such as metallic denture bases, complex partial denture structures and certain types of bridgework. The question whether the use of such alloys is more advantageous than the use of gold alloys for the same purpose is definitely controversial. Certainly, the cobalt-chrome alloys are lighter in weight, and they are as corrosion resistant as the gold alloys because of the passivating effect of the chromium.

A disadvantage of this type of alloy is its technical complexity in the production of dental appliances. The high fusing temperature of the alloys precludes the use of the usual gas-air flame for casting. Its extreme hardness requires the use of a sandblasting unit for cleaning and smoothing the work after casting. These and similar procedures not generally adaptable to a laboratory in a dental office have generally limited the technical production of such castings to the commercial dental laboratory. Consequently, only those factors will be discussed in detail which are of importance to the dentist in evaluating and directing the work of the technician.

It is a matter of interest that one of these alloys, originally developed for dental use, is now used extensively in bone surgery and in the construction of intricate parts of airplane engines for jet propulsion. Not only do these alloys exhibit high strength, hardness and resistance to tarnish and corrosion at room temperature, but also at high temperatures the alloys are stable and inert. These alloys are classified metallurgically as *stellite*.

**Composition.** The compositions of 14 cobalt-chromium alloys are presented in Table 34–1. The first six compositions designated by letters represent the compositions employed in typical American alloys;[1] the next five are the compositions of alloys employed in England and Europe.[2] The last five alloys are designated by "stellite numbers,"[3] and are industrial alloys.

These latter alloys were developed mainly during World War II for industrial use.[4] It is interesting to note that stellite No. 21 is the industrial version of the dental alloy *D*. Although all of these alloys

*Table 34–1.*   *Composition of Typical Cobalt-Chromium Alloys*

| ALLOY NO.* | CHROMIUM (%) | COBALT (%) | NICKEL (%) | MOLYB-DENUM (%) | TUNG-STEN (%) | MAN-GANESE (%) | SILICON (%) | IRON (%) | CARBON (%) |
|---|---|---|---|---|---|---|---|---|---|
| A† | 21.6 | 43.5 | 20.1 | 7.0 | — | 3.0 | 0.35 | 0.25 | 0.05 |
| B | 30.3 | 59.4 | 1.5 | 5.8 | 0.35 | 0.34 | 0.55 | 0.7 | ** |
| C | 22.3 | 29.7 | 0.7 | 3.3 | — | 0.9 | 1.7 | 40.0 | ** |
| D†* | 26.2 | 62.6 | 2.3 | 5.0 | 1.2 | 0.16 | 0.55 | 1.0 | 0.25 |
| E | 27.6 | 51.6 | 2.3 | 5.3 | — | 0.8 | †† | 1.6 | †† |
| F*** | 35.0 | 65.0 | — | 4.0 | — | — | — | — | — |
| I | 26.0 | 66.0 | — | 6.1 | — | — | 0.4 | 1.6 | 0.2–0.4 |
| II | 24.0 | 66.0 | — | 5.1 | — | — | 0.6 | 4.0 | 0.2–0.4 |
| III | 27.3 | 66.7 | — | — | 5.0 | 0.4 | 0.2 | 0.05 | 0.2–0.4 |
| IV | 26.0 | 66.0 | — | 5.6 | — | — | 1.0 | 1.6 | 0.2–0.4 |
| V | 26.0 | 65.0 | — | 8.0 | — | — | 0.1 | 0.8 | 0.2–0.4 |
| 21 | 27.0 | 62.6 | 2.0 | 6.0 | — | 0.6 | 0.6 | 1.0 | 0.2 |
| 23 | 23.0 | 67.4 | 2.0 | — | 5.0 | 0.6 | 0.6 | 1.0 | 0.4 |
| 27 | 23.0 | 36.4 | 32.0 | 6.0 | — | 0.6 | 0.6 | 1.0 | 0.4 |
| 30 | 23.0 | 52.4 | 16.0 | 6.0 | — | 0.6 | 0.6 | 1.0 | 0.4 |
| 31 | 23.0 | 57.6 | 10.0 | — | 7.0 | 0.6 | 0.6 | 1.0 | 0.4 |

* Lettered designations, Taylor, Leibfritz, and Adler, *J.A.D.A.*, March, 1958; Roman numeral designations, Earnshaw, R., Thesis, University of Manchester (Eng.); Arabic numeral designations, Metals Handbook, 1948 edition.

† Contains copper 3.5%, beryllium 0.9%.

** Not determined.

†* Contains copper 0.20%.

†† Silicon, carbon, aluminum content, 1.0%.

*** Unspecified content, 1.0%.

probably could be used for dental casting, so far as is known, they are not used at the present time. They are included only for purposes of comparison and study.

**Contributions of Alloy Constituents.**    The constitution of these alloys is essentially a solid solution of about 70 per cent cobalt and 30 per cent chromium. Any considerable departure from this ratio without the substitution of comparable metals generally results in lowered mechanical properties and decreased tarnish resistance.[5]

The chief contribution of the chromium is to insure that the alloy will resist tarnish and corrosion by virtue of its passivating effect.

The cobalt contributes strength, rigidity and hardness, particularly at elevated temperatures. As indicated particularly in the case of alloys A and 27 in Table 34–1, the cobalt can be replaced with nickel. It is interesting to note that none of the European alloys contain nickel.

As noted in connection with the wrought cobalt-chromium alloys in the previous chapter, the nickel and iron supplement each other in improving the ability of the alloy to be cold worked, with the nickel generally being in greater amount than the iron. As can be noted from Table 34–1, most of the alloys contain iron, generally in small amount.

Again as noted in the previous chapter, the molybdenum, tungsten, manganese and silicon are all hardeners and are generally used sparingly in these alloys. The molybdenum is the best hardener and strengthener of the four metals and it is generally credited with the production of a smaller grain size. Tungsten can be substituted for molybdenum with a slight reduction in strength.

Although manganese and silicon act to a slight degree as strengtheners, their chief function is to act as deoxidizers or "scavengers" while the metal is being cast. However, their content is usually kept less than 1 per cent because they tend to make the alloy brittle.

The function of the beryllium in alloy A (Table 34–1) is possibly to reduce the fusion temperature of the alloy as indicated in Table 34–2, although it might aid in strengthening the alloy and the refinement of grain structure[6] as well.

*Table 34–2.*    *Liquidus Temperatures of Cobalt-Chromium Alloys*\*

| ALLOY | LIQUIDUS TEMPERATURE | |
|:-----:|:----:|:----:|
| NO.† | °C. | °F. |
| A | 1290 | 2355 |
| B | 1480 | 2605 |
| D | 1415 | 2575 |
| E | 1450 | 2650 |
| F | 1400 | 2560 |

\* Taylor, Leibfritz and Adler, *J.A.D.A.*, March, 1958.
† Composition given in Table 34–1.

Of all the constituents, the carbon content is the most critical. Small variations may have a pronounced effect on the strength, hardness and ductility of the alloy. Carbon can form carbides with any of the metallic constituents, and, as has been noted in connection with other similar alloys, such formations can alter the physical properties quite markedly. Such carbides appear to form spontaneously as finely dispersed globules, since the solubility of the carbon in the cobalt-chromium solid solution is very limited.[5]

The control of the carbon content is difficult during both the manufacture and casting procedures. Particularly when a flame is used, carbon is likely to be incorporated during casting. Complete control of the applied heat is extremely important at this stage.

By virtue of the carbide precipitations, the carbon content affects both the strength and the ductility of the metal.

**Metallography.** A typical metallographic structure[5] of a cobalt-chromium dental alloy is shown in Figure 34–1. The matrix is the solid solution of cobalt and chromium, whereas the core is formed of islands of the metallic carbides as previously discussed. The pattern of the carbide formation is influenced by the dendritic crystallization, since the carbide phases solidify at the grain boundaries of the dendrites. Such a structure introduces increased slip interference at the grain boundaries and thus increases the strength and hardness properties but it reduces the ductility.[5] Although the increase in carbon content generally results in a more brittle alloy, the distribution and surface contour of the carbide islands as shown in Figure 34–1 are also important in their effect on the mechanical properties.

It should be evident from Figure 34–1 that the arrangement of the islands as shown, regularly and fairly widely spaced, would allow more slip with greater ductility as a consequence, than if the islands

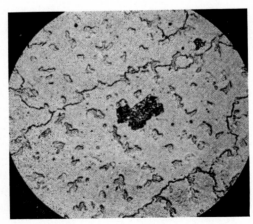

Fig. 34–1. Photomicrograph of a dental cobalt-chromium alloy as cast. ×150 (Earnshaw, *Brit. D.J.*, Aug. 7, 1956.)

were more irregular both in form or spacing. As the carbon content is increased, the islands become larger and more irregular until the structure becomes continuous. At this stage, the alloy will likely be too brittle for dental use.

As with any metal, the more slowly the alloy cools during solidification, the larger will be the grain size. The dental castings made with stellite alloys are likely to have a coarse grain size because of the very hot molds employed. It has been shown that the grain size of such castings increases as either the mold temperature or the alloy casting temperature is increased, whereas the carbide spacing increases only with the mold temperature. Consequently, it follows that, although a high mold temperature may result in a reduction in strength because of the larger grain size, it may also cause an increase in ductility because of the increased carbide spacing.[5] These two factors should be carefully balanced during the actual casting of the dental appliance. Usually because of the high strength values inherent in the alloy, the ductility of the appliance is generally to be favored over a slight sacrifice of strength properties.

**Fusion Temperature.** The fusion temperature of these alloys (Table 34–2) is considerably higher than that of the casting gold alloys (p. 416). The alloys cannot be melted with the ordinary gas-air torch. A mixture of oxygen and acetylene gases is usually employed as a fuel although other types of fuel can be used as well. Electrical sources of melting are often used to advantage, such as carbon arcs, argon arcs, high-frequency induction or silicon-carbide resistance furnaces.[5]

**Physical Properties.** The density of the cobalt-chromium alloys is between 8 and 9 grams per cubic centimeter, a value which is less than half that of many of the gold alloys.

These alloys are harder than most gold alloys even though the latter are age hardened.[1] All of the stellites are very difficult to cut, grind or finish. The lower carbon content alloys with a lower hardness number are more difficult to abrade or machine than are the harder, more brittle alloys.[5] So far as dental finishing processes are concerned, special hard, high-speed finishing tools are necessary for cutting, smoothing or trimming such alloys.

The greater hardness of these alloys as compared to enamel has led to the frequent statement that partial denture clasps made from these materials might produce abrasion of the underlying tooth structure. The problem is accentuated by the high modulus of elasticity which might contribute to wear on the tooth surface during removal and insertion of the appliance. However, according to experimental evidence,[7] the partial denture clasp, regardless of the type of alloy used, produces no abrasion of the enamel. Apparent abrasion or erosion that is commonly seen under clasps can be attributed to other causes, such as unhygienic conditions on the clasp or tooth, areas of decalcification and possible dissolution of enamel because of galvanic currents.

All dental stellites work harden very easily when they are cold worked. Consequently, regardless of the percentage elongation in the "as-cast" condition, as indicated in Table 34–3, the adjustment of clasp arms is difficult, if not impossible, within a certain factor of safety. Even though the clasp arm may not be fractured during the actual adjustment, it may later fail in service because of the strain hardening received initially.[5] Even a slight increase in the original ductility of the alloy may prevent such a failure. It is for this reason that some of the strength in a dental stellite can be sacrificed for a corresponding increase in ductility. In general, the percentage elongation of the dental stellites is comparable to that of a type D gold alloy after age hardening.

The modulus of elasticity of these alloys is greater than that of the gold alloys. Consequently, it can be expected that the stellite dental appliances may be stiffer than those made with gold alloys. Actually, however, advantage can be taken of this fact to decrease the thickness of the stellite appliance and thus decrease its weight. Since the specific gravity of the cobalt-chromium appliance is about one-half that of a comparable gold alloy appliance, the net decrease in weight may be considerable. Whether the weight of a dental appliance is significant within the range indicated is not known.

Such a change in design should be done conservatively, however, since the proportional limit of the stellite (as well as its strength) may be less than that of a comparable age hardened gold-base alloy.[5] As a result, the modulus of resilience of the structure may be reduced to the extent that its resistance to impact may be lowered in comparison to that of a gold alloy.

According to the current American Dental Association Specification No. 14 for Dental Cobalt-Chromium Casting Alloy, the tensile strength of a dental stellite should be greater than 6300 kilograms per square centimeter (90,000 pounds per square inch) when tested with a cast circular rod 2.3 millimeters (0.09 inch) in diameter. The minimum value for the percentage elongation is given as 1.5 per cent.

It should be noted that the diameter of the test specimen should be stated in connection with the tensile testing of all cast alloys and particularly in the case of a stellite. Not only are thin castings apt to be less sound than thicker castings, but also the characteristically coarse grain structure of these alloys would favor the test results with the thicker specimen. For this reason, the tensile properties (excepting possibly the modulus of elasticity) of the dental stellites A, B, C, D, E and F given in Table 34–3 cannot be compared directly with those of the industrial alloys with stellite numbers. In the first instance, rods 2.3 millimeters (0.09 inch) were used and in the second case the test rods were 6.4 millimeters (0.75 inch) in diameter.

However, in the interpretation of the results in Table 34–3 it should

*Table 34-3.* Physical Properties of Cobalt-Chromium Alloys

| ALLOY NO.* | ULTIMATE TENSILE STRENGTH (KG./CM.²) | (LB./IN.²) | YIELD STRENGTH (KG./CM.²) | (LB./IN.²) | MODULUS OF ELASTICITY (KG./CM.²) | (LB./IN.²) | ELONGATION (%) | DENSITY (GM./CM.³) |
|---|---|---|---|---|---|---|---|---|
| A | 7,600 | 108,500 | 4,470 | 64,000 | 1,960,000 | 28,000,000 | 3.4 | — |
| B | 7,500 | 107,500 | 4,260 | 61,000 | 2,060,000 | 29,500,000 | 3.2 | — |
| C | 7,250 | 104,000 | 3,460 | 49,500 | 1,820,000 | 26,000,000 | 2.7 | — |
| D | 5,900 | 84,500 | 3,920 | 56,000 | 1,920,000 | 27,500,000 | 6.0 | — |
| E | 7,150 | 102,500 | 4,360 | 62,400 | 2,000,000 | 28,500,000 | 1.9 | — |
| F | 7,350 | 105,100 | 4,200 | 60,000 | 2,030,000 | 29,000,000 | 1.9 | — |
| 21 | 7,100 | 101,300 | 5,750 | 82,300 | 2,500,000 | 36,000,000 | 8.2 | 8.3 |
| 23 | 7,360 | 105,400 | 4,080 | 58,400 | 2,000,000 | 29,000,000 | 7.0 | 8.5 |
| 27 | 5,770 | 82,500 | 3,280 | 46,900 | 1,900,000 | 28,000,000 | 7.0 | 8.2 |
| 30 | 6,860 | 98,100 | 3,860 | 55,100 | 2,300,000 | 33,000,000 | 5.0 | 8.3 |
| 31 | 7,060 | 101,000 | 5,180 | 74,100 | 1,900,000 | 28,000,000 | 11.0 | 8.6 |

* Lettered designations, Taylor, Leibfritz, and Adler, *J.A.D.A.*, March, 1958. Numbers are "stellite numbers," Metals Handbook, 1948 edition. Compositions as given in Table 34-1.

Note: Smaller size test bars were used for testing the alloys designated by letters than for the "stellite number" alloys. Testing with the larger test bars would result in higher values for the tensile properties with the possible exception of the modulus of elasticity.

be borne in mind that the properties indicated for the dental alloys are probably more characteristic of the properties of dental appliances. Clasps, saddles, bars, etc., are thin and not bulky. On the other hand, if it is desired to determine the tensile properties of the alloys as influenced by metallographic considerations only, the results obtained with the larger test bars are more reliable.

**Casting Shrinkage.** As in the case of the cast gold alloys, a casting shrinkage occurs for the same reasons (p. 422) with the cobalt-chromium alloys during solidification. As might be expected, because of their high fusion temperatures, the casting shrinkage of the dental stellites is greater than that of the gold casting alloys. The casting shrinkages of the European alloys with the compositions shown in Table 34–1 are presented[8] in Table 34–4.

According to the theory of casting shrinkage presented on page 423 for gold alloy castings, it is to be expected that the greater the surface area of a casting in comparison to its volume, the less will be its casting shrinkage. As indicated in Table 34–5, such a theory is true for the dental stellites as well as the gold alloys.[8] The lengths of the cast rods were kept constant, only the diameters were varied. As can be noted, the greater the diameter of the rod, the greater is the casting shrinkage.

It has been shown[5] that for large castings, the strength of the investment may also affect the casting shrinkage. In castings of irregular

*Table 34–4.*  *Casting Shrinkage of Dental Cobalt-Chromium Casting Alloys\**

| ALLOY NO.† | CASTING SHRINKAGE (%) |
|:---:|:---:|
| I | 2.24 |
| II | 2.23 |
| III | 2.14 |
| IV | 2.15 |
| V | 2.13 |

\* Earnshaw, *Austral. D. J.*, June, 1958.
† Compositions as given in Table 34–1.

*Table 34–5.*  *Influence of the Surface Area of the Casting on the Casting Shrinkage\**

| DIAMETER OF CAST ROD (MM.) | (INCH) | CASTING SHRINKAGE (%) |
|:---:|:---:|:---:|
| 3.18 | 0.125 | 2.25 |
| 6.36 | 0.250 | 2.33 |
| 9.54 | 0.375 | 2.39 |

\* Earnshaw, *Austral. D. J.*, June, 1958.

shape, the casting shrinkage may be reduced to some extent when a strong investment is used as compared to that obtained with a weak investment. Presumably, the strong investment is more resistant to the early casting shrinkage than is the weaker investment.

**Investment.** The properties of the investment employed for casting the cobalt-chromium alloys are quite similar to those for casting gold alloys, except that the binder in the former must be able to withstand the much higher temperature of the molten stellite alloy.

The refractory in the investment is either quartz or cristobalite, and the large expansion at the inversion temperatures of the two forms of silica is expected to provide part of the mold compensation as in the case of the gypsum investments for gold castings. The chief differences in composition between the two types of investment are in the binder employed.

*Gypsum Bonded Investments.* As with other dental investments, $\alpha$-hemihydrate can be used as a binder if the fusion temperature of the cobalt-chromium alloy is sufficiently low (*e.g.*, alloy A, Tables 34–1 and 34–2). The primary objection to the use of a gypsum binder is the danger of embrittlement of the casting from the sulfur trioxide evolved by the breakdown of the gypsum in contact with the molten stellite.[5] For use with the lower fusing stellites, this objection can be minimized by the incorporation of an oxalate in the investment.[2, 9] During the heating, the oxalate decomposes to form carbon dioxide in the mold which protects the molten metal from the sulfur trioxide.[5]

*Phosphate Binders.* A binder consisting of a phosphate and a metallic oxide can be employed.[10, 11] For example, primary ammonium phosphate ($NH_4H_2PO_4$) can be made to react in solution with magnesium oxide (MgO) to form a hard mass, probably according to the following reaction:

$$MgO + NH_4H_2PO_4 \rightarrow MgNH_4PO_4 + H_2O$$

The crystals of magnesium ammonium phosphate provide the "green" strength to the investment before it is heated. The amount and crystal size of the quartz or cristobalite powder added determine to a considerable extent the setting and thermal expansion of the investment.

The investments of this type can withstand the impact of any of the molten dental stellites without any important amount of decomposition or loss of strength. At the high elimination temperatures, probably complex silicophosphates are formed to give the investment greater strength.

*Silica Bonded Investments.* In this case, the binder is a silica gel which reverts to silica (cristobalite) on heating.

A colloidal silicic acid is first formed by hydrolyzing ethyl silicate in the presence of hydrochloric acid, ethyl alcohol and water. In its simplest form, the reaction can be expressed as:

$$Si(OC_2H_5)_4 + 4H_2O \rightarrow Si(OH)_4 + 4C_2H_5OH$$

Since a polymerized form of ethyl silicate is actually used, a colloidal sol of polysilicic acids is to be expected instead of the simpler silicic acid sol shown in the reaction.

The sol is then mixed with the quartz or cristobalite to which is added a small amount of finely powdered magnesium oxide to render the mixture alkaline. A coherent gel of polysilicic acid then forms accompanied by a *setting shrinkage*. This soft gel is dried at a temperature less than 200° C. (334° F.).[5] During the drying, the gel loses alcohol and water to form a concentrated, hard gel.[5] As might be expected, a volumetric contraction accompanies the drying, which reduces the size of the mold. This contraction is known as "green shrinkage" and it occurs in addition to the setting shrinkage.

The above gelation process is apt to be slow and time consuming. An alternative and faster method for the production of the silica gel can be employed. Amines of certain types can be added to the solution of ethyl silicate so that hydrolysis and gelation occur simultaneously.

It follows that with an investment of this type the mold enlargement before casting must compensate not only for the casting shrinkage of the metal, but also for the "green shrinkage" and the setting shrinkage of the investment.

As can be noted from Figure 34–2, the thermal expansion of such an investment is likely to be quite high since both the binder and the refractory are forms of silica which exhibit inversion (see page 448) during heating. The "green shrinkage" is shown at *G* and a third shrinkage is shown at *F*. This shrinkage occurs at the temperature at which the polysilicic acid gel is changed to silica (above 680° C.).[5] Generally there is not a great deal to be gained by heating the mold much above 700 to 800° C. (1292 to 1472° F.),[5] at which temperature sufficient mold compensation can be obtained for most dental appliances. As with other investments, the thermal expansion can be controlled by the amount, particle size and type of silica filler employed.

**Preparation for Investing.**   As previously noted, in the United States the actual investing and casting procedures are usually completed in the commercial dental laboratory by a trained technician. Although the casting technic for large castings is basically the same as for the small inlay or crown, there are certain variables to be controlled in the former case which need not be considered with the small castings.

The technician is furnished with a stone-cast reproduction of the patient's mouth including all of the tooth preparations. The first stage is to reproduce the original stone cast, or *master cast*, as it is generally called, with the casting investment to be used. Usually a reversible hydrocolloid is used for purposes of duplication. An agar-base material can be used if a gypsum-base investment is employed. Otherwise, a gelatin base gel is used. Neither the phosphate bonded nor the silica

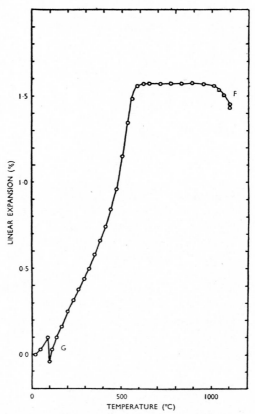

Fig. 34–2. Thermal expansion of a silica-bonded investment. The "green shrink-age" is shown at *G*, and the firing shrinkage at *F*. (Earnshaw, *Brit. D. J.*, Aug. 7, 1956.)

bonded investments will set properly in contact with the agar-base gels.

The duplicating material is poured around the master cast and al-lowed to gel. The master cast is then removed and the investment is poured into the gel mold formed by the master cast. Any hygroscopic setting expansion occurring at this stage with gypsum bonded invest-ments is apt to cause a distortion.[12] A special duplicating flask is em-ployed to minimize syneresis of the gel.

Once a hard investment model is obtained, the wax pattern of the appliance is formed on this model. The wax pattern should be accurate and smooth in every detail in order to minimize any necessary finish-ing procedures on the tough metal after casting.

**Spruing.** As a general rule, wax sprue formers are used through-out. The spruing of a large casting is likely to be a complicated proce-dure both as to the design and size of the sprue former and as to its position of attachment on the pattern. Not only should the investment surface be protected from the inrushing metal, but also the soundness and accuracy of the casting may be affected by the spruing technic.

**Porosity.**     The cobalt-chromium castings are subject to the same types of porosity previously described for the gold castings (p. 424). Furthermore, the danger of oxide and other inclusions during casting is much greater than with gold castings. As with the gold castings, porosity can be avoided by the proper design of sprue formers, the proper direction of the flame and similar factors.

Back pressure porosity, as shown in Figure 34–3, is apt to be particularly troublesome with the casting of cobalt-chromium alloys be-

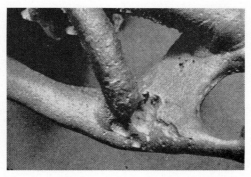

Fig. 34–3.   Back pressure porosity in a partial denture casting, because of trapped gases in the mold. (Earnshaw, *Brit. D. J.*, Aug. 7, 1956.)

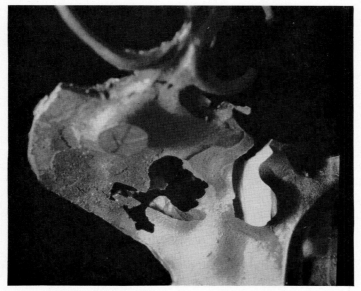

Fig. 34–4.   Incomplete casting owing to entrapment of gas in the mold. (Peyton, *D. Clin. North America*, November, 1958.)

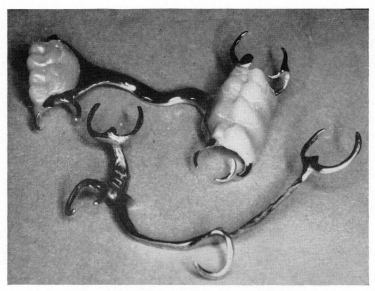

Fig. 34–5.   Finished partial denture appliances cast with dental cobalt-chromium alloy. The appliance in the foreground is a skeleton framework to which the acrylic resin "ridge" and artificial teeth will be attached, as shown in the finished appliance behind. (Peyton, *D. Clin. North America*, November, 1958.)

cause of the lack of venting in the investment mold, particularly when silica-bonded investments are used. Furthermore, an incomplete casting may result[6] as can be noted in Figure 34–4.

In order to enable the gases trapped ahead of the molten metal to escape, vents can be resorted to by attaching wax sprues at strategic areas before the case is invested. Presumably, the gases will collect in the vent areas and will not affect the accuracy or the contour of the casting.

**Investing and Casting.**    Both the investment model and the pattern are invested together in a large ring or *casting flask*. The investing procedure is similar to that described for small gold castings.

The high heat casting technic is used, and the wax is eliminated as the investment is heated. At the time of casting, the mold temperature may be as high as 1100° C. (2000° F.) although as previously stated, 800° C. is usually sufficiently high.

As previously noted, the metal is melted by flame or by electricity. Usually a centrifugal machine is employed for casting.

The flask is usually cooled slowly and the casting is separated from the investment. As previously described, the surface is smoothed by sand blasting. Any adjustments are made with special abrasive wheels and disks revolving at a high speed. The appliance is then given a high polish which it maintains indefinitely if the proper technical procedures have been followed. Two finished cast partial denture appliances are shown[6] in Figure 34–5.

## *Literature*

1. Taylor, D. F., Leibfritz, W. A. and Adler, A. G.: *Physical Properties of Chromium-Cobalt Dental Alloys.* J.A.D.A., *56*:343–351 (March), 1958.
2. Earnshaw, R.: *The Casting Shrinkage of Some Dental Cobalt-Chromium Alloys and Its Compensation by Investment Expansion.* A thesis presented to the Victoria University of Manchester (England) for the degree of Doctor of Philosophy (1957).
3. Subcommittee on Heat-Resistant Castings: *Heat Resistant Castings—Cobalt Base Alloys.* Metals Handbook, Cleveland, American Society for Metals, 1948, pp. 578–581.
4. Anonymous: *Secret Wartime High Temperature Alloys Now Available for Peacetime Use.* Machinery, *52*:183–187 (July), 1946.
5. Earnshaw, R.: *Cobalt Chromium Alloys in Dentistry.* Brit. D. J., *101*:67–75 (Aug. 7), 1956.
6. Peyton, F. A.: *Cast Chromium-Cobalt Alloys.* D. Clin. North America, November, 1958, pp. 759–771.
7. Phillips, R. W. and Leonard, L. J.: *A Study of Enamel Abrasion as Related to Partial Denture Clasps.* J. Pros. Den., *6*:657–671 (Sept.), 1956.
8. Earnshaw, R.: *The Casting Shrinkage of Cobalt-Chromium Alloys.* Austral. D. J., *3*:159–179 (June), 1958.
9. Moore, T. E.: *Dental Investment Material.* U.S. Patent No. 2,222,787 (Nov. 26), 1940.
10. Moore, T. E. and Watts, C. H.: *Investment Material.* U.S. Patent No. 2,479,504 (Aug. 16), 1949.
11. Prosen, E. M.: *Refractory Investment.* U.S. Patent No. 2,209,035 (July 23), 1940.
12. Osborne, J. and Skinner, E. W.: *Physical Properties of Gypsum Model Investments.* J.A.D.A., *59*:708–715 (Oct.), 1959.

# CHAPTER 35

# Abrasion and Polishing.

# Dentifrices.

Before any dental restoration or appliance is placed permanently in the mouth of a patient, it should be highly polished. Not only is a rough surface on a restoration, denture, orthodontic appliance, etc., uncomfortable, but also food and other débris will cling to it. Such a restoration or appliance will become unclean and in some cases a tarnish or corrosion may occur.

Rough surfaces are likely to occur unavoidably during the construction of an appliance. For example, in spite of all the care possible, an acrylic denture base may exhibit minor surface roughnesses which will need to be removed before the denture is polished.

**Abrasion.** The term *abrasion* in the strict sense of the word connotes a wearing of one surface against another by friction. Such abrasion is destructive in nature and is to be avoided. The type of abrasion under consideration is useful in order to smooth a roughened surface in preparation for *polishing*. It is actually a cutting action obtained by the passing of sharp particles of *abrasive* over a surface. In a grinding wheel, for example, not just a few blades are present as in a cutting tool, but rather thousands of sharp abrasive points pass over the work during every revolution and cut as individual blades. Each "blade" removes a chip or shaving of the material as it contacts the work.

For example, rough nodules on a denture base can be removed with an abrasive. They can be removed with a file, sandpaper, emery arbor or a grinding wheel. In each case, the teeth on the file or the "teeth" formed by the abrasive particles can remove the rough spots as they move over the surface. Most abrasives are in the form of small particles such as the sand particles impregnated on sandpaper. The sand can, of course, be used as an abrasive by itself by simply rubbing it over the surface with the hand, or it can be impregnated in a rapidly revolving cloth wheel which is brought into contact with the work. Usually in dentistry, the abrasive is impregnated on paper or a plastic in the form of disks which can be attached to the dental handpiece.

Coarse abrasives leave scratches in the surface, which must be removed with finer abrasives. Finally, the abrasive can be so fine that a surface condition results which is so smooth that it reflects light regularly, and the surface is said to be *polished*.

The subject of abrasion will be discussed first, to be followed by the theory and technic of polishing.

**Types of Abrasives.** There are many abrading and polishing agents available, but only those which can be used in dentistry will be discussed.

*Emery.* Emery consists of a natural oxide of aluminum, called *corundum*. There are various impurities present, such as iron oxide, which may also act as an abrasive.

*Aluminum oxide.* Pure aluminum oxide is manufactured from *bauxite*, an impure aluminum oxide. It can be produced in various grain sizes, and has, to some extent, replaced the use of emery for abrasive purposes.[1]

Extremely fine particles of aluminum oxide can be obtained by a water floatation process. In this form it is known as *levigated alumina* and it is used extensively for polishing metallographic specimens.

*Garnet.* This term includes a number of different minerals which possess similar physical properties and crystalline form. The minerals comprise the silicates of any combinations of aluminum, cobalt, magnesium, iron and manganese. Garnet is usually coated on paper or cloth with glue or a similar binder. It is one of the common abrasives used in denture abrasive disks as operated with the dental handpiece and engine.

*Pumice.* Pumice is a highly siliceous material of volcanic origin, and it is suitable for use either as an abrasive or as a polishing agent, according to its particle size. It is used in dentistry quite extensively for many operations, from the smoothing of denture bases to the polishing of teeth in the mouth.

*Kieselguhr.* Kieselguhr is composed of the siliceous remains of minute aquatic plants known as *diatoms*. The coarser form is called "diatomaceous earth," which is used as a filler in many dental materials such as the hydrocolloid impression materials. It is excellent as a mild abrasive and polishing agent.

*Tripoli.* This mild abrasive and polishing agent is often confused with kieselguhr, which is often substituted for it. True tripoli originates from certain porous rocks, first found in northern Africa near Tripoli, for which it was named.

*Rouge.*     Rouge is a fine red powder composed of iron oxide ($Fe_2O_3$). It is usually employed in cake form. It may be impregnated on paper or cloth, known as "crocus cloth." It is an excellent polishing agent for gold and precious metal alloys, but it is likely to be dirty to handle.

*Tin Oxide.*     Tin oxide, or "putty powder," is used extensively as a polishing agent for teeth and metallic restorations in the mouth. It is mixed with water, alcohol or glycerin and used as a paste. It is a pure white powder, made by treating the product of a reaction between tin and concentrated nitric acid at a high temperature.

*Chalk.*     Chalk is calcium carbonate prepared by a precipitation method. There are various grades and physical forms of calcium carbonate available for different polishing technics. It is the polishing agent often employed in dentifrices. Other polishing agents used in dentifrices are various varieties of *magnesia, calcium phosphate, sodium phosphate, calcium sulfate, sodium bicarbonate,* and *sodium chloride.*

*Chromium oxide* is often used as a polishing agent, particularly for stainless steel.

*Sand.*     Sand and other forms of quartz are used as abrasive agents. Its use in sandpaper is a common example. It is also used as a powder in sandblasting equipments. When a less abrasive material is desired, ground *walnut shells* may be used instead.

*Carbides.*     Various carbides are employed effectively as abrading agents, such as silicon carbide (SiC) and boron carbide (BoC). Both of these products are manufactured by heating silicon and boron at a very high temperature to effect their union with the carbon. The silicon carbide is sintered, or pressed with a binder, into grinding wheels or disks. Most of the stone burs employed for the cutting of tooth structure are made of silicon carbide.

*Diamond.*     The hardest and most effective abrasive for tooth enamel is composed of diamond chips. The chips are impregnated in a binder to form the diamond "stones" and disks so popular with the dental profession.

**Abrasive Action.**     As previously noted, the action of the abrasive as it moves over a surface is essentially a cutting action. Each tiny abrasive particle presents a sharp edge which cuts through the surface in a manner similar to a sharp pointed chisel. A shaving is formed which immediately crushes to a fine powder and often clogs the abrasive tool so that frequent cleaning is necessary.

In the abrading of metals, the crystalline structure of the surface is disturbed, sometimes to a depth of 10 microns. The grains become disoriented in much the same manner as they are during strain hardening. The greater the amount of abrasion, the greater the disorientation.

Some of the crystals fracture and the minute powder-like particles may remain in the surface. Many of these minute particles may be removed by washing the work with soap and water; such a cleansing should always be done before a polishing operation. Strain hardening also accompanies the disorientation, and the superficial hardness of the surface is increased.

The surface effect varies with different metals. For example, in the case of a ductile metal, such as gold, less of the surface may be removed by the abrasive than in the case of a brittle metal. In a ductile metal, the scratch left by the abrasive may display a ridge of metal on either side, much like the soil on either side of a plowed furrow. In other words, the abrasive particle has merely "plowed" through the surface, without actually removing much of it. Such a theory accounts for the finding that many of the gold alloys with a high Brinell hardness number may be less resistant to abrasion than are some of the softer alloys.[2]

The surface disturbance of a resin, as in a denture base, undoubtedly includes the introduction of surface stresses which may cause a distortion if the abrasion is too rigorous. The generation of heat during the abrasion will relieve such stresses to some extent, but if it is too great it may relieve processing strains so that a general warpage results, as well as an actual melting of the surface of the resin.

**Desirable Characteristics of an Abrasive.**     In the first place, the abrasive should be irregular in shape, so that it presents a sharp edge. Round, smooth particles of sand, such as are found on the seashore, would possess poor abrasive properties. Also, the impregnation of sandpaper with cubical particles which would always present a flat face to the work would not be so effective in abrasion as would irregular jagged particles.

Secondly, the abrasive should be harder than the work it abrades.[3] If the abrasive cannot indent the surface to be abraded, it cannot remove any of it. In such a case, the abrasive dulls or wears. The Knoop hardness numbers of a number of abrasives are presented in Table 35–1.

A third desirable property of an abrasive is that it should possess a high impact strength or *body strength.*[3] For example, when a grinding wheel is applied against a metal, the abrasive particle strikes the work

*Table 35–1.    Knoop Hardness Numbers of Abrasives\**

| ABRASIVE | K.H.N. |
|---|---|
| Sand | 800 |
| Emery | 2000 |
| Silicon carbide | 2500 |
| Boron carbide | 2800 |
| Diamond | >7000 |

\* Wayner, *Welding Engineer*, Nov., 1950.

suddenly as it moves along the circumference of the wheel. If it shatters the instant it contacts the work, it will be ineffective. On the other hand, if it never fractures, its edge may become dull in time, and the efficiency of the abrasive will be reduced. Ideally, the abrasive should fracture rather than dull, so that a sharp edge is always present. Fracture of the abrasive is also helpful in shedding the débris accumulated from the work. Although diamond "stones" will cut almost any type of tooth structure or restorative material, the diamond particles do not fracture; rather they lose substance at the tip. Furthermore, they are likely to become clogged when ductile or soft substances are abraded. They are most effective when they are used on the very hard and brittle tooth enamel.

The rating of the body strengths of the abrasives listed in Table 35–1 is in the same order as their hardness.[3]

A fourth quality of an abrasive is that it possess an *attrition resistance* so that it will not wear or dull. An example of attrition is the normal wear of chalk on a blackboard or a pencil on paper. Attrition or dulling is not always the result of wear, however. The abrasive may be "dissolved" or impregnated into the work by a chemical action. For example, silicon carbide will dull more rapidly on steel than will aluminum oxide because it is soluble in steel.[3]

**Grading of Abrasive and Polishing Agents.**     Abrasives are graded on the basis of the fineness of the standard sieve through which they will pass. For example, an abrasive graded as number 8 will pass through a sieve with 8 meshes to the inch, but it will not pass through a sieve finer than this. Different types of abrasives are graded differently. For example, a silicon carbide abrasive is graded[4] as 8, 10, 12, 14, 16, 20, 24, 30, 36, 46, 60, 70, 80, 90, 100, 120, 150, 180, 220 and 240. Finer abrasives are designated as powders or flours and are graded in increasing fineness as F, FF, FFF, etc., or, in the case of impregnated papers, as 0, 00, 000, etc.

**Binder.**     In abrasive wheels and disks, the abrasive particles are held together by means of a binder of some nature. A ceramic bond is used in many cases, particularly for binding diamond chips in dental diamond tools, although an electroplating process to provide a metallic binder may also be used. For "soft grade" disks, rubber or shellac may be used. The latter types, as might be expected, wear rapidly, but they are useful in some dental operations where delicate abrasion is required.

The type of binder is intimately related to the life of the tool in use. In the case of most abrasives, the binder is impregnated throughout with an abrasive of a certain grade so that as a particle is wrenched from the binder during use, another will take its place as the binder wears. Furthermore, the abrasive should be so spaced that the surface of the tool wears evenly, particularly if the disk or wheel is used for cutting along its periphery.

Such is not the case with a dental diamond tool. The diamond chips are too expensive for this purpose. Furthermore, they dull very slowly in comparison to other abrasives. One manufacturer's idea for the placing of the diamond chips on a dental tool is shown in Figure 35–1. The arrangement in Figures 35–1 A and B provides for smooth cutting with little tool vibration. In Figure 35–1C, the points protrude farther from the binder and are more widely spaced. This tool will cut faster but the scratches on the surface will be deeper. It is intended for coarse cutting. The wide spaces between the points provide room for the débris resulting from the cutting with less chance for packing or clogging.

The heterogeneous arrangement of the diamond chips in Figure 35–1D provides a rough contour to the tool surface. Not only is there a

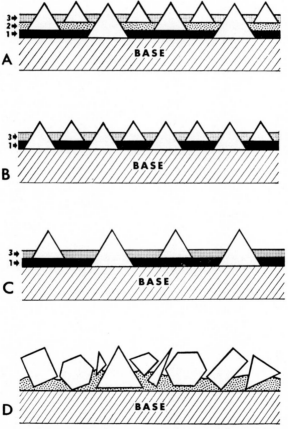

Fig. 35–1.   Diagrammatic arrangement of diamond chips on a dental abrasive tool in cross section. A, A sturdy 3-layer construction using 3 grades of diamond chips attached with a ceramc binder to a metal base. B, A thinner arrangement with 2 grades of chips. C, A coarse cutting tool with two grades of chips. D, Miscellaneous sizes in one layer of band, poorly arranged. (Courtesy of Densco, Inc.)

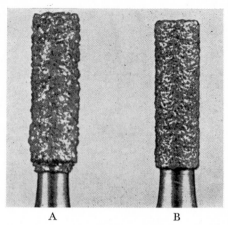

A                    B

Fig. 35–2.   Two dental diamond abrasive tools somewhat enlarged to show the effect of irregularly arranged chips (A) in comparison to the use of a regular arrangement (B). (Courtesy of Densco, Inc.)

greater chance that the chips will be removed from the binder during use, but also the tool may vibrate, or "chatter," causing excessive heat generation and generally inefficient cutting. Furthermore, the control of cutting by the operator will be more difficult. The surface contour of such a diamond tool can be seen in Figure 35–2A in contrast to the regular outline of the tool at the right, Figure 35–2B.

**Factors Affecting the Rate of Abrasion.**     Assuming that the abrasive possesses the proper characteristics as outlined in the previous section, the size of the abrasive particle will be a potent factor in the rate at which the surface is abraded. The larger the particle, the deeper the scratches in the surface will be, and the faster the surface will be worn away.

The choice of the size of an abrasive is largely a matter of judgment. If there are many large nodules and similar coarse rough spots on the surface of the work, the use of a coarse abrasive is indicated. However, a coarse abrasive will introduce deep scratches which must subsequently be removed by progressively finer abrasives. On the other hand, it would be a waste of time and material to start with a fine abrasive on a coarse surface, simply to avoid the deep scratches.

A second factor to be considered is the pressure of the work against the abrasive. This factor is best illustrated in the case of a grinding wheel or an abrading tool that the dentist might use with a dental engine. If the work is pressed tightly against the grinding wheel, the scratches will be deeper and the abrasion will be more rapid. Such an observation does not, however, take into account the force on the abrasive particle. As the particle passes over the work, the back pressure of the work tends to dislodge or fracture the abrasive. Obviously, the greater the pressure of the work on the wheel, the deeper is the scratch, and the greater is the tendency for the abrasive particle to be dislodged or fractured. The efficiency of the abrasive operation is greatly reduced under such circumstances, and the grinding wheel is worn away.

A third and very important factor in the control of the rate of the abrasion is the speed with which the particle travels across the work. The faster the wheel turns, the more times per unit of time the particle contacts the surface. Increasing the speed of the wheel is the logical method for increasing the rate of abrasion with a given abrasive without wearing away the abrasive tool. With many particles of abrasive passing across the work at a rapid rate, the pressure of the work against the wheel can be decreased without a decrease in the rate of abrasion.

**Rotational Speed and Linear Speed.**     The speed with which the particle passes over the work is its linear speed. The linear speed of an abrasive wheel is related to its rotational speed according to the size of the wheel. For example, if the abrasive particle is on the circumference of the wheel, when the wheel turns around once, the particle will travel the length of the circumference, which is, of course, $\pi$ times the diameter of the wheel. If the wheel turns at the rate of $n$ revolutions per minute, the linear speed of the particle will be given by the mathematical relation:

$$v = \pi dn$$
Where $d$ = diameter of the wheel
and     $n$ = revolutions per minute (r.p.m.)
$v$ = linear speed

The unit generally employed for the linear speed is meters or feet per minute.

Different abrasives require different speeds for their maximum efficiency, and such optimum speeds are determined largely by experience. A linear speed of 1500 meters (5000 feet) per minute has been suggested[5] as an average value for the optimum speed. On such a basis, the motor speed of a lathe should be 6300 revolutions per minute for an abrasive wheel 8 centimeters (3 inches) in diameter. Since most dental lathes operate at two rotational speeds, 1750 and 3400 revolutions per minute, such abrasive wheels cannot be operated at their optimum speeds under such circumstances.

An interesting calculation is to determine the optimum rotational speed of a dental stone (silicon carbide) bur used in the preparation of teeth for the reception of gold inlays. An inverted cone silicon carbide "stone" has a maximum diameter of approximately 4.8 millimeters ($\frac{3}{16}$ inch). On the basis of the above calculation, the bur should turn at a speed of 120,000 revolutions per minute to obtain its maximum efficiency in operation.

It is evident from the above calculations that the abrasive wheels and rotating tools used in dentistry must be specially constructed if they are to be efficient in dental operations. Unfortunately, many of the dental abrasive tools are not efficient, and they wear out quite rapidly. The use of the diamond abrasive tool has greatly improved the effectiveness of cutting or abrading tooth enamel. The diamond particle is so hard, strong and resistant to attrition, that the only way in which such a tool can wear is for the diamond to be pulled from the binder.

Another factor which has increased the effectiveness of the use of abrasives for dental operations is the increase in rotational speed now employed to a considerable extent. Rotational speeds as high as 200,000 to 300,000 revolutions per minute are being used in many dental offices. Such a speed encourages the dentist to employ a low pressure when the tool is applied to the tooth, with no increase in the time spent on the operation.

**Polishing.** Metallographically speaking, polishing connotes the production of a smooth, mirror-like surface on a metal without the use of a film. A surface can be made to "shine" with a wax, for example, but such a method of "polishing" is not included in the present discussion.

As previously described, the surface crystals become more disoriented as the abrasion proceeds. With finer abrasives, the small particles formed during the disorientation become much finer. Finally, they become so small that the surface of the metal appears to be a layer of amorphous material, referred to as the *polish layer* or the *Beilby layer*, named after the scientist who first postulated the presence of such a layer. It was formerly thought that the polish layer was completely amorphous, but modern investigations indicate that it is composed of extremely minute crystallites or disoriented atomic spacings, similar to the condition described for the intergranular substance (p. 296).

The presence of such a layer can explain the phenomenon sometimes observed in metallographic polishing. The fine scratches shown in the copper specimen in Figure 35–3 are shown partially removed in Figure 35–4 after the specimen had been partially polished. If the specimen shown in Figure 35–4 is etched, the scratches will generally reappear. A similar technic is employed in the preparation of metallographic specimens, except that all of the scratches are removed with fine abrasives before the polishing. When the polish layer is etched in this case, the grain structure appears.

The optimum speeds for polishing are somewhat higher than for abrading. Linear speeds as high as 3000 meters (10,000 feet) per minute may be used. The optimum linear speed varies with different polishing agents, but the average speed is in the neighborhood of 2300 meters (7500 feet) per minute. Very little of the surface is removed during polishing, not more than 50 microns (0.0002 inch).[6]

**Burnishing.**      Burnishing is somewhat related to polishing and abrading in that the surface is drawn or moved to a greater depth. If a round steel point is rubbed over the margin of a gold inlay (type I or II gold alloy), the metal may be moved so that any small discrepancy between the inlay and the tooth is closed. The dentist may use this method, or he may employ a special bur revolving at high speed.

It is important that the burnishing instrument not be of such material that it will adhere to or dissolve in the surface of the burnished metal. The use of a brass instrument would undoubtedly impregnate copper atoms into the surface of the gold inlay. The reverse practice is sometimes used commercially for "gold plating." For example, a gold

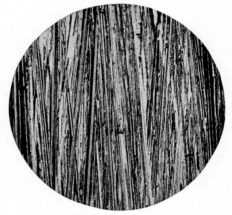

Fig. 35–3.   Scratches on copper produced by grinding with emery. ×200. (Dresch, *The Chemistry of Solids*, Cornell University Press.)

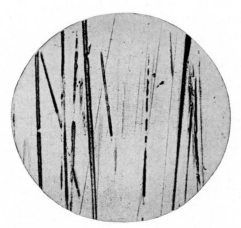

Fig. 35–4.   Scratches on copper partly removed by polishing ×200. (Dresch, *The Chemistry of Solids*, Cornell University Press.)

layer can be placed on a brass or copper surface by burnishing it with a rapidly revolving gold-wire brush.

**Technical Considerations.**    The technics to be described are to be used in the dental laboratory on large pieces. The technics for use in the mouth are best considered in the dental technic courses. The general principles of the two technics are the same fundamentally.

The first smoothing of the work can be done with a coarse abrasive or a bur, both of which leave large scratches. These scratches are removed with a finer abrasive, but the difference in fineness should not be too great. The use of too fine an abrasive after a relatively coarse abrasive is not economical in time, and it is likely to cause an appearance of streaking or a formation resembling fish tails in the final surface.

After changing to a finer abrasive, the direction of the abrasion should be changed if possible, so that the new scratches will appear at right angles to the coarser scratches. A more uniform abrasion will thus result.

When the scratches are no longer visible to the eye, the preliminary polishing can be accomplished with a pumice flour applied with a canvas buff wheel. Such a procedure is especially valuable in polishing an acrylic resin denture.

The work is cleansed thoroughly with soap and water, to remove all traces of abrasive and as many of the particles of the material removed by the abrasive as possible. The bench should be cleaned as well.

A paste is formed by mixing the pumice with water to a sticky "muddy" consistency. As any water evaporates or is otherwise lost, it should be replenished. The buff wheel should turn at a high speed toward the operator from its top side. The work is grasped firmly in one hand, and some of the pumice paste is applied to the work with the other. The work is then carried into the revolving wheel at its bottom side, and immediately removed. The process is repeated again and again, over the entire surface to be polished, until the surface appears bright and reasonably well polished. It should be stressed that the paste is applied *to the work* and not to the wheel. The wheel will not hold the pumice. As it revolves, the water and pumice are thrown off by the rotational forces involved.

The work should again be cleansed thoroughly. One grain of abrasive remaining at this stage may roughen the surface to the extent that the entire polishing procedure may need to be repeated. The canvas wheel is replaced with a felt or cotton flannel buff wheel. The wheel should rotate as before at the highest speed available. A polishing agent in cake form, with a grease of some sort as a binder, can be used. The cake is held against the wheel until the latter is thoroughly impregnated. The grease aids in holding the polishing agent on the wheel, and at the same time it cushions the action of the polishing agent so that a more uniform finish and luster are attained.[6] The work is held against the wheel and turned so that all of the surfaces are polished uniformly. A light pressure should be used in contacting the work with the wheel so that too much heat will not be generated. Such a precaution should be especially observed when a resin denture is polished.

The final polish should be complete in its smoothness and luster. Under such a condition, the patient will be more comfortable and the appliance will be more resistant to tarnish and corrosion.

## DENTIFRICES

No discussion of the action of abrasives or polishing agents in dentistry would be complete without some mention of the effect of dentifrices on tooth surfaces. In addition to flavoring oils, detergents and sweetening agents, tooth powders and pastes contain certain abrasives.[7] The function of the abrasive is to remove débris and stain from the teeth and to polish the tooth surface. The abrasive ideally then should effect maximum cleansing with a minimum of abrasion.

People vary in their need for an abrasive in a dentifrice.[8] Some individuals may prevent stain formation by use of only a brush and water while others require a more vigorous agent. For those individuals where only a slight degree of abrasion is necessary, a mixture of baking soda and table salt or baking soda alone will suffice.

**Composition.** The most widely used abrasives in commercial dentifrices are calcium carbonate, anhydrous dibasic calcium phosphate, tricalcium phosphate, insoluble sodium metaphosphate and hydrated alumina. The precipitated calcium carbonate may occur in the following grades, all of which have different characteristics: light, medium, dense and extra dense.

The information concerned with the abrasiveness of dentifrices is comparatively meager. This is owing in part to the fact that the other ingredients commonly found in the dentifrice may alter the behavior of the abrasive itself. For example, the abrasiveness of a calcium carbonate slurry is reduced one-half when a certain amount of sodium alkyl sulfate is present.[9] It is known that the particle size, shape and the presence of impurities influence the behavior of the abrasive. Very abrasive substances are usually hard and have sharp projections. Harder substances always abrade, but the softer and rounded particles will not abrade as rapidly as will the sharp ones.

**Measurement of Abrasiveness.** There is no relationship between abrasive action of the agent and its ability to produce a smooth tooth surface. For example, levigated alumina is quite effective in producing a highly polished surface, yet it is so abrasive that it cannot be used alone in a dentifrice.

Various technics have been employed for measuring dentifrice and dentifrice ingredient abrasiveness, such as height[10, 11] and weight loss[12] measurements on tooth structure. Because of the inherent variables in individual tooth surfaces, various metals have been tried as a substitute for the tooth structure itself. The weight loss or dimensional change of blocks of antimony, copper and silver after brushing with dentifrices have all been measured.[13] Although antimony showed the most promise, there is adequate evidence that there is no good correlation between the amount of abrasion on metal plates and that produced on enamel. To date the only good way of determining abrasiveness of a dentifrice is on tooth structure itself.

A shadowgraphic method has been used for measuring dentin wear.[14] It was this study that showed that the abrasion of exposed cementum was greater than that of either dentin or enamel when teeth were brushed across the long axis of the tooth rather than parallel to it. The cervical erosion that is often observed clinically may be owing in part to the abrasive effect of the dentifrice and brush. Dentin abrades approximately 25 times faster than enamel, and cementum 35 times more rapidly than enamel. Also using teeth, other investigators[15, 16] have demonstrated the deleterious effects of certain impurities that may be present in the dentifrice. For example, small amounts of silica will greatly increase the abrasiveness of calcium carbonate.

In view of the pronounced effect of impurities that could be present in dentifrices, a qualitative test has been devised to determine the presence of small percentages of highly abrasive particles.[17] The dentifrice is placed on a clean glass slide and rubbed with a metal instrument comparable to a five-cent coin. If a dentifrice powder is used, distilled water is added to produce a slurry. The instrument is rubbed over the slide for 100 double strokes under a load of 16 ounces. A lubricant control, such as glycerol, is used on an adjacent part of the slide. The glass is cleaned with acid to remove any metal particles and the residue is viewed in both transmitted and reflected light. If the test shows greater scratching when the dentifrice is used as compared to the lubricant control, the dentifrice is considered unduly abrasive.

Although this test is not designed to determine quantitatively the relative abrasiveness of commercial products, it is useful in detecting the presence of traces of highly abrasive materials. As little as 0.0156 per cent flour of pumice or 0.0037 per cent silica may be detected[18] in this manner.

The abrasion of tooth enamel in terms of depth of surface loss by various abrasives is shown in Table 35–2. It is to be noted that enamel loss with most of the abrasives commonly used in dentifrices (calcium carbonate, calcium phosphates and sodium metaphosphate) is markedly less than with other abrasives such as flour of pumice and levigated alumina.

**Effect on Tooth Luster.**     The primary purpose of a dentifrice is to

Table 35–2.    *Relative Abrasiveness of Various Compounds on Tooth Enamel**

| ABRASIVE | ABRASION LOSS (mm.) |
|---|---|
| Calcium carbonate, extra dense | 0.012 |
| Light chalk, USP | 0.003 |
| Extra light chalk, USP | 0.003 |
| Bentonite | 0.006 |
| Flour of pumice | 0.300 |
| Levigated alumina | 0.300 |
| Hydrated alumina | 0.002 |
| Dibasic calcium phosphate, dihydrate | 0.001 |
| Dibasic calcium phosphate, anhydrous | 0.021 |
| Tribasic calcium phosphate | 0.001 |
| Stannic oxide, CP | 0.083 |
| Zinc oxide | 0.003 |
| Calcium pyrophosphate | 0.005 |
| Magnesium trisilicate | 0.009 |
| Insoluble sodium metaphosphate and dibasic calcium phosphate, dihydrate (1:1) | 0.001 |

*Gershon, *Cosmetics Science and Technology, 15:* 296, 1957.

assist the toothbrush in freeing the accessible surfaces of the teeth of the newly deposited débris and stain. However, even when done effectively, the teeth may be relatively clean yet still exhibit a dull appearance, or low luster. Such a tooth is esthetically undesirable since the abraded surface reflects less light and appears dull. A second function of a dentifrice, then, should be to polish the tooth.

There is a difference in the effect of various abrasives and commercial dentifrices upon the luster of the tooth surface. Some such agents actually abrade enamel, leaving a dull surface, while others polish the enamel and produce a brighter appearing tooth. Abrasives such as extra heavy calcium carbonate will dull a polished tooth, while a combination of insoluble sodium metaphosphate and tricalcium phosphate will rapidly polish a dull tooth.[19] Still other abrasives and commercial dentifrices are apparently quite inert and have little effect on the enamel surface.

An example of the effect of representative abrasive compounds may be seen in Figures 35–5 and 35–6. In Figure 35–5, a photograph of a tooth crown is shown after brushing half of each side with two commercial dentifrices, one containing extra dense calcium carbonate as its principal abrasive agents, and the other containing insoluble sodium metaphosphate. The abrasive and dulling action of the extra dense calcium carbonate is quite different from the polishing effect of the dentifrice containing insoluble sodium metaphosphate seen at the right. The difference is even more pronounced in the photomicrograph, Figure 35–6.

There is another advantage of a highly polished tooth surface other

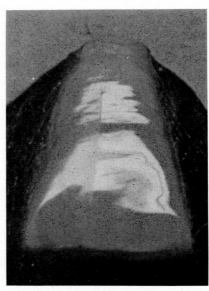

Fig. 35–5.   Tooth crown. Right side brushed with a dentifrice containing insoluble sodium metaphosphate, whereas the dull left side was brushed with a dentifrice containing extra dense calcium carbonate.

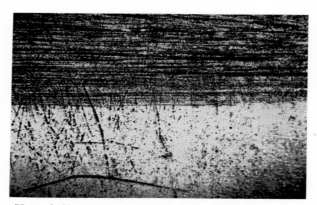

Fig. 35–6.   Upper half—enamel surface brushed with a dentifrice containing extra dense calcium carbonate. Lower half—dentifrice containing insoluble sodium metaphosphate. ×50.

than a cosmetic effect. The smoother the surface of a metallic restoration, the less will be the tendency for it to discolor. In addition, it has been demonstrated[20] that bacteria will accumulate to a greater degree, per unit of time, on a rough, abraded enamel surface than upon a highly polished surface. Furthermore, the bacteria are retained in greater numbers by the rough surfaces even after vigorous brushing.

Thus it appears that a dentifrice which produces a smooth surface,

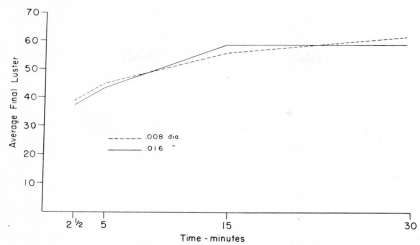

Fig. 35–7. Effect of two different diameter nylon toothbrushes on surface luster (arbitrary units) of enamel. Although the same dentifrice was employed, no difference is evident.

all other factors being equal, would be clinically advantageous. Such a surface will appear better and it will stay cleaner longer.

The exact polishing mechanism is still obscure. Electron diffraction studies[21] indicate that there may be a disorientation of the apatite crystals in the enamel, comparable to the Beilby layer formed during the polishing of metals. Surface changes occur in enamel, with an amorphous-like appearance after polishing when viewed in a microscope.

**Effect of the Toothbrush.**     The toothbrush itself, whether it be nylon or natural bristle, has little or no abrasive effect on enamel or dentin.[22] Abrasion of tooth structure is independent of the stiffness or composition of the bristle. It depends almost entirely on the properties of the dentifrice used in conjunction with the toothbrush. For example, a medium abrasive tooth powder will increase the abrasive action of any toothbrush by several hundred per cent.[22]

The diameter of the bristle does not influence the effect which a given dentifrice will produce on the enamel surface.[23, 24] This fact is demonstrated in Figure 35–7 where two nylon brushes of widely varying bristle diameters were used in conjunction with a dentifrice which tends to polish the enamel surface.[23] The change in luster varies little with either brush. Furthermore, the effect of the polishing agent is neither impaired or enhanced by the wetness of the bristle.

### Literature

1. Lewis, K. B.: *The Grinding Wheel.* Greendal, Massachusetts, The Grinding Wheel Institute, 1951, pp. 11–12.
2. Skinner, E. W. and Lasater, R. L.: *Abrasion of Dental Gold Alloys.* J. D. Res., *21:*103–106 (Feb.), 1942.

3. Wayner, H. W.: *New Concepts of Abrasive Properties.* Welding Engr., *35:*No. 11, 40–42 (Nov.), 1950.
4. Lewis, K. B., *loc. cit.* p. 18.
5. Jacobs, F. B.: *The Abrasive Handbook.* Cleveland, The Penton Publishing Co., 1928, p. 364.
6. Lindsey, J. H.: *Polishing and Buffing.* Plating, *37:*1143–1148 (Nov.), 1950.
7. *Accepted Dental Remedies,* 24th edition. American Dental Association, Chicago, Ill., 1959.
8. Kitchin, P. C. and Robinson, H. B. G.: *How Abrasive Need a Dentifrice Be?* J. D. Res., *27:*501–506 (Aug.), 1948.
9. Epstein, S. and Tainter, M. L.: *Abrasion of Teeth by Commercial Dentifrices.* J.A.D.A., *30:*1036–1045 (July), 1943.
10. Head, J.: *Modern Dentistry.* Philadelphia, W. B. Saunders Co., 1917, pp. 60–64.
11. van der Merwe, S. W.: *Some Aspects of Modern Dentifrices.* J. D. Res., *7:*327–335, 1927.
12. Carney, H. J.: *Comparative Abrasive Qualities of Five Dentifrices.* J. D. Res., *3:*cxxxiii–cxxxvi, 1921.
13. Tainter, M. L. and Epstein, S.: *Use of Metal Plates for Testing the Abrasiveness of Dentifrices.* J. D. Res., *22:*381–389 (Oct.), 1943.
14. Manly, R. S.: *Factors Influencing Tests on the Abrasion of Dentin by Brushing with Dentifrices.* J. D. Res., *23:*59–72 (Feb.), 1944.
15. Smith, R. W.: *Machine for Testing Dentifrice Abrasion.* Ind. Eng. Chem., Anal. Ed., *12:*419 (July 15), 1940.
16. Tainter, M. L. and Epstein, S.: *A Standard Procedure for Determining Abrasion by Dentifrices.* J. Am. Col. Den., *9:*353–379 (Dec.), 1942.
17. Souder, W. and Schoonover, I. C.: *A Specification for Tooth Paste.* J.A.D.A., *24:* 1817–1821 (Nov.), 1937.
18. Epstein, S. and Tainter, M. L.: *Glass Slide Procedure for Detecting Undue Abrasion of Dentifrices.* J.A.D.A., *30:*1591–1594 (Oct.), 1943.
19. Phillips, R. W. and Van Huysen, G.: *Dentifrices and the Tooth Surface.* Am. Perf. & Essential Oil Rev., *50:*33–37 (Jan.), 1948.
20. Swartz, M. L. and Phillips, R. W.: *Comparison of Bacterial Accumulations on Rough and Smooth Enamel Surfaces.* J. Periodont., *28:*304–307 (Oct.), 1957.
21. Skinner, E. W., Osborne, J., Copeland, P. L. and Fiegel, L. J.: *Surface Structure of Enamel and Apatite—a Progress Report.* I.A.D.R., *35:*26, 1957. Abstract.
22. Manly, R. S. and Brudevold, F.: *Relative Abrasiveness of Natural and Synthetic Toothbrush Bristles on Cementum and Dentin.* J.A.D.A., *55:*779–780 (Dec.), 1957.
23. Phillips, R. W. and Swartz, M. L.: *Effects of Diameter of Nylon Bristles on Enamel Surface.* J.A.D.A., *47:*20–26 (July), 1953.
24. Mooser, M.: *Abrasive Action of Toothbrushes with Natural and Synthetic Bristles and of Tooth Pastes.* Parodontol., *13:*131–133 (Oct.), 1959.

# CHAPTER 36

# Dental Burs.

# Mechanics of Cutting.

# Power Sources.

In the preceding chapter, the theory and use of abrasives were discussed at some length. As noted, abrasive tools are often employed to cut tooth structure. The abrasive tool is actually a cutting tool, but the efficiency of the cutting operation is not entirely under the control of the operator because of the heterogeneous arrangement of the abrasive particles, or cutting "blades." In other words, the amount, or depth, of the surface cut varies from one abrasive particle, or "blade," to the next.

In the case of a cutting tool, the blade can cut through the work at a predetermined rate which is controlled by many factors. Unfortunately, studies in the cutting of tooth structure have been meager compared to those completed in industrial cutting. Also, the design of dental tools has not kept pace with the design of those employed in machine shop practice. Consequently, the principles of dental cutting must, to some extent, be presented as analogous to those employed in industrial cutting.

Such analogies should be made with reservation, however. In dental cutting the biologic factors are paramount to all other considerations. For example, the generation of excessive heat in industrial cutting is to be avoided on the basis of tool wear and possible reduction in the physical properties of the work. In dental cutting, the heat generation may cause irreversible injury to the dental pulp as well as severe discomfort to the patient. Temperatures involved in cutting teeth must be kept much lower than in metal cutting for this reason.

Another difference between industrial cutting and dental cutting is the method of applying the cutting tool. In metal work, the work is usually carried or *fed* to the tool at a constant rate, whereas the dentist carries the tool to the work. He regulates the force and cutting of the tool according to his own judgment.

A third difference is that the force applied to the dental tool is much less than is ordinarily employed in industrial cutting; less material is removed per unit of time by the dentist.

## DENTAL BURS

Dental burs are essentially miniature milling cutters as used in industry. Occasionally industrial cutters are used which are as small as a dental bur, although they usually have shanks of greater diameter.

**Types.** There are many shapes and sizes of dental burs available for various purposes in the preparation and finishing of cavities and restorations. A few of the typical shapes are shown in Figure 36–1. The names of the burs from left to right are: straight fissure crosscut, straight fissure, spiral fissure, inverted cone, and round bur, respectively. Bur nomenclature and shape will be studied in detail in the course in Operative Dentistry.

**Composition and Manufacture.** Dental burs can be classified by their composition. One type is made from hypereutectoid steel with certain hardening agents added in minor amount as described in Chapter 32. Burs of this type are generally called *carbon steel burs* or merely *steel burs. Tungsten carbide burs*, or, simply, *carbide burs*, are a second type.

The steel bur is usually cut from blank stock by means of a rotating cutter that cuts parallel to the axis of the bur as, for example, the straight fissure bur[1] (Fig. 36–1). The bur is then hardened[2] and tempered.

There is a definite economic factor involved in the manufacture of steel burs. The dentist is accustomed to a certain price level in purchasing the bur, and it is only natural that with an increase in price a better performance is expected. Unfortunately, so far, any improvements in manufacturing processes involving greater cost have not demonstrated any important improvement in cutting ability.

Regardless of the bur design, whenever a steel bur contacts tooth enamel during cutting, its edges are turned, chipped and worn almost immediately. So long as the cutting is in dentin, the steel tool cuts quite effectively, but the junction of the dentin and the enamel is so irregular in outline in reference to the tooth contour that it is virtually impossible to cut dentin without contacting an irregular contour of enamel. The Vickers hardness number of the tempered steel bur[2] is approximately 800, whereas that of enamel is 260 to 300.

The tungsten carbide bur is a product of *powder metallurgy*. Powder metallurgy refers to a process of alloying in which complete fusion of the constituents does not occur. For example, if a tungsten carbide powder is mixed with powdered cobalt in proportion of 90 parts to 10 parts, placed under pressure in a vacuum, and heated to approximately 1350° C. (2460° F.), a partial alloying, or sintering, of the metals takes place. Presumably, a eutectic alloy is formed which becomes the bond, or matrix, for the particles of tungsten carbide not previously attacked.[3]

A typical microstructure of such a cobalt-tungsten carbide alloy is shown[3] in Figure 36–2. As previously noted, the core is formed by the tungsten carbide with the cobalt-tungsten carbide mixture as the matrix, or bond. The composition of the dental tungsten carbide bur ranges from 5 to 10 per cent cobalt with the remainder being tungsten carbide and possibly small amounts of iron (approximately 0.2 per cent), nickel (0.15 to 0.25 per cent), titanium (0.01 to 0.1 per cent) and/or silicon (approximately 0.1 per cent).[3] Very likely, most of the dental tools contain not more than 5 to 7 per cent cobalt. The Vickers hardness number of the carbide bur is given[3] as 1650 to 1700.

A blank is formed and the tungsten carbide bur is cut with diamond tools. The cutting process is better controlled than with the steel bur. As might be expected, the cost per tool is higher than that of the steel bur.

The cutting head is fastened to a steel shank either by soldering or (mainly) by electric butt welding.[3]

**Design of Dental Burs.** As previously stated, the dental bur is a small milling cutter. The possible tooth designs[4] of such tools are shown in Figure 36–3.

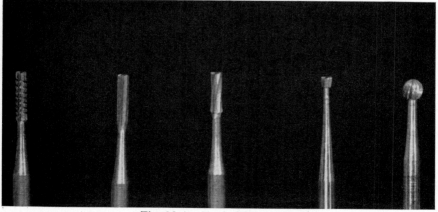

Fig. 36–1. Typical bur types.

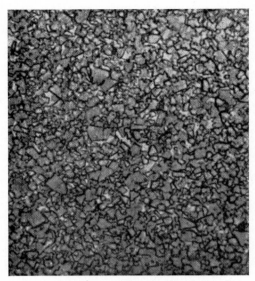

Fig. 36–2. Microstructure of a cobalt-tungsten carbide alloy bur. ×1500. (Lammie, *D. Record*, December, 1952.)

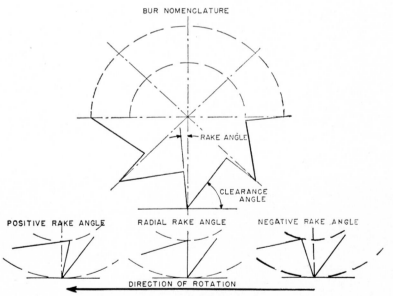

Fig. 36–3. Bur tooth designs and nomenclature. (Henry and Peyton, *J. D. Res.*, April, 1954.)

It should be noted in the diagram that the tool is turning clockwise. The upper drawing indicates a portion of the tool with its teeth in outline. The *blade,* or *cutting edge,* is in contact with the horizontal line or *work.* The side of the tooth ahead of the cutting edge in the direction of rotation is known as the *tooth face;* the opposite or following surface is called the *back,* or *flank,* of the tooth.

It can be noted that the face of the bur tooth is at an angle with the radial line from the center to the cutting edge. This angle is known as the *rake angle.* In this instance, the face is beyond or leading the radial line in reference to the direction of rotation. The angle thus formed between the face and the radial line is called a *negative rake angle.* As can be noted in the drawing immediately below the large drawing, the radial line and the face contour correspond. In this case, the rake angle is zero. In such an instance, the bur tooth is said to have a *zero* or *radial rake angle.* If the radial line leads the face so that the rake angle is on the inside of the radial line, the rake angle is said to be *positive.*

The angle between the back of the tooth and the work is known as the *clearance angle* (Fig. 36–3). An outline of a possible cutter, rotating counterclockwise in this case, is shown[2] in Figure 36–4. The plane surface immediately following the cutting edge is called the *land,* and the angle it makes with the work is known as the *primary clearance.* The angle between the back and the work is called the *secondary clearance.* Although many milling cutters are of this type, so far as is known this design is not employed with dental burs owing to the mechanical difficulties and manufacturing expense incurred with such a small cutter. This design has been included for purposes of comparison only.

The *tooth angle* is measured between the face and the back, or, if a land is present, between the face and the land. The space between successive teeth is known as the *flute* or *chip space.*

The number of teeth in a dental bur is usually six or eight. An eight-tooth bur is shown in cross section in Figure 36–5, whereas the

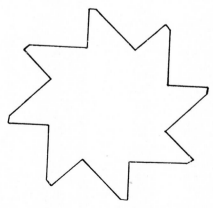

Fig. 36–4.   Possible design for a dental bur. (Osborne, Anderson and Lammie, *Brit. D. J.,* May 1, 1951.)

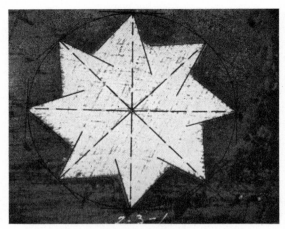

Fig. 36–5.   Eight-tooth bur. (Henry and Peyton, *J. D. Res.*, April, 1954.)

burs in Figures 36–6 to 36–8 have six teeth. As a rule, dental burs are provided with negative rake angles, although the bur designs shown in Figures 36–7 and 36–8 are exceptions. In the case of the bur cross section in Figure 36–7, the rake angle is very nearly zero and was possibly intended to be so by the manufacturer. The bur cross section shown in Figure 36–8 is that of a carbide bur with a radial rake angle.

The clearance angle of most of the burs is straight and clearly defined as noted in Figures 36–5 and 36–6. Where the back surface of the tooth is curved, the clearance is said to be *radial* as illustrated in Figures 36–7 and 36–8.

**Rake Angles.**    In industrial cutting, a positive rake angle is used wherever possible.[5] One advantage is that it improves the flow of the metal along the face of the tool. The smaller the positive rake angle, the greater is the resistance to cutting. This fact is illustrated in Figures 36–9 and 36–10. It has been demonstrated* that the dental bur shown in Figure 36–8 with a radial rake angle cuts more effectively in tusk ivory than do the other designs with negative rake angles under the same conditions of load and rotational speed. Tusk ivory has been shown to be equivalent to tooth dentin in its "machinability" by dental burs.[6]

With a negative rake angle, the chip moves directly away from the edge and is often fractured into small bits or dust. A cutting edge with a negative rake angle is shown in Figure 36–11 as it cuts tusk ivory. As can be observed, the chip is in the form of a shaving, but, instead of sliding along the face of the cutter as in Figures 36–9 and 36–10, it moves directly away from the edge in the direction of motion.[7] In the case of the more brittle enamel, the chip is always small and irregular[8, 9] as shown in Figure 36–12.

* Unpublished data.

There are practical objections to the use of positive rake angles in dental burs, particularly with steel burs. For example, the small tooth angles of the bur teeth in Figure 36–7 would be turned or flattened more easily in the case of a steel bur than the teeth shown in Figures 36–5 or 36–6 because of the smaller bulk at the cutting edge in the former case. The use of a positive rake angle would reduce the bulk at the edge even more. On the basis of such an argument, it is evident that in the case of a steel bur, the use of a zero or negative rake is necessary and it is further desirable in all bur designs.

The design shown in Figure 36–8 can be used successfully with a tungsten carbide bur, where the greater hardness and strength of the

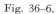

Fig. 36–6.

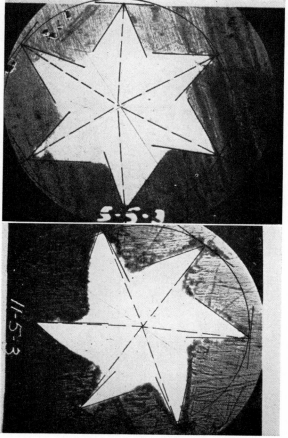

Fig. 36–7.

Fig. 36–6.  Six-tooth bur. (Henry and Peyton, *J. D. Res.*, April, 1954.)
Fig. 36–7.  Six-tooth bur with radial rake angle. (Henry and Peyton, *J. D. Res.*, April, 1954.)

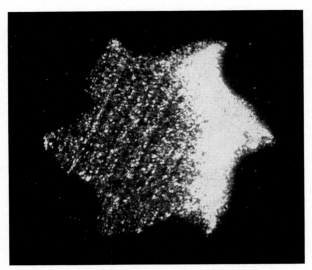

Fig. 36–8.   Six-tooth bur with a radial clearance.

material allow a certain amount of sacrifice of bulk to obtain a more efficient cutting edge, based on recognized milling principles. However, the design in Figure 36–13 is more nearly the rule.[2] The negative rake angle together with the radial clearance and short tooth height provide maximum strength to the teeth and possibly contribute to a longer bur life.

**Clearance Angles.**   The purpose of the clearance angle is, as its name implies, to provide clearance between the work and the cutting edge in order to prevent the tool back from rubbing on the work. There is always a frictional force component on any cutting edge as it rubs against the surface following the dislodgment of the chip. It logically follows that the frictional energy, or heat, will be less, the smaller the area of contact at the cutting edge. The clearance angle of the milling cutters in Figures 36–9 and 36–10 is very small but nevertheless evident. In Figures 36–8 and 36–13, radial clearances are provided.

Theoretically, the clearance angle should be small so as to provide additional bulk at the cutting edge,[10] as previously mentioned. Not only is strength provided for the cutting edge, but also more metal is present to dissipate the heat generated during cutting. However, the clearance should not be so small as to negate its original purpose, *i.e.*, to prevent rubbing the work by the tooth back. It should be noted that any dulling or flattening of the tooth edge may provide a plane surface which will rub against the surface of the work and partially negate the usefulness of the clearance.

This particular effect is likely to be very important in the case of the dental bur. It is estimated that only about 1 micron (0.00004

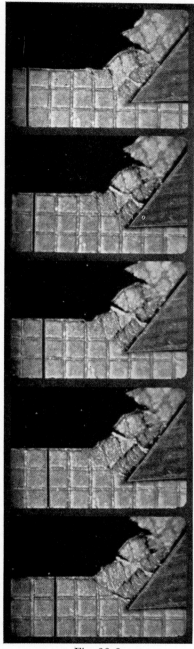

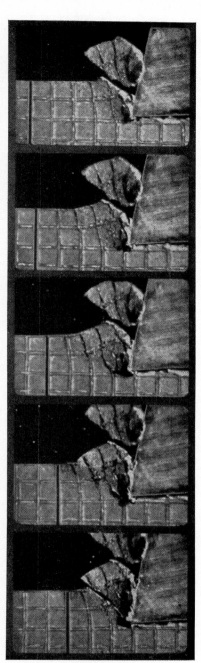

Fig. 36–9.             Fig. 36–10.

Fig. 36–9.    Steel chip formed with positive rake angle of 35 degrees. Note that the metal slides along the tool face with little discontinuity. (*A Treatise on Milling and Milling Machines*, Cincinnati Milling Machine Co.)

Fig. 36–10.    Chip formed in steel with positive rake angle of 15 degrees. Note greater deformation of metal in cutting. (*A Treatise on Milling and Milling Machines*, Cincinnati Milling Machine Co.)

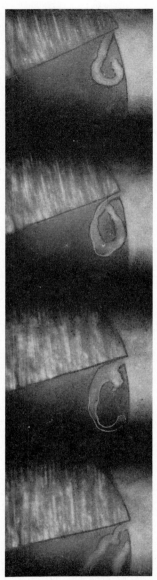

Fig. 36–11.   Chip formed in tusk ivory with a negative rake angle.

inch) of the cutting edge is effective in cutting tooth dentin. The depth of the effective cutting edge in enamel is possibly reduced tenfold[1] in comparison. It should be evident that any slight wear of the cutting edge will increase the dulling perceptibly. It is possible that the large clearance angles employed many times with steel burs (Figs. 36–5 to 36–7) may result in less rapid dulling on this basis.

**Number of Teeth.**     As previously noted, the number of teeth in a dental bur is usually limited to six or eight. When it is considered that the diameter of the bur head may be as small as 0.5 millimeter (0.02 inch), the dimensions of the teeth may be quite small.

The number of blades on the bur and the size of the flutes are definitely related. If too many blades are present, there will not be sufficient space for chip removal, and the bur will clog. Actually, however, it has been shown by motion picture studies that any dental bur

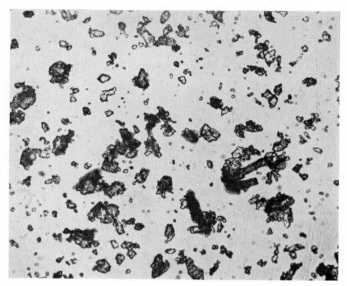

Fig. 36–12.   Enamel chips produced by a tungsten carbide bur. ×335. (Lammie, *Brit. D. J.*, May 15, 1951.)

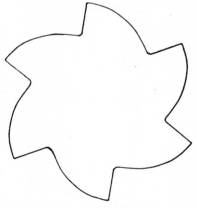

Fig. 36–13.   A typical cross section design, in outline, of a tungsten carbide bur. (Osborne, Anderson and Lammie, *Brit. D. J.*, May 1, 1951.)

is likely to clog repeatedly as it is used, but with proper flute design, it unclogs within two or three revolutions.[7]

Theoretically, a greater speed of cutting should result with more teeth in the tool, other factors held constant. In practice, the difference in speed of cutting tusk ivory, for example, with a six-tooth, as compared with an eight-tooth, dental bur is unimportant.[11]

As might be expected, the smaller the number of teeth, the greater is the tendency for vibration. However, if there are two or more blades in contact with the work at one time, this effect should not be of great importance, particularly as related to the difference between a six-tooth and an eight-tooth dental bur.

If the bur teeth are crosscut (Fig. 36–1, first bur from the left), the general effect is to increase the number of teeth. Presumably, the crosscuts reduce the friction in cutting and provide more chip space. In any event, the crosscut bur generally cuts more effectively than its prototype without the crosscuts.[12] This type of bur is very popular with dentists.

**Run Out.**     *Run out* is the eccentricity or maximum displacement of the bur head from its axis of rotation as the bur turns. Even the most precise tool exhibits a certain amount of run out, since it is impossible to center a tool perfectly on its shank. It is usually measured by rotating the bur in a precision chuck or a V-shaped block in contact with a dial indicator. According to one study,[13] the run out of 80 commercial burs was from 0 to 0.05 millimeter (0 to 0.002 inch), with an average value of approximately 0.025 millimeter (0.001 inch).

The run out will depend not only on the eccentricity of the bur itself, but also on the precision of the dental handpiece. If the shaft or collet attached to the bur wobbles during rotation, the effect will be magnified at the bur head according to the length of the bur shank.

The run out of a bur is definitely related to its efficiency in cutting. If the bur moves away from the tooth periodically, all of the blades will not cut equally. For example, a study of the motion picture frames in Figure 36–14 indicates that not all of the teeth are cutting.

If the dentist senses this lack of cutting, he will probably exert a greater force on the bur. The result will be, at one stage of the revolution, that the bur and tooth will tend to be pushed apart only to be driven together at the next half wobble. The result is a vibration, which is disagreeable to the patient.

So far as the rate of removal of the tooth structure is concerned, although it may appear to be increased during such vibration, the structure is removed by a shattering process rather than by cutting. Such a method of tooth removal is inefficient and inaccurate and increases heat generation.

**Bur Life.**     The life, or length of use, of a bur depends upon many factors, some of which are not under the control of the dentist. The influence of the design of the bur on the preservation of its cutting edge has already been discussed. The speed of rotation is a factor which the dentist can control, but its influence on the life of the bur is not entirely clear.

The probable life history of a dental bur during cutting is presented graphically[3] in Figure 36–15. A dental tungsten carbide bur was ar-

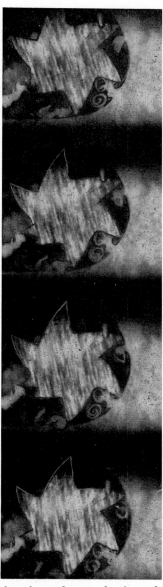

Fig. 36–14.   Successive motion picture frames of a six-tooth spiral bur cutting in ivory.

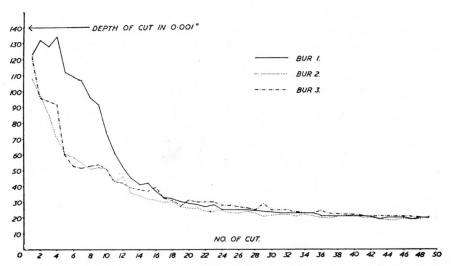

Fig. 36–15. Graph showing the relation of the depth of cut in optical glass by a tungsten carbide bur to the number of successive cuts. (Lammie, *D. Record*, December, 1952.)

ranged to cut for successive 15 second periods directly into a plate of optical glass, under water. The depth of cut during each period was noted and plotted as a function of the number of cuts.

Generally, such a *life function curve* indicates a rapid decrease in cutting with distance or number of cuts as indicated by burs Nos. 1 and 2 in Figure 36–15. As can be noted, the cutting rate finally tends to become constant with further cutting.[13]

Occasionally, a dental bur exhibits an increase in cutting rate before it begins to dull (bur No. 1, Fig. 36–15). The reason for such a phenomenon is not entirely understood. However, it might be because of an irregularity of the height of the bur teeth as a result of the manufacturing process. If one or two of the teeth were slightly higher than the others, it is possible that as the blades on the higher teeth dull, more blades would be brought into action, and an increased cutting rate would result.[13]

So far as is known, the life function curve is independent of the speed of rotation, but as the rotational speed increases, the rate of cutting increases also. However, in industrial cutting, it is expected that the tool life will decrease as the rotational speed increases, other factors being equal.[14]

**Influence of Load.** The force, or *load*, exerted by the dentist on a bur during cutting is related to the rotational speed of a bur of a given design. The exact amount of force generally employed is not known, but it has been estimated as being equivalent to a maximum of 1000 grams (2 pounds) for low rotational speeds, and from 60 grams (2 ounces) to 120 grams (4 ounces) at high rotational speeds.[15] Actually, the dentist operates according to his judgment as influenced by his tactile sense, and the force exerted will change according to the variables encountered.

It should be noted that the discussion is concerned with the force, or load, exerted by the dentist on the tool head and *not* the pressure or stress induced in the tooth during cutting. The latter quantity is related to the force divided by the area of contact of the bur during the cutting, and such an area, in turn, will vary according to the type of bur employed[16] and the material cut.

With a given load the rate of cutting increases with the rotational speed, but the increase is not in direct proportion. The rate of increase in cutting at rotational speeds above 30,000 revolutions per minute is greater than that below this speed.[17] However, it has been found[15] at very high speeds (100,000 to 150,000 revolutions per minute) that the time required for the removal of the same weight of tooth structure is very nearly the same as at still higher speeds. Such a conclusion appears to indicate that no time is saved by the dentist when rotational speeds are employed higher than 150,000 revolutions per minute.

There is, however, a minimum rotational speed for a given load below which the bur will not cut. The greater the load, the lower is this minimum rotational speed.[15] The correlation between the load and the minimum rotational speed depends upon whether enamel or dentin is being cut, the design and composition of the bur and similar factors.[18] Here again, the tactile sense of the dentist acquired by experience is the controlling factor under clinical conditions of cutting.

**Coolants.** It has been shown that the effect of a coolant applied to the bur reduces the heat generated during cutting[19] and also increases its cutting rate.[20] The chief purposes of the coolant are to reduce the temperature during cutting and to aid in the removal of débris.

There are three types of coolant available to the dentist: (1) air, (2) water, and (3) water spray (air and water combined). All three coolants are effective in reducing the temperature during cutting. The water stream is the most effective, water spray, second, and air blown on the bur during cutting, third.[19]

According to one investigation,[20] when an air-water mist was employed as a coolant, the bur tended to clog during the cutting of dentin, and the cutting rate was reduced. On the other hand, the presence of a water spray increased the cutting rate of the bur ten times when cutting enamel in comparison to the cutting rate when no coolant was used. No noticeable difference could be noted when a water stream was substituted for the water spray.

**Heat Generation.** During cutting, heat is generated by (1) the internal friction of the material being deformed in the process of forming the chip, (2) the friction between the face of the tooth and

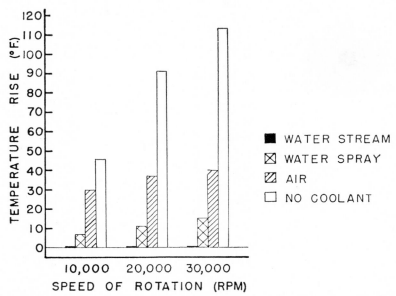

Fig. 36–16.   Effect of rotational speed and type of coolant on the temperature rise during tooth cutting. (Peyton, *J.A.D.A.*, May, 1958.)

the chip as it is sheared from the work, and (3) the friction of the blade as it moves across the work. This heat can be dissipated (1) by conduction through the tool, (2) by conduction through the work, (3) by the chip itself, as it is removed, and (4) by a coolant. Although the life of the bur, particularly if it is a steel bur, may be reduced markedly by the first method, the most important factor from the dental standpoint is the heat absorbed by the tooth. If the temperature of the tooth becomes too great, irreversible pulp damage may occur.

It has been demonstrated[9, 19] that cutting with a tungsten carbide bur reduced the amount of heat generated during cavity preparation in comparison to that generated with a steel bur. Even under water, the heat generated by the steel bur increased during the cutting of enamel whereas that produced by the tungsten carbide bur remained constant.[9]

The steel bur dulls rapidly during the cutting of enamel, whereas the tungsten carbide bur does not. It follows that as the bur dulls, the friction of the cutting edge increases, and less material is removed. The result is that most of the heat is dissipated into the tooth itself.

The use of a coolant greatly reduces the amount of heat generated regardless of the rotational speed of the bur, as indicated by the bar graphs[19] shown in Figure 36–16. The tooth structure was cut with a carbide bur under a load of 228 grams (8 ounces). Apparently, the water stream provided the most effective cooling. However, the use of the more convenient air-water spray in dental practice is sufficiently efficient so that the temperature increase is not clinically significant.

It can be further noted from Figure 36–16 that an increase in temperature occurs with an increase in rotational speed. When the rotational speed is increased above approximately 10,000 revolutions per minute, the use of an adequate coolant becomes a necessity, since temperatures are generated which might cause an irreversible pulp reaction without a coolant.

The less the applied load on the dental bur, the less is the amount of heat generated. For example, with speeds of 8000 revolutions per minute or less, it has been shown that temperatures of 16° C. (30° F.) to 27° C. (48° F.) may be generated in a tooth using a steel bur under a load of 228 grams (8 ounces) with intermittent cutting.[21] However, as previously noted, the force exerted by the dentist generally increases as the rotational speed decreases. If the estimated load of 1000 grams (2 pounds) is applied at speeds of 6000 revolutions per minute, or lower, the temperature rise without a coolant may be as high as 70° C. (125° F.). It follows, therefore, that the use of a coolant is desirable as a safety factor while cutting tooth structure regardless of the rotational speed employed.

Another important factor is the period of time the bur is applied to the tooth. Intermittent cutting at intervals of a few seconds should be the rule. Removing the bur from the tooth intermittently for even a few seconds can reduce the heat generation considerably. Even though the temperature is kept comparatively low, a sustained application may result in greater pulp damage than would result if a higher temperature were applied for a short time.

Actually, the greatest protecting factor against pulp damage is the low thermal conductivity of the dentin itself. If it were not for this factor, the preparation of a tooth cavity would be a serious problem even under optimum conditions of temperature control.

**Mechanics of Cutting.** A great many of the conclusions presented in the previous discussion can be summarized and accounted for on the basis of a theory of cutting. The elementary description of this theory to be presented is based on a more elaborate and mathematical presentation.[22]

Let it be assumed that a dental bur is rotating as diagrammed in Figure 36–3. As one of the teeth rotates into position to contact the work, a compressive stress is first induced as the blade forces its way into the work. If cutting results, the blade essentially fractures or shears the surface; it gradually becomes parallel with the surface of the work and it pushes the material ahead along the tooth face to form the chip. The chip is subjected to compressive stress and the material behind the blade is under tension. However, it can be seen that the material at the cutting edge is subjected to a shearing stress predominantly as it is removed from the surface of the work.

Although the stresses are complex, nevertheless they can be categorized by analysis into the three stress types. Furthermore, both elasticity and permanent deformation of the work are involved. If such is the case, it follows that the stress-strain relationships as related to the stress-strain curve presented in Chapter 2 should be applicable.

For example, as the rotating bur tooth contacts the work, the first stress introduced is elastic in nature. If the force at the cutting edge is sufficient, the stress will soon exceed the proportional or elastic limit of the material and a permanent deformation and then fracture will occur.

On the other hand, if the force exerted by the blade in rotation is insufficient to cause the induced stresses to exceed the elastic limit of the material, only elastic deformation will occur as the blade moves across the work, with no cutting or chip formation. This explanation accounts for the fact, as previously discussed, that for any rotational speed there is a minimum load which can be exerted to produce cutting. When such a situation occurs in practice, the dentist merely exerts more force on the handpiece so that cutting will occur.

It can be reasoned, therefore, that the greater the load, the more the blade "bites" into the work, and the greater is the amount of material removed. There is a limit, however, to the magnitude of the load which can be exerted on a given bur tooth at a constant rotational speed. For example, the friction of the cutting edge against the work increases with the load, and excessive heat may be generated as well as a dulling and chipping of the cutting edge. Even more important, particularly with modern dental handpieces, the bur will stall because of insufficient torque, particularly at very high rotational speeds.

When the load is held constant, the rate of cutting can be increased by increasing the rotational speed. One reason for this fact is, of course, that more blades contact the work per unit of time. On the other hand, the increase in cutting rate is not directly proportional to the increase in rotational speed.

This latter effect can be explained on the basis of the rate of recovery or relaxation of the work after deformation. After the material cut has been permanently deformed, time must elapse for relaxation. If one blade follows another in cutting so rapidly that there is not sufficient time for the stressed material to recover, the amount of deformation of the work produced by the succeeding blade will be less. In other words, the following blade will likely contact the work while it is permanently deformed from the previous blade so that energy need not be expended for the initial elastic deformation. Thus, the total efficiency of the cutting is increased. Consequently, the amount of material removed per tooth at the higher speeds is greater than at the lower speeds under the same conditions of loading. Therefore, the rate of cutting at the higher speeds is greater in proportion to the cutting rate at lower speeds as previously concluded from the experimental data.

## POWER SOURCES

As might be expected, the power source for rotating the bur is extremely important in relation to its torque and rotational speed. Traditionally, the rotation is effected by means of a belt and pulley arrangement attached to an electric motor, the speed of which is regulated by a rheostat controlled by a foot pedal. Such equipment is known as a "dental engine," a term which is now obsolete in engineering circles.

It is necessary that the bur be able to cut at any angle, as guided by the hand of the dentist. For this reason, the collet, or chuck, holding the bur must be contained in a slender handpiece which can be easily grasped by the dentist.

Although the removal of tooth structure is generally effected by the use of a rotating tool, other means have been tried with some success, and two of these technics will be described.

**Airbrasive Technic.** Tooth structure can be removed by a process similar to that of sandblasting. Particles of aluminum oxide are directed toward the tooth by means of a high pressure gas stream (carbon dioxide). The abrasive is emitted from a small tungsten carbide nozzle, 9.5 millimeters (0.375 inch) in length and 0.46 millimeter (0.018 inch) in diameter. The abrasive stream diverges from the nozzle at an average angle of 3.5 degrees. The velocity of the particles at the time they leave the nozzle is said to be 300 meters (1000 feet) per second.[23]

By virtue of the divergence of the abrasive stream, the operator can control its width and, therefore, the width of the cut, according to the distance of the nozzle tip from the tooth. By turning the handpiece, the angle of the abrasive stream to the tooth can be controlled.

The patient acceptance of this device was very good since the pain and discomfort was considerably reduced in comparison to that incurred during the dental operations of the period of its invention (*circa* 1945).

As has been repeatedly stated, the dentist's control of the removal of tooth structure is greatly guided by his tactile sense. In the case of this particular equipment, no tactile sense was present, and the operation was completed by direct vision only. Probably this difference was the principal reason why this method never became popular.

A few dentists have acquired the necessary skill and are still using this technic at the present time.[24]

**Ultrasonic Technic.** When a suitable tip is provided, tooth structure can be removed by ultrasonic vibration with the aid of an abrasive. In practice, the tip is energized with vibrations in the neighborhood of 29,000 cycles per second. A slurry of the abrasive is propelled against the tip in contact with the tooth. The abrasive employed is aluminum oxide. Various shaped tips are provided for different orientations and design of the various cavity forms.

The chief advantage of this method for the removal of tooth structure appears to be patient comfort. It is the least painful method for cavity preparation yet devised.[25]

The disadvantages as listed by the dentist are many. Although a certain amount of tactile sense is present, the abrasive slurry completely obscures the operating area while cutting. Like the airbrasive unit, the initial cost of the ultrasonic unit is considerable.

It might be conjectured that if this instrument had been introduced prior to the advent of the modern high speed rotary tools, it might have been more popular. The time required for the preparation of a cavity with the ultrasonic unit is approximately twice that of the high speed rotary instruments.

Ultrasonic instrumentation has been successfully employed in prophylactic treatment for scaling operations[26] and for the condensation of amalgam.[27]

**Rotary Type Instruments.**    The traditional method for the removal of tooth structure is by rotating tools. It is not the purpose of this discussion to explain the mechanics and construction of the various power units and equipment available to the dentist, but rather to describe each briefly and finally to compare them as to effectiveness and patient acceptance. The instrumentation in this field is likely to be in a state of flux for a considerable period of time and consequently a detailed discussion might be only of passing interest.

**Classification.**    The available rotary instruments can be classified on the basis of their rotational speeds. For example, the older belt driven handpiece is equipped with a motor and pulley system to deliver a rotational speed of 500 to 6000 revolutions per minute at the bur. Such equipment can be called a *low speed* unit.

A *medium speed* pulley system allows the unit to deliver approximately 10,000 to 20,000 revolutions per minute. If the rotational speed is 20,000 to 60,000 revolutions per minute, the range can be called *high speed.* Any speed above 60,000 revolutions per minute is designated as *ultra high speed.*

The units can be further classified as *belt driven* and *turbine driven.* The turbine driven units are subdivided into air turbine units and water turbine units. The belt driven units can deliver a maximum rotational speed of approximately 180,000 revolutions per minute, whereas the rotational speed of some air turbine units can approach 300,000 revolutions per minute. Such speeds assume no load. Under load the rotation of the bur will be decreased according to the magnitude of the load and the type of tool. The turbine units are more sensitive in this respect than are the belt driven units.[28]

**Belt Driven Handpieces.** Aside from the cutting tool itself, the handpiece is the most important part of the unit so far as efficient handling is concerned. It cannot be bulky in any part, otherwise it would hamper the dentist in handling and guiding it, and it could not be inserted into all parts of the mouth with ease. At the same time, it should have precision bearings and proper lubrication to prevent vibration caused either by improper construction or by wear. The bearings should be completely protected from dust, water and saliva.

A typical ball-bearing belt driven handpiece is shown in Figure 36–17. The bur can be inserted at the end of the straight handpiece or in the part to the right, known as the *contra-angle*. The contra-angle part can be inserted into the straight handpiece and a *contra-angle handpiece* is formed. The contra-angle in this handpiece is gear driven. The handpiece with the contra-angle can be used at rotational speeds up to 25,000 revolutions per minute.

The type of bearings employed in a dental handpiece vary from friction bearings of glass or hard metal to ball bearings. In general, the gear driven contra-angles and friction bearing handpieces are used only in the low and medium speed ranges.

At higher speeds, a belt driven contra-angle is usually employed. The contra-angle handpiece shown in Figure 36–18 contains two belts. The tube, or cable, leading to the handpiece supplies the coolant. The handpiece and contra-angle are a single unit in this instrument. Separate belt driven contra-angles can be obtained to fit high speed straight handpieces if desired.

The instrument shown in Figure 36–18 can be operated by belt drive at speeds ranging from 20,000 to 150,000 revolutions per minute.

**Air Turbine.** A typical air turbine is shown in Figure 36–19. The gauge on the panel indicates the air pressure as controlled by the knob at the right. The left knob is to control the coolant. The hose leading

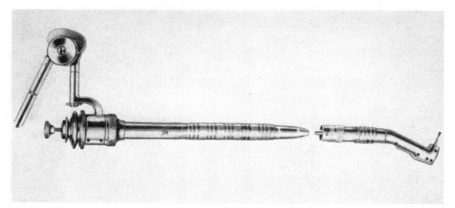

Fig. 36–17. A typical modern handpiece with contra-angle attachment. (Kilpatrick, *High Speed and Ultra Speed in Dentistry.*)

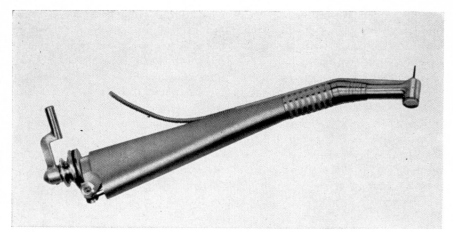

Fig. 36–18. A belt-driven contra-angle handpiece. (Kilpatrick, *High Speed and Ultra Speed in Dentistry.*)

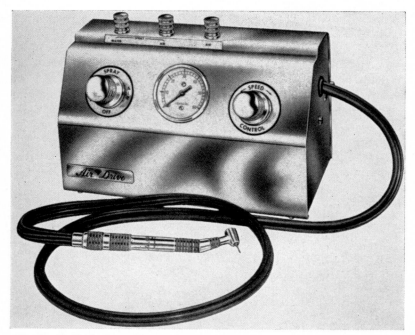

Fig. 36–19. Typical air turbine equipment with handpiece. (Kilpatrick, *High Speed and Ultra Speed in Dentistry.*)

to the handpiece carries both the air and the coolant to the instrument head.

The handpiece is a contra-angle type. Very few air turbines include a straight handpiece.

The construction of the air turbine power unit is very simple, as illustrated in Figure 36–20. The cartridge containing the rotor, or turbine, is inserted into the head of the handpiece so that the intake hole is opposite the air supply. The chuck is attached to the rotor and the bur to the chuck. No belts or electric motors are needed. The units typically operate at air pressures from 1400 grams per square centimeter (20 pounds per square inch) to 2400 grams per square centimeter (35 pounds per square inch). The greater the pressure, the higher is the rotational speed and torque. However, owing to the sensitivity of the torque to changes in air pressure, as a rule it is not feasible to regulate the rotational speed over too wide a range by changing the air pressure.

**Water Turbine.**    A turbine contra-angle handpiece is available which is driven by a water stream.[29] A typical unit is illustrated in Figure 36–21. An electrically driven pump is inclosed in the cabinet which forces the water against the blades of the turbine located in the head of the contra-angle as in the case of the air turbine (Fig. 36–20). The water is then returned to the tank inside the cabinet for recirculation.

The unit can be used at a single rotational speed of 55,000 revolutions per minute. It has a very low torque and cannot be employed with dental burs. Its use is limited to diamond stones and similar abrading tools. The inventor considers the diamond tools less harmful to tooth structure at high speeds than are the bur type instruments.[30]

**Coolant Application.**    A coolant of some nature should be used at all times when cutting tooth structure. There are a number of nozzle devices available which can be fastened to the handpiece or contra-angle as indicated in Figure 36–22. The tube carrying the coolant can be adapted close to the handpiece as shown so as not to inconvenience the dentist during the operation. A flexible tube connects the handpiece tube with the water or air source. In the case of a

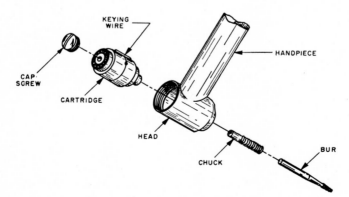

Fig. 36–20.   Parts of an air turbine power unit. (Kilpatrick, *High Speed and Ultra Speed in Dentistry.*)

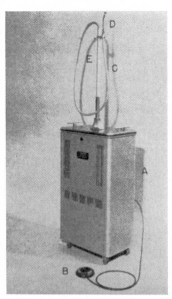

Fig. 36–21. Water turbine equipment. *A*. Cabinet containing pump. *B*. Foot control switch. *C*. Tubing for water supply. *D*. Handpiece. *E*. Flexible arm for support of tubing. (Nelsen and Nelsen, *J.A.D.A.*, Jan., 1959.)

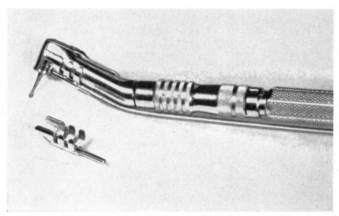

Fig. 36–22. The tube for the coolant is clipped to the contra-angle as shown. (Kilpatrick, *High Speed and Ultra Speed in Dentistry*.)

belt driven unit, it may follow the belt arm arrangement as shown in Figure 36–23.

The turbine equipment is supplied with coolant through the same cable that supplies the air or water pressure (Figs. 36–19 and 36–21).

Most of the units are capable of delivering either water, air-water spray or air coolant. Convenient controls are supplied so that the dentist can easily change the type of coolant while working.

It is important that the coolant strike the bur in a direction which will effect the greatest amount of cooling. In milling practice, the stream of coolant is directed toward the location where the tooth leaves the work.[31] It is at this stage that the cutter is at the maximum temperature. Furthermore, the chip is cooled at the same time. In a dental operation, the coolant should saturate the entire area of cutting.

The air-water spray is generally effective clinically, although the water stream produces more cooling. The air-water spray does not obscure the vision. When a water stream is employed, the entire area, including the clothes of the patient, is apt to be sprayed. Furthermore, the removal of the water may be a problem. However, if the dental tool tends to clog, the use of a water stream is indicated to remove the débris more rapidly.

**Comparison.** There are two important factors which predominantly influence a dentist in the selection of equipment for the removal of tooth structure. One is the acceptance by the patient with regard to comfort and to the minimization of pain and traumatic effects. The second factor is the speed with which the operation can be completed.

The most objective clinical study regarding these factors was concerned with the belt driven handpiece, the water turbine and ultrasonic equipment.[25] Vibrations transmitted to the bones of the skull were recorded by means of an oscilloscope arrangement.

In addition, each patient was questioned as to his reaction to the particular handpiece employed. These data were combined to estimate

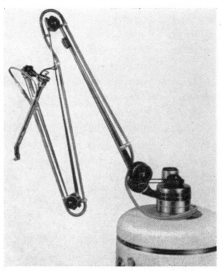

Fig. 36–23. A flexible tube, clamped to the belt arms, delivers the coolant to the tube arrangement on the handpiece. (Kilpatrick, *High Speed and Ultra Speed in Dentistry.*)

*Table 36–1.* *Patient Acceptance and Time to Cut Cavity**

| ROTATIONAL SPEED (R.P.M.) | ANNOYANCE FACTOR | PATIENTS REQUESTING ANESTHESIA (PER CENT) | TIME TO CUT CAVITY (MINUTES) |
|---|---|---|---|
| 4,500–6,000 | 10 | 100 | 3.4 |
| 12,000–16,000 | 8 | 50 | 2.3 |
| 45,000‡ | 4 | 0 | 2.0 |
| 80,000–120,000 | 5 | 0 | 1.7 |
| Ultrasonic | 2 | 0 | 3.3 |

*Data summarized from Hartley, *J. Pros. Den.*, Jan., 1958.
‡Water turbine equipment used.

an "annoyance factor," which was rated from 10 to 1. The factor of 10 represented the greatest discomfort and highest vibration or noise experienced by the patient. Annoyance factors lower than 10 indicated less discomfort and better patient acceptance in proportion to 10. The patient was allowed to request a local anesthetic at any time during the operation. The time for the cutting of the cavity was recorded automatically in each case. The average annoyance factors and times for cutting intracoronal cavities are presented in Table 36–1.

As can be noted from the Table, the use of low speeds (4500 to 6000 revolutions per minute) was definitely contraindicated so far as patient acceptance was concerned. The fact that all of the patients requested anesthesia indicated that the pain was severe. The vibrations recorded were the highest in amplitude of any of the procedures employed.

Although the time of cutting was reduced with the higher speeds of 12,000 to 16,000 revolutions per minute, the patient acceptance was not good, although it was better than for the low speeds.

The use of the water turbine equipment resulted in the best patient acceptance of any of the rotary instruments employed. The chief factor was its comparatively quiet action and lack of noise. As previously noted, only diamond stones could be employed in this case.

At the ultra high speeds (80,000 to 120,000 revolutions per minute), the patients complained of the noise of the instrument, but the vibrations recorded were the lowest in amplitude of the entire series of rotating instruments. None of the patients requested anesthesia. It was noted that the pitch, or frequency, of the vibrations was annoying to both the patient and the dentist.

So far as the average time of cutting is concerned (Table 36–1), the differences are not of importance at any of the speeds above 12,000 revolutions per minute.

The vibration of the bur at any speed can be reduced if the unit is properly cared for. The bearings in the handpiece should be replaced when worn. In a belt driven handpiece, any loosening of the pulley bearings, belt slippage and similar factors, all contribute to vibration effects. The bearings should be cleaned and oiled frequently.

Apparently none of the cutting methods result in any type of irreversible pulp disturbance.[32] Although the frequency ranges of the sound vibrations from some of the air turbine handpieces are in the pathologic auditory range, no permanent damage to the hearing of the dentist has been demonstrated.[33, 34]

The force exerted by the dentist at the ultra speeds is much less than that required at lower speeds. In fact, at the ultra speeds, the sensation incurred by the dentist during cutting appears to be that he is using a brush to remove tooth structure,[25] the required force is so small. Such an observation indicates that more skill and training are required by the dentist at these speeds in order that the cutting will not be more extensive than is necessary or desired, particularly in relation to the possibility of an unintentional pulp exposure.

In general, the belt driven instruments appear to be more versatile in relation to their stalling force. Usually, any force on the tool greater than 100 to 200 grams (4 to 7 ounces) will stall the bur in an air turbine handpiece, whereas forces greater than 450 grams (16 ounces) are required to stall the bur in a belt driven handpiece.[35] From the standpoint of operating safety, however, perhaps the instruments with the lower torque are to be preferred.

## Literature

1. Henry, E. E.: *The Influence of Design Factors on the Performance of the Inverted Cone Bur.* J. D. Res., *35:*704–713 (Oct.), 1956.
2. Osborne, J., Anderson, J. N., and Lammie, G. A.: *Tungsten Carbide and Its Application to the Dental Bur.* Brit. D. J., *90:*229–235 (May 1), 1951.
3. Lammie, G. A.: *A Study of Some Different Tungsten Carbide Burs.* Den. Record., *72:*285–300 (Dec.), 1952.
4. Henry, E. E., and Peyton, F. A.: *The Relationship between Design and Cutting Efficiency of Dental Burs.* J. D. Res., *33:*281–292 (April), 1954.
5. *A Treatise on Milling and Milling Machines.* Cincinnati, The Cincinnati Milling Machine Co., 1951, pp. 112–113.
6. Bryton, B., Skinner, E. W., Lindenmeyer, R. S., and Lasater, R. L.: *The Cutting Effectiveness of a Dental Bur as Related to Its Design.* J. D. Res., *33:*693 (Oct.), 1954. Abstract.
7. Skinner, E. W., Lasater, R. L., Lindenmeyer, R. S., and Rigas, T. J.: *Dental Bur Research.* Report to the Office of the Surgeon General, Department of the Army, 1955, p. 107.
8. Hartley, J. L., Hudson, D. C., Sweeney, W. T., and Richardson, W. P.: *Cutting Characteristics of Dental Burs.* U. S. Armed Forces Med. J., *8:*209–218 (Feb.), 1951.
9. Lammie, G. A.: *A Comparison of the Cutting Efficiency and Heat Production of Tungsten Carbide and Steel Burs.* Brit. D. J., *90:*251–259 (May 15), 1951.
10. Reference 5, p. 129.
11. Reference 7, p. 70.
12. Skinner, E. W., Lasater, R. L., Lindenmeyer, R. S., and Bryton, B.: *Dental Bur Research.* Report to the Office of the Surgeon General, Department of the Army, 1954, pp. 64–69.
13. Skinner, E. W., Lasater, R. L., Lindenmeyer, R. S., and Bryton, B.: *Dental Bur Research.* Report to Office of the Surgeon General, Department of the Army, 1953.

14. Reference 5, p. 193.
15. Peyton, F. A.: *Current Developments in Tooth Cutting Instruments.* New York J. Den., *28:*187–191 (May), 1958.
16. Morrison, A. H., and Grinnell, H. W.: *The Theoretical and Functional Evaluation of Higher Speed Rotary Instrumentation.* J. Pros. Den., *8:*297–314 (March), 1958.
17. Skinner, E. W., Lindenmeyer, R. S., Lasater, R. L., and Osterman, P.: *Mechanics of Cutting with Rotary Dental Instruments.* Report to the Office of the Surgeon General, Department of the Army, 1960.
18. Reference 12, p. 27.
19. Peyton, F. A.: *Effectiveness of Water Coolants with Rotary Cutting Instruments.* J.A.D.A., *56:*604–675 (May), 1958.
20. Skinner, E. W., Lasater, R. L., Lindenmeyer, R. S., Rigas, T. J., and Rigas, D. J.: *Dental Bur Research.* Final Report to the Office of the Surgeon General, Department of the Army, 1957, pp. 114–139.
21. Peyton, F. A.: *Response to Shaping Cavities with Modern High Speed Instruments.* New York J. Den., *28:*262–267 (Aug.–Sept.), 1958.
22. Reference 20, pp. 144–162.
23. Black, R. B.: *Airbrasive: Some Fundamentals.* J.A.D.A., *41:*701–710 (Dec.), 1950.
24. Peyton, F. A., and Morrant, G. A.: *High Speed and Other Instruments for Cavity Preparation.* Internat. D. J., *9:*309–329 (Sept.), 1959.
25. Hartley, J. L.: *Comparative Evaluation of Newer Devices and Techniques for the Removal of Tooth Structure.* J. Pros. Den., *8:*170–182 (Jan.), 1958.
26. Wilson, J. R.: *The Use of Ultrasonics in Periodontal Treatment.* J. Pros. Den., *8:161–166* (Jan.), 1958.
27. Skinner, E. W., and Mizera, G. T.: *Condensation of Amalgam with Ultrasonic Vibration.* J. Pros. Den., *8:*183–194 (Jan.), 1958.
28. Kilpatrick, H. C.: *High Speed and Ultra Speed in Dentistry.* Philadelphia, W. B. Saunders Company, 1959, p. 274.
29. Nelsen, R. J., Pelander, C. E., and Kumpula, J. W.: *Hydraulic Turbine Handpiece.* J.A.D.A., *47:*324–329 (Sept.), 1953.
30. Nelsen, R. J., and Nelsen, A. E.: *The Patient, the Tooth and the Dentist: A Modern Perspective of Tooth Preparation.* J.A.D.A., *58:*1–15 (Jan.), 1959.
31. Reference 5, p. 264.
32. Lefkowitz, W., Robinson, H. B. G., and Postle, H. H.: *Pulp Response to Cavity Preparation.* J. Pros. Den., *8:*315–324 (March), 1958.
33. Rapp, G. W.: *Physiologic Responses to High-Speed Handpiece Sounds.* Paper presented at the 38th General Meeting of the I.A.D.R., 1960.
34. Brenman, A. K., Brenman, H. S., Erulkar, S., and Ackerman, J. L.: *The Effect of Noise Producing Dental Instruments on the Auditory Mechanism.* Paper presented at the 38th General Meeting of the I.A.D.R., 1960.
35. Kilpatrick, *op. cit.*, p. 275.

# Index